ACP | MKSAP® 17
Medical Knowledge Self-Assessment Program®

Hematology and Oncology

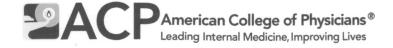

American College of Physicians®
Leading Internal Medicine, Improving Lives

Welcome to the Hematology and Oncology Section of MKSAP 17!

In these pages, you will find updated information on hematopoietic stem cell disorders, multiple myeloma, bleeding disorders, hematologic issues in pregnancy, and other hematologic topics. Also addressed are issues in oncology; breast, ovarian, and cervical cancers; gastroenterological malignancies; lung cancer; lymphoid malignancies; cancer of unknown primary site; melanoma; and other topics in oncology. The effects of cancer therapy and survivorship are discussed, as well. All of these topics are uniquely focused on the needs of generalists and subspecialists *outside* of hematology and oncology.

The publication of the 17th edition of Medical Knowledge Self-Assessment Program (MKSAP) represents nearly a half-century of serving as the gold-standard resource for internal medicine education. It also marks its evolution into an innovative learning system to better meet the changing educational needs and learning styles of all internists.

The core content of MKSAP has been developed as in previous editions—newly generated, essential information in 11 topic areas of internal medicine created by dozens of leading generalists and subspecialists and guided by certification and recertification requirements, emerging knowledge in the field, and user feedback. MKSAP 17 also contains 1200 all-new, psychometrically validated, and peer-reviewed multiple-choice questions (MCQs) for self-assessment and study, including 149 in Hematology and Oncology. MKSAP 17 continues to include *High Value Care* (HVC) recommendations, based on the concept of balancing clinical benefit with costs and harms, with links to MCQs that illustrate these principles. In addition, HVC Key Points are highlighted in the text. Also highlighted, with blue text, are *Hospitalist*-focused content and MCQs that directly address the learning needs of internists who work in the hospital setting.

MKSAP 17 Digital provides access to additional tools allowing you to customize your learning experience, including regular text updates with practice-changing, new information and 200 new self-assessment questions; a board-style pretest to help direct your learning; and enhanced custom-quiz options. And, with MKSAP Complete, learners can access 1200 electronic flashcards for quick review of important concepts or review the updated and enhanced version of Virtual Dx, an image-based self-assessment tool.

As before, MKSAP 17 is optimized for use on your mobile devices, with iOS- and Android-based apps allowing you to sync your work between your apps and online account and submit for CME credits and MOC points online.

Please visit us at the MKSAP Resource Site (mksap.acponline.org) to find out how we can help you study, earn CME credit and MOC points, and stay up to date.

Whether you prefer to use the traditional print version or take advantage of the features available through the digital version, we hope you enjoy MKSAP 17 and that it meets and exceeds your personal learning needs.

On behalf of the many internists who have offered their time and expertise to create the content for MKSAP 17 and the editorial staff who work to bring this material to you in the best possible way, we are honored that you have chosen to use MKSAP 17 and appreciate any feedback about the program you may have. Please feel free to send us any comments to mksap_editors@acponline.org.

Sincerely,

Philip A. Masters, MD, FACP
Editor-in-Chief
Senior Physician Educator
Director, Content Development
Medical Education Division
American College of Physicians

Hematology and Oncology

Associate Editor

Richard S. Eisenstaedt, MD, MACP[1]
Clinical Professor of Medicine
Temple University School of Medicine
Chair, Department of Medicine
Abington Memorial Hospital
Abington, Pennsylvania

Hematology Committee

Peter M. Voorhees, MD, Section Editor[2]
Associate Professor of Medicine
Division of Hematology/Oncology
University of North Carolina School of Medicine
Lineberger Comprehensive Cancer Center
Chapel Hill, North Carolina

Christian T. Cable, MD, MHPE, FACP[1]
Associate Professor of Medicine
Hematology/Oncology
Baylor Scott & White Health
Texas A&M College of Medicine
Temple, Texas

Rebecca Kruse-Jarres, MD, MPH[2]
Associate Professor of Medicine
Division of Hematology
University of Washington
Seattle, Washington

Alice D. Ma, MD[2]
Associate Professor of Medicine
Division of Hematology/Oncology
University of North Carolina School of Medicine
Chapel Hill, North Carolina

Stephan Moll, MD[2]
Professor of Medicine
Division of Hematology/Oncology
University of North Carolina School of Medicine
Chapel Hill, North Carolina

Oncology Committee

Bernard A. Mason, MD, FACP, Section Editor[1]
Clinical Professor of Medicine
Perelman School of Medicine at the University of
　Pennsylvania
Philadelphia, Pennsylvania

Caroline C. Block, MD[2]
Associate Clinical Professor of Medicine
Tufts University School of Medicine
New England Hematology/Oncology
Vernon Cancer Center
Newton-Wellesley Hospital
Newton, Massachusetts

Lee Hartner, MD[1]
Clinical Associate Professor of Medicine
Perelman School of Medicine at the University of
　Pennsylvania
Abramson Cancer Center at Pennsylvania Hospital
Philadelphia, Pennsylvania

Andrew L. Pecora, MD, FACP, CPE[2]
Vice President Cancer Services and Chief Innovations Officer
John Theurer Cancer Center at Hackensack University
　Medical Center
President, Regional Cancer Care Associates
Professor of Medicine and Oncology
Georgetown University
Hackensack, New Jersey

Leonard B. Saltz, MD[2]
Professor of Medicine
Weill Medical College of Cornell University
Chief, Gastrointestinal Oncology Service
Memorial Sloan Kettering Cancer Center
New York, New York

Editor-in-Chief

Philip A. Masters, MD, FACP[1]
Director, Clinical Content Development
American College of Physicians
Philadelphia, Pennsylvania

Director, Clinical Program Development

Cynthia D. Smith, MD, FACP[2]
American College of Physicians
Philadelphia, Pennsylvania

Hematology Reviewers

John K. Chamberlain, MD, MACP[1]
Duane R. Hospenthal, MD, FACP[1]
Robert T. Means, Jr., MD, FACP[2]
Joseph Padinjarayveetil, MD[1]

Andrew L. Pecora, MD, FACP, CPE
Board member
Cancer Genetics
Other
GlaxoSmithKline, Novartis
Research Grants/Contracts
Bristol-Myers Squibb, Derma
Stock Options/Holdings
NeoStem, Amorcyte, TetraLogics

Leonard Saltz, MD
Consultantship
Roche, Genentech, Pfizer, Boehringer Ingelheim, Sanofi,
  Abbott Pharmaceuticals, Bristol-Myers Squibb, ImClone,
  Merck, Bristol-Myers Squibb
Research Grants/Contracts
Amgen, Taiho Pharmaceuticals
Honoraria
Johnson & Johnson

Cynthia D. Smith, MD, FACP
Stock Options/Holdings
Merck and Co.; spousal employment at Merck

Peter M. Voorhees, MD
Consultantship
GlaxoSmithKline, MedImmune, Novartis, Millennium
  Pharmaceuticals, Celgene, Array BioPharma,
  Oncopeptides
Research Grants/Contracts
Centocor Ortho Biotech, Acetylon Pharmaceuticals,
  Prolexys Pharmaceuticals, Merck & Co., Pfizer, Onyx
  Pharmaceuticals, GlaxoSmithKline, Oncopeptides,
  Millennium Pharmaceuticals

Peter Wiernik, MD
Honoraria
Novartis, Celgene, Teva

Acknowledgments

The American College of Physicians (ACP) gratefully acknowledges the special contributions to the development and production of the 17th edition of the Medical Knowledge Self-Assessment Program® (MKSAP® 17) made by the following people:

Graphic Design: Michael Ripca (Graphics Technical Administrator) and WFGD Studio (Graphic Designers).

Production/Systems: Dan Hoffmann (Director, Web Services & Systems Development), Neil Kohl (Senior Architect), Chris Patterson (Senior Architect), and Scott Hurd (Manager, Web Projects & CMS Services).

MKSAP 17 Digital: Under the direction of Steven Spadt, Vice President, Digital Products & Services, the digital version of MKSAP 17 was developed within the ACP's Digital Product Development Department, led by Brian Sweigard (Director). Other members of the team included Dan Barron (Senior Web Application Developer/Architect), Chris Forrest (Senior Software Developer/Design Lead), Kara Kronenwetter (Senior Web Developer), Brad Lord (Senior Web Application Developer), John McKnight (Senior Web Developer), and Nate Pershall (Senior Web Developer).

The College also wishes to acknowledge that many other persons, too numerous to mention, have contributed to the production of this program. Without their dedicated efforts, this program would not have been possible.

MKSAP Resource Site (mksap.acponline.org)

The MKSAP Resource Site (mksap.acponline.org) is a continually updated site that provides links to MKSAP 17 online answer sheets for print subscribers; the latest details on Continuing Medical Education (CME) and Maintenance of Certification (MOC) in the United States, Canada, and Australia; errata; and other new information.

ABIM Maintenance of Certification

Check the MKSAP Resource Site (mksap.acponline.org) for the latest information on how MKSAP tests can be used to apply to the American Board of Internal Medicine for Maintenance of Certification (MOC) points.

Royal College Maintenance of Certification

In Canada, MKSAP 17 is an Accredited Self-Assessment Program (Section 3) as defined by the Maintenance of Certification (MOC) Program of The Royal College of Physicians and Surgeons of Canada and approved by the Canadian Society of Internal Medicine on December 9, 2014. Approval extends from July 31, 2015 until July 31, 2018 for the Part A sections. Approval extends from December 31, 2015 to December 31, 2018 for the Part B sections.

Fellows of the Royal College may earn three credits per hour for participating in MKSAP 17 under Section 3. MKSAP 17 also meets multiple CanMEDS Roles, including that of Medical Expert, Communicator, Collaborator, Manager, Health Advocate, Scholar, and Professional. For information on how to apply MKSAP 17 Continuing Medical Education (CME) credits to the Royal College MOC Program, visit the MKSAP Resource Site at mksap.acponline.org.

The Royal Australasian College of Physicians CPD Program

In Australia, MKSAP 17 is a Category 3 program that may be used by Fellows of The Royal Australasian College of Physicians (RACP) to meet mandatory Continuing Professional Development (CPD) points. Two CPD credits are awarded for each of the 200 *AMA PRA Category 1 Credits*™ available in MKSAP 17. More information about using MKSAP 17 for this purpose is available at the MKSAP Resource Site at mksap.acponline.org and at www.racp.edu.au. CPD credits earned through MKSAP 17 should be reported at the MyCPD site at www.racp.edu.au/mycpd.

Continuing Medical Education

The American College of Physicians (ACP) is accredited by the Accreditation Council for Continuing Medical Education (ACCME) to provide continuing medical education for physicians.

The ACP designates this enduring material, MKSAP 17, for a maximum of 200 *AMA PRA Category 1 Credits*™. Physicians should claim only the credit commensurate with the extent of their participation in the activity.

Up to 22 *AMA PRA Category 1 Credits*™ are available from July 31, 2015, to July 31, 2018, for the MKSAP 17 Hematology and Oncology section.

Learning Objectives

The learning objectives of MKSAP 17 are to:
- Close gaps between actual care in your practice and preferred standards of care, based on best evidence
- Diagnose disease states that are less common and sometimes overlooked or confusing
- Improve management of comorbid conditions that can complicate patient care
- Determine when to refer patients for surgery or care by subspecialists
- Pass the ABIM Certification Examination
- Pass the ABIM Maintenance of Certification Examination

Target Audience

- General internists and primary care physicians
- Subspecialists who need to remain up-to-date in internal medicine and in areas outside of their own subspecialty area
- Residents preparing for the certification examination in internal medicine
- Physicians preparing for maintenance of certification in internal medicine (recertification)

Earn "Instantaneous" CME Credits Online

Print subscribers can enter their answers online to earn instantaneous Continuing Medical Education (CME) cred-its. You can submit your answers using online answer sheets that are provided at mksap.acponline.org, where a record of your MKSAP 17 credits will be available. To earn CME credits, you need to answer all of the questions in a test and earn a score of at least 50% correct (number of correct answers divided by the total number of questions). Take any of the following approaches:

1. Use the printed answer sheet at the back of this book to record your answers. Go to mksap.acponline.org, access the appropriate online answer sheet, transcribe your answers, and submit your test for instantaneous CME credits. There is no additional fee for this service.

2. Go to mksap.acponline.org, access the appropriate online answer sheet, directly enter your answers, and submit your test for instantaneous CME credits. There is no additional fee for this service.

3. Pay a $15 processing fee per answer sheet and submit the printed answer sheet at the back of this book by mail or fax, as instructed on the answer sheet. Make sure you calculate your score and fax the answer sheet to 215-351-2799 or mail the answer sheet to Member and Customer Service, American College of Physicians, 190 N. Independence Mall West, Philadelphia, PA 19106-1572, using the courtesy envelope provided in your MKSAP 17 slipcase. You will need your 10-digit order number and 8-digit ACP ID number, which are printed on your packing slip. Please allow 4 to 6 weeks for your score report to be emailed back to you. Be sure to include your email address for a response.

If you do not have a 10-digit order number and 8-digit ACP ID number or if you need help creating a user name and password to access the MKSAP 17 online answer sheets, go to mksap.acponline.org or email custserv@acponline.org.

Disclosure Policy

It is the policy of the American College of Physicians (ACP) to ensure balance, independence, objectivity, and scientific rigor in all of its educational activities. To this end, and consistent with the policies of the ACP and the Accreditation Council for Continuing Medical Education (ACCME), contributors to all ACP continuing medical education activities are required to disclose all relevant financial relationships with any entity producing, marketing, re-selling, or distributing health care goods or services consumed by, or used on, patients. Contributors are required to use generic names in the discussion of therapeutic options and are required to identify any unapproved, off-label, or investigative use of commercial products or devices. Where a trade name is used, all available trade names for the same product type are also included.

If trade-name products manufactured by companies with whom contributors have relationships are discussed, contributors are asked to provide evidence-based citations in support of the discussion. The information is reviewed by the committee responsible for producing this text. If necessary, adjustments to topics or contributors' roles in content development are made to balance the discussion. Further, all readers of this text are asked to evaluate the content for evidence of commercial bias and send any relevant comments to mksap_editors@acponline.org so that future decisions about content and contributors can be made in light of this information.

Resolution of Conflicts

To resolve all conflicts of interest and influences of vested interests, the American College of Physicians (ACP) precluded members of the content-creation committee from deciding on any content issues that involved generic or trade-name products associated with proprietary entities with which these committee members had relationships. In addition, content was based on best evidence and updated clinical care guidelines, when such evidence and guidelines were available. Contributors' disclosure information can be found with the list of contributors' names and those of ACP principal staff listed in the beginning of this book.

Hospital-Based Medicine

For the convenience of subscribers who provide care in hospital settings, content that is specific to the hospital setting has been highlighted in blue. Hospital icons (H) highlight where the hospital-based content begins, continues over more than one page, and ends.

High Value Care Key Points

Key Points in the text that relate to High Value Care concepts (that is, concepts that discuss balancing clinical benefit with costs and harms) are designated by the HVC icon (HVC).

Educational Disclaimer

The editors and publisher of MKSAP 17 recognize that the development of new material offers many opportunities for error. Despite our best efforts, some errors may persist in print. Drug dosage schedules are, we believe, accurate and in accordance with current standards. Readers are advised, however, to ensure that the recommended dosages in MKSAP 17 concur with the information provided in the product information material. This is especially important in cases of new, infrequently used, or highly toxic drugs. Application of the information in MKSAP 17 remains the professional responsibility of the practitioner.

The primary purpose of MKSAP 17 is educational. Information presented, as well as publications, technologies, products, and/or services discussed, is intended to inform subscribers about the knowledge, techniques, and experiences of the contributors. A diversity of professional opinion exists, and the views of the contributors are their own and not those of the American College of Physicians (ACP). Inclusion of any material in the program does not constitute endorsement or recommendation by the ACP. The ACP does not warrant the safety, reliability, accuracy, completeness, or usefulness of and disclaims any and all liability for damages and claims that may result from the use of information, publications, technologies, products, and/or services discussed in this program.

Publisher's Information

Unauthorized Use of This Book Is Against the Law

MKSAP 17 ISBN: 978-1-938245-18-3
(Hematology and Oncology) ISBN: 978-1-938245-22-0

Printed in the United States of America.

For order information in the United States or Canada call 800-523-1546, extension 2600. All other countries call 215-351-2600, (M-F, 9 AM – 5 PM ET). Fax inquiries to 215-351-2799 or email to custserv@acponline.org.

Errata

Errata for MKSAP 17 will be available through the MKSAP Resource Site at mksap.acponline.org as new information becomes known to the editors.

Table of Contents

Hematology and Oncology High Value Care Recommendations

The American College of Physicians, in collaboration with multiple other organizations, is engaged in a worldwide initiative to promote the practice of High Value Care (HVC). The goals of the HVC initiative are to improve health care outcomes by providing care of proven benefit and reducing costs by avoiding unnecessary and even harmful interventions. The initiative comprises several programs that integrate the important concept of health care value (balancing clinical benefit with costs and harms) for a given intervention into a broad range of educational materials to address the needs of trainees, practicing physicians, and patients.

HVC content has been integrated into MKSAP 17 in several important ways. MKSAP 17 now includes HVC-identified key points in the text, HVC-focused multiple choice questions, and, for subscribers to MKSAP Digital, an HVC custom quiz. From the text and questions, we have generated the following list of HVC recommendations that meet the definition below of high value care and bring us closer to our goal of improving patient outcomes while conserving finite resources.

High Value Care Recommendation: A recommendation to choose diagnostic and management strategies for patients in specific clinical situations that balance clinical benefit with cost and harms with the goal of improving patient outcomes.

Below are the High Value Care Recommendations for the Hematology and Oncology section of MKSAP 17.

- Management of aplastic anemia with hematopoietic growth factors is ineffective.
- Myelodysplastic syndrome should be managed based on risk stratification, with patients with low-risk disease requiring no treatment (see Item 72).
- Observation alone is safe for patients with essential thrombocythemia at low risk for thromboembolic complications, whereas platelet-lowering therapy is indicated for patients at high risk.
- Patients with a clear cause of secondary erythrocytosis such as hypoxemia should be managed with treatment of the underlying problem and do not require bone marrow biopsy, *JAK2 V617F* testing, or phlebotomy (see Item 18).
- Serum and urine protein electrophoresis for plasma cell dyscrasias (PCDs) should be restricted to situations in which a symptomatic PCD requiring intervention or an asymptomatic PCD at high risk of progression to a clinically symptomatic condition is suspected

- Measurement of erythropoietin levels is not useful in diagnosing the anemia of kidney disease.
- Inflammatory anemia typically requires no treatment other than for the underlying condition (see Item 45).
- α-Thalassemia trait (or α-thalassemia minor), which is associated with mild anemia, microcytosis, hypochromia, target cells on the peripheral blood smear, and, in adults, normal hemoglobin electrophoresis results, requires no treatment (see Item 61).
- Methylmalonic acid and total homocysteine levels are helpful in differentiating cobalamin deficiency (both levels are elevated) from folate deficiency (elevated homocysteine but normal methylmalonic acid level); bone marrow biopsy is not necessary and can be confusing.
- In patients with sickle cell disease, including pregnant patients, transfusion is not indicated for uncomplicated pregnancy, routine painful episodes, minor surgery not requiring anesthesia, or asymptomatic anemia (see Item 34).
- Expert opinion recommends that pregnant patients should receive the same treatment for acute vaso-occlusive crisis as nonpregnant patients with sickle cell disease (see Item 65).
- An elevated transferrin saturation remains the most sensitive and cost-effective initial screening test for hemochromatosis.
- Universal screening for hereditary hemochromatosis is not recommended and should be reserved for first-degree relatives of patients with classic *HFE*-related hemochromatosis, those with active liver disease, and patients with abnormal iron study results.
- No diagnostic test can identify immune-mediated thrombocytopenia, and antiplatelet antibody testing is not recommended because of its low sensitivity and specificity.
- Patients with immune thrombocytopenic purpura without evidence of bleeding and platelet counts greater than 30,000 to 40,000/µL (30-40 × 10⁹/L) have less than a 15% chance of developing more severe thrombocytopenia requiring treatment and can be managed with careful observation (see Item 23).
- Assessing the pretest probability of heparin-induced thrombocytopenia by using a risk scoring system, such as the 4T score, is helpful in guiding therapy in patients at low risk for it (see Item 39).
- In hospitalized patients without symptoms or end-organ damage, a restrictive treatment strategy for hemoglobin levels less than 7 g/dL (70 g/L) and targeting 7 to 9 g/dL (70-90 g/L) is appropriate (see Item 40).

- Patients with mild coagulopathy requiring central venous catheter insertion do not need to receive fresh frozen plasma or other transfusions before the procedure (see Item 41).
- Fresh frozen plasma is ineffective for treating mild coagulopathies characterized by an INR of 1.85 or less.
- Platelet clumping signifies pseudothrombocytopenia, which will resolve if blood is redrawn using a citrated or heparinized tube (see Item 42).
- Clinically stable patients with chemotherapy-induced thrombocytopenia who are not bleeding do not benefit from platelet transfusion when the platelet count is 10,000/μL (10×10^9/L) or greater (see Item 20).
- Routine extensive screening for underlying cancer in all patients with unprovoked venous thromboembolism is not recommended.
- A low-probability Wells score with a negative D-dimer blood test rules out venous thromboembolism.
- A blood D-dimer test using a moderately or highly sensitive assay should be the first step in the diagnosis of deep venous thrombosis in a patient with low pretest probability (see Item 52).
- The preferred initial diagnostic test to perform in a pregnant patient with possible pulmonary embolism is lower extremity venous duplex ultrasonography to assess for the presence of deep venous thrombosis, which, if present, would obviate the need for radiation and contrast exposure associated with other diagnostic studies (see Item 14).
- Outpatient anticoagulation management is possible for patients with pulmonary embolism, unless they require supplemental oxygen, intravenous pain medications, or management of comorbid conditions that may contribute to rapid clinical deterioration or if home circumstances make outpatient therapy unfeasible (see Item 63).
- Thrombophilia testing is not indicated in patients who develop a venous thromboembolism in the setting of a major transient risk factor (major surgery or trauma or prolonged immobility), because results would not influence duration or intensity of anticoagulation therapy (see Item 12).
- Routine testing for factor V Leiden (FVL) mutation in offspring of a patient with FVL is not indicated (see Item 30).
- The only clear indication for an inferior vena cava filter is in patients with acute pelvic or proximal leg DVT who cannot be anticoagulated because of active bleeding or a very high risk for bleeding
- Although prophylactic transfusions during pregnancy can reduce pain crises in patients with sickle cell disease, neither transfusion nor exchange transfusion has been shown to reduce pregnancy-related morbidity or mortality, and increased risk for alloantibody production in this population must be considered.
- During staging of patients with cancer, tests with a very low yield should not be ordered in the absence of specific directing symptoms.
- Less toxic regimens or no chemotherapy may be warranted in patients with cancer and a poor performance status and for whom supportive, comfort-oriented care may be most appropriate.
- Supportive, comfort-oriented care is appropriate for a frail patient with metastatic cancer, significant medical comorbidities, and a poor performance status (see Item 81).
- The goal of personalized medicine is to direct therapeutic approaches that are optimally beneficial to an individual patient through a better understanding of the molecular makeup of the individual and the tumor.
- Imaging studies to identify occult metastatic disease are not needed in patients with stage I and II breast cancer unless worrisome symptoms or the following poor prognostic features are present: hormone receptor–negative cancer, *HER2* overexpression, large tumor size, high tumor grade, positive lymph nodes, and the presence of extensive lymphovascular invasion.
- After completion of treatment, follow-up monitoring in patients with early-stage breast cancer should occur every 3 to 6 months for 2 years, every 6 months during years 2 through 5, and then annually, with annual mammography for all survivors, and MRI of the breast reserved for those at high risk for recurrence.
- In asymptomatic patients with a history of early breast cancer, routine imaging studies (excluding annual mammography) or blood tests, including tumor marker studies, are not beneficial (see Item 126).
- Women at average risk for ovarian cancer should not receive ovarian cancer screening; the predictive value of serum CA-125 testing and ultrasonography are each less than 3% and lead to a high rate of false-positive results and unnecessary surgeries (see Item 114).
- Follow-up for patients who have completed treatment for ovarian cancer includes a periodic history, physical examination, and pelvic examination for 5 years after treatment; routine monitoring of CA-125 levels, other laboratory testing, and imaging studies does not improve survival and should be reserved for addressing specific clinical concerns.
- The human papillomavirus vaccine, given before infection develops, is 90% effective at preventing infection and 97% to 100% effective at preventing cervical intraepithelial neoplasia and invasive cervical cancer.
- PET scans have not been demonstrated to improve preoperative staging in patients with colorectal cancer and should not be routinely used.
- Treatment of small-volume, widely metastatic, but asymptomatic, disease discovered on surveillance has not been associated with improved outcomes and may subject patients to significant treatment toxicity.
- PET scanning should not be used for routine surveillance of patients with colorectal cancer but may be used to further evaluate an equivocal finding on CT scans in some patients.

- Because well-differentiated neuroendocrine tumors are so indolent, patients often can be effectively managed with expectant observation and serial imaging using triple-phase contrast-enhanced CT scanning or MRI with gadolinium.
- Appropriate management for a patient with an incidental finding of a metastatic low-grade carcinoid tumor that is asymptomatic and hormonally nonfunctional consists of expectant observation and repeat imaging studies several times each year to determine whether the disease is progressing (see Item 135).
- Metastatic non–small cell lung cancer (stage IV) is not curable and treatment is palliative; the benefit of systemic therapy in this patient population is confined to those with adequate performance status.
- Patients with metastatic non–small cell lung cancer and adequate performance status should be treated with systemic therapy selected based on the pattern of metastatic spread and the results of histologic and molecular assessment.
- Patients with lung cancer and poor performance status do not benefit from chemotherapy and should undergo a palliative care assessment (see Item 138).
- Early palliative care has shown to improve symptom control and survival in patients with non–small cell lung cancer and associated poor performance status (see Item 149).
- In patients with prostate cancer, imaging studies to assess for possible metastatic disease or regional lymph node involvement are only indicated for men with poor-risk features (typically men with intermediate, high, or very high–risk cancer).
- Imaging studies are not indicated for men with newly diagnosed early-stage prostate cancer in the absence of symptoms or other high-risk features (see Item 107).
- Active surveillance, with the use of serum prostate-specific antigen measurement, digital rectal examination, and repeat prostate biopsy, is appropriate only for men with very low–risk or low-risk prostate cancer who have a life expectancy of at least 10 years.
- Observation is the appropriate management for an elderly man with newly diagnosed, low-risk prostate cancer and medical comorbidities that significantly limit life expectancy (see Item 132).
- Patients with small, soft, freely moveable lymph nodes that are limited to one or two adjacent sites and who have no other significant history or physical examination findings can be followed with serial examinations and require no laboratory studies or imaging.

- Patients with asymptomatic grade 1 and 2 follicular lymphoma should be observed and only treated when they become symptomatic; treatment is not curative and does not improve survival (see Item 102).
- The initial treatment of a patient with gastric mucosa-associated lymphoid tissue (MALT) lymphoma associated with *Helicobacter pylori* infection is antimicrobial therapy plus a proton pump inhibitor (see Item 121).
- Asymptomatic patients with low-stage chronic lymphocytic leukemia (stage 0 to II) can be observed without therapy for decades.
- The clinical evaluation in patients with cancer of unknown primary site should not involve an exhaustive search for a primary tumor because finding an asymptomatic and occult primary site does not improve outcome.
- In patients with cancer of unknown primary site, measurement of serum tumor marker levels, such as carcinoembryonic antigen, CA-19-9, CA-15-3, and CA-125, is rarely helpful and virtually never diagnostic.
- Although PET scans may sometimes suggest the location of a primary tumor, these findings are rarely definitive and do not improve long-term outcome in patients with cancer of unknown primary site.
- In the follow-up care of patients with melanoma, routine blood tests are not recommended, and the value of screening chest radiography, CT scanning, or PET/CT scanning is questionable.
- Hematopoietic growth factors, including granulocyte colony-stimulating factor and granulocyte-macrophage colony-stimulating factor, can decrease the severity and duration of neutropenia but due to expense and only modest effect on outcomes, they should be reserved for patients at high risk for neutropenia-associated infection.
- Platelet growth factors such as thrombopoietin are not considered standard therapeutic practice for patients with chemotherapy-induced thrombocytopenia and are reserved for those with immune-mediated thrombocytopenia.
- Close observation is the standard of care for patients following surgical resection for nonmetastatic renal cell carcinoma, as no studies to date have identified an adjuvant therapy that improves survival in these patients (see Item 115).
- Active surveillance is the recommended management strategy for patients with stage I seminoma diagnosed after radical inguinal orchiectomy; other options are adjuvant single-agent carboplatin or para-aortic lymph node irradiation (see Item 123).

Hematology and Oncology

Hematopoietic Stem Cells and Their Disorders

Overview

Hematopoiesis is the orderly formation of all recognizable blood elements from a pluripotent stem cell in the bone marrow. Hematopoietic stem cells (HSCs) can self-renew and differentiate (**Figure 1**) but can also transdifferentiate into mesenchymal tissues. Hematopoietic growth factors, bone marrow stroma, and adequate nutrients are all key ingredients in normal blood production. Disorders of the blood may occur at the HSC level or with any of the more differentiated descendants such as the myeloid, lymphoid, or erythroid progenitors.

Pure red cell aplasia (PRCA) and isolated neutropenia often reflect the response of the blood to autoimmunity or viral infection. Similarly, isolated thrombocytopenia is rarely caused by bone marrow failure. Its mechanism usually involves peripheral consumption and immune-mediated causes. Pancytopenia, in contrast, indicates failure of the bone marrow or severe peripheral sequestration, most often associated with cirrhosis and hypersplenism.

Aplastic anemia and myelodysplastic syndrome (MDS) are contrasting marrow-failure disorders presenting with pancytopenia and very different findings within the bone marrow. The myeloproliferative neoplasms (MPNs) are clonal myeloid conditions in which blood production is deregulated and independent of hematopoietic growth factors.

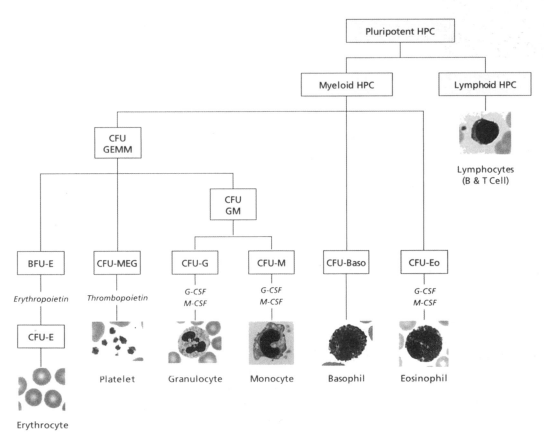

FIGURE 1. Regulation of hematopoiesis. The process of hematopoiesis is regulated by lineage-specific cytokines. These cytokines stimulate the proliferation and/or differentiation of pluripotent stem cells to committed mature peripheral blood cells. The pluripotent HPC is also known as an HSC.

BFU-E = burst-forming unit-erythrocyte; CFU-Baso = colony-forming unit-basophil; CFU-E = colony-forming unit-erythrocyte; CFU-Eo = colony-forming unit-eosinophil; CFU-G = colony-forming unit-granulocyte; CFU GEMM = colony-forming unit-granulocyte, erythrocyte, megakaryocyte, monocyte; CFU GM = colony-forming unit-granulocyte, monocyte; CFU-M = colony-forming unit-monocyte; CFU-MEG = colony-forming unit-megakaryocyte; G-CSF = granulocyte colony-stimulating factor; HPC = hematopoietic progenitor cell; M-CSF = macrophage colony-stimulating factor.

Cell images courtesy of Deepty Bhansali, MD; Baylor Scott & White Health.

Acute leukemias of myeloblastic (AML) or lymphoblastic (ALL) origin can arise de novo or from a pre-existing MDS or MPN. They are often initially managed emergently. The clinical use of hematopoietic growth factors and HSC transplantation (HSCT) can be very helpful in the management of these diseases.

Bone Marrow Failure Syndromes

Aplastic Anemia

The normal adult bone marrow contains blood-making elements and fat in a ratio inversely related to age. Aplastic (without formation) anemia (AA) is a condition characterized by pancytopenia, with associated neutropenia, anemia, and thrombocytopenia, and a severely hypocellular bone marrow (<10%). Isolated cytopenias are uncommon despite the designation of anemia. The severity of the condition is defined by the degree of neutropenia, thrombocytopenia, or reticulocytopenia and has important implications for treatment and prognosis (**Table 1**). AA is usually acquired and is caused by toxic, viral, or autoimmune mechanisms.

Although many medications may cause dose-related suppression of the bone marrow, true AA is rare. Marrow suppression caused by NSAIDs, β-lactam antibiotics, antiepileptic drugs, and psychotropic medications will usually resolve with discontinuation of the medication. Finding a definitive medication or viral association with AA, however, is uncommon. Autoimmunity is the dominant cause of adult AA. Autoreactive T cells attack pluripotent HSCs and cause aplasia. Therefore, immunosuppression with cyclosporine and antithymocyte globulin is first-line therapy and leads to disease control in 70% of adult patients. Allogeneic HSCT is a potentially curative therapy and should be considered for those younger than 50 years who have compatible donors. Treatment with hematopoietic growth factors is ineffective. **H**

AA, paroxysmal nocturnal hemoglobinuria (PNH), and MDS are all acquired defects of the HSC, so clinical overlap is considerable. PNH is an acquired disorder in which erythrocytes lack membrane proteins CD55 and CD59 required to stabilize complement, leading to episodic intravascular hemolysis (see Erythrocyte Disorders). Screening patients with AA reveals that up to 50% have erythrocytes lacking CD55 and CD59; however, this is usually without evidence of overt hemolysis or thrombosis. A hypoplastic variant of MDS exists that can be difficult to distinguish from AA. Clues indicating the former can include cytogenetic abnormalities or dysplastic hematopoietic cells in the marrow. Up to 10% of patients with AA will develop typical MDS or AML within 10 years.

KEY POINTS

- Immunosuppression with cyclosporine and antithymocyte globulin leads to disease control in 70% of adult patients with aplastic anemia.
- Allogeneic hematopoietic stem cell transplantation is a potentially curative therapy for aplastic anemia and should be considered for patients younger than 50 years who have compatible donors.
- Management of aplastic anemia with hematopoietic growth factors is ineffective. **HVC**

Pure Red Cell Aplasia

The cardinal clinical feature in PRCA is isolated, severe anemia without an adequate reticulocyte response. Examination of the bone marrow shows an absence of erythrocyte precursors. Known causes and associations of PRCA are listed in **Table 2**. Similar to AA, the mechanism of action is predominantly T cell autoimmunity (pregnancy, thymoma, malignancy) or direct toxicity to erythrocyte precursors (viral, medications).

In patients with chronic, compensated hemolytic anemia such as sickle cell anemia, parvovirus B19 infection can cause PRCA and a severe anemic crisis. Such patients rely on high levels of reticulocytosis and can lose all reserve with infection. Intravenous immune globulin (IVIG) may hasten viral clearance by providing adopted immunity to parvovirus and can be helpful in immunocompromised patients. Immunocompetent patients and those without chronic hemolytic anemia are less vulnerable to PRCA from this infection and may recover without IVIG.

Bone marrow examination is required to diagnose PRCA and is useful for excluding secondary causes such as chronic lymphocytic leukemia or other indolent non-Hodgkin

TABLE 1.	Classification of Aplastic Anemia
Classification	**Characteristics**
Very severe aplastic anemia	ANC <200/μL (0.2 × 10⁹/L)
Severe aplastic anemia	Two or more of the following:
	ANC 200-500/μL (0.2-0.5 × 10⁹/L)
	Platelet count <20,000/μL (20 × 10⁹/L)
	Absolute reticulocyte count <40,000/μL (40 × 10⁹/L)
ANC = absolute neutrophil count.	

TABLE 2.	Causes of Acquired Pure Red Cell Aplasia
Parvovirus B19 infection
Thymoma
Autoimmune disease
Lymphoid leukemias and lymphomas
Solid tumors
Drugs (phenytoin, isoniazid)
Pregnancy
Anti-EPO antibodies in patients receiving EPO
EPO = erythropoietin.

CONT.

lymphomas. Leukemias and lymphomas cause PRCA by immune-mediated mechanisms rather than direct ablation of erythrocyte precursors. A particular T-cell lymphoproliferative disorder, large granular lymphocytosis, can be associated with PRCA and is associated with rheumatoid arthritis in one third of patients. It is diagnosed by peripheral blood smear and lymphocyte CD57 positivity on flow cytometry. It can be treated with methotrexate and has clinical overlap with Felty syndrome, which is the clinical triad of rheumatoid arthritis, splenomegaly, and neutropenia. Thymoma is excluded by CT scan of the chest for patients in whom infectious or marrow-based causes are not apparent.

Idiopathic cases of PRCA are presumed to have an autoimmune cause and are treated primarily with immunosuppression. Prednisone, either administered alone or with cyclosporine or cyclophosphamide, can lead to improvement within 1 to 3 months.

KEY POINTS

- Diagnosis of pure red cell aplasia requires bone marrow examination, which can also exclude secondary causes such as lymphoproliferative disorders.

- Treatment of patients with idiopathic pure red cell aplasia primarily consists of immunosuppression, with prednisone as monotherapy or in combination with cyclosporine or cyclophosphamide, leading to improvement in 1 to 3 months.

Neutropenia

Isolated neutropenia usually has a hereditary, toxic, or immune cause. Patients of African and Middle Eastern heritage often have lower neutrophil counts with no clinical consequence. A large U.S. population-based study demonstrated that mild neutropenia (1000-1500/μL [1-1.5 × 10⁹/L]) was present in about 4% of healthy black persons. Neutropenia of greater severity (500-1000/μL [0.5-1 × 10⁹/L]) was seen in 1% of healthy persons. An absolute neutrophil count less than 500/μL (0.5 × 10⁹/L) is less likely to be a normal variant and more likely to be associated with increased risk for bacterial and fungal infections.

Toxicity to neutrophil precursors can be caused by viral or bacterial infections or by medications. Acute HIV, cytomegalovirus, and Epstein-Barr virus infection may all lead to isolated neutropenia. Rickettsial infection or overwhelming bacterial infection can similarly manifest with isolated leukopenia as opposed to leukocytosis. Neutropenia is an expected toxicity of many cytotoxic chemotherapies. More common medications associated with neutropenia are NSAIDs, carbamazepine, phenytoin, propylthiouracil, cephalosporins, trimethoprim-sulfamethoxazole, and psychotropic drugs. Reactions to these agents tend to be idiosyncratic rather than dose dependent. Drug-induced neutropenia usually resolves with removal of the offending medication alone and is diagnosed by history, appropriate timing, and exclusion of other causes.

Immune-mediated neutropenia is frequently associated with connective tissue diseases such as systemic lupus erythematosus and rheumatoid arthritis. Treatment with antirheumatic drugs often alleviates neutropenia. Similar to PRCA, populations of large granular lymphocytes may be identified in clinically diagnosed Felty syndrome.

Neutropenia can be a presenting sign of nutritional deficiencies such as vitamin B₁₂ or folate deficiency. Likewise, MDS may present with neutropenia in isolation, although both are much more likely to be associated with other cytopenias, especially anemia.

Therapy for neutropenia attempts first to correct the underlying cause. An offending drug can be removed and growth factor support with granulocyte colony-stimulating factor (G-CSF) can shorten the duration of neutropenia associated with chemotherapy. Viral infections are usually treated supportively. Immune-associated neutropenia related to frequent infections is treated with immunosuppressive therapy.

KEY POINT

- Drug-induced neutropenia, diagnosed by history, appropriate timing, and exclusion of other causes, usually resolves with removal of the offending medication.

The Myelodysplastic Syndromes

In distinction to AA, the dysplastic (difficult formation) marrow of MDS is most commonly hypercellular. A full bone marrow yields low blood counts because the cells are ineffectively formed and have limited survival. MDS can be associated with past radiation or chemotherapy exposure, but is more commonly a primary process. MDS ranges in severity from an asymptomatic disease characterized by mild normocytic or macrocytic anemia to a transfusion-dependent anemia heralding conversion to AML. The World Health Organization (WHO) classification of MDS and the frequency of each subtype are presented in **Table 3**.

The incidence of MDS increases with age. The diagnosis should be suspected in patients with macrocytic anemia or pancytopenia in whom vitamin B₁₂ and folate deficiency have been excluded. Abnormal erythrocyte forms with basophilic stippling or Howell-Jolly bodies and dysplastic neutrophils with decreased nuclear segmentation and granulation may be present. Increased myeloblasts can be seen in more advanced disease. Diagnosis and prognosis require bone marrow biopsy and aspiration with cytogenetic studies. Many older adult patients have mild stable macrocytic anemia that probably represents mild MDS. These patients do not generally require consultation. The revised International Prognostic Scoring System (IPSS-R) presented in **Table 4** weighs percentage of marrow blasts, cytogenetics of the marrow, and peripheral blood cytopenias to assign prognosis and inform therapy.

Treatment has two goals. The first is to relieve transfusion dependence. Many patients with low-risk MDS require no treatment at all or infrequent transfusions. In 25% of

TABLE 3. World Health Organization Classification of MDS

Category	Frequency	Marrow Blasts	Other Features
Refractory cytopenia with unilineage dysplasia	20%	<5%	Single cell line dysplasia (usually erythrocytes)
Refractory cytopenia with multilineage dysplasia	30%	<5%	Dysplasia in ≥2 lineages
MDS associated with isolated 5q–	Uncommon	<5%	Increased hypolobated megakaryocytes
Refractory anemia with ring sideroblasts	10%	<5%	Erythroid dysplasia, ≥15% ring sideroblasts
RAEB-1	40%	5%-9%	Unilineage or multilineage dysplasia
RAEB-2	40%	10%-19%	Unilineage or multilineage dysplasia
MDS, unclassified	Uncommon	<5%	Does not fit other categories

MDS = myelodysplastic syndrome; RAEB-1/2 = refractory anemia with excess blasts, type 1 or 2.

TABLE 4. International Prognostic Scoring System-Revised (IPSS-R) for Myelodysplastic Syndromes

Variable	Points						
	0	0.5	1	1.5	2	3	4
Bone marrow blasts (%)	<2		>2 to <5		5-10	>10	
Cytogenetics[a]	Very good		Good		Intermediate	Poor	Very poor
Hemoglobin (g/dL [g/L])	>10 (100)		8-10 (80-100)	<8 (80)			
Platelet count (cells/μL [× 10⁹/L])	>100,000 (100)	50,000-100,000 (50-100)	<50,000 (50)				
ANC (cells/μL [× 10⁹/L])	>800 (0.8)	<800 (0.8)					

Risk Group	IPSS-R Score	Median Survival (yrs)
Very low	≤1.5	8.8
Low	>1.5-3	5.3
Intermediate	>3-4.5	3
High	>4.5-6	1.6
Very high	>6	0.8

ANC = absolute neutrophil count.

[a]Cytogenetics: Very good: -Y, del 11q. Good: Normal, del(5q), del(12p), del(20q)
Intermediate: del(7q), +8, +19, i(17q), any other single or double independent clones.
Poor: -7, inv(3)/t(3q)/del(3q), double including -7/del(7q), complex: 3 abnormalities.
Very poor: Complex: >3 abnormalities.

Adapted with permission of the American Society of Hematology, from Greenberg PL, Tuechler H, Shanz J, et al. Revised International Prognostic Scoring System for myelodysplastic syndromes. Blood. 2012 Sep 20;120(12):2458. [PMID: 22740453]; permission conveyed through Copyright Clearance Center, Inc.

CONT.

patients needing more frequent transfusions, erythropoiesis-stimulating agents (ESAs) can decrease transfusion burden. The second goal of therapy is to prevent transformation to AML, a complication that is uniformly resistant to treatment and associated with short survival. In reviewing the IPSS-R, it is apparent that a patient with complex cytogenetics and a marrow blast count of greater than 10% has a median time to AML progression and death of less than 1 year. Patients considered high or very high risk by IPSS-R criteria require treatment at diagnosis. Therapies include allogeneic HSCT in fit younger patients with a compatible donor or hypomethylating chemotherapy such as azacytidine and decitabine. Both agents can reduce transfusion requirements and delay transformation to AML. However, both also worsen blood counts initially and may take up to 6 months to show an effect.

Transfusion support and antibiotics for infection are required until an effect or lack thereof is apparent. **H**

KEY POINTS

- Diagnosis and prognosis of myelodysplastic syndrome require bone marrow biopsy and aspiration with cytogenetic studies.
- Many patients with low-risk myelodysplastic syndrome require no treatment at all or infrequent transfusions. **HVC**

Myeloproliferative Neoplasms

The MPNs are caused by acquired genetic defects in myeloid stem cells and are characterized by deregulated production of leukocytes, erythrocytes, or platelets. Although each disorder is named according to the dominant cell line affected, all can cause an elevation in several cell lines. The MPNs may present with unusual thromboses, massive splenomegaly, or constitutional symptoms such as fever, chills, weight loss, and drenching night sweats. Each has a chronic phase that may progress at varying frequency to AML. For this reason, MPNs are considered myeloid neoplasms, albeit with widely varying prognoses. Long-standing MPNs can also cause secondary fibrosis of the bone marrow, likely as a result of fibroblasts responding to activated HSC growth factors.

Chronic Myeloid Leukemia

Chronic myeloid leukemia (CML) remains the classic MPN with regard to pathophysiology, diagnosis, and targeted therapy. CML may be diagnosed incidentally on a complete blood count (CBC) obtained for another reason or based on the constitutional symptoms and splenomegaly shared by other MPNs. Granulocytic leukocytosis is present on CBC, and earlier myeloid forms such as metamyelocytes, myelocytes, and less than 5% blasts are present on peripheral blood smear review (**Figure 2**). Eosinophilia or basophilia may also be present. The main indicator for extreme granulocytic leukocytosis (leukocyte count >50,000/μL [50 × 10⁹/L]) is the leukemoid reaction. When sepsis occurs, the bone marrow responds by releasing early cells into circulation, and a leukemoid reaction may be difficult to distinguish from CML in an acutely ill patient. However, very few patients with typical sepsis, even gram-negative bacillary bacteremia, develop such counts. *Clostridium difficile* is the most common hospital-based cause. Blasts and basophils are much less likely with a leukemoid reaction.

CML is caused by the Philadelphia chromosome, an acquired translocation of chromosomes 9 and 22 [t(9;22)] in an HSC, that leads to development of a fusion gene called

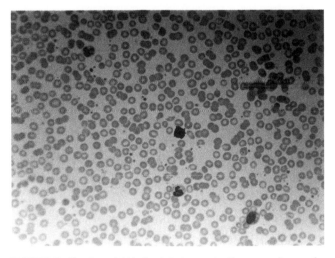

FIGURE 2. Chronic myeloid leukemia is characterized by a preponderance of mature granulocytes (*upper left*) as well as less mature myeloid cells such as myelocytes (*bottom right*) and metamyelocytes (*top right*). Basophils (*center*) are helpful in differentiating the myeloproliferative neoplasms from reactive processes.

Figure courtesy of Deepty Bhansali, MD; Baylor Scott & White Health.

BCR-ABL. The *BCR-ABL* gene encodes a mutant, activated tyrosine kinase that leads to constant downstream proliferative signaling. Discovery of the Philadelphia chromosome in 1960 was the first example of a cancer having a defining molecular event. The t(9;22) is both necessary and sufficient for diagnosing CML. The presence of *BCR-ABL* and t(9;22) may be verified in less than 24 hours with reverse transcriptase polymerase chain reaction (PCR) or fluorescence in situ hybridization (FISH), respectively, performed on peripheral blood. Standard cytogenetic studies by karyotype take several days to complete but are able to reveal more complex cytogenetic abnormalities that may influence prognosis.

CML is usually diagnosed in the chronic phase. Therapy is required at diagnosis, as opposed to management of essential thrombocytosis (ET) and primary myelofibrosis (PMF) in which observation for patients with minimal symptoms may be appropriate. CML can enter a transitional accelerated phase or progress to an overt blast crisis, which is a secondary form of acute leukemia. Of the acute leukemias arising from CML, 80% are myeloid (AML) and 20% are lymphoid (ALL). Both types harbor the *BCR-ABL* mutation. Effective therapy has made accelerated phase and blast crisis transformation of CML less common.

Tyrosine kinase inhibitors (TKIs) target the protein product of the *BCR-ABL* gene, decreasing tumor cell proliferation; imatinib was the first-in-class drug of this type. TKI therapy revolutionized CML treatment, but also heralded a host of specific inhibitors to come in the next decade, many as a result of the Human Genome Project. Before 2000, the 8-year overall survival for CML diagnosed in the chronic phase was approximately 50%. Since 2001, this number has increased to 87%. Allogeneic HSCT for CML is now rare.

Either imatinib or second-generation TKIs such as nilotinib or dasatinib may be used as first-line therapy. Although second-generation agents lead to quicker molecular remission, they have not been demonstrated to improve overall survival. All TKIs can prolong the QT interval, and careful attention to drug interactions and periodic electrocardiographic monitoring are recommended. Dasatinib has a unique association with pericardial and pleural effusions and has been more recently associated with pulmonary arterial hypertension. No TKI is considered safe in pregnancy. Therapeutic options include close observation without therapy or interferon alfa.

Progression of CML is usually a result of medication nonadherence or mutation of the BCR-ABL tyrosine kinase that causes resistance to TKI therapy. A new TKI, ponatinib, which overcomes some resistance to previous TKIs, was recently FDA approved. However, ponatinib has been associated with severe thromboembolic complications and requires strict safety measures mandated by the FDA in its approval.

All commercially available TKIs for the treatment of CML cost approximately $100,000/year. Multidisciplinary support, including social work, is required to help patients obtain the treatment. The benefit of these medications is that a uniformly fatal disease has been transformed into a chronic illness with modest toxicity.

Polycythemia Vera

Polycythemia vera (PV) is a disorder of the myeloid/erythroid stem cell that causes erythropoietin-independent proliferation of erythrocytes. Analogous to the Philadelphia chromosome in CML, an activating mutation of *JAK2* (*JAK2 V617F*) is present in 97% of PV. PV is suspected with a hemoglobin level greater than 18.5 g/dL (185 g/L) in men or greater than 16.5 g/dL (165 g/L) in women after secondary causes are excluded. Activation of *JAK2* has been implicated in the thrombotic risk of PV, but the mechanism is not completely understood. Erythrocyte elevations secondary to other causes must be excluded to implicate PV. Most causes of secondary erythrocytosis share the mechanism of an elevated erythropoietin level. Most commonly, this is driven by hypoxemia, but can be due to ectopic production of growth factor. **Table 5** compares and contrasts the primary and secondary causes of erythrocytosis with regard to symptoms and examination and laboratory findings.

The clinical features that help differentiate secondary erythrocytosis from the MPNs include pruritus after a warm bath or shower; intermittent heat, redness, and pain of the palms and soles (erythromelalgia); hepatosplenomegaly; a concomitant elevation of the leukocyte and platelet counts; and a propensity for unusual thromboses. Basophilia is a strong predictor of PV instead of a reactive state. Elevated serum vitamin B_{12} levels, caused by increased levels of transcobalamin III produced in proliferating leukocytes, and hyperuricemia as a consequence of DNA turnover in the marrow are classic for PV. A rational evaluation begins with a consideration of the clinical features of secondary erythrocytosis. Pulse oximetry should be conducted with ambient air as well as palpation of the abdomen to detect splenomegaly. Review of the peripheral blood smear is required to evaluate the presence of basophils or immature myeloid forms. Determination of serum erythropoietin level and JAK2 will

TABLE 5. Causes of Secondary Erythrocytosis

Disorders	Symptoms	Physical Examination	Laboratory Studies
Polycythemia vera (primary)	Pruritus after a warm shower	Splenomegaly	Low erythropoietin
	Erythromelalgia	Plethora	Basophilia
	Transient ischemic attack		Leukocytosis
	Deep venous thrombosis/pulmonary embolism		Thrombocytosis
			JAK2 positive
Mediated by hypoxemia	Thrombosis	Plethora	High erythropoietin
COPD	Transient ischemic attack	No splenomegaly	No basophilia
Sleep apnea	Erythromelalgia unlikely		No leukocytosis
Congenital heart disease	Pruritus unlikely		*JAK2* negative
Intrapulmonary shunting			
Elevated altitude			
Renal artery stenosis			
Mediated by ectopic or excessive erythropoietin	Thrombosis possible	Plethora	High erythropoietin
	Transient ischemic attack unlikely	No splenomegaly	Microscopic hematuria
Renal cell carcinoma	Erythromelalgia unlikely		No basophilia
Hepatocellular carcinoma	Pruritus unlikely		Leukocytosis possible
Uterine fibroids			*JAK2* negative
Unusual causes	Thrombosis	Plethora	High erythropoietin
High oxygen affinity hemoglobin	Transient ischemic attack	No splenomegaly	No basophilia
	Erythromelalgia unlikely		No leukocytosis
	Pruritus unlikely		*JAK2* negative

complete the evaluation and lead to a diagnosis in most patients. A patient with no apparent cause for secondary erythrocytosis and a low or undetectable erythropoietin level likely has PV. The *JAK2* mutation confirms the diagnosis.

PV may be diagnosed in the latent phase, proliferative phase, or, more rarely, the spent phase that mimics PMF. The latent phase may present with symptoms of erythrocytosis but does not pose the same thrombotic risks as the proliferative phase. Unusual clots, especially portal or splanchnic clots, are classic for MPNs in general and PV specifically. Diagnosis of hepatic vein thrombosis (the Budd-Chiari syndrome) or portal vein thrombosis should prompt consideration of PV. Interestingly, in approximately 50% of young women taking oral contraceptive pills who develop Budd-Chiari syndrome, the *JAK2* mutation is present without other features of MPN.

As with CML, therapy for PV is required at diagnosis. Low-dose aspirin (<100 mg/d) decreases arterial and venous clot risk in PV and should be initiated unless strong contraindications exist. Phlebotomy is the mainstay of therapy and may be safely applied in addition to aspirin in patients younger than 60 years without a previous thromboembolic event. The goal of phlebotomy is to attain a hematocrit level of less than 45%. This may be achieved by weekly phlebotomy and may be maintained with intermittent treatments. Hydroxyurea, an antimetabolite chemotherapeutic agent, can be used in conjunction with phlebotomy in patients older than 60 years or those with previous thromboembolic events. Use of hydroxyurea decreases thrombotic risk independently of its effect on lowering hemoglobin.

PV may remain stable with therapy (70%), enter a spent or burned out phase (20%), or evolve into secondary AML (10%). In the spent phase, secondary fibrosis occurs in the bone marrow and extramedullary hematopoiesis leads to progressive splenic and hepatic enlargement. A patient with decreasing phlebotomy or hydroxyurea requirements and increasing splenomegaly may be entering this fibrotic stage. A leukoerythroblastic blood smear (teardrop cells, nucleated erythrocytes, and immature myeloid forms) similar to that seen with PMF and other myelophthisic processes that displace normal marrow elements will result (**Figure 3**).

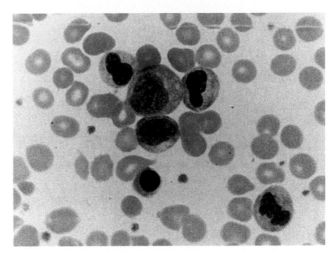

FIGURE 3. Leukoerythroblastic blood smear. Left-shifted granulopoiesis and nucleated and teardrop-shaped erythrocytes define a crowded myelophthisic marrow such as is seen in primary myelofibrosis or other secondary processes such as metastatic carcinoma.

KEY POINTS

- The evaluation of erythrocytosis includes pulse oximetry, examination of the peripheral blood smear, measurement of the serum erythropoietin level, and evaluation for *JAK2* mutation.

- Low-dose aspirin and phlebotomy comprise initial therapy for most patients with polycythemia vera; hydroxyurea can be combined with phlebotomy for patients older than 60 years or those with a higher risk of thromboembolism.

Essential Thrombocythemia

Essential thrombocythemia (ET) is suspected when a platelet count of greater than 600,000/µL (600 × 10⁹/L) is detected on two occasions at least 1 month apart in the absence of secondary causes. Iron deficiency anemia is the most common cause of secondary thrombocytosis followed by reactive states due to infection or inflammation. The *JAK2* mutation is present in 50% of patients with ET, so a negative test does not exclude the diagnosis. The Philadelphia chromosome must also be excluded, because CML may present with thrombocytosis alone.

Most patients will be asymptomatic, but symptoms from digital ischemia, erythromelalgia, transient ischemic attack, visual disturbances, venous thromboembolism, or bleeding (due to dysfunctional platelets) may be present. In contrast to CML and PV, many patients with ET may be observed. By using the International Prognostic Score for ET (**Table 6**) and other observations from large series, patients at low risk may be defined as meeting all these criteria: younger than 60 years, no previous thrombosis, and leukocyte count less than 11,000/µL (11 × 10⁹/L). Such patients may be safely observed without platelet-lowering therapy. Low-dose aspirin does not increase bleeding risk in such patients and does reduce erythromelalgia.

Platelet-lowering therapy is indicated for any patient at high risk. Hydroxyurea was compared with anagrelide, an agent that inhibits megakaryocyte budding, and was found to be superior in preventing thrombosis and bleeding regardless of platelet count achieved. Anagrelide may cause fluid retention and exacerbation of chronic heart failure. By contrast, hydroxyurea is well tolerated in older adult patients and is considered first-line therapy for nonpregnant patients. Interferon alfa is the only platelet-lowering agent safe in pregnancy. Plateletpheresis may be employed emergently to temporarily decrease platelet counts in symptomatic patients with extreme thrombocytosis (generally greater than 1,000,000/µL [1000 × 10⁹/L]).

TABLE 6. International Prognostic Score for Essential Thrombocytosis

Factor	Points
Age ≥60 years	2
Leukocyte count >11,000/μL (11 × 10⁹/L)	1
History of thrombosis	1

Applying Score to Prognosis		
Score	Median Overall Survival	10-Year Thrombosis-free Survival
0 — Low Risk	Not reached	89%
1 or 2 — Intermediate Risk	24.5 years	84%
3 or 4 — High Risk	13.8 years	69%

Adapted with permission of the American Society of Hematology, from Passamonti F, Thiele J, Girodon F, et al. A prognostic model to predict survival in 867 World Health Organization-defined essential thrombocythemia at diagnosis: a study by the International Working Group on Myelofibrosis Research and Treatment. Blood. 2012 Aug 9;120(6):1198. [PMID: 22740446]; permission conveyed through Copyright Clearance Center, Inc.

ET is the least likely MPN to progress to AML or secondary fibrosis, and the least likely to present with symptomatic splenomegaly or constitutional symptoms.

KEY POINTS

HVC
- Observation alone is safe for patients with essential thrombocythemia at low risk for thromboembolic complications, whereas platelet-lowering therapy is indicated for patients at high risk.

Primary Myelofibrosis

PMF is an MPN that does not present with a dominant blood count elevation. Rather, it is a clonal myeloid disorder characterized by abnormal, proliferating megakaryocytes that produce excess fibroblast growth factor. This causes marrow fibrosis and leads to extramedullary hematopoiesis. The classic leukoerythroblastic peripheral blood smear of PMF is not distinguishable from fibrosis of secondary cause or myelophthisic processes of different origin (see Figure 3). An attempt at bone marrow aspiration in PMF is often described as a "dry tap." Markers of increased cell turnover such as lactate dehydrogenase and uric acid are frequently elevated. The *JAK2* mutation is present in 50% of patients.

Sites of extramedullary hematopoiesis, caused as HSCs seek refuge from a fibrotic marrow, include the spine or lymph nodes. Cytokine-mediated symptoms such as fever, chills, night sweats, and malaise may predominate in PMF. Early satiety, weight loss, and abdominal discomfort from splenomegaly are also common, because the splenomegaly may be massive, with the spleen descending to the pelvic brim.

Although the presentation of PMF may be dramatic, it can also be indolent. Initial and sometimes prolonged observation is possible. Treatment is required for symptomatic splenomegaly,

worsening cytopenias, and constitutional symptoms. With the exception of allogeneic HSCT, which can be applied in younger patients, treatment is palliative. Splenectomy in PMF is a perilous procedure with a higher risk of complication and death than expected from other indications.

Hydroxyurea may be used to alleviate splenomegaly and constitutional symptoms. The first JAK2 inhibitor, ruxolitinib, has demonstrated an ability to relieve symptoms in PMF. Risk of thrombosis and AML conversion are not affected. Interestingly, palliative benefit is independent of *JAK2* mutation. It is most effective in patients with severe symptoms and may yield relief of constitutional symptoms and a 33% reduction in spleen volume. Ruxolitinib has not been found effective in the treatment of PV or ET.

KEY POINTS

- With the exception of allogeneic hematopoietic stem cell transplantation, which can be applied in younger patients, treatment for primary myelofibrosis is palliative.

Eosinophilia and Hypereosinophilic Syndromes

The general differential diagnosis of eosinophilia has long been described by the mnemonic CHINA (**Table 7**). A careful history, including current and past medications, and a physical examination, including dermatologic and lymphatic assessment, are critical for evaluation of atopy, asthma, and malignancy. Helminthic infections are common causes of eosinophilia around the world; they are less common within the United States, but coccidioidomycosis is endemic in much of the country. *Strongyloides* is well described in the evaluation of chronic diarrhea associated with eosinophilia.

Hypereosinophilic syndromes (HESs) are diseases characterized by eosinophilia with a count greater than 1500/μL (1.5 × 10⁹/L) and eosinophilic infiltrates of the tissues (skin, lungs, heart, liver, spleen, lymph nodes) resulting in organ damage in addition to systemic symptoms such as fever, chills, night sweats, and weight loss. HES may be primary or have a reactive cause. Primary, or neoplastic, HES is characterized as an MPN with molecular activation of platelet-derived growth factor receptor (PDGFR) α or β or without a known stimulating factor. Reactive, or secondary, HES results from polyclonal expansion in response to an identified stimulus such as a parasitic infection.

TABLE 7. Causes of Eosinophilia

C	Collagen vascular disease (eosinophilic granulomatosis with polyangiitis [formerly known as Churg-Strauss syndrome])
H	Helminthic (parasitic worm) infection (*Strongyloides*)
I	Idiopathic hypereosinophilic syndrome (cause unknown after extensive evaluation)
N	Neoplasia (lymphomas most common)
A	Allergy, atopy, asthma (also drug induced: carbamazepine, sulfonamides)

Glucocorticoids have a dramatic lytic effect on peripheral and tissue eosinophils, but long-term use in patients with HES is problematic. Likewise, steroid-refractory HESs are common; for those with activating mutations of PDGFR α or β, imatinib leads to durable and dramatic responses.

- Glucocorticoids have a dramatic lytic effect on peripheral and tissue eosinophils, and imatinib leads to durable and dramatic responses in steroid-refractory primary hypereosinophilic syndrome with activation mutations of platelet-derived growth factor receptors α or β.

Acute Leukemias

Acute Myeloid Leukemia

 AML is an acquired, malignant HSC disorder that may manifest de novo or arise from preceding MDS or MPN. Age is the greatest risk factor, with a mean age at presentation of 67 years. Leukemic blasts divide on an hourly basis, and the typical patient becomes ill over days to weeks. Diagnosis requires 20% or more myeloblasts in either the peripheral blood or the marrow. Symptoms of anemia, thrombocytopenia, and neutropenia prevail. In adults, 90% of acute leukemia is myeloblastic and 10% is lymphoblastic. The incidence reverses for children and adolescents. Within the first 24 hours of a suspected acute leukemia, a few key decisions must be made (**Table 8**). In practice, urgent consultation with a hematologist and pathologist is required when acute leukemia is suspected. For patients with greater than 50,000 circulating myeloid blasts, a hyperleukocytosis syndrome including hypoxemia and mental status changes can be caused by stasis of the immature cells in small capillary networks. Removal of the cells by leukapheresis is a life-saving, but temporizing, measure until specific chemotherapy is administered.

Especially in older patients, leukemia may present with pancytopenia rather than with leukocytosis and circulating blasts. Bone marrow examination will demonstrate a hypercellular marrow with 20% or more blasts. Underlying dysplasia may be assessed in other cell lines as a clue to the primary or secondary nature of the process. The greatest influence on survival in AML is the genetic profile of the leukemic cells. Traditional risk factors and the modifications provided by newer molecular markers are presented in **Table 9**.

A type of AML, acute promyelocytic leukemia (APL), must be quickly recognized and promptly treated. Disseminated intravascular coagulation is the defining clinical clue to this subtype of AML characterized by t(15;17). All-*trans* retinoic acid (ATRA) allows prompt resolution of disseminated intravascular coagulation and is the backbone of specific therapy. Recently, ATRA in combination with arsenic trioxide (ATO) was found to be equivalent to ATRA plus chemotherapy in low- to intermediate-risk APL. This non-chemotherapy-containing regimen may be safely administered to older patients with the intention of cure. ATRA and ATO can cause a differentiation syndrome characterized by hypoxemia, pulmonary infiltrates, and fever. Prompt initiation of glucocorticoids and brief interruption of the medications are effective in treatment. Monitoring for QT prolongation and careful attention to drug interactions are required with ATO usage.

TABLE 8. Acute Leukemia Decisions

Task	Method
Suspected Acute Leukemia: Early Decisions[a]	
Confirm acute leukemia	Exclude leukemoid reaction, atypical monocytosis, and chronic leukemias: peripheral blood smear review, flow cytometry
AML vs. ALL	Auer rod on blood smear suggests AML, confirmed with flow cytometry; different treatment paths
Exclude APL	Clinically suspected with DIC, classically with promyelocytes and prominent Auer rods, microgranular variant evaluated by flow cytometry (within 24 hours is ideal, but not possible at all institutions), FISH for t(15;17). Administer ATRA if suspected; do not await confirmation.
AML — not APL	Begin induction therapy with cytosine arabinoside and an anthracycline
ALL	Philadelphia chromosome positivity or negativity (determination within 24 hours is ideal, but not possible at all institutions) decides TKI therapy during induction; adolescents/young adults benefit from more intensive pediatric regimens
Acute Leukemia: Later Decisions	
Allogeneic HSC consolidation	Based on fitness of patient and risk of leukemia, predominantly determined by cytogenetic and molecular risk profile
Chemotherapy consolidation	Lower risk leukemia, older or less fit patient

ALL = acute lymphoblastic leukemia; AML = acute myeloid leukemia; APL = acute promyelocytic leukemia; ATRA = all-*trans* retinoic acid; DIC = disseminated intravascular coagulation; FISH = fluorescence in situ hybridization; HSC = hematopoietic stem cell; TKI = tyrosine kinase inhibitor.

[a]Consultation with an experienced hematologist is recommended in early determinations of suspected acute leukemia.

TABLE 9. Acute Myeloid Leukemia Genetic Risk Profile and Effect on 5-Year Survival		
Cytogenetic Category	Age ≤55 Years	Age >55 Years
Favorable t(8;21), inv(16), t(15;17)	65%	34%
Intermediate neither favorable nor high	41%	13%
High complex (≥5 abnormalities), -5,-7,del(5q), 3q abnormal	14%	2%

Molecular modifications to traditional risk profile: Favorable: *c-kit* mutation worsens prognosis of t(8;21) and inv(16); Intermediate: *Flt3* internal tandem duplication mutation worsens prognosis; Intermediate: *NPM1* mutation improves prognosis.

Non-APL AML is treated with a 7-day course of cytarabine and a 3-day course of an anthracycline in fit patients. Patients older than 70 years or ill younger adults do not tolerate this therapy well. A less toxic alternative for older patients is a hypomethylating agent such as azacitidine or decitabine administered on an outpatient basis with transfusion support. Less fit older patients are best served by palliative care.

KEY POINTS

- Disseminated intravascular coagulation is the defining clinical clue to promyelocytic leukemia characterized by t(15;17), and all-*trans* retinoic acid allows prompt resolution of disseminated intravascular coagulation.

Acute Lymphoblastic Leukemia

ALL is less common in adult patients. The clinical presentation is similar to AML, although in contrast, frequent involvement of the central nervous system requires staging by cerebrospinal fluid analysis and prophylaxis with intrathecal chemotherapy. The presence of 25% lymphoblasts in the blood or bone marrow defines the diagnosis. Lymphoid blasts are usually terminal deoxynucleotidyl transferase positive and myeloperoxidase negative. Like AML, risk stratification in ALL relies on clinical and cytogenetic factors. Predictors of poor outcome include advanced age, B-cell versus T-cell disease, more than 30,000 blasts at diagnosis, and poor-risk cytogenetics. *MLL* gene rearrangement and hypodiploidy are adverse risk factors. The Philadelphia chromosome, t(9;22), also portends a poor prognosis, but now offers an attractive target to the TKI dasatinib. This is especially true in older patients in whom traditional chemotherapy is more toxic and less effective.

Young adults, up to the age of 30 years, have better results if they are treated with intensive pediatric regimens containing asparaginase. Therapy for ALL involves induction, intensification, and up to 2 years of maintenance therapy. Alternatively, for fit patients with high-risk disease, allogeneic HSCT can be used to consolidate remission. Overall prognosis for adults with ALL is poor, with 30% to 40% of patients cured by chemotherapy-based approaches.

KEY POINTS

- Otherwise healthy patients with high-risk acute lymphoblastic leukemia can be treated with allogeneic hematopoietic stem cell transplantation to consolidate remission.

- Patients with Philadelphia chromosome–positive acute lymphoblastic leukemia can be treated with the tyrosine kinase inhibitor, dasatinib.

Hematopoietic Growth Factors

At each stage of hematopoietic development, cytokine growth factors stimulate production of mature blood cells. Two recombinant growth factors are in common clinical use. G-CSF is used to stimulate production of neutrophils in autoimmune neutropenia, to hasten neutrophil recovery after cytotoxic chemotherapy, and for HSC mobilization. In the more common chemotherapy regimen, it is usually administered in a pegylated formulation that has activity for several weeks.

Recombinant erythropoietin, an ESA, is indicated for treatment of anemia of chronic kidney disease in the dialysis or predialysis population if iron, vitamin B$_{12}$, and folate levels are replete. Targets before treatment include transferrin saturation greater than 20% and serum ferritin level greater than 100 ng/mL (100 µg/L). Erythropoietin can lead to arterial and venous thrombosis when normal hemoglobin levels are reached. Current guidelines for use in anemia of chronic kidney disease target a hemoglobin level of no more than 11 g/dL (110 g/L).

Another indication for erythropoietin is to hasten recovery in chemotherapy-associated anemia. In several clinical trials using erythropoietin during potentially curative chemotherapy, overall mortality worsened as higher hemoglobin levels were obtained. Current guidelines allow initiation of erythropoietin for chemotherapy-associated anemia for symptomatic anemia with an initial hemoglobin level less than 10 g/dL (100 g/L) only in noncurative regimens. In practice, judicious transfusion may be preferable. Erythropoietin is also used in MDS to reduce transfusion requirements.

KEY POINTS

- Granulocyte colony-stimulating factor is used to stimulate production of neutrophils in autoimmune neutropenia and to hasten neutrophil recovery after cytotoxic chemotherapy.

- Recombinant erythropoietin is indicated for treatment of anemia of chronic kidney disease if iron, vitamin B$_{12}$, and folate levels are replete and to hasten recovery in chemotherapy-associated anemia.

Hematopoietic Stem Cell Transplantation

In theory, allogeneic HSCT can cure any benign or malignant bone marrow failure syndrome. On the level of case series, this is true. In practice, allogeneic HSCT is most helpful in treating AA, high-risk MDS, and acute leukemias. In an allogeneic HSCT, an HLA-matched sibling or matched unrelated donor undergoes HSC collection by apheresis after G-CSF mobilization.

Patients undergoing allogeneic HSCT are immunosuppressed to allow donor HSCs to engraft. Unlike solid organ transplants, this immunosuppression can be tapered over 3 months to 1 year. Chemotherapy preceding modern allogeneic HSCT is generally less intense (reduced intensity conditioning), which has led to decreased short-term morbidity and mortality. HSCs from the donor (graft) are infused by peripheral blood and begin to proliferate in the patient (host). Cure of many bone marrow disorders is possible with this therapy because the blood and immune system of the donor replace that of the patient. Donor immune cells recognize the patient's cancer cells as foreign and mount a T-cell/NK-cell–mediated attack. This is referred to as a graft-versus-leukemia effect and is the goal of HSCT.

Opportunistic infection and graft-versus-host disease (GVHD) are major risks to allogeneic transplantation. Common bacterial infections, viral infections with cytomegalovirus or varicella-zoster virus, and invasive fungal disease such as aspergillosis are common. Infectious morbidity has decreased with improved methods to detect and treat such infections. Acute GVHD occurs when graft T cells recognize the patient's normal gut, skin, and liver sinusoids as foreign. Severe GVHD is life threatening and is treated with high-dose glucocorticoids. Varying second-line immunosuppressants are used for steroid-refractory disease but none have emerged as superior. Therapy for GVHD can be tapered as the disease burns out, generally after 1 year of treatment. With improved supportive care, outcomes with unrelated donor transplants have approached those of sibling transplants. Despite risks of infection and GVHD, the primary cause of mortality after HSCT for malignant disease is relapse of the original disease. H

KEY POINTS

- Allogeneic hematopoietic stem cell transplantation is most helpful in treating aplastic anemia, high-risk myelodysplastic syndrome, and acute leukemias.
- Life-threatening acute graft-versus-host disease occurs when graft T cells recognize the patient's normal gut, skin, and liver sinusoids as foreign; treatment is high-dose glucocorticoids.

Multiple Myeloma and Related Disorders

Overview

Plasma cell dyscrasias (PCDs) are clonal plasma or lymphoplasmacytic cell disorders characterized by the production of monoclonal antibody (M protein) detectable in the serum or urine (Table 10). PCDs produce an M protein consisting of a heavy chain (IgG, IgA, IgD, or IgM) complexed with a κ or λ light chain or of κ or λ free light chains (FLCs) without a heavy chain component. These disorders may be asymptomatic. Alternatively, pathogenic antibodies or proliferation of the abnormal clone may produce clinical manifestations that require treatment.

Evaluation for Monoclonal Gammopathies

Monoclonal gammopathy of undetermined significance (MGUS) is common and usually does not evolve into a condition requiring treatment. Therefore, testing should be restricted to situations in which a symptomatic PCD requiring intervention or an asymptomatic PCD at high risk of progression to a clinically symptomatic condition is suspected. PCDs are more common with advancing age, and other common diseases may share similar clinical features. Table 11 outlines appropriate clinical scenarios for testing.

TABLE 10. Disorders Associated with Monoclonal Gammopathies
Plasma Cell Disorders
Monoclonal gammopathy of undetermined significance[a]
Multiple myeloma
Immunoglobulin light-chain (AL) amyloidosis
Monoclonal immunoglobulin deposition disease
Proximal tubulopathy (with or without Fanconi syndrome)
Solitary plasmacytoma
Solitary plasmacytoma of bone
Solitary extramedullary plasmacytoma
POEMS syndrome[b]/Osteosclerotic myeloma
B-cell Disorders
Waldenström macroglobulinemia/lymphoplasmacytic lymphoma
Marginal zone lymphoma
Chronic lymphocytic leukemia/small lymphocytic lymphoma
Heavy chain disease

[a]Many diseases may be associated with monoclonocal gammopathy of undetermined significance, including but not limited to connective tissue diseases, hepatitis C, HIV, cryoglobulinemia, and cold agglutinin disease.

[b]Polyneuropathy, Organomegaly, Endocrinopathy, presence of M protein, and Skin changes.

TABLE 11. Common Clinical Scenarios for Consideration of Plasma Cell Dyscrasia Testing[a]

Clinical Scenario	Disease Considerations	Disease Characteristics	Associated PCDs/ Lymphoproliferative Disorders	Additional Investigative Evaluation[b]
Lytic bone lesions or hypercalcemia	MM	Osteolytic bone lesions, PTH-independent hypercalcemia	MM	Standard investigative evaluation
Age-inappropriate bone loss[c]	MGUS, MM	Osteopenia or osteoporosis with or without associated fractures	MGUS, MM	Standard investigative evaluation
Peripheral neuropathy	AL amyloidosis	Sensorimotor axonal polyneuropathy	MGUS, MM, WM (rare)	Tissue aspirate/biopsy for amyloid
	POEMS syndrome	Sensorimotor inflammatory demyelinating polyneuropathy, hepatosplenomegaly, endocrinopathies (hypogonadism, adrenal insufficiency), hyperpigmentation, hypertrichosis, multicentric Castleman disease, osteosclerotic bone lesions	MGUS, MM, solitary plasmacytoma of bone	VEGF, endocrine evaluation (e.g., testosterone level)
	Anti-MAG neuropathy	Sensory demyelinating polyneuropathy	IgM MGUS, WM	Anti-MAG antibodies
	Cryoglobulinemic vasculitis	Sensory or sensorimotor polyneuropathy, mononeuropathy multiplex	MGUS, MM, B-cell non-Hodgkin lymphoma (e.g., WM)	Cryoglobulins, complement levels
Kidney disease	Cast nephropathy	Acute kidney injury, nonalbumin proteinuria (monoclonal FLCs), bland urine sediment	MM	Kidney biopsy
	AL amyloidosis	Nephrotic syndrome	MGUS, MM	Tissue aspirate/biopsy for amyloid
	MIDD	Proteinuria (sometimes nephrotic range), acute kidney impairment, hepatomegaly/impairment (rare), cardiomyopathy (rare)	MGUS, MM	Kidney biopsy
	Proximal tubulopathy +/− Fanconi syndrome	Normal anion gap, hyperchloremic metabolic acidosis, hypophosphatemia, hypouricemia, renal glucosuria, amino aciduria	MGUS, MM	Kidney biopsy, serum phosphorus and uric acid, urinalysis
	Cryoglobulinemic vasculitis	Membranoproliferative glomerulonephritis with proteinuria and active urinary sediment	IgM MGUS, B-cell non-Hodgkin lymphoma (e.g., WM)	Cryoglobulins, complement levels
Anemia	Cold agglutinin disease	Normocytic anemia, jaundice, dark urine, acrocyanosis	IgM MGUS, B-cell non-Hodgkin lymphoma (e.g., WM)	Reticulocyte count, lactate dehydrogenase, total bilirubin, direct antiglobulin (Coombs) test, cold agglutinin titer
	MM	Normocytic (occasionally macrocytic) anemia	MM	Standard investigative evaluation

AL amyloidosis = immunoglobulin light-chain amyloidosis; FLC = free light chain; MAG = myelin-associated glycoprotein; MGUS = monoclonal gammopathy of undetermined significance; MIDD = monoclonal immunoglobulin deposition disease; MM = multiple myeloma; POEMS = Polyneuropathy, Organomegaly, Endocrinopathy, M protein, and Skin changes; PTH = parathyroid hormone; VEGF = vascular endothelial growth factor; WM = Waldenström macroglobulinemia.

[a]This is not an all-inclusive list; other less common conditions can be associated with plasma cell dyscrasias.

[b]Evaluation beyond the standard evaluation for a monoclonal gammopathy.

[c]Premenopausal women or men <65 years of age with no additional risk factors for bone loss.

Available tests for detection of PCDs include serum or urine protein electrophoresis (SPEP and UPEP), serum or urine immunofixation, and serum FLC testing (**Figure 4**). SPEP and UPEP detect the presence of and quantify M proteins but do not determine their isotype. UPEP is more sensitive at detecting monoclonal FLCs than SPEP. Serum and urine immunofixation assays identify the isotype of an M protein and are more sensitive than SPEP and UPEP. The serum FLC test is an antibody-based assay that measures the amount of free κ and λ light chains not complexed to heavy chains and is the most sensitive test for detecting monoclonal FLC gammopathies. FLCs are usually reported as the ratio of κ to λ FLCs. An increased amount of either κ or λ FLCs, with the increased component termed the "involved" light chain, will skew the ratio of κ to λ light chains outside of the normal range and indicates the presence of a PCD. With advancing kidney impairment, the basal levels of serum FLCs increase, κ more than λ, leading to an increased serum κ to λ FLC ratio. As such, a corrected normal reference range has been proposed for those with advanced kidney dysfunction. Generally, a combination of SPEP and serum FLCs detects most PCDs. A serum immunofixation and 24-hour UPEP and urine immunofixation may also be needed if SPEP and serum FLC testing are negative and suspicion of a clinically significant PCD persists. The specific-

ity and cost effectiveness of these approaches in different clinical scenarios have not been rigorously assessed.

Many PCDs cause clinical disease, not all of which are associated with multiple myeloma or B-cell lymphomas. As such, an investigative evaluation of a confirmed monoclonal gammopathy requires not only an assessment of possible multiple myeloma or lymphoma but of the other PCDs (see Table 10). Tests that should be considered in all patients with a confirmed monoclonal gammopathy include a complete blood count (CBC); serum chemistries, including creatinine, calcium, and albumin; urinalysis; SPEP, 24-hour UPEP, serum and urine immunofixation, and serum FLC tests (if not already done); and quantitative immunoglobulins (serum IgG, IgA, and IgM). Other laboratory testing is dictated by the suspected disease entity and should be guided by a thorough history and physical examination (see Table 11). For non-IgM gammopathies, a skeletal survey (plain radiographs of the skeleton) is performed to assess for the presence of lytic bone lesions or osteopenia that might be seen with multiple myeloma. IgM gammopathies are more likely associated with B-cell lymphomas, and CT scans of the chest, abdomen, and pelvis should be performed in patients with appropriate signs and symptoms (unexplained fever or weight loss, drenching sweats, lymphadenopathy, or hepatosplenomegaly). A bone marrow biopsy is performed in many cases, but patients with an IgG

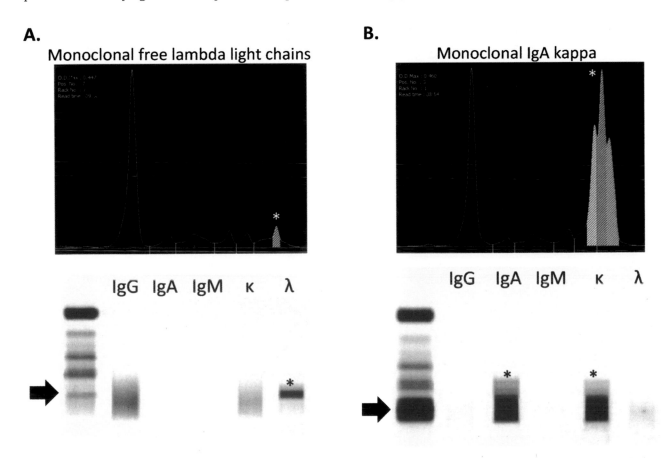

FIGURE 4. Serum protein electrophoresis (SPEP, *top panels*) and immunofixation testing (*bottom panels*) in a patient with free λ light chain (*A*) and IgA κ (*B*) multiple myeloma. The top panels represent serum protein fractions separated by capillary gel electrophoresis. The *white asterisks* denote the monoclonal protein. The bottom panels show patient sera run on multiple lanes of a gel, with each lane stained using anti-IgG, -IgA, -IgM, -κ or –λ antibodies. The first lanes are the SPEP results for that patient. The *black arrows* denote the monoclonal protein band identified by SPEP and the *black asterisks* the isotype specificity of the monoclonal protein by immunofixation testing.

gammopathy measuring less than 1.5 g/dL, a normal serum FLC ratio, and no evidence of disease-specific end-organ damage can safely defer testing.

KEY POINTS

HVC
- Serum and urine protein electrophoresis for plasma cell dyscrasias (PCDs) should be restricted to situations in which a symptomatic PCD requiring intervention or an asymptomatic PCD at high risk of progression to a clinically symptomatic condition is suspected

- The serum free light chain (FLC) assay can detect monoclonal FLCs before they are detectable by urine protein electrophoresis and is the most sensitive test for detecting monoclonal FLC gammopathies.

(Continued)

KEY POINTS *(continued)*

- A combination of serum protein electrophoresis, serum immunofixation, and serum free light chain testing detects almost all plasma cell dyscrasias.

Monoclonal Gammopathy of Undetermined Significance

MGUS is defined as an M protein level less than 3 g/dL (or less than 500 mg/24 hr of urinary monoclonal FLCs), clonal plasma cells comprising less than 10% of the bone marrow cellularity, and the absence of PCD-related signs or symptoms (**Table 12**). MGUS is common, with a prevalence of 5.3% for persons aged 70 years or older.

TABLE 12. Diagnostic Criteria for the Plasma and Lymphoplasmacytic Cell Dyscrasias

Diagnosis	M Protein	Bone Marrow Clonal Plasma Cells or Lymphoid Cells	Disease-specific Signs/Symptoms
MGUS			
Non-IgM (IgG, IgA)	<3 g/dL	<10%	No
IgM	<3 g/dL	<10%	No
Light chain[a]	Affected serum FLC increased and serum FLC ratio increased	<10%	No
	Urinary M protein <500 mg/24 hr		
Smoldering myeloma[b]	IgG or IgA ≥3 g/dL or κ or λ urinary FLC M protein ≥500 mg/24 hr	10%-59%	No
Smoldering WM[b]	IgM ≥3 g/dL	≥10%	No
Multiple myeloma requiring therapy	Present (absent in nonsecretory disease)	≥10% or biopsy evidence of a bony or extramedullary plasmacytoma	Yes
WM requiring therapy	Present	≥10%	Yes

CRAB Criteria for Myeloma-related Signs and Symptoms

Hypercalcemia. Serum calcium >11 mg/dL (2.8 mmol/L) or >1 mg/dL (0.3 mmol/L) higher than the upper limit of normal

Renal failure. Serum creatinine >2 mg/dL (177 μmol/L) or creatinine clearance <40 mL/min

Anemia. Hemoglobin <10 g/dL (100 g/L) or 2 g/dL (20 g/L) below the lower limit of normal

Bone disease. ≥1 lytic bone lesions on imaging studies

Myeloma-defining Biomarkers for Myeloma-related Signs and Symptoms

≥60% clonal plasma cells on bone marrow examination

Involved: uninvolved serum FLC ratio ≥100

≥1 focal lesion on MRI

WM-related Signs and Symptoms

Systemic symptoms: Fatigue, B symptoms (fevers, night sweats, weight loss), neuropathy, hyperviscosity

Physical examination findings: Symptomatic lymphadenopathy or hepatosplenomegaly

Laboratory findings: Cytopenias (anemia, thrombocytopenia)

AL amyloidosis = immunoglobulin light-chain amyloidosis; FLC = free light chain; MGUS = monoclonal gammopathy of undetermined significance; WM = Waldenström macroglobulinemia.

[a]Light-chain MGUS does not have a heavy-chain component.

[b]Smoldering myeloma or WM may have the diagnostic M protein level WITH OR WITHOUT the percentage of bone marrow clonal plasma or lymphoid cells.

Data from Rajkumar SV, Dimopoulos MA, Palumbo A, et al. International Myeloma Working Group updated criteria for the diagnosis of multiple myeloma. Lancet Oncol. 2014 Nov;15(12):e538-48. [PMID: 25439696]

Non-IgM MGUS, IgM MGUS, and light-chain MGUS transform into multiple myeloma or another PCD at 1%, 1.5%, and 0.3% per year, respectively. Patients with non-IgM and light-chain MGUS are more likely to develop multiple myeloma, whereas patients with IgM MGUS are more likely to develop Waldenström macroglobulinemia or other B-cell non-Hodgkin lymphoma. MGUS may infrequently transform to immunoglobulin light-chain (AL) amyloidosis. The presence of an IgA or IgM gammopathy, an M protein level of 1.5 g/dL or more, and an abnormal serum FLC ratio are predictive of progression to multiple myeloma or other PCD in non–light-chain MGUS (**Table 13**).

Patients with MGUS are reassessed 6 months after initial diagnosis, and, if stable, yearly thereafter. Patients with IgG MGUS, an M protein level less than 1.5 g/dL, and a normal serum FLC ratio may undergo follow-up once every 2 to 3 years. Evaluation should include a CBC, serum calcium and creatinine levels, and repeat M protein testing. Additional testing should be guided by history and physical examination. Imaging is not recommended in the absence of symptoms. The clinical value and economic impact of MGUS surveillance strategies have not been rigorously assessed. Patients with an increasing M protein level or new findings of a clinically symptomatic PCD (such as progressive anemia or kidney impairment) require additional evaluation. Patients with MGUS are at increased risk of osteoporosis and associated skeletal complications, most notably vertebral body compression fractures (hazard ratio 2.37) and should be considered for bone mineral density testing.

Multiple Myeloma

Multiple myeloma is a plasma cell malignancy involving the bone marrow. Patients may have smoldering (asymptomatic) disease or have symptomatic disease presenting with significant morbidity. Prompt recognition of symptomatic multiple myeloma is critical, because delayed diagnosis is associated with increased complications.

Clinical Manifestations and Findings

Smoldering myeloma is characterized by an M protein level of 3 g/dL or more (or ≥500 mg/24 hr of urinary monoclonal FLCs) or clonal plasma cells comprising 10% or more of the marrow cellularity and no evidence of myeloma-related signs or symptoms requiring therapy. It is typically diagnosed as part of an evaluation for an elevated serum total protein level on routine laboratory studies. Symptomatic myeloma is defined by the presence of an M protein, clonal plasma cells comprising 10% or more of the marrow cellularity, and myeloma-related end-organ damage (see Table 12).

For patients with symptomatic disease, fatigue and a normocytic anemia are common. Blood smear review may reveal rouleaux formation. Leukopenia and suppression of normal immunoglobulin production, from neoplastic plasma cell proliferation that replaces bone marrow precursors and normal plasma cells, can lead to frequent, sometimes life-threatening infections, particularly of the respiratory tract. Significant thrombocytopenia is uncommon.

Skeletal manifestations may include bone pain and nonvertebral or vertebral body compression fractures. A skeletal survey may reveal lytic bone lesions or osteopenia (**Figure 5**). Hypercalcemia due to osteolysis is common at diagnosis. Of those without initial bone complications, 25% will develop a skeletal-related event during the course of their disease.

Kidney dysfunction is found in 29% of patients, often due to cast nephropathy (also termed myeloma kidney), a condition in which excess monoclonal FLCs precipitate in the distal tubules and incite tubulointerstitial damage. Hypercalcemia and exposure to nephrotoxic agents are other frequent causes of kidney dysfunction, whereas AL amyloidosis, monoclonal immunoglobulin deposition disease, cryoglobulinemic glomerulonephritis, and proximal tubulopathy (with or without Fanconi syndrome) are less common.

TABLE 13. Risk of MGUS Progression to a Clinically Symptomatic Plasma Cell Dyscrasia

Diagnosis	Risk Factors	Progression
Non-light chain MGUS (IgG, IgA, IgM)	M protein ≥1.5 g/dL	At 20 years:
	Non-IgG M protein	3 RFs: 58%
	Abnormal serum FLC ratio	2 RFs: 37%
		1 RF: 21%
		0 RFs: 5%
Smoldering myeloma	M protein ≥3 g/dL	At 5 years:
	Bone marrow plasma cells ≥10%	3 RFs: 76%
		2 RFs: 51%
	Serum FLC ratio <0.125 or >8 mg/dL	1 RF: 25%

FLC = free light chain; MGUS = monoclonal gammopathy of undetermined significance; RF = risk factor.

Data adapted from: Rajkumar SV, Kyle RA, Therneau TM, et al. Serum free light chain ratio is an independent risk factor for progression in monoclonal gammopathy of undetermined significance. Blood. 2005 Aug 1;106(3):812-7. [PMID: 15855274]; and Dispenzieri A, Kyle RA, Katzmann JA, et al. Immunoglobulin free light chain ratio is an independent risk factor for progression of smoldering (asymptomatic) multiple myeloma. Blood. 2008 Jan 15;111(2):785-9. [PMID: 17942755].

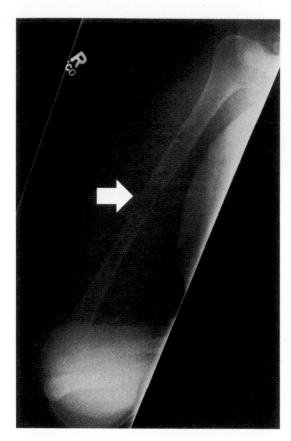

FIGURE 5. Lytic bone lesions in a patient with multiple myeloma. The *arrow* denotes an oblique pathologic fracture through a mid humerus lytic lesion. Other lesions can be seen both proximal and distal to the fracture.

KEY POINTS

- Smoldering multiple myeloma is characterized by a serum M protein level of 3 g/dL or greater (or ≥500 mg/24 hr of urinary monoclonal free light chains) or bone marrow plasma clonal cells of 10% or greater and no evidence of myeloma-related signs or symptoms requiring therapy.

- Symptomatic multiple myeloma is characterized by the presence of serum M protein, bone marrow plasma clonal cells of 10% or greater, and end-organ damage (hypercalcemia, kidney injury, anemia, bone disease).

Diagnosis and Prognosis

Criteria for diagnosing smoldering myeloma and multiple myeloma requiring treatment are outlined in Table 12. In addition to the initial testing noted previously (see Evaluation for Monoclonal Gammopathies), further diagnostic evaluation may be required to distinguish between the two. A skeletal survey is an important part of the initial evaluation of multiple myeloma, but more than 30% of trabecular bone loss must occur before lytic bone lesions are evident. An MRI or CT is more sensitive at detecting bone lesions than plain radiographs and should be considered when bone pain is present and radiographs are unrevealing. MRI should also be performed to assess for spinal cord impingement if back pain is present or a compression fracture is seen on radiographs. Bone scans are insensitive for detection of myeloma bone lesions. The role of whole body PET-CT in the initial evaluation of multiple myeloma and as a tool for assessing response to treatment is an area of active investigation. A kidney biopsy may be required when multiple myeloma–related kidney dysfunction is suspected if the results will impact treatment decisions. AL amyloidosis is found in 10% of patients with multiple myeloma, and appropriate testing should be pursued if clinically suspected (see Immunoglobulin Light-Chain Amyloidosis).

Most smoldering myeloma progresses to symptomatic myeloma or AL amyloidosis, the former being far more common; 51% and 66% of patients progress to symptomatic disease at 5 and 10 years, respectively, with a median time to progression of 4.8 years. Risk factors for progression include a high M protein level, a large burden of clonal plasma cells, and an abnormal serum FLC ratio (see Table 13). Additionally, markers of imminent progression include plasma cells comprising 60% or more of the bone marrow cellularity, more than one focal bone lesion on MRI, or a serum FLC ratio of 0.01 or less or 100 or more; these patients are not considered to have smoldering myeloma and should be considered for early treatment. Management of most patients with smoldering myeloma consists of evaluation every 3 to 6 months. Testing includes a CBC, serum calcium and creatinine levels, and repeat M protein assessment; other testing should be guided by history and physical examination.

After a diagnosis of multiple myeloma requiring treatment is established, additional testing can help determine prognosis and appropriate treatment. The serum β_2-microglobulin and albumin levels determine the stage of disease, which has prognostic significance.

KEY POINT

- Management of most patients with smoldering multiple myeloma consists of evaluation every 3 to 6 months, including a complete blood count, serum calcium and creatinine levels, and repeat M protein assessment.

Treatment

Studies evaluating the use of chemotherapy for patients with high-risk smoldering myeloma have been completed or are ongoing and will clarify whether early intervention can alter the course of the disease with acceptable toxicity. Pamidronate and zoledronic acid have no impact on time to progression to multiple myeloma requiring treatment or overall survival.

Patients with multiple myeloma requiring treatment are initially treated with induction chemotherapy, including some combination of a proteasome inhibitor (bortezomib), an immunomodulatory agent (thalidomide or lenalidomide), a glucocorticoid (prednisone or dexamethasone), or an

CONT.

alkylating agent (melphalan or cyclophosphamide). Autologous hematopoietic stem cell transplantation (HSCT) using high-dose melphalan after initial induction therapy is associated with improved progression-free and, in some studies, overall survival. The use of lenalidomide maintenance therapy after an initial course of treatment improves progression-free survival and may impact overall survival after autologous HSCT. Patients who relapse are typically treated with regimens containing the drug classes noted. Carfilzomib, a second-generation proteasome inhibitor, and the immunomodulatory agent pomalidomide in combination with dexamethasone are also effective in patients with relapsed and refractory disease.

Bortezomib and thalidomide are associated with a high risk of peripheral neuropathy. Patients taking thalidomide-, lenalidomide-, or pomalidomide-based therapy are at increased risk of venous thromboembolism (VTE). Patients with additional risk factors for VTE, including myeloma-related risk factors (concomitant use of dexamethasone, anthracyclines, or erythropoietin; immobilization; hyperviscosity), should be considered for prophylaxis with aspirin, low-molecular-weight heparin, or warfarin. Lenalidomide used as a maintenance therapy immediately after melphalan-based treatment is associated with an increased risk of secondary malignancies. The use of low-dose melphalan as part of initial chemotherapy for multiple myeloma may compromise future collection of hematopoietic stem cells and should be avoided in patients eligible for autologous HSCT.

Surgical stabilization may be required for established or impending pathologic fractures. Palliative therapy includes radiation therapy for bone pain from lytic bone lesions. Pamidronate reduces the risk of skeletal-related complications in symptomatic myeloma. Zoledronic acid protects against skeletal-related events, even in patients without evidence of bone disease on skeletal survey, and improves median overall survival. Guidelines recommend pamidronate or zoledronic acid once every 3 to 4 weeks for a minimum of 2 years in all newly diagnosed patients with symptomatic myeloma.

Cast nephropathy is managed with intravenous fluids, avoidance of nephrotoxic agents, and immediate initiation of chemotherapy to reduce the monoclonal FLC burden. Plasmapheresis clears FLCs inefficiently, and its role remains controversial. Hypercalcemia is managed with intravenous fluids and bisphosphonates.

Annual influenza vaccination is recommended. For adults with multiple myeloma, pneumococcal vaccination utilizing the 13-valent pneumococcal conjugate vaccine (PCV-13) and 23-valent pneumococcal polysaccharide vaccine (PPSV-23) should be performed in accordance with Advisory Committee on Immunization Practices guidelines (see MKSAP 17 General Internal Medicine). Intravenous immune globulin therapy may be used in select patients with low immunoglobulin levels and recurrent severe infections.

KEY POINTS

- The treatment of choice for patients with smoldering multiple myeloma at lower risk for progression is expectant management with monitoring every 3 to 6 months.

- For eligible patients with multiple myeloma requiring therapy, autologous hematopoietic stem cell transplantation with high-dose melphalan after initial induction therapy is associated with improved progression-free and, in some studies, overall survival.

Immunoglobulin Light-Chain Amyloidosis

The amyloidoses are characterized by the extracellular deposition of low-molecular-weight proteins in a β-pleated sheet configuration. The various types are outlined in **Table 14**. Proper identification of the amyloid type is critical and guides appropriate therapy. AL amyloidosis is the most common type

TABLE 14. The Amyloidoses		
Type	**Disease Association**	**Amyloid Protein**
AL amyloidosis	Plasma cell dyscrasias (MGUS, multiple myeloma), Waldenström macroglobulinemia (rare)	Monoclonal free λ or κ light chains
Hereditary amyloidosis	Inherited	Mutated transthyretin (TTR), fibrinogen α chain[a]
AA amyloidosis	Rheumatoid arthritis, inflammatory bowel disease, familial Mediterranean fever, chronic infection	Serum amyloid A protein
Age-related (senile) amyloidosis	Age	Wild type TTR
Dialysis-related amyloidosis	Dialysis for any reason	β$_2$-microglobulin

AA = secondary amyloidosis; AL = immunoglobulin light-chain amyloidosis; MGUS = monoclonal gammopathy of undetermined significance.

[a]Not an all-inclusive list.

and is a PCD-related disease characterized by end-organ damage related to tissue deposition of monoclonal free λ or κ light-chain fibrils. Clinical symptoms and manifestations vary and are dictated by the tissue tropism of the amyloidogenic light chain (**Table 15**).

H AL amyloidosis is diagnosed by an abdominal fat pad aspirate and bone marrow biopsy in most cases, although a more invasive biopsy of a clinically affected organ may be required if these tests are negative and clinical suspicion persists. Amyloid deposits in the biopsy sample demonstrate apple green birefringence under polarized light with Congo red staining. If amyloid deposits are identified, other types of amyloidosis should be excluded by typing, which can be done by κ/λ light-chain immunohistochemistry or immunofluorescence of a biopsy sample or mass spectroscopy–based protein sequencing of the amyloid deposits. A clonal plasma cell disorder should be confirmed, as defined by the presence of an M protein on serum or urine testing or the presence of clonal plasma cells in the marrow.

For patients with confirmed AL amyloidosis, in addition to the standard diagnostic tests noted previously (see Evaluation for Monoclonal Gammopathies), further studies should be conducted to assess organ involvement and establish a baseline for subsequent follow-up. Specific testing includes (1) serum troponin T, serum N-terminal proB-type natriuretic peptide (NT-proBNP), chest radiography, transthoracic echocardiography, and electrocardiography to assess cardiac involvement; (2) serologic liver tests, especially alkaline phosphatase, and abdominal ultrasonography to screen for hepatic amyloid; and (3) prothrombin and activated partial thromboplastin times to evaluate the presence of a coagulopathy (and, if abnormal, factor X level measurement). Pulmonary function tests, electromyography with nerve conduction studies, and gastric emptying studies should be considered for patients with symptoms of dyspnea, peripheral neuropathy, and gastroparesis, respectively. **H**

The prognosis of systemic AL amyloidosis is driven by the extent of cardiac involvement and levels of affected serum FLCs. A prognostic model incorporates an elevated serum troponin T level or NT-proBNP level and a significant difference in the involved to uninvolved serum FLC level; patients with 0, 1, 2, or 3 risk factors have a median overall survival of 94.1, 40.3, 14.0, or 5.8 months, respectively.

Treatment algorithms are similar to those used in multiple myeloma. Retrospective studies have demonstrated high hematologic response rates, improvement in organ function, and durable progression-free and overall survival with autologous HSCT in carefully selected patients. Patients not eligible for HSCT are considered for chemotherapy, which commonly consists of low-dose melphalan with dexamethasone.

TABLE 15. Clinical Manifestations of AL Amyloidosis by Organ System		
Organ System	**Clinical Manifestations**	**Findings**
Kidney	Anasarca, lower extremity edema, foamy urine	Nephrotic range proteinuria with bland urine sediment, hypoalbuminemia, elevated creatinine, nephromegaly on kidney ultrasonography
Gastrointestinal	Gastrointestinal bleeding, dysphagia, early satiety, abdominal distention, steatorrhea	Anemia, iron deficiency, submucosal hematomas on endoscopy, hypoalbuminemia, delayed gastric emptying, intestinal pseudo-obstruction, malabsorption, small bowel bacterial overgrowth
Liver	Weight loss, abdominal pain, features of chronic liver disease and portal hypertension	Cholestatic liver test abnormalities, hepatosplenomegaly, ascites, varices, evidence of portal hypertension
Neurologic	Distal numbness, paresthesias, neuropathic pain, weakness, autonomic nerve dysfunction	Distal sensorimotor polyneuropathy on electromyography/nerve conduction studies, autonomic neuropathy
Cardiac	Chest pain, symptoms from chronic heart failure or arrhythmia	Echocardiographic changes (ventricular hypertrophy with granular appearance, restrictive cardiomyopathy with diastolic heart failure greater than systolic heart failure), electrocardiographic changes (low voltages, pseudoinfarct pattern, conduction system changes, arrhythmias), abnormal cardiac MRI (late gadolinium enhancement)
Coagulation	Bleeding diathesis, periorbital purpura	Factor X deficiency with prolonged PT and aPTT, prolonged PT and aPTT from advanced liver impairment, blood vessel fragility from vascular amyloid deposition
Musculoskeletal	Macroglossia, muscle pseudohypertrophy, symmetric arthropathy, submandibular gland enlargement, carpal tunnel syndrome	Carpal tunnel syndrome on electromyography/nerve conduction studies, joint space widening on plain radiographs, periarticular soft tissue and muscle infiltration on MRI

aPTT = activated partial thromboplastin time; PT = prothrombin time.

Bortezomib-based and immunomodulatory drug–based therapy have shown encouraging results in small studies. The treatment goal is attainment of complete hematologic response (undetectable M protein), because this is associated with a higher likelihood of improvement in organ function.

KEY POINTS

- AL amyloidosis is diagnosed by the presence of amyloid deposits in the tissue biopsy sample (whether from abdominal fat pad aspirate or bone marrow or organ biopsy), proof that amyloid deposits are monoclonal free light chains, and confirmation of a clonal plasma cell disorder.

- Treatment with autologous hematopoietic stem cell transplantation in select patients with AL amyloidosis has demonstrated high hematologic response rates, improved organ function, and durable progression-free and overall survival.

Waldenström Macroglobulinemia

Waldenström macroglobulinemia is an indolent B-cell non-Hodgkin lymphoma characterized by production of an IgM κ or λ M protein. Smoldering (asymptomatic) Waldenström macroglobulinemia is defined as a neoplastic infiltrate consisting of clonal lymphocytes, plasmacytoid lymphocytes, plasma cells, and immunoblasts comprising 10% or more of the bone marrow cellularity or an M protein level of 3 g/dL or more and the absence of disease-related signs, symptoms, or organ dysfunction. Waldenström macroglobulinemia requiring therapy is similarly defined, but symptoms are present (see Table 12).

Patients with symptomatic disease may experience fatigue, and anemia is common. Systemic symptoms, commonly referred to as "B symptoms," include unexplained drenching sweats, fever, and weight loss. A bleeding diathesis is present in one quarter of patients at diagnosis, attributable to hyperviscosity, qualitative platelet dysfunction, or, less commonly, dysfibrinogenemia. Symptoms attributable to hyperviscosity may include headache, blurred vision, hearing loss, tinnitus, dizziness, altered mental status, and nasal and oropharyngeal bleeding. Funduscopic evaluation may reveal hyperviscosity-related findings, including dilated retinal veins, papilledema, and flame hemorrhages. Lymphadenopathy, hepatomegaly, and splenomegaly are often found on physical examination. Twenty percent of patients have a distal sensorimotor polyneuropathy that is commonly caused by antimyelin-associated glycoprotein activity of the M protein. Other rare manifestations of Waldenström macroglobulinemia include amyloidosis, cryoglobulinemia, and cold agglutinin disease.

In addition to the initial diagnostic evaluation outlined previously (see Evaluation for Monoclonal Gammopathies), a prothrombin time, activated partial thromboplastin time, and thrombin time should be performed to screen for dysfibrinogenemia in those with a bleeding diathesis not attributable to

hyperviscosity. Measurement of serum viscosity should be performed in those with symptoms or characteristic retinal findings. Patients with suspected cold agglutinin disease or cryoglobulinemia should have cold agglutinin titers or serum cryoglobulins and complement levels assessed. Assessment of serum β_2-microglobulin, albumin, and lactate dehydrogenase levels helps determine prognosis.

Symptomatic hyperviscosity is a medical emergency and requires immediate institution of plasmapheresis. Initial therapy may consist of rituximab as monotherapy or in combination with chemotherapy, which may consist of an alkylating agent (chlorambucil, cyclophosphamide, bendamustine) or a purine analog (fludarabine, cladribine) with or without a glucocorticoid. Autologous HSCT has been used in some patients. Bortezomib-based therapy may be used but is associated with high rates of peripheral neuropathy. ⊞

KEY POINTS

- Symptoms attributable to hyperviscosity, a medical emergency requiring immediate institution of plasmapheresis, are seen in 31% of patients with Waldenström macroglobulinemia and may include headache, blurred vision, hearing loss, tinnitus, dizziness, altered mental status, and nasal and oropharyngeal bleeding.

- In patients with Waldenström macroglobulinemia, funduscopic evaluation may reveal hyperviscosity-related findings, including dilated retinal veins, papilledema, and flame hemorrhages.

Cryoglobulinemia

Cryoglobulins are proteins that precipitate from serum at temperatures less than 37.0 °C (98.6 °F) and dissolve with warming. Cryoglobulins may cause no symptoms or lead to complications of hyperviscosity and thrombosis or manifestations of a small- to medium-vessel vasculitis. Cryoglobulinemias are classified by the composition of the cryoglobulin into types I, II, and III. Types II and III cryoglobulinemia are commonly referred to as mixed cryoglobulinemia. Type I cryoglobulinemia results from an underlying PCD or lymphoproliferative disorder (B-cell non-Hodgkin lymphoma), whereas mixed cryoglobulinemia can be caused by chronic infection, a PCD or lymphoproliferative disorder, or a systemic autoimmune disease. The most common disease associated with mixed cryoglobulinemia is hepatitis C. Although manifestations of vascular occlusion are more common in type I cryoglobulinemia, and vasculitis is common in mixed cryoglobulinemia, overlap is considerable. The clinical manifestations and disease associations for the various cryoglobulinemias are presented in **Table 16**.

Serologic testing for cryoglobulins should be performed using syringes and tubes prewarmed to 37.0 °C (98.6 °F) to avoid false-negative results. Rheumatoid factor and complement levels should be obtained. Additional testing may include evaluation for underlying disease states associated

TABLE 16. The Cryoglobulinemias

Type	Cryoglobulin Characteristics	Disease Associations	Clinical Manifestations
I	Monoclonal immunoglobulin (IgG, IgM, or IgA) with no RF activity	PCDs and lymphoproliferative disorders (MGUS, multiple myeloma, Waldenström macroglobulinemia, B-cell non-Hodgkin lymphoma, CLL)	Acrocyanosis, digital ischemia, livedo reticularis, skin ulcers and necrosis, lower extremity purpura, peripheral neuropathy (more common with types II and III), hyperviscosity, arthralgia, membranoproliferative glomerulonephritis (more common with types II and III)
II[a]	Polyclonal immunoglobulins + monoclonal immunoglobulin (IgM, IgA) with RF activity	Infection (hepatitis C), connective tissue disease (Sjögren syndrome, SLE), lymphoproliferative disorders (Waldenström macroglobulinemia, B-cell non-Hodgkin lymphoma, CLL)	Acrocyanosis; digital ischemia; fatigue; arthralgia; lower extremity purpura; skin ulcers and necrosis; peripheral neuropathy; membranoproliferative glomerulonephritis; pulmonary, CNS, and gastrointestinal vasculitis
III[a]	Polyclonal immunoglobulins with RF activity	Connective tissue disease, lymphoproliferative disorders	Same as type II

CLL = chronic lymphocytic leukemia; CNS = central nervous system; MGUS = monoclonal gammopathy of undetermined significance; PCD = plasma cell dyscrasia; RF = rheumatoid factor; SLE = systemic lupus erythematosus.

[a]Types II and III are mixed cryoglobulinemias.

Data from Terrier B, Karras A, Kahn JE, et al. The spectrum of type I cryoglobulinemic vasculitis: new insights based on 64 cases. Medicine. 2013 Mar;92(2):61-8. [PMID: 23429354] and Terrier B, Krastinova E, Marie I, et al. Management of noninfectious mixed cryoglobulinemia vasculitis: data from 242 cases included in the CryoVas survey. Blood. 2012 Jun 21;119(25):5996-6004. [PMID: 22474249]

CONT.

with cryoglobulinemia, such as hepatitis C antibody testing in a patient with type II cryoglobulinemia or a bone marrow biopsy in a patient with a suspected PCD or lymphoproliferative disorder.

Treatment of type I cryoglobulinemia includes plasmapheresis for those with symptomatic hyperviscosity and treatment of the underlying PCD or lymphoproliferative disorder. Management of mixed cryoglobulinemia consists of treatment of the underlying disease and immunosuppressive therapy for patients with more severe manifestations of vasculitis (rituximab or cyclophosphamide with a short course of glucocorticoids). H

KEY POINTS

- The most common disease associated with mixed cryoglobulinemia is hepatitis C.

- Type I cryoglobulinemia with hyperviscosity is managed with plasmapheresis and treatment of the underlying plasma cell dyscrasia or lymphoproliferative disorder.

- Mixed cryoglobulinemia is managed by treating the underlying disease and immunosuppressive therapy for patients with more severe manifestations of vasculitis.

Erythrocyte Disorders
Approach to Anemia

The primary function of erythrocytes is to deliver oxygen to tissues. Anemia, defined as decreased circulating red blood cell mass or hemoglobin, can limit oxygen delivery and result in symptoms of fatigue, dizziness, shortness of breath, and palpitations. Anemia itself is not a diagnosis, but a sign of an underlying condition. Although a good medical and family history is essential, it may not always explain the cause of the anemia. A targeted laboratory evaluation is often a window into understanding the underlying disorder.

When considering a patient with anemia, it is important to first establish chronicity. This provides insight into potential inherited versus acquired conditions. Anemia generally results from blood loss or underproduction or destruction of erythrocytes. Gross blood loss can usually be ruled out by history, but microscopic or factitious (patient mediated) loss must be considered, especially when iron deficiency is present.

Underproduction can be distinguished from destruction by the reticulocyte count, a measure of bone marrow production of erythrocytes, which is typically low in underproduction and elevated in destruction. Reticulocytes are immature erythrocytes, and their count is reported as the absolute reticulocyte count. The corrected reticulocyte count adjusts for the patient's hematocrit value. Reticulocytes usually mature into erythrocytes within 24 hours of release into the circulation. In times of severe anemia, reticulocytes can be released into the circulation earlier and will take longer to mature into erythrocytes (2-3 days). This correction for immature reticulocytes is adjusted by the reticulocyte production index.

The mean corpuscular volume (MCV) reflects erythrocyte size and can characterize certain anemias (**Table 17**). Red cell distribution width (RDW), which is a measure of the variation in size of the circulating erythrocytes relative to the MCV, provides additional information for characterizing the cause of anemia. An elevated RDW usually reflects the presence of

TABLE 17. Characterization of Anemia by Mean Corpuscular Volume		
Microcytic (MCV <80 fL)	**Normocytic**	**Macrocytic (MCV >100 fL)**
Iron deficiency	Inflammatory anemia[a]	Cobalamin (vitamin B_{12}) or folate deficiency
Thalassemia	Anemia of kidney disease	Autoimmune hemolytic anemia[b]
	Hereditary spherocytosis	Liver disease
	Sickle cell disease	Hypothyroidism
		Myelodysplastic syndrome[c]
		Sideroblastic anemia[d]
		Alcohol
		Drugs (e.g., HU, ZDV)

HU = hydroxyurea; MCV = mean corpuscular volume; ZDV = zidovudine.

[a]Inflammatory anemia can occasionally be microcytic.

[b]Autoimmune hemolytic anemia can occur because of reticulocytosis.

[c]Myelodysplastic syndrome can present with a normocytic anemia.

[d]Either congenital or acquired (e.g., by lead poisoning, copper deficiency, or drugs such as isoniazid, chloramphenicol, cycloserine, and linezolid).

erythrocytes of different sizes and may indicate a mixed process. For example, concomitant iron deficiency (microcytic) anemia and vitamin B_{12} (macrocytic) anemia would result in a normal MCV but an elevated RDW. Examination of the peripheral blood smear will reveal possible causes by characteristic morphologies.

KEY POINTS

- Anemia generally results from blood loss or underproduction or destruction of erythrocytes; underproduction can be distinguished from destruction by the reticulocyte count, which is typically low in the former and elevated in the latter.

Anemia Due to Erythrocyte Underproduction or Maturation Defects

Iron Deficiency

Iron is absorbed in the duodenum by enterocytes, which release it to the circulation destined for the bone marrow for incorporation into the hemoglobin molecule during erythropoiesis. Iron is transported in the plasma in its ferric form by the transport protein transferrin. Any excess iron is stored in the liver and reticuloendothelial system as ferritin for release as needed. Hepcidin, a peptide hormone produced in the liver, is a main regulator of iron homeostasis. It decreases intestinal iron absorption and release of iron stores by down-regulating the ferroportin-mediated release of iron from enterocytes, hepatocytes, and macrophages. Hepcidin is produced by hepatocytes when iron is abundant and in inflammatory anemia; it is suppressed in iron deficiency anemia (**Figure 6**).

Iron deficiency is the most common nutritional deficiency worldwide and is highly prevalent in developing countries. In the United States, it particularly affects children aged 1 to 2 years (7%-9% of toddlers) and girls and women aged 12 to 49 years (9%-16% of girls and women). The prevalence in the United States is higher in non-Hispanic black and Mexican American women (19%-22%). When diagnosing iron deficiency, it is crucial to consider, diagnose, and treat the underlying causes.

Approximately two thirds of iron is in the heme form and is incorporated into erythrocytes. The other one third is stored as ferritin or hemosiderin. A significant amount of iron is recycled from senescent erythrocytes. Dietary iron (1-2 mg/d) replaces natural losses of iron in urine, sweat, and stools. Insufficient dietary intake to replace this required amount and any additional loss (such as blood loss) will result in anemia over the course of a few months to years. Additionally, intestinal malabsorption of iron can lead to deficiency. Common causes of iron deficiency anemia are listed in **Table 18**.

Typical features of iron deficiency are identical to those of any symptomatic anemia but may be subtle owing to an insidious onset of the condition. Headache and pica (craving for typically undesirable items such as ice, dirt, clay, paper, and laundry starch) are frequently associated symptoms; other less common symptoms include restless legs syndrome and hair loss.

Recent blood transfusion or iron replacement may interfere with the accurate evaluation of iron deficiency. The hallmark of iron deficiency is a microcytic hypochromic anemia (**Figure 7**). However, this is usually only seen in advanced iron deficiency, and anemia tends to precede morphologic changes in the cells. On the other hand, abnormalities in iron studies typically precede the anemia. Serum iron concentrations tend to be low, but may be normal. Total iron-binding capacity (TIBC), a measure of the amount of transferrin in the plasma, is usually elevated. The transferrin saturation is a percentage calculated as serum iron/TIBC.

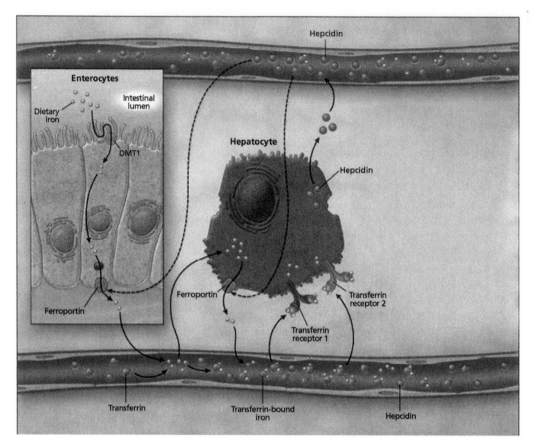

FIGURE 6. Dietary iron is absorbed from the gut (mainly the duodenum) into the blood stream via enterocytes (*inset*). This is facilitated by the divalent metal transporter-1 (DMT1) protein on the gut and the ferroportin on the vessel surface. Iron entering the vascular space is rapidly bound by transferrin and mostly transported to erythrocytes where it gets incorporated as hemoglobin. Excess iron is stored in the liver in hepatocytes and Kupffer cells utilizing transferrin receptors and ferroportin to transport it across the membrane. This transmembrane transport in the enterocyte and hepatic cells is down regulated by hepcidin, a hormone produced by hepatocytes in response to increased iron stores and inflammation.

TABLE 18.	Causes of Iron Deficiency Anemia
Loss of iron	
Bleeding	
Menstruation	
Phlebotomy	
Gastrointestinal bleeding (can be microscopic)	
Genitourinary bleeding (can be microscopic)	
Other blood loss (overt, microscopic, or factitious)	
Decreased intake	
Nutritional deficiency	
Decreased intake	
Decreased absorption	
After gastric/duodenal surgery	
Celiac disease	
Helicobacter pylori infection	
Autoimmune atrophic gastritis	
Increased iron requirements	
Pregnancy	
Lactation	

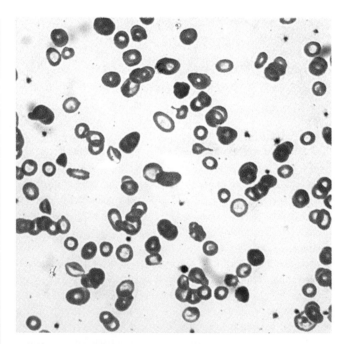

FIGURE 7. Iron deficiency anemia is characterized by microcytic (small) and hypochromic (pale-appearing) erythrocytes. The cells are often of various shapes and sizes as seen in this peripheral blood smear.

Transferrin saturation is usually less than 15% in iron deficiency anemia. Serum ferritin levels, as a measure of total body iron, are typically no more than 12 ng/mL (12 µg/L) in iron deficiency anemia and may be slightly higher in iron deficiency without anemia. Serum ferritin levels can be in the normal range when an associated inflammatory condition exists (for example, rheumatoid arthritis, malignancy, Gaucher disease). In inflammatory states, a serum ferritin level of greater than 100 ng/mL (100 µg/L) usually excludes iron deficiency. It is important to distinguish iron deficiency anemia from inflammatory anemia.

The presence of reticulocytes reflects the bone marrow response to anemia. In iron deficiency, the reticulocyte count is typically low, although occasionally it can be normal or even elevated.

Iron deficiency is managed by treating the underlying causes and by replacing iron. In premenopausal women, iron deficiency can result from menstrual blood loss, which need not imply any uterine or hormonal pathology and does not require further investigation. Further evaluation is warranted in all other persons with unexplained blood loss, and older men and women especially should be evaluated with colonoscopy, because a significant proportion will have colon cancer or premalignant polyps. Replacement can be achieved through oral supplementation, erythrocyte transfusion, or intravenous infusion (**Table 19**). One unit of packed red blood cells contains 225 to 250 mg of iron. Transfusion is an effective way to replace iron but is only indicated if the patient is profoundly anemic and symptomatic. Various oral replacement preparations are available.

They should provide 30 to 100 mg of elemental iron (in the ferrous form) per dose and should be given two to three times per day to provide an approximate total of 150 to 200 mg of iron. The least expensive, ferrous sulfate, is as effective as any of the more expensive oral preparations; more costly oral preparations that are reported to cause fewer adverse effects typically do so by exposing the patient to less absorbed iron. Enteric-coated preparations can have decreased absorption. In general, oral iron supplementation is well tolerated but is commonly accompanied by gastrointestinal symptoms (nausea, vomiting, dark stools, constipation) and a metallic taste.

Iron deficiency seemingly refractory to oral iron supplementation may indicate a subclinical underlying *Helicobacter pylori* infection; treatment of the infection may lead to improved iron absorption. In patients with subclinical hypothyroidism, adding levothyroxine may improve the response to oral iron replacement.

In persons who cannot tolerate or adequately absorb oral iron, intravenous replacement is indicated. To determine adequate iron absorption, an oral challenge can be given (check a fasting serum iron level and compare it to a level 1-2 hours after giving 60 mg of oral elemental iron; an increase of >100 µg/dL [17.9 µmol/L] suggests adequate oral absorption). Several parenteral iron-carbohydrate complexes are available. Iron dextran has been associated with anaphylactic reactions and a test dose should be administered (see Table 19).

In patients with chronic heart failure, iron deficiency is common and is associated with more severe disease and

TABLE 19.	Approach to Iron Replacement		
	Packed Red Blood Cell Transfusion	**Oral Replacement**	**Intravenous Replacement**
Dose	220-250 mg of iron/unit	Ferrous sulfate: 65 mg per 325-mg tablet Ferrous gluconate: 36 mg per 300-mg tablet Ferrous fumarate: 33 mg per 100-mg tablet	Ferric gluconate: 12.5 mg/mL Iron dextran: 50 mg/mL[a] Iron sucrose: 20 mg/mL Ferumoxytol: 30 mg/mL
Indication	Severe, symptomatic anemia Hemodynamically unstable patients End-organ damage	Iron deficiency not due to impaired intestinal absorption	GI malabsorption Inability to tolerate oral iron Poor response to oral iron Patients undergoing kidney dialysis receiving ESAs
Benefits	Rapid replacement of iron and lost blood	Inexpensive and readily available outpatient treatment	More rapid replacement, works in malabsorption, usually given in outpatient infusions
Side effects	Possible transfusion reaction	Often takes many months to fully replace stores, GI side effects	More expensive, allergic reactions

ESA = erythropoiesis-stimulating agent; GI = gastrointestinal.

[a]Requires test dose.

higher mortality. Treatment with iron was shown to alleviate symptoms and improve functional capacity and quality of life in these patients regardless of the degree of anemia.

- The hallmark of iron deficiency is a microcytic hypochromic anemia, but anemia tends to precede morphologic changes in the cells, and abnormalities in iron studies typically precede the anemia.

- Transferrin saturation is usually less than 15% in iron deficiency anemia, and the serum ferritin level is typically no more than 12 ng/mL (12 μg/L).

- The least expensive iron replacement is ferrous sulfate, which is as effective as any of the more expensive oral preparations.

Inflammatory Anemia

Inflammatory anemia, also referred to as anemia of chronic disease, is the most common anemia found in hospitalized patients. It is caused by underlying proinflammatory states such as infection, cancer, and autoimmune disease and other conditions, including chronic heart failure and diabetes mellitus, not traditionally characterized as proinflammatory. Pathophysiologically, these proinflammatory states result in dysregulation of iron homeostasis, impaired erythropoiesis, and blunted erythropoietin response. H

Hepcidin is upregulated in iron overload states as well as in inflammatory conditions, and proinflammatory cytokines such as interleukin-6, interleukin-1, and interferon-γ have been shown to induce hepcidin production. These inflammatory cytokines also blunt the erythropoietin response to anemia.

Inflammatory anemia is relatively mild, with most patients experiencing symptoms related to their underlying disease rather than the anemia. Inflammatory anemia and iron deficiency anemia can present with low serum iron levels but can be distinguished by other laboratory values (**Table 20**).

Most significantly, inflammatory anemia is usually normocytic and has a low TIBC.

As with iron deficiency anemia, management includes maximizing treatment of or eliminating the underlying disorder. Studies targeting the hepcidin-ferroportin axis are ongoing and could present promising future treatment modalities. H

- Inflammatory anemia is usually normocytic with a low serum iron level and total iron-binding capacity.

- Management of inflammatory anemia includes maximizing treatment of or eliminating the underlying disorder.

Anemia of Kidney Disease

Underproduction anemia is a very common association of chronic kidney disease (CKD) and affects about 90% of patients with a glomerular filtration rate (GFR) less than 25 to 30 mL/min/1.73 m^2; however, anemia can occur with higher GFR levels. The anemia is usually normochromic and normocytic and demonstrates a low reticulocyte count. In advanced kidney disease, typical echinocyte or "burr cell" morphology can be seen on peripheral blood smears. Although the primary cause of this anemia is decreased erythropoietin production by the failing kidney, erythropoietin levels measured in plasma do not accurately reflect functional or absolute erythropoietin deficiency and may appear normal. Measuring erythropoietin levels is thus not useful in diagnosing the anemia of kidney disease. Additional factors contributing to anemia are decreased lifespan of the erythrocytes, bone marrow suppression (from uremic toxins), and blood loss/destruction during hemodialysis. Diseases associated with kidney injury can also produce anemia by other mechanisms (for example, microangiopathic hemolytic anemia associated with hemolytic uremic syndrome–thrombotic thrombocytopenic purpura [see Platelet Disorders]). Anemia in kidney disease is discussed further in MKSAP 17 Nephrology.

Finding	Type of Anemia		
	Inflammatory Anemia	**Iron Deficiency Anemia**	**IDA with Inflammation**
MCV	72-100 fL	<80 fL	<100 fL
MCHC	<36 g/dL (360 g/L)	<32 g/dL (320 g/L)	<32 g/dL (320 g/L)
Serum iron	<60 μg/dL (11 μmol/L)	<60 μg/dL (11 μmol/L)	<60 μg/dL (11 μmol/L)
TIBC	<250 μg/dL (45 μmol/L)	>400 μg/dL (72 μmol/L)	<400 μg/dL (72 μmol/L)
TIBC saturation	2%-20%	<15% (usually <10%)	<15%
Ferritin	>35 ng/mL (35 μg/L)	<15 ng/mL (15 μg/L)	<100 ng/mL (100 μg/L)
Serum soluble transferrin receptor concentration	Normal	Increased	Increased
Stainable iron in bone marrow	Present	Absent	Absent

TABLE 20. Laboratory Characteristics of Inflammatory Anemia, Iron Deficiency Anemia (IDA), and IDA with Inflammation

MCHC = mean corpuscular hemoglobin concentration; MCV = mean corpuscular volume; TIBC = total iron-binding capacity.

- Underproduction anemia affects approximately 90% of patients with a glomerular filtration rate less than 25 to 30 mL/min/1.73 m^2; the anemia is usually normochromic and normocytic and demonstrates a low reticulocyte count.

- Measurement of erythropoietin levels is not useful in diagnosing the anemia of kidney disease.

Cobalamin (Vitamin B$_{12}$) Deficiency

Cobalamin (vitamin B$_{12}$) deficiency can result in a macrocytic underproduction anemia as well as a demyelinating nervous system disease.

Cobalamin is a cofactor needed by two enzymes in human cells: L-methylmalonyl–coenzyme A mutase and methionine synthase (**Figure 8**). Deficiency of cobalamin will thus cause increased methylmalonic acid and homocysteine levels and affect myelopoiesis as well as myelination of the central nervous system. Dyssynchronous development of the cytoplasm and the nucleus results in macrocytosis, hemolysis of erythrocytes within the bone marrow, and hypersegmentation in granulocytes.

Cobalamin deficiency is caused by insufficient intake or impaired absorption. Foods containing cobalamin are of animal origin, so vegetarians are at higher risk for cobalamin deficiency. Insufficient absorption can be caused by gastric, bariatric, or ileal surgery; inflammatory bowel disease; or pernicious anemia (autoimmune gastritis). Pernicious anemia is the most common cause of severe deficiency affecting all age groups, but especially older adults. It results in the destruction of gastric parietal cells, which synthesize intrinsic factor needed for cobalamin absorption. Because cobalamin is efficiently stored, and bile losses are effectively recycled by the enterohepatic circulation, it takes 2 to 3 years of insufficient intake or impaired absorption before cobalamin deficiency ensues.

Symptoms are those of anemia, hemolysis, or neurologic dysfunction. Common neurologic findings are symmetric paresthesias, numbness, decreased vibratory sense, and gait problems, and even neuropsychiatric symptoms, which can occur in the absence of anemia or other hematologic findings. Other associated symptoms include glossitis, hyperpigmentation, and infertility.

A thorough history to elicit potential causes of cobalamin deficiency and a neurologic examination must accompany laboratory evaluation. Patients with pernicious anemia often have other autoimmune disorders (for example, thyroid disease, diabetes mellitus, vitiligo).

Laboratory evaluation typically reveals macrocytic anemia and decreased reticulocyte count. Peripheral blood smears show large oval erythrocytes, hypersegmented neutrophils (≥6 lobes) (**Figure 9**), and possible pancytopenia. Measurement of the cobalamin level has poor sensitivity and specificity and can vary greatly between laboratories, especially in patients with anti-intrinsic factor antibodies. A reasonable first step in evaluating suspected vitamin B$_{12}$ deficiency is a serum cobalamin level, with levels greater than 300 pg/mL (221 pmol/L) making deficiency unlikely and levels less than 200 pg/mL (148 pmol/L) strongly suggesting deficiency. If diagnostic uncertainty exists, methylmalonic acid and homocysteine measurement may be helpful. Both are elevated in 98% of patients with cobalamin deficiency, even in patients with neurologic symptoms without anemia. Levels should be measured before repletion therapy is initiated. Methylmalonic acid levels can be mildly elevated in kidney injury, but levels greater than 500 nmol/L are reasonably specific for cobalamin deficiency. Homocysteine levels are less specific and can be elevated in folate deficiency as well. Methylmalonic acid and total homocysteine levels are helpful in differentiating cobalamin deficiency (both levels are elevated) from folate deficiency (elevated homocysteine but normal methylmalonic acid level).

Bone marrow biopsy is not necessary to diagnose cobalamin deficiency and can be confusing, showing hypercellular, dysplastic changes that could be mistaken for myelodysplastic syndrome or an acute myeloid leukemia.

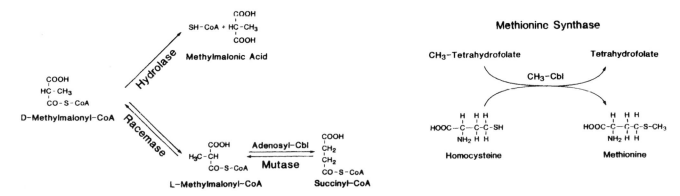

FIGURE 8. The two cobalamin (vitamin B$_{12}$)-dependent enzymes, L-methylmalonyl-CoA mutase (*left*) and methionine synthase (*right*).

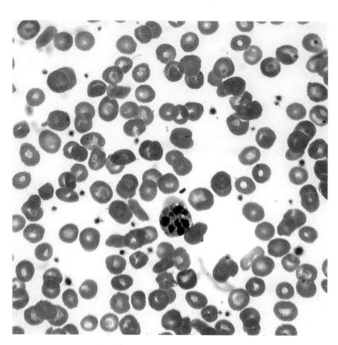

FIGURE 9. Cobalamin deficiency is often accompanied by macrocytic (large) erythrocytes and hypersegmented neutrophils with six or more nuclear lobes as shown in the image.

 A bone marrow examination might be helpful if these disorders are suspected and the patient is not responding to replacement therapy. **H**

Parietal cell antibody levels are sensitive for pernicious anemia, but can also be positive in chronic gastritis. Antibodies to intrinsic factor are more specific. Patients with unexplained cobalamin deficiency should be tested for pernicious anemia.

Deficiency resulting from insufficient dietary intake is rare and requires chronic, long-standing nutritional deficiency. It can be prevented by foods enriched with vitamin B_{12} and/or oral supplementation of more than 2 µg/d in persons with low dietary cobalamin intake. Malabsorption must be overcome with either high-dose oral supplementation or injections.

High-dose oral supplementation of 1000 to 2000 µg/d is usually as effective as parenteral administration, even in patients with intrinsic factor insufficiency, and should be the initial therapy for most patients.

In patients with severe anemia, neurologic dysfunction, or those not responding to oral replacement, cobalamin injections (intramuscular or subcutaneous) ensure adequate delivery, usually with 1000 µg several times per week for 1 to 2 weeks, then weekly until symptom relief or improved findings. Monthly injections thereafter are indicated if the underlying cause persists (for example, pernicious anemia).

The hematologic recovery is usually quick, with an increased reticulocyte count in 1 week and correction of megaloblastic anemia in 6 to 8 weeks. Neurologic recovery depends on the duration of symptoms before treatment, can include transient worsening, and may take weeks to months. **H**

KEY POINTS

- Methylmalonic acid and total homocysteine levels are helpful in differentiating cobalamin deficiency (both levels are elevated) from folate deficiency (elevated homocysteine but normal methylmalonic acid level); bone marrow biopsy is not necessary and can be confusing. **HVC**

- High-dose oral vitamin B_{12} supplementation of 1000 to 2000 µg/d is usually as effective as parenteral administration, even in patients with intrinsic factor insufficiency, and should be the initial therapy for most patients.

Folate Deficiency

Like cobalamin deficiency, folate deficiency leads to impaired DNA synthesis resulting in a megaloblastic anemia (MCV >100 fL). The bone marrow is characterized by erythroid hyperplasia with abnormal (megaloblastic) morphology.

Folate is available from animal and nonanimal sources (including asparagus, broccoli, spinach, lemons, mushrooms, fortified grains). Despite that, most folate deficiency is dietary in nature and particularly affects older adults, patients in nursing homes, and persons who consume large amounts of alcohol. Other causes of deficiency include malabsorption from entities such as celiac disease, inflammatory bowel disease, or short gut syndrome; medications accelerating folate metabolism, including phenytoin, trimethoprim, and methotrexate; and conditions requiring higher folate intake, including pregnancy, lactation, states of chronic hemolysis, and exfoliant dermatitis. Compared with cobalamin, folate is not well stored, and deficiency can occur in weeks rather than months. Symptoms of folate deficiency are usually related to the anemia, and neurologic deficits do not manifest.

Laboratory findings are similar to cobalamin deficiency (macrocytic anemia, hypersegmented neutrophils). Likewise, homocysteine levels are elevated in folate deficiency, although in contrast, methylmalonic acid levels will not be elevated. Serum folate levels have short-range fluctuations and are a poor measure of deficiency. Serum levels can normalize after a single folate-containing meal. However, they can be a good screening tool, especially if they are low in the absence of recent folate ingestion.

Folate deficiency can be treated with oral folic acid, 1 to 5 mg/d, until complete hematologic recovery; oral therapy is effective even in malabsorption conditions. Cobalamin deficiency should be excluded before initiating therapy, because large doses of folic acid may lead to improved hematopoiesis despite cobalamin deficiency, thus leaving patients vulnerable to central and peripheral nervous system injury from vitamin B_{12} deficiency. **H**

- Folate deficiency can be treated with oral folic acid, 1 to 5 mg/d, until complete hematologic recovery; oral therapy is effective even in malabsorption conditions.

- Cobalamin deficiency should be excluded before initiating folate deficiency therapy, because large doses of folic acid may lead to improved hematopoiesis despite cobalamin deficiency, leaving patients vulnerable to central and peripheral nervous system injury from vitamin B_{12} deficiency.

TABLE 22. Causes of Hemolytic Anemia Determined by Peripheral Blood Smear

Finding on Peripheral Blood Smear	Associated Disease State
Spherocytes	Hereditary spherocytosis
	Autoimmune hemolytic anemia
Target cells	Thalassemia
	Hemoglobin C
	Liver disease
Schistocytes	Microangiopathic hemolytic anemia
Bite cells	Glucose-6-phosphate dehydrogenase deficiency

Hemolytic Anemias

Overview

Hemolytic anemias are characterized by early destruction of erythrocytes secondary to lysis. This happens within the circulatory system (intravascular); in the spleen, liver, or bone marrow (extravascular); or both. It can be due to an inherited defect (erythrocyte membrane or enzymatic defect, abnormal hemoglobin synthesis) or an acquired disorder (immune or nonimmune) (**Table 21**).

Hemolytic processes are characterized by compensatory increases in erythrocyte production (reticulocytosis) in many, but not all, cases; signs of erythrocyte destruction (elevated indirect bilirubin and lactate dehydrogenase [LDH]); and free hemoglobin secretion (hemosiderinuria, hemoglobinuria). If erythrocyte destruction and production do not balance, anemia results. A peripheral blood smear can be very useful in distinguishing different causes (**Table 22**).

Symptoms of hemolytic anemia depend on the severity and chronicity. Besides the usual symptoms of anemia, jaundice can be seen with acute hemolytic anemia and cholelithiasis can develop with chronic hemolysis. In severe cases, extramedullary hematopoiesis can occur and result in hepatosplenomegaly or lymphadenopathy that develops over years. ▯

Congenital Hemolytic Anemias

Hereditary Spherocytosis

Hereditary spherocytosis (HS) is a common form of inherited anemia in people of Northern European descent. It is usually autosomal dominant (75% of patients), but can also be recessive. Mutations causing deficiencies or dysfunction in five erythrocyte membrane proteins (α-spectrin, β-spectrin, ankyrin, band 3, and protein 4.2) have been identified. These will adversely affect the interaction between the lipid bilayer and cytoskeleton layer of the erythrocyte wall, reducing surface-to-volume ratio. Ultimately, this results in osmotically fragile spherocytes (hemolysis) and splenic sequestration (splenomegaly).

Symptoms of HS range from asymptomatic carrier states to severe hemolysis. Symptomatic patients usually present with anemia, jaundice, and splenomegaly and may have pigmented (bilirubin) gallstones.

Typical laboratory findings include spherocytes on peripheral blood smear and varying degrees of anemia, reticulocytosis, and bilirubin elevation. An increased mean corpuscular hemoglobin concentration reflecting membrane loss and erythrocyte dehydration is characteristic. Patients with representative

TABLE 21. Examples of Congenital and Acquired Causes of Hemolytic Anemia

Congenital Hemolytic Anemias	Examples
Defects in the erythrocyte membrane	Hereditary spherocytosis
Deficiencies in erythrocyte metabolic enzymes	Glucose-6-phosphate dehydrogenase deficiency
Defects in hemoglobin structure or synthesis	Sickle cell disease, α- and β-thalassemia

Acquired Hemolytic Anemias	Examples
Autoimmune hemolytic anemia	Warm autoimmune hemolytic anemia, cold agglutinin disease
Microangiopathic hemolytic anemias	Thrombotic thrombocytopenic purpura, disseminated intravascular coagulation
Paroxysmal nocturnal hemoglobinuria	
Infectious, chemical, and physical agents	*Plasmodium* species, *Babesia microti*, *Clostridium perfringens* (formerly *C. welchii*), *Bartonella bacilliformis*, copper, thermal injury, venoms and toxins (brown recluse spider bites)

clinical and laboratory findings, especially if they have a family history of HS, do not require additional testing for the diagnosis. In less obvious presentations, the cryohemolysis test and eosin-5-maleimide binding test are effective screening tests with high predictive value, although they are not readily available at most hospitals. Additionally, the osmotic fragility test has not performed well as a screening test.

As in other hemolytic anemias, folate is consumed during active hemolysis, which could lead to a megaloblastic anemia. Folic acid supplementation is recommended in moderate and severe forms of HS. Splenectomy is effective in reducing hemolysis and should be considered in severe conditions. Partial splenectomy can be effective, especially in children in whom preserved splenic immune function is desired. It is important to appropriately vaccinate patients against encapsulated organisms such as *Streptococcus pneumoniae*, *Haemophilus influenzae*, and *Neisseria meningitidis* before splenectomy.

Glucose-6-Phosphate Dehydrogenase Deficiency

Glucose-6-phosphate dehydrogenase (G6PD) deficiency is an X-linked disorder, thus primarily affecting men. Women can be affected in the rare event of homozygous disease, lyonization with preference of expression of the defective gene, and in XO karyotypes. It is the most common enzyme deficiency in humans, with about 140 identified gene mutations. These affect the enzyme G6PD, the first enzyme in the pentose phosphate pathway, a crucial step in nicotinamide adenine dinucleotide phosphate reduction (NADP to NADPH), which is essential for cells to counterbalance oxidative stress. G6PD deficiency occurs most commonly in people of African, Asian, Mediterranean, and Middle Eastern descent.

It can cause various clinical phenotypes and presents with neonatal jaundice or acute hemolysis in response to a "trigger." Certain medications (sulfonamides, some antimalarials, rasburicase), naphthalene in mothballs, fava beans, and infection can trigger hemolysis within 24 to 72 hours. Clinical manifestations can range from asymptomatic mild hemolysis to severe hemolysis. The most common G6PD mutation found in blacks typically results in a very mild defect that may or may not lead to clinically relevant hemolysis following use of oxidative drugs or other stress. Some patients may have chronic nonspherocytic hemolysis. Patients often report fatigue, jaundice, shortness of breath, and dark urine. Typical laboratory markers for hemolysis are present and peripheral blood smears show typical bite cells (**Figure 10**) and Heinz bodies (**Figure 11**), which are denatured oxidized hemoglobin visualized as intranuclear inclusions seen on supravital stain. Severe hemolysis can lead to acute kidney injury and dialysis; chronic hemolysis can lead to cholelithiasis.

A fluorescent spot screening test for G6PD activity detects the formation of NADPH and is reliable in men who are not experiencing an acute hemolytic episode. This test is less useful in acute episodes, with reticulocytosis (young cells produce higher levels of enzyme), and in women (chimerism); measuring

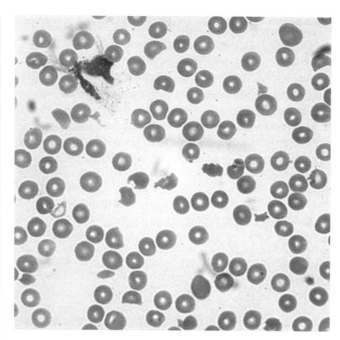

FIGURE 10. Bite cells seen at the center of this slide are typical findings in glucose-6-phosphate dehydrogenase (G6PD) deficiency and are characterized by a membrane defect that appears as though a semicircular bite has been taken out of the erythrocyte. The defect is caused by removal of denatured hemoglobin by macrophages in the spleen.

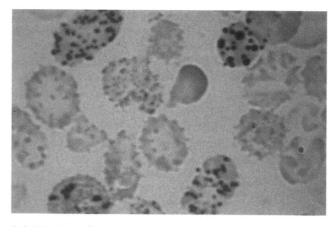

FIGURE 11. Erythrocytes with Heinz bodies in a patient with glucose-6-phosphate dehydrogenase (G6PD) deficiency, a type of hemolytic anemia.

quantitative G6PD enzyme activity can provide a more specific diagnosis.

The most effective management of G6PD deficiency is prevention of hemolytic episodes by avoiding offending agents. When hemolysis occurs, treatment is supportive, with blood transfusions reserved for severe cases. The use of antioxidants such as vitamin E and selenium is controversial.

Thalassemia

The hemoglobin molecule in normal erythrocytes is made up of two α- and two β-globin subunits ($\alpha_2\beta_2$). Thalassemia is a common genetic disorder caused either by a mutation in the α globin (chromosome 16) or the β globin (chromosome 11) that leads to a quantitative deficiency in the synthesis of that globin chain. The imbalance in globin chain synthesis leads to impaired production of hemoglobin and ineffective erythropoiesis, with intramedullary hemolysis. Severity of the associated microcytic anemia depends on how many globin chains are affected and the severity of the mutation. Of the world population, 1% to 5% has a mutation in at least one β chain; mutations in an α chain are even more common. This incidence of thalassemia is especially high in Mediterranean countries, the Middle East, tropical and subtropical regions of Africa, Asia, and Southeast Asia.

Unlike iron deficiency, the overall erythrocyte count is normal to elevated in α- and β-thalassemia, and iron studies are in the normal range. Decreased β-chain synthesis leads to impaired production of hemoglobin A $(\alpha_2\beta_2)$ and resultant increased synthesis of hemoglobin A_2 $(\alpha_2\delta_2)$ and/or hemoglobin F $(\alpha_2\gamma_2)$. The hemoglobin electrophoresis in α-thalassemia shows a normal pattern and cannot be differentiated from that of a person without thalassemia.

α-thalassemia

Duplication of the α-globin chain on chromosome 16 results in 4 α-globin genes (αα/αα); α-thalassemia results from deletion of one or more of these. The diagnosis is suspected in individuals with microcytic anemia not consistent with iron deficiency anemia and normal hemoglobin A_2 levels on electrophoresis.

The absence of one α gene (-α/αα) results in an asymptomatic carrier state. Absence of two α genes (-α/α- or -/αα) results in a mild microcytic anemia (α-thalassemia trait or α-thalassemia minor). Deletion of three α genes (-/-α), known as hemoglobin H disease, results in moderate microcytic anemia with hemoglobin levels of 8 to 10 g/dL (80-100 g/L), some hemolysis, and splenomegaly. α-Thalassemia trait and hemoglobin H disease are easily confused with iron deficiency anemia because of their microcytic nature. The complete absence of α-globin chains results in hydrops fetalis and intrauterine fetal demise.

Patients with α-thalassemia trait do not require treatment or further monitoring, but should be well educated regarding the condition to prevent unnecessary treatment with iron supplementation in the future. In hemoglobin H disease, blood transfusions occasionally become necessary if the patient is significantly symptomatic from the anemia, predisposing the patient to iron overload. As with any other hemolytic anemia, oral folic acid at 1 mg/d should be given.

β-thalassemia

More than 200 mutations in the β-globin chain have been described and may result in mild to severe reduction of β-chain expression (β⁺-thalassemia) or complete gene deletion (β⁰-thalassemia). This translates into a range of clinical diseases based on the degree of β-chain expression, classified into phenotypic subtypes of thalassemia minor, intermedia, and major.

Heterozygous gene mutations result in β-thalassemia trait (minor) characterized by an asymptomatic, microcytic (MCV 60-70 fL) mild anemia (hemoglobin 10-13 g/dL [100-130 g/L]), which is often confused with iron deficiency anemia. Homozygous or compound heterozygous (different mutations affecting the two genes) mutations result in more severe disease, depending on the type of mutation, and result in overstimulation of the bone marrow, ineffective erythropoiesis, and potential iron overload. Mild to moderate forms of β-thalassemia (intermedia) are associated with moderate hemolytic anemia, maintaining hemoglobin levels (>7 g/dL [70 g/L]) without transfusion support. Patients usually present during childhood with varying degrees of hemolytic anemia. Relatively normal growth without blood transfusions is common, but patients may require transfusions during periods of worsened and symptomatic anemia (such as aplastic crisis during infection). Complications from chronic hemolysis, such as folate deficiency and cholelithiasis, can occur. Folic acid supplementation is indicated. As in α-thalassemia, patients are often mistakenly diagnosed with iron deficiency anemia because of microcytosis, but iron replacement is only indicated if true iron deficiency can be demonstrated. Severe β-thalassemia (major) presents early in life with pallor, failure to thrive, severe hemolytic anemia, erythroid hyperplasia in the bone marrow, associated bone deformities, and massive hepatosplenomegaly due to extramedullary hematopoiesis. These patients, if untreated, usually die in the first or second decade of life.

Monthly erythrocyte transfusion should be initiated for hemoglobin levels less than 7 g/dL (70 g/L). Other contributing causes of anemia must be excluded (such as G6PD deficiency), and folic acid supplementation is required. However, risks of chronic transfusions include iron overload with subsequent cardiomyopathy, hepatic fibrosis, and endocrine dysfunction. Even patients not receiving transfusions are at risk for iron overload because of increased iron absorption as a result of ineffective erythropoiesis. Close monitoring and iron chelation therapy (if indicated) are crucial in all patients with thalassemia intermedia and major.

Subcutaneous desferrioxamine or an oral iron chelation agent (deferasirox, deferiprone), as monotherapy or combined, have shown good efficacy in reducing liver and myocardial iron load.

Allogeneic hematopoietic stem cell transplantation (HSCT) can be curative and should be considered with severe forms, preferably before the onset of end-organ damage.

Sickle Cell Syndromes

Sickle cell disease (SCD) is a recessively inherited hemoglobinopathy characterized by a single point mutation in the β-globin chain resulting in abnormal hemoglobin. This abnormal hemoglobin S (Hb S) results in polymerization of hemoglobin molecules under oxidative stress, leading to a formational change of the erythrocyte to a sickle shape and subsequent obstruction of the circulation as well as resultant hemolysis. Adhesion of cells to the endothelium, inflammation, decreased nitric oxide (due to binding with free hemoglobin released from lysing erythrocytes), and resulting vasoconstriction contribute to this complex pathophysiology.

Because most gene mutations are of African origin, most patients with homozygous sickle cell anemia (Hb SS) in the United States are black and about 1/200 blacks has sickle cell trait. The Hb S mutation can be coinherited with other hemoglobinopathies, resulting in differentiating values on hemogram and hemoglobin electrophoresis (**Table 23**).

Interestingly, these single point mutations causing Hb SS can result in a wide array of phenotypic expression in SCD, potentially affecting any organ system and leading to significantly decreased life expectancy.

Sickle Cell Disease Complications and Their Management

SCD results in a chronic hemolytic anemia, and maintenance of blood counts is dependent on a chronic, brisk reticulocytosis that is vulnerable to infections (particularly parvovirus B19) and vitamin deficiencies (folate deficiency). The three common disease-altering strategies are allogeneic HSCT, prophylactic transfusions, and hydroxyurea therapy. The timing and patient population for whom HSCT should be considered have not been clarified. Patients not considered for HSCT or prophylactic transfusions should be evaluated to receive hydroxyurea if they experience one or two vaso-occlusive episodes per year. Hydroxyurea therapy has been shown to decrease vaso-occlusive episodes and acute chest syndrome (ACS), to decrease transfusion requirements and hospitalizations, and to prolong overall survival.

The management of sickle cell complications is complex, benefits from a comprehensive care model, and must include preventive, acute, and chronic treatment approaches (**Table 24**).

Painful episodes are the hallmark of SCD resulting from vaso-occlusive ischemic episodes. Although most of these episodes seem to be spontaneous, precipitating factors (dehydration, temperature/climate changes, physical or emotional stress, infection, asthma, acidosis, sleep apnea, pregnancy) can cause them. The pain can occur anywhere in the body and take place only a few times over a lifetime or up to several episodes per month. Acute pain often requires treatment with scheduled narcotics with the exception of meperidine, which has been associated with a lower seizure threshold and is not recommended. **H**

Chronic pain is common in SCD and is poorly understood. The pain tends to be constant, lasting for months and years and can affect any body part. It is often triggered by frequent, severe, acute painful episodes and is thought to be a hypersensitization to normal environmental stimuli. Chronic pain is often accompanied by depression, anxiety, insomnia, and chronic narcotic use and dependency. Patients benefit from a multidisciplinary, multimodality approach (for example, opioids, NSAIDs, antidepressants, relaxation techniques, massage, acupuncture, biofeedback).

ACS results from vaso-occlusive involvement of the pulmonary vasculature and is diagnosed by new pulmonary infiltrates involving at least one complete lung segment that is consistent with alveolar consolidation with either chest pain, fever (>38.5 °C [101.3 °F]), tachypnea, wheezing, or cough. It is crucial to consider and rule out other causes that may present similarly, including infectious pneumonia, fat or bone marrow embolism, or more traditional venous thromboembolism.

Infection, particularly with encapsulated bacteria such as pneumococcus, was previously the primary cause of death in SCD. It has now been surpassed by cardiopulmonary causes (pulmonary hypertension, pulmonary thromboembolism,

TABLE 23.	Characteristics of Adult Sickle Cell Syndromes						
Disease Type	**Hb (g/dL)**	**MCV (fL)**	**Hb S (%)**	**Hb A (%)**	**Hb A$_2$ (%)**	**Peripheral Blood Smear Findings**	**Clinical Severity[a] 0 to +++**
Sickle trait (AS)	NL	NL	40	60	<3.5	NL	0
Hb SS	6-8	NL	>90	0	<3.5	Sickle cells	+++
Sβ$^+$-Thalassemia	9-12	70-75	>60	10-30	>3.5	Rare sickle cells Target cells	+ to ++
Sβ^0-Thalassemia	7-9	65-70	>80	0	>3.5	Sickle cells Target cells	+++
SCD	10-15	75-NL	50	0	Hb A$_2$ = 0 Hb C = 50[b]	Fat sickle cells Target cells	+ to ++

Hb = hemoglobin; Hb SS = homozygous sickle cell anemia; MCV = mean corpuscular volume; NL = normal; Sβ$^+$ = sickle β$^+$; Sβ^0 = sickle β^0; SCD = sickle cell disease.

[a]Clinical severity is variable within each genotype.

[b]Note that Hb C comigrates with Hb A$_2$ on standard alkaline cellulose acetate electrophoresis but will separate on citrate agar electrophoresis.

NOTE: Hb percentages may not total 100% because Hb F is not included in this table.

TABLE 24. Common Complications and Treatments in Adults with Sickle Cell Disease

Complications	Treatment
Vaso-occlusive pain episode	**Acute:** rest, relaxation, warmth, NSAIDs, oral and IV hydration, narcotic analgesia
	Recurring: HU, avoidance of triggers, nonnarcotic or narcotic analgesia
Acute chest syndrome	**Acute:** oxygen, incentive spirometry, analgesics, empiric antibiotics, IV fluids, simple or erythrocyte exchange transfusions
	Preventive: HU, incentive spirometry
Aplastic crisis	**Acute:** supportive care, blood transfusions as needed
Infection	**Acute:** Appropriate and immediate antibiotic management (particular concern for encapsulated bacteria)
	Prevention: Influenza, pneumococcal, and meningococcal vaccines
Hyperhemolytic crisis	**Acute:** supportive care, avoid further blood transfusions, immunosuppression might be helpful
	Preventive: avoid blood transfusions if possible, extended antibody screen can lessen but not eliminate recurrence
Multiorgan failure	**Acute:** Erythrocyte exchange transfusions
Ischemic stroke	**Acute:** Erythrocyte exchange transfusions, aspirin
	Preventive: Chronic simple transfusions or erythrocyte exchange transfusions (target Hb S <30%-50%)
Hepatic crisis	**Acute:** Supportive, transfusion or exchange transfusion if anemia is symptomatic
Cholelithiasis	**Acute:** If symptomatic, cholecystectomy with preoperative transfusions to hemoglobin of 10 g/dL (100 g/L)
Chronic kidney disease/ proteinuria	**Preventive:** good blood pressure control to <130/80 mm Hg
	Secondary preventive: ACE inhibitor or ARB
Priapism	**Acute:** relaxation, hydration, narcotic analgesics, aspiration of blood from corpora cavernosa and irrigation with dilute epinephrine, transfusions, shunt procedure
	Preventive: oral α-adrenergic agonists, HU. The role of leuprolide and sildenafil is not clear.
Pulmonary hypertension	No proven therapy established for prevention or treatment
Retinopathy	Annual ophthalmologic examination, laser phototherapy as needed
Osteopenia/osteoporosis	Supplementation with calcium and vitamin D
Avascular necrosis	Chronic narcotic analgesia, arthroplasty
Foot and leg ulcers	**Acute:** early aggressive treatment, debridement, bandage impregnated with zinc oxide
	Preventive: proper footwear to prevent pressure points

ARB = angiotensin receptor blocker; Hb S = hemoglobin S; HU = hydroxyurea; IV = intravenous.

pulmonary microthrombi, sudden cardiac death) but remains a major factor in morbidity and mortality. In febrile patients, especially with leukocyte counts above baseline, infection with encapsulated bacteria must always be considered (even in vaccinated persons) and must be treated immediately.

Pulmonary hypertension can be a chronic and severe complication of SCD, and about 25% to 30% of persons with Hb SS or Hb Sβ⁰-thalassemia will have suggestive abnormalities on echocardiogram. Of those, 25% of patients will have confirmed pulmonary hypertension on right heart catheterization. In patients with confirmed pulmonary hypertension, an increased tricuspid regurgitation velocity on Doppler echocardiography has been associated with increased mortality. Advanced age; a history of leg ulcers; higher LDH, creatinine, alkaline phosphatase, and N-terminal proB-type natriuretic peptide levels; and a higher New York Heart Association func-

tional class scoring are associated with increased mortality risk. No proven therapy is available for the prevention or treatment of pulmonary hypertension.

Persons with SCD are at increased risk for ischemic stroke during childhood and with advancing age. The Hb SS subtype is more affected than Hb SC, and stroke is rare in Hb Sβ⁰-thalassemia subtypes. In children, transcranial Doppler (TCD) ultrasonography of the middle cerebral arteries (to assess for increased velocity) has been shown to be a strong predictor of stroke risk, and prophylactic transfusion or exchange transfusion is proven to reduce this risk. Switching from transfusion to hydroxyurea therapy in these patients to lessen the risk of iron overload from overtransfusion increases the risk for ischemic stroke without improving iron concentration. Approximately 30% of patients with Hb SS or Sβ⁰-thalassemia without overt stroke may have silent infarcts. Lower hemoglobin levels, male sex, and higher blood pressure may be predisposing factors. Transfusion protocols to prevent or treat silent strokes have not been established.

Differing from strokes during childhood, strokes in the third and fourth decades of life tend to be hemorrhagic and are often attributable to underlying moyamoya disease (arterial narrowing at the basal ganglia and resulting fragile collateral circulation). ᴴ

Adults with sickle cell anemia have lower neurocognitive performance than matched controls. This decreased neuro-cognitive performance (memory, processing speed, and executive function) is related to lower baseline hemoglobin levels (especially in older patients), but does not correlate with abnormal findings on MRI. No preventive measures have been established for decreasing neurocognitive function.

Hepatic crisis is characterized by right upper quadrant pain, elevated liver enzyme levels, and an enlarged liver. Hepatic crisis due to vaso-occlusive sickle cell episodes usually has a sudden onset and is self-limiting. It can be associated with hepatic sequestration typified by a rapid enlargement of the liver and decrease in hemoglobin level. Transfusion or exchange transfusion is the treatment of choice to support symptomatic anemia. Other causes such as acute or chronic hepatitis, liver involvement from hemosiderosis, and chole-lithiasis should not be overlooked.

Nephropathy caused by decreased medullary blood flow, microinfarct, and papillary necrosis can result in CKD in SCD. Proteinuria is associated with progressively declining GFR and is evidence of glomerular injury. Impaired ability to concentrate urine, hematuria, urinary tract infections, and limited renal acidification and potassium secretion are common. Patients must be monitored periodically (serum creatinine level and testing for proteinuria every 3-6 months) for declining kidney function and require strict blood pressure control. Proteinuria should be treated with an ACE inhibitor or an angiotensin receptor blocker. Progression of kidney disease despite these measures may require dialysis and kidney transplantation. ᴴ

Priapism is an unwanted, painful, sometimes recurrent penile erection lasting for hours to days. It is a common (35% of men with SCD) and often understated complication of SCD in young men and can lead to erectile dysfunction and impotence. The pathophysiology is not fully understood, but obstruction of venous outflow seems to be a contributing factor.

Decreased bone density is common in SCD and may be a result of vitamin D deficiency, increased bone resorption, or bone necrosis due to vaso-occlusion. Treatment with vitamin D, calcium, and bisphosphonates has not been studied. Avascular necrosis is common and poses a major problem because it presents with daily pain in children and young adults. It is uncertain what the best timing is for joint replacement in this relatively young population.

Spontaneous or traumatic leg ulcers are common in SCD, are related to impaired circulation, and are often complicated by prolonged wound healing. They are often located on the lower legs, particularly the medial and lateral ankle. Lower hemoglobin and increased hemolytic markers are associated with increased risk of skin ulcers.

Allogeneic HSCT to at least achieve chimerism between the donor and recipient (production of donor cells while retaining production of some recipient cells) has been investigated, and a small study in adults showed significant reduction in Hb S, increase in baseline hemoglobin level, and decrease in hemolysis in patients who received a nonmyeloablative transplant from a matched sibling. All of these patients were alive 1 year after the transplant and none had developed graft-versus-host disease.

Erythrocyte Transfusions in Sickle Cell Disease

Persons with SCD typically have baseline hemoglobin levels of 6 to 7 g/dL (60-70 g/L) in Hb SS and 8 to 10 mg/dL (80-100 g/L) in Hb SC; however, they have physiologically adjusted to this anemia. Transfusion to achieve hemoglobin levels of persons without SCD can be dangerous and lead to hyperviscosity. Therefore, persons with SCD should not receive transfusions unless they have significant symptoms from their anemia (dizziness, shortness of breath, chest pain that is significantly worse than their typical vaso-occlusive symptoms) or they have signs of end-organ failure (such as acute neurologic symptoms, ACS, multiorgan failure). Transfusions for simple vaso-occlusive pain are generally not indicated. ᴴ

Transfusions may have significant adverse effects. The risk of infection was highlighted in the 1980s and 1990s with blood product contamination by HIV and hepatitis C virus. Patients who received transfusions in those years should be screened for these viruses. Better donor screening and disease surveillance have minimized, but not eliminated, this risk. Another significant risk is alloimmunization (see Transfusion), and as many as 18% of patients with SCD who undergo transfusion develop alloantibodies. This particularly affects women of childbearing age. Phenotypic matching for the C, E, and K antigens can decrease alloimmunization significantly and is done at some, but not all, institutions. Antibody formation may be immediate, but can cause delayed hyperhemolytic reactions (significant hemolysis with precipitous drop in hemoglobin level and increase in hemolytic markers such as LDH and indirect bilirubin) occurring 2 to 19 days after transfusion, presenting a significant, life-threatening challenge. Additionally, because mechanisms for eliminating iron are limited, erythrocyte transfusions carry an increasing cumulative risk of iron overload. This primarily results in liver damage, and close surveillance and iron chelation are indicated. In patients receiving regular transfusions (such as for stroke prevention), erythrocyte exchange transfusions can lessen the iron burden by removing some of the patient's erythrocytes.

Patients undergoing surgery should be transfused before their procedure to avoid complications. Transfusion to a hemoglobin level of 10 g/dL (100 g/L) has been shown to be equivalent to exchange transfusions in low- to medium-risk surgeries (low-risk surgery includes adenoidectomy,

CONT.

inguinal-hernia repair; medium-risk surgery includes cholecystectomy, joint replacement). **H**

Other Hemoglobinopathies

More than 1000 mutations of the globin chains have been identified. Besides the most common hemoglobinopathies (sickle cell anemia and thalassemia), several rarer types can occur.

Hemoglobin C is a common mutation in black patients. Those with homozygous disease may have mild microcytic anemia and demonstrate numerous target cells on peripheral blood smear. Sickling only occurs if it is coinherited with Hb S, which typically leads to a milder form of SCD.

KEY POINTS

- Patients with chronic hemolytic anemias should receive folic acid supplementation and pneumococcal (13- and 23-valent), *Haemophilus influenzae* type b, influenza, and meningococcal immunizations.

- Acute hemolysis caused by glucose-6-phosphate dehydrogenase deficiency is characterized by typical laboratory markers for hemolysis and peripheral blood smears showing bite cells and Heinz bodies.

- The thalassemias are characterized by microcytosis, target cells, normal iron studies, and an elevated or normal erythrocyte count; electrophoresis in β-thalassemia shows slightly increased hemoglobin A_2 levels and fetal hemoglobin levels, whereas in α-thalassemia it shows a normal pattern.

- The three common disease-altering strategies in congenital hemolytic anemias are hematopoietic stem cell transplantation, prophylactic transfusions, and hydroxyurea therapy.

(Continued)

KEY POINTS *(continued)*

- In patients with sickle cell disease, hydroxyurea therapy has been shown to decrease vaso-occlusive episodes, acute chest syndrome, transfusion requirements, and hospitalization and to prolong overall survival.

- Persons with sickle cell disease should not receive transfusions unless they have symptomatic anemia or signs of end-organ damage.

HVC

Acquired Hemolytic Anemias

Immune-Mediated Hemolysis

The mechanism underlying immune-mediated hemolysis involves antibodies binding to erythrocytes, with or without the activation of complement, leading to erythrocyte destruction. Antibodies causing hemolysis can be divided into two categories, warm and cold, referring to the optimal temperature for antibody-erythrocyte interaction. Antibodies reacting to erythrocytes at body temperature lead to warm autoimmune hemolytic anemia; those reacting at less than normal body temperature lead to a form of autoimmune hemolytic anemia also termed cold agglutinin disease. The characteristics of these conditions are listed in (**Table 25**). The hallmark of immune-mediated hemolytic anemia is the direct antiglobulin (Coombs) test, which tests for either IgG or C3 bound to erythrocytes.

Warm Autoimmune Hemolytic Anemia

In warm autoimmune hemolytic anemia, pathogenic IgG antibodies are directed against erythrocyte surface membrane molecules. IgG-coated membrane fragments are engulfed by macrophages in the reticuloendothelial system through Fc receptors, leading to loss of erythrocyte surface area, causing the erythrocytes to become progressively more spherocytic. Warm autoimmune hemolytic anemia can manifest as a primary disorder or

TABLE 25.	Characteristics of Warm Autoimmune Hemolytic Anemia (WAIHA) and Cold Agglutinin Disease	
	WAIHA	**Cold Agglutinin Disease**
Temperature for optimal antibody binding to erythrocytes	37.0 °C (98.6 °F)	<37.0 °C (98.6 °F)
Immunoglobulin class	IgG	IgM
Typical AGT pattern	IgG positive, C3 positive or negative	IgG negative, C3 positive
Peripheral blood smear findings	Spherocytes	Erythrocyte agglutination
Clinical manifestations[a]	Anemia, fatigue, dyspnea, jaundice, splenomegaly	Anemia, fatigue, dyspnea, jaundice, acrocyanosis, splenomegaly
Associated conditions	Autoimmune, lymphoproliferative (chronic lymphocytic leukemia, B-cell non-Hodgkin lymphomas), drug-induced[b]	Infectious (*Mycoplasma* and mononucleosis), lymphoproliferative (IgM MGUS, Waldenström macroglobulinemia, other B-cell non-Hodgkin lymphomas)
Treatment	Glucocorticoids, splenectomy, immunosuppression, treatment of underlying condition	Cold avoidance, rituximab, plasmapheresis, treatment of underlying condition

AGT = antiglobulin (Coombs) test; MGUS = monoclonal gammopathy of undetermined significance.

[a]Manifestations in cold agglutinin disease are worse upon exposure to the cold. Lymphadenopathy in either entity should raise suspicion of a lymphoproliferative disorder.

[b]Cephalosporins, penicillins, NSAIDs, isoniazid, procainamide, methyldopa, levodopa.

can be a complication of another disorder such as an autoimmune condition or a lymphoproliferative disorder such as chronic lymphocytic leukemia. It can also be induced by certain medications (see Drug-induced Immune Hemolytic Anemia).

The severity of anemia symptoms depends on the rate of hemolysis and the compensatory rise in erythrocyte production. Patients may notice "tea-colored" urine. Clinical findings can include pallor, jaundice, and splenomegaly. Laboratory findings may reveal evidence of ongoing hemolysis, including an increased reticulocyte count, but more consistently reveal an elevated bilirubin level, decreased or absent haptoglobin, and increased LDH level. The direct antiglobulin test is positive, and spherocytes are seen on the peripheral blood smear.

Treatment is based on immunosuppression to halt immune-mediated erythrocyte destruction and allow the patient's own bone marrow to regenerate the erythrocytes, if possible. The physician must judge how well the patient tolerates the anemia and how the patient's marrow is responding. These two factors determine if the patient should receive erythrocyte transfusion. If erythrocytes must be transfused, it is recommended to give a single unit of blood at a time, assessing the patient's status after each unit. Because the autoantibody typically reacts against all erythrocytes, a completely cross-match-compatible unit may be impossible to find. The presence of autoantibodies can mask the presence of underlying alloantibodies that can lead to further hemolytic transfusion requirements, and these scenarios typically require consultation between a hematologist and a transfusion medicine physician. Nonetheless, if the patient is deemed to require additional oxygen-carrying capacity, transfusion of type-specific, cross-match-incompatible blood should be ordered. Patients should also receive glucocorticoids, either orally or parenterally. An inadequate response to glucocorticoids may indicate the need for splenectomy or alternative immunosuppression. Folic acid supplementation is indicated in all patients. [H]

Cold Agglutinin Disease
Pathogenic IgM molecules bind best in colder temperatures, typically in the fingers, toes, and nose. IgM-coated erythrocytes will agglutinate and clump in the microvasculature, leading to cyanosis and ischemia in the cold extremities. IgM also fixes to complement, leading to erythrocyte destruction, either by completion of the complement cascade with intravascular hemolysis or by phagocytosis through complement receptors on macrophages. This disease can be primary, with no other underlying disorders, but may be associated with lymphoproliferative disorders such as Waldenström macroglobulinemia, other B-cell non-Hodgkin lymphomas, and IgM monoclonal gammopathy of undetermined significance. Cold agglutinin disease may also be precipitated by infections, typically *Mycoplasma pneumoniae* or Epstein-Barr virus.

The mainstay of treatment is cold avoidance and treatment of the underlying lymphoproliferative disorder, when appropriate. Treatment with rituximab has been effective, and plasmapheresis should be considered for those with more severe disease manifestations. Unlike in warm autoimmune hemolytic anemia, therapy with glucocorticoids or splenectomy is usually ineffective.

Drug-induced Immune Hemolytic Anemia
Medications can lead to an immune-mediated hemolytic anemia by one of two pathways. Erythrocyte antigens are altered, leading to the development of antibodies with cross-reactivity to unaltered erythrocyte antigens, or antierythrocyte antibodies develop, directed against antigenic drug-protein complexes on the erythrocyte cell surface. The former mechanism can occur with methyldopa, levodopa, or procainamide. Hemolysis ensues within a few weeks to months following therapy initiation and subsides within several months of discontinuing the implicated agent. The latter mechanism is commonly seen with cephalosporins, penicillins, NSAIDs, quinine, quinidine, and isoniazid; occurs within days of starting the drug; and subsides within days of stopping the medication.

Diagnosis is made on clinical grounds and requires a thorough medication history. The direct and indirect antiglobulin tests are typically positive with the former pathway, whereas the indirect antiglobulin test will only be positive with incubation in the presence of the offending agent with the latter pathway. Treatment consists of stopping the offending agent. [H]

Nonimmune Hemolytic Anemia
Nonimmune hemolytic anemia may occur as the result of mechanical trauma to erythrocytes by a microangiopathic mechanism, abnormalities in the heart and large vessels leading to abnormal shear forces from flow through a large pressure gradient (such as in a leaky prosthetic aortic valve or a ventricular septal defect), or direct trauma (as in march hemoglobinuria) (see later section). Infections may lead to hemolysis either through direct infection of the erythrocytes or toxin-mediated membrane damage. Lastly, drugs, chemicals, and venoms may lead to hemolysis.

Microangiopathic Hemolytic Anemia
Microangiopathic hemolytic anemia (MAHA) represents shear damage to erythrocytes as the result of endothelial cell activation or endothelial cell damage. The hallmark of disease is the presence of schistocytes on the peripheral blood smear, typically accompanied by an elevated LDH level and other clues of intravascular hemolysis. Various disorders can cause MAHA and are listed in **Table 26**. Treatment is directed toward the underlying disorder. Thrombotic thrombocytopenic purpura is a catastrophic disorder manifested by MAHA and thrombocytopenia that may be associated with development of other symptoms, including fever, kidney failure, and neurologic findings. It is discussed further in the Platelet Disorders chapter. [H]

Paroxysmal Nocturnal Hemoglobinuria
Paroxysmal nocturnal hemoglobinuria (PNH) is an acquired disease in which an abnormal progenitor cell clone develops, resulting in erythrocytes, leukocytes, and platelets that are missing

TABLE 26.	Causes of Microangiopathic Hemolytic Anemia
Cause	
Thrombotic thrombocytopenic purpura	
Hemolytic uremic syndrome	
Disseminated intravascular coagulation	
Malignant hypertension	
Vasculitis	
Eclampsia	
HELLP (Hemolysis, Elevated Liver enzymes, Low Platelets) syndrome	
Antiphospholipid antibody syndrome	
Scleroderma renal crisis	
Metastatic cancer	
Calcineurin inhibitors	
Solid organ transplant rejection	

proteins normally attached to the cell surface by a glycophosphatidylinositol (GPI) anchor. The progenitor cell clone is defective in the gene *PIG-A*, which encodes the enzyme normally responsible for attaching these proteins to the cell surface via the GPI anchor. Among these proteins are CD55 and CD59, which are responsible for inactivating complement on the surface of erythrocytes. PNH cells are therefore more susceptible to complement-mediated lysis. Because complement-mediated lysis occurs more readily at lower pH levels, hemolysis typically occurs at night as the P_{CO_2} rises, so patients may report hematuria in the morning. For reasons that have not been fully explained, patients are at increased risk for developing thrombosis, especially at unusual sites. Arterial and venous clots are seen with increased frequency, including the Budd-Chiari syndrome (see Hematopoietic Stem Cell Disorders). Patients can also develop pancytopenia, which results from bone marrow hypoplasia. PNH may evolve into aplastic anemia and acute myeloid leukemia in some patients. Conversely, PNH clones may develop in patients with existing aplastic anemia or myelodysplastic syndrome (see Hematopoietic Stem Cell Disorders). Patients require folate repletion because of chronic hemolysis. Iron supplementation or transfusion may be necessary because of urine iron losses or symptomatic anemia, respectively. Eculizumab, a monoclonal antibody that binds C5 and inhibits activation of the terminal component of the complement cascade, decreases hemolysis and the need for erythrocyte transfusions and improves quality of life.

KEY POINTS

- Diagnosis of warm autoimmune hemolytic anemia includes physical and laboratory findings of pallor, jaundice, splenomegaly, increased reticulocyte count, elevated bilirubin level, decreased or absent haptoglobin, increased lactate dehydrogenase level, positive antiglobulin (Coombs) test, and spherocytes on the peripheral blood smear.

(Continued)

KEY POINTS (continued)

- The mainstay treatments for warm autoimmune hemolytic anemia and cold agglutinin disease are glucocorticoids and cold avoidance, respectively.

Other Causes of Hemolysis

Macroangiopathic Hemolytic Anemia

Abnormalities within the heart and the large vessels can cause shear damage to erythrocytes. Disorders can include problems with heart valves (especially mechanical heart valves), intracardiac tumors, or rupture of either chordae tendineae or an aneurysm of the sinus of Valsalva. This also produces schistocytes. Patients can become iron deficient because of chronic iron loss through hemosiderin in the urine. Development of hemolysis from a cardiac defect may require surgical correction.

March Hemoglobinuria

This disorder is caused by repetitive trauma to the soles of the feet or palms of the hands and can be provoked by marching, running, hand-drum playing, karate, or head banging. Many individuals who run long distances develop this condition. The Prussian blue stain for urine hemosiderin will be positive.

Hemolysis Associated with Chemical and Physical Agents

Arsenic, especially arsine gas used in the manufacture of semiconductors, can cause severe hemolysis. Elevated copper levels in the serum, either owing to Wilson disease or from copper contamination of dialysis fluid, can lead to hemolysis.

Insect and spider bites, especially the bite of the brown recluse spider, may cause severe intravascular hemolysis. Severe burns cause hemolysis through direct thermal injury to erythrocytes.

Hemolysis from Infections

Malarial infection invariably leads to hemolysis. At least part of the life cycle of all malarial forms occurs within the erythrocyte, requiring lysis to exit. *Babesia microti* is an intracellular parasite carried by the same tick as Lyme disease and leads to hemolysis. *Clostridium perfringens* (the agent of gas gangrene) toxin causes severe hemolysis; the bacteria produce a lysolecithinase, which attacks the membrane bilayer. *Bartonella bacilliformis*, the agent of Oroya fever, is an extracellular bacterium that can cause dramatic hemolytic episodes.

KEY POINTS

- Macroangiopathic hemolytic anemia can be caused by disorders of the heart valves (especially mechanical heart valves), intracardiac tumors, or rupture of chordae tendineae.

- March hemoglobinuria can be caused by repetitive trauma to the soles of the feet or palms of the hands, such as with marching or running.

(Continued)

- *Plasmodium* species, *Babesia microti*, *Clostridium perfringens*, and *Bartonella bacilliformis* infections can cause hemolytic anemia.

Iron Overload Syndromes

Introduction

Despite iron's importance to living cells, it is toxic when present in excess. Excess iron may arise from increased absorption, related to mutations in iron regulatory genes; from chronic hemolytic states with ineffective erythropoiesis (such as thalassemia major); or from chronic transfusion therapy in diseases such as sickle cell anemia, aplastic anemia, and myelodysplasia.

Primary/Hereditary Hemochromatosis

Hereditary hemochromatosis affects approximately 1 in 400 persons of Northern European ancestry. It results from an autosomal recessive defect in the *HFE* gene, which leads to increased absorption of dietary iron. Two main defects in *HFE*, the *C282Y* and *H63D* mutations, account for most of the genotypic and phenotypic expression of hereditary hemochromatosis. Neither mutation is common in blacks or Asians with iron overload. Homozygosity for *C282Y* is found in 85% to 90% of phenotypically affected persons, and the likelihood of developing disease depends on many factors, including iron intake and rates of blood loss (women do not develop overt iron overload until after menopause). Only 10% of those homozygous for *C282Y* develop symptoms. Persons with one copy of *C282Y* and one copy of *H63D*, known as compound heterozygotes, are at much lower risk for iron overload than those who are homozygous for *C282Y*. Because other gene mutations or alternative causes may exist, approximately 5% to 10% of patients with iron overload have a negative hemochromatosis gene test. Therefore, the absence of *C282Y* does not eliminate the diagnosis of an iron overload disorder.

Most patients with hereditary hemochromatosis are diagnosed in the presymptomatic phase when iron test results are abnormal. In patients with symptoms, clinical presentation varies and often includes nonspecific findings such as chronic fatigue, weakness, nonspecific abdominal pain, arthralgia, and mildly elevated liver enzymes. A predilection for developing arthropathy is seen, especially in the second and third metacarpophalangeal joints. Endocrine organs are commonly affected, and diabetes mellitus, hypothyroidism, and gonadal failure may occur. Patients may present with heart failure or arrhythmias. An increased frequency of depression has been noted. As the disease advances and iron deposition goes untreated, hepatic fibrosis and cirrhosis may develop. When cirrhosis develops, a 200-fold increased risk of hepatocellular carcinoma has been documented.

Early diagnosis is essential to alter the disease course and avoid end-organ complications. The most sensitive and cost-effective initial diagnostic study in patients with suspected hemochromatosis is measurement of the fasting serum transferrin saturation. A consensus does not exist for transferrin saturation cut-off levels for diagnosis of hemochromatosis, with some guidelines recommending a value of greater than 60% in men or greater than 50% in women, and others suggesting a level of greater than 55% for all patients. Serum ferritin level measurement is indicated in patients with an elevated transferrin saturation; a markedly elevated level further supports the diagnosis and predicts the development of symptoms.

Universal screening for hereditary hemochromatosis is not recommended, but testing should be performed in first-degree relatives of patients with classic *HFE*-related hemochromatosis, those with evidence of active liver disease, and in patients with abnormal iron study results obtained for other indications. Screening for hepatocellular carcinoma is reserved for those with hereditary hemochromatosis and cirrhosis.

Patients who are *C282Y* homozygous but have a normal serum ferritin level can be monitored without treatment. In patients with abnormal ferritin levels, prompt and aggressive treatment with phlebotomy before end-organ complications occur will prevent subsequent morbidity and mortality. One unit of blood should be removed at weekly intervals until ferritin levels decrease to 10 to 50 ng/mL (10-50 µg/L), provided the hematocrit is maintained at greater than 30%. Subsequently, life-long maintenance phlebotomy is required. Iron chelation should be considered only rarely for patients in whom phlebotomy is contraindicated.

The risks of eating raw seafood or undercooked pork should be communicated, because the incidence of *Vibrio vulnificus* and *Yersinia enterocolitica* infections is increased in iron overload conditions. Patients with iron overload are also at risk for infection with mucormycosis, especially as they begin iron reduction therapy.

- An elevated transferrin saturation remains the most sensitive and cost-effective initial screening test for hemochromatosis. **HVC**

- Universal screening for hereditary hemochromatosis is not recommended and should be reserved for first-degree relatives of patients with classic *HFE*-related hemochromatosis, those with active liver disease, and patients with abnormal iron study results. **HVC**

- Prompt and aggressive treatment with phlebotomy before end-organ complications occur will prevent subsequent morbidity and mortality in patients with hemochromatosis.

Secondary Iron Overload

In most cases, secondary iron overload occurs in patients with severe anemia who require chronic transfusion therapy. Because iron excretion has no regulated mechanism, multiple transfusions (for anemias not stemming from blood loss or iron deficiency) lead to iron overload, with subsequent secondary organ damage. If these anemias resolve (either from hematopoietic stem cell transplantation or remission from leukemias), phlebotomy should be initiated. When anemia is ongoing, iron chelation is required, for which deferoxamine, deferiprone, or deferasirox may be used. These agents are relatively toxic, leading to potential kidney and liver damage, agranulocytosis, or ocular and ophthalmic disorders.

KEY POINT

- Iron chelation is required in patients with secondary iron overload with ongoing anemia.

Platelet Disorders

Normal Platelet Physiology

Platelets are normally made in the bone marrow from stem cells known as megakaryocytes. The lifespan of a normal platelet is approximately 10 days, and every day one tenth of the total platelet population is replaced. A normal platelet count ranges from 150,000 to 440,000/µL (150-440 × 10⁹/L). The most important hormonal stimulus for platelet production is thrombopoietin.

Platelets play an important role in hemostasis and thrombosis. Platelets form the initial plug at the site of vascular injury in three coordinated steps: adhesion, aggregation, and secretion. At sites of vascular injury, von Willebrand factor (vWF) attaches to subendothelial collagen. Under shear conditions, the vWF exposes binding sites for glycoprotein Ib-IX-V complex on the platelet surface that allow it to become tethered to the vessel wall. Exposure to a variety of agonist agents arising from the injured vessel wall, damaged erythrocytes, and other activated platelets converts glycoprotein IIb-IIIa on the platelet surface to its activated state, allowing it to bind fibrinogen, which can thus aggregate numerous platelets together by providing binding sites for other platelets. Platelets activated by platelet agonists release the contents of their granules, including fibrinogen, epinephrine, and platelet agonists such as adenosine diphosphate, vWF, and factor V, thus propagating the platelet response. Additionally, platelets also serve as the phospholipid scaffold upon which other coagulation reactions occur, including generation of factor Xa and thrombin.

Approach to the Patient with Thrombocytopenia

In diagnosing thrombocytopenia, pseudothrombocytopenia, or platelet clumping, must be excluded. In some patients, platelets will clump in vitro when the anticoagulant ethylenediaminetetraacetic acid (EDTA) is present. The platelet count is thus spuriously low. This can be recognized by viewing platelet clumps on the peripheral blood smear. Drawing blood into a citrated tube frequently eliminates the clumping. No physiologic consequence to this finding exists, and it needs no treatment.

The next step in evaluating thrombocytopenia is to determine if the patient is experiencing symptoms related to the low platelet count. Severe thrombocytopenia leads to mucocutaneous bleeding (that is, epistaxis, gum bleeding, heavy menses, easy bruising, and petechiae). These symptoms are seldom seen at platelet counts greater than 30,000/µL (30 × 10⁹/L). In general, patients with platelet counts greater than 100,000/µL (100 × 10⁹/L) are asymptomatic. Patients with platelet counts between 50,000 and 100,000/µL (50-100 × 10⁹/L) are generally able to undergo abdominal surgery without risk of abnormal bleeding. However, patients with platelet counts less than 10,000/µL (10 × 10⁹/L) are at risk for spontaneous intracranial hemorrhage.

The history should focus on previous platelet counts, if known. A careful list of all newly prescribed and over-the-counter medications should be obtained in patients with a new thrombocytopenia, because many medications can cause thrombocytopenia. A history of autoimmunity may point to immune thrombocytopenic purpura (ITP), and a history of fever, headache, hematuria, or abdominal pain may indicate thrombotic thrombocytopenic purpura (TTP). Physical examination should focus on the presence or absence of mucocutaneous bleeding. Stigmata of liver disease may point to the cause of thrombocytopenia, because splenomegaly can cause platelet sequestration.

Laboratory evaluation requires peripheral blood smear **H** assessment, looking for schistocytes, which must be seen to diagnose TTP and may be seen in disseminated intravascular coagulation (DIC) and other causes of microangiopathic hemolytic anemia (MAHA) associated with thrombocytopenia. Prothrombin and activated partial thromboplastin times, fibrinogen level, and D-dimer measurement can be ordered if DIC is suspected. Thyroid function should be checked because both hyper- and hypofunction of the thyroid can lead to thrombocytopenia. It is recommended that antibodies to HIV and hepatitis C virus be determined in all patients being evaluated for thrombocytopenia. Other laboratory evaluations should be guided by the disease entity suspected. **H**

Thrombocytopenic Disorders

The differential diagnoses for thrombocytopenia can be broadly attributed to three causes: disorders of underproduction, splenic sequestration, or peripheral destruction.

Underproduction thrombocytopenias are characterized by inadequate megakaryocyte numbers in the bone marrow. Other blood cell lines are usually decreased, as well. **Table 27**

TABLE 27. Causes of Platelet Underproduction

Cause	Result
Marrow failure	Aplastic anemia
	Myelodysplasia
	Vitamin B$_{12}$/folate deficiency
	Fanconi anemia
Marrow invasion	Leukemias
	Tumors (small cell lung cancer metastatic to marrow)
	Granulomatous diseases (sarcoidosis)
	Fibrosis (primary myelofibrosis)
Marrow injury	Drugs (especially alcohol, chemotherapy)
	Radiation
	Infections (hepatitis C virus, HIV)
Congenital	Wiskott-Aldrich syndrome
	Thrombocytopenia absent radius (TAR) syndrome
	May-Hegglin anomaly
	Gray platelet syndrome
	Bernard-Soulier syndrome

includes some examples of conditions associated with inadequate platelet production.

Platelet sequestration in the spleen leads to decreases in the circulating platelet count. Unlike erythropoietin, which increases synthesis to increase the erythrocyte count in response to anemia, thrombopoietin synthesis is static in splenic sequestration. Circulating thrombopoietin binds to the surface of megakaryocytes and platelets and is internalized; thus, free thrombopoietin levels are negatively regulated by an increased platelet mass, including the platelets sequestered in an enlarged spleen. Therefore, the body is unable to mount a compensatory increase in platelet production in this clinical setting.

Thrombocytopenias due to peripheral destruction are classified as those being caused by either immune or nonimmune mechanisms.

Non-Immune-Mediated Thrombocytopenia

Nonimmune mechanisms of platelet destruction are typically microangiopathic (shear damage to erythrocytes and platelets as the result of endothelial cell activation or endothelial cell damage). This category encompasses three classic syndromes: DIC, TTP, and the hemolytic uremic syndrome (HUS). See the Bleeding Disorders chapter for a discussion of DIC.

Thrombotic Thrombocytopenic Purpura

TTP is characterized by abnormal activation of platelets and endothelial cells, deposition of fibrin in the microvasculature, and peripheral destruction of erythrocytes and platelets. The diagnosis is clinical and requires the presence of thrombocytopenia and MAHA in the absence of other causes of these findings such as malignant hypertension or scleroderma renal crisis. Additionally, patients may have fever, kidney disease, neurologic findings such as mental status changes or stroke, or abdominal pain. The most common cause of TTP is sporadic and is due to a deficiency in the protease ADAMTS-13, which cleaves the high-molecular-weight multimers of vWF. This deficiency can be congenital or produced by an autoantibody. The decrease in ADAMTS-13 activity leads to accumulation of clumps of ultra-large-molecular-weight vWF multimers, which bind to masses of platelets, leading to microvascular occlusion and thrombocytopenia. Schistocytes form as erythrocytes are damaged by these tangles of vWF and platelets. TTP can also be triggered by medications, especially quinine, ticlopidine, cyclosporine, and gemcitabine; with the latter two drugs, the cause may be endothelial cell damage rather than formation of antibodies against ADAMTS-13. MAHA leads to an increase in lactate dehydrogenase and bilirubin levels. Schistocytes are invariably seen on the peripheral blood smear. The blood urea nitrogen and creatinine levels may be elevated. Abdominal pain, with or without an increase in amylase level, is also a prevalent clinical feature.

Prompt and accurate diagnosis is critical, because TTP is fatal in 90% of patients without therapy. Patients require emergent treatment with plasma exchange, a form of therapeutic apheresis in which native plasma is removed and replaced with fresh frozen plasma. In a randomized clinical trial, plasma exchange was shown to be superior to simple plasma infusions. Platelet levels rarely decrease to less than 10,000/µL (10 × 10^9/L), and routine platelet transfusions are contraindicated, because transfusion of platelets can potentially precipitate microvascular occlusion.

Hemolytic Uremic Syndrome

HUS frequently overlaps in clinical presentation with TTP; however, HUS occurs more frequently in children and has more kidney and fewer neurologic manifestations. HUS can be precipitated by infectious diarrheal illnesses, especially *Escherichia coli* O157:H7 and others elaborating Shiga toxin. Plasma exchange is the standard of care for HUS in adults. Atypical HUS is a congenital syndrome that differs from typical HUS in that it is not preceded by a diarrheal illness. Rather, it is a disorder caused by overwhelming complement activation. The distinction between TTP and typical and atypical HUS is difficult but important to make, because atypical HUS is effectively treated by infusions of eculizumab, a monoclonal antibody directed against the terminal components of the complement cascade. ◨

- Clinical diagnosis of thrombotic thrombocytopenic purpura requires the presence of thrombocytopenia and microangiopathic hemolytic anemia in the absence of other causes of these findings and may include fever, kidney disease, neurologic findings, or abdominal pain.

- Atypical hemolytic uremic syndrome is effectively treated by infusions of eculizumab.

Immune-Mediated Thrombocytopenia

The pathophysiologic mechanism underlying immune-mediated thrombocytopenia involves antibodies binding to platelets, with platelet destruction mediated through Fc receptors on macrophages within the reticuloendothelial system.

Unlike autoimmune hemolytic anemia, there is no diagnostic test for immune-mediated thrombocytopenia. Antiplatelet antibody testing is not recommended because of low sensitivity and specificity. Like immune-mediated hemolytic anemia, certain medications can provoke immune-mediated thrombocytopenia. The mechanisms of drug-induced thrombocytopenia are identical to drug-induced hemolysis, including direct stimulation of antiplatelet antibodies and a hapten mechanism.

Immune Thrombocytopenic Purpura

ITP should be considered in patients with isolated new-onset thrombocytopenia. Unless the patient has been bleeding, the hemoglobin level and leukocyte count should be normal. The peripheral blood smear should show large platelets and no schistocytes. Splenomegaly and thyroid disease should be ruled out as causes of the thrombocytopenia (hypo- and hyperthyroidism can be causative). All new and unnecessary medications, supplements, and herbal therapies should be stopped. ITP may be a primary disorder or may be associated with any autoimmune conditions or lymphoproliferative disorders (such as chronic lymphocytic leukemia or Hodgkin and non-Hodgkin lymphomas). It may also present in pregnancy (see Hematologic Issues in Pregnancy). Certain viral illnesses may induce ITP, and for this reason, HIV and hepatitis C virus testing is warranted in patients with new-onset thrombocytopenia.

Specific therapy should be reserved for platelet counts less than 30,000/µL (30×10^9/L) or if the patient is bleeding. Initial therapy with glucocorticoids should be initiated with either prednisone, 1 mg/kg followed by a slow taper over the course of weeks, or dexamethasone, 40 mg/d for 4 days. Following a course of glucocorticoids, 25% of patients respond and never relapse, but the remainder do not respond or relapses after glucocorticoid taper. Intravenous immune globulin (IVIG) and anti-D immune globulin are other therapeutic first-line options, but anti-D immune globulin is effective only in Rh-positive patients. Second-line therapy is controversial and may include either splenectomy, use of off-label rituximab, or use of a thrombopoietin mimetic agent (either eltrombopag or romiplostim).

Patients with platelet counts less than 10,000/µL (10×10^9/L) or those with life-threatening bleeding may require more robust therapy. IVIG should be added and platelets transfused if bleeding is present. Routine transfusion of platelets is not recommended, because they are rapidly consumed, but their use for bleeding is not disputed.

- No diagnostic test can identify immune-mediated thrombocytopenia, and antiplatelet antibody testing is not recommended because of its low sensitivity and specificity. **HVC**

- Patients with immune thrombocytopenic purpura may require therapy if the platelet count is less than 30,000/µL (30×10^9/L) or if bleeding is present.

Heparin-Induced Thrombocytopenia

Heparin-induced thrombocytopenia (HIT) is a specific, drug-induced thrombocytopenia in which the antigen is a complex between platelet factor 4 (PF4) and heparin. Antibodies directed against the heparin/PF4 complex can activate platelets via Fc receptors on platelets, leading to thrombocytopenia and, paradoxically in some patients, thrombosis. Risk factors for development of HIT include heparin treatment for more than 4 days, surgery, and treatment with unfractionated instead of low-molecular-weight heparin (LMWH); however, cases of HIT have been reported after use of LMWH, and LMWH should not be used in patients with a history of HIT. Platelet counts decrease by at least 50% 5 to 10 days after treatment with heparin. A scoring system for determining the pretest probability of a patient having HIT is shown in **Table 28**.

Diagnostic testing involves serologic testing (usually by enzyme-linked immunosorbent assay) for anti-heparin/PF4 antibodies and functional assays to determine platelet activation, of which the serotonin release assay is the gold standard. Serologic testing, although widely available, is limited by lack of specificity, which can be increased by testing for IgG rather than all anti-heparin/PF4 antibodies. Functional assays are more specific but are not readily available at all centers. As soon as HIT is suspected, heparin should be stopped, argatroban therapy should be initiated, and diagnostic testing ordered. Baseline Doppler ultrasound studies of all four extremities should be obtained, because the risk of thrombosis in HIT is more than 30%. Warfarin therapy should not be started until the platelet count normalizes because of the risk of developing warfarin skin necrosis. Platelet administration is relatively contraindicated. Anticoagulation should be continued at least until the platelet count is greater than 150,000/µL (150×10^9/L) in patients without thrombosis. Patients with thrombosis should complete the course of anticoagulation needed to treat their clot.

TABLE 28.	The 4T Scoring System for Predicting Heparin-Induced Thrombocytopenia and Thrombosis (HIT/T)		
4 Ts	2 Points	1 Point	0 Points
Thrombocytopenia	Platelet count decrease >50% and platelet nadir ≥20,000/μL (20 × 10⁹/L)	Platelet count decrease 30%-50% or platelet nadir 10,000-19,000/μL (10-19 × 10⁹/L)	Platelet count decrease <30% or platelet nadir <10,000/μL (10 × 10⁹/L)
Timing of platelet count decrease	Clear onset between days 5-10 or platelet count decrease ≤1 day (with heparin exposure within 30 days)	Consistent with platelet count decrease between days 5-10, but unclear (e.g., missing platelet counts); onset after day 10; or decrease ≤1 day (heparin exposure 30-100 days ago)	Platelet count decrease <4 days without recent exposure
Thrombosis or other sequelae	New thrombosis (confirmed); skin necrosis; acute systemic reaction after intravenous unfractionated heparin bolus	Progressive or recurrent clot; nonnecrotizing (e.g., erythematous) skin lesions; suspected thrombosis (not proved)	None
Other causes for thrombocytopenia	None apparent	Possible	Definite

High probability: 6-8 points

Intermediate probability: 4-5 points

Low probability: 0-3 points

- Diagnostic testing for heparin-induced thrombocytopenia includes serologic testing with the enzyme-linked immunosorbent assay and the functional assays, of which the serotonin release assay is the gold standard.

Qualitative Platelet Disorders

Acquired Platelet Dysfunction

Even if they are normal in number, dysfunctional platelets may lead to mucocutaneous bleeding. A qualitative platelet defect should be suspected in patients with clinical bleeding (suggesting a defect in hemostasis) whose platelet count, prothrombin time, and activated partial thromboplastin time are normal. A list of diagnoses leading to qualitative platelet disorders is given in **Table 29**. In general, platelet function defects are usually mild and unlikely to trigger bleeding without additional vascular injury or other hemostatic abnormalities. Some of these disorders may respond to desmopressin, whereas others require transfusion to treat or prevent bleeding.

Platelet Function Testing

Diagnostic evaluation starts with an abnormal bleeding time or Platelet Function Analyzer-100 (PFA-100®) result. In the PFA-100® test, whole citrated blood is aspirated through a small aperture into a microcapillary membrane infused with a mixture of collagen and either epinephrine or adenosine diphosphate. The shear stress produced by the rapid aspiration mimics arterial shear, leading to vWF binding to collagen. Platelets are activated by either collagen or epinephrine, and blood flow slows and eventually stops as platelets and erythrocytes obstruct the microcapillaries. If warranted, more specific platelet function assays such as platelet aggregation, flow cytometry, or electron microscopy can be performed at a specialized center.

Platelet function testing has been used to evaluate resistance to antiplatelet agents such as aspirin and clopidogrel. One such instrument, the Verifynow®, is a point-of-care instrument using the principle that fibrinogen-coated polystyrene beads will agglutinate in proportion to the number of glycoprotein IIb-IIIa receptors activated by specific agonists. Various cartridges use specific stimuli to monitor various antiplatelet drugs. Monitoring for aspirin therapy uses arachidonic acid as the platelet agonist and is given in aspirin-response units. Monitoring for clopidogrel uses adenosine diphosphate as the platelet agonist and is given in P2Y12 response units. Monitoring for glycoprotein IIb-IIIa inhibitors uses a peptide that activates the thrombin receptor. Although this test is currently available, guidelines recommend against routine monitoring of antiplatelet therapy with platelet function testing.

- A qualitative platelet defect should be suspected in patients with clinical bleeding (suggesting a defect in hemostasis) whose platelet count, prothrombin time, and activated partial thromboplastin time are normal.

TABLE 29. Causes of Platelet Dysfunction

	Comments	Severity	Treatment
Congenital Platelet Defects			
Glanzmann thrombasthenia	Defect in glycoprotein IIb-IIIa	Severe	Platelets or recombinant factor VIIa, ε-aminocaproic acid
Bernard-Soulier syndrome	Defect in glycoprotein Ib-IX	Severe	Platelets, ε-aminocaproic acid
Wiskott-Aldrich syndrome	Triad of eczema, thrombocytopenia, immunodeficiency	Moderate	Platelets, ε-aminocaproic acid
Gray platelet syndrome	Patients may develop myelofibrosis	Moderate	Platelets, ε-aminocaproic acid
Storage pool disease		Moderate to mild	Platelets, ε-aminocaproic acid; some may respond to desmopressin
Acquired Platelet Defects			
Uremia		Mild	Dialysis, desmopressin, ε-aminocaproic acid
Liver disease	Also associated with hyperfibrinolysis and coagulopathy	Mild to severe	Platelets, ε-aminocaproic acid
Myeloproliferative neoplasms	If platelet count is >1-1.5 million/μL (1000-1500 × 10⁹/L), may be associated with acquired von Willebrand disease	Mild to severe	Before surgical procedures, normalize the platelet count. Platelet transfusion may be necessary if bleeding occurs
Post-cardiac bypass		Mild	Platelets, if necessary
Antiplatelet drugs			
IIb-IIIa inhibitors		Severe	Platelets
Aspirin	Irreversible	Mild	Platelets, if necessary
Clopidogrel	Irreversible	Mild	Platelets, if necessary
NSAIDs	Temporary	Mild	None usually needed
Other drugs and herbs (β-lactams, vitamin E, ginkgo, turmeric, garlic, Chinese tree fungus)		Mild	None usually needed

Bleeding Disorders

Normal Hemostasis

Hemostasis encompasses the orderly, tightly regulated processes that occur in response to vascular injury to prevent bleeding. Primary hemostasis refers to the interaction between the injured vessel wall, von Willebrand factor (vWF), and platelets. Platelet adhesion, aggregation, and secretion were described previously in the section on platelets. Activated platelets also serve as the scaffold on which the series of proteolytic clotting factor reactions take place that culminate in the formation of a stable fibrin clot.

The "waterfall" model was initially used to describe hemostasis, but this model is now useful only to delineate the clotting factors necessary for testing prothrombin time (PT) and activated partial thromboplastin time (aPTT) (**Figure 12**). In this model, clotting factors X, V, II, and fibrinogen are

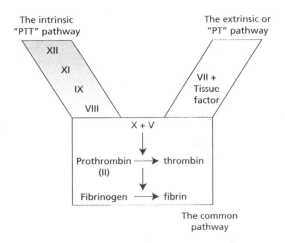

FIGURE 12. The "waterfall" model of hemostasis is useful for teasing out coagulation disorders affecting the prothrombin time (PT) and the activated partial thromboplastin time (aPTT). In this model, factors common to the PT and the aPTT are X, V, II, and fibrinogen. Factor VII is unique to the PT, and factors XII, XI, VIII, and IX are unique to the aPTT.

common to the PT and the aPTT pathways; factor VII is unique to the PT pathway; and factors XII, XI, IX, and VIII are unique to the aPTT pathway. Limitations in the waterfall model have led to the development of a cell-based model of hemostasis, which characterizes the phases of coagulation as initiation, priming, and propagation (**Figure 13**). Thus, hemophilia A and B are understood to be defects in thrombin generation on the surface of activated platelets, and the hemorrhagic consequences are more clearly understood.

Table 30 lists the differential diagnoses for patients experiencing bleeding who have specific abnormalities in clotting assays.

Evaluation of Patients with Suspected Bleeding Disorders

The evaluation of a patient experiencing bleeding episodes is aimed at determining the likelihood that the patient has an underlying hemorrhagic disorder and at treating future bleeding episodes. Although the history and physical examination can increase suspicion for the presence of a bleeding disorder, laboratory confirmation is required for precise diagnosis and treatment.

A detailed history of bleeding episodes, including family history, is critical in elucidating whether a bleeding diathesis is present. The history should include an orderly description of bleeding episodes during infancy and childhood. Bleeding with dental procedures, including wisdom tooth removal, should be

TABLE 30. Differential Diagnoses for Patients Experiencing Bleeding	
Clotting Assay Abnormality	**Differential Diagnoses**
Prolonged PT, normal aPTT	Factor VII deficiency
	DIC
	Liver disease
	Vitamin K deficiency
	Warfarin ingestion
Normal PT, prolonged aPTT	Deficiency of factors VIII, IX, XI, or XII
	von Willebrand disease (if severe and factor VIII level is quite low)
	Heparin exposure
Prolonged PT and aPTT	Deficiency of factors V, X, II, or fibrinogen
	Severe liver disease, DIC, vitamin K deficiency, warfarin use
	Heparin overdose
Normal PT and aPTT	Platelet dysfunction (acquired and congenital)
	von Willebrand disease (if mild and factor VIII level is not too low)
	Scurvy
	Ehlers-Danlos syndrome
	Hereditary hemorrhagic telangiectasia
	Deficiency of factor XIII

aPTT = activated partial thromboplastin time; DIC = disseminated intravascular coagulation; PT = prothrombin time.

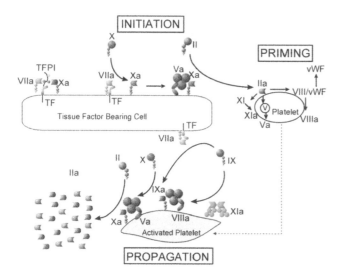

FIGURE 13. The cell-based model of hemostasis is useful for understanding coagulation as it occurs in vivo. The initiation of coagulation takes place on the surface of a tissue factor–bearing cell, such as a macrophage, tumor cell, or an activated endothelial cell. Tissue factor (TF) and a small amount of factor VIIa generate factor Xa, which joins with factor Va to form a small amount of thrombin (factor II). In the priming step, this small amount of thrombin proceeds to activate platelets and factor VIII, which joins with factor IX to generate factor Xa. On the platelet surface, the prothrombinase complex can generate a large thrombin burst in the propagation step, allowing for cleavage of fibrinogen into fibrin.

TFPI = tissue factor pathway inhibitor; vWF = von Willebrand factor.

explored. Epistaxis may be a presenting symptom of von Willebrand disease (vWD) or hereditary hemorrhagic telangiectasia, and is especially notable if it does not stop with pressure and requires either cautery or an emergency department visit.

Other bleeding episodes, whether spontaneous or provoked, should be explored. Bleeding into muscles and joints is characteristic of disorders of humoral clotting factors (hemophilia), whereas mucosal bleeding is more common in disorders of primary hemostasis (vWD, thrombocytopenia of any cause). Easy bruisability is reported by many patients without underlying bleeding disorders, but certain historical features are worth noting. The new onset of bruising can herald a new thrombocytopenic disorder such as immune thrombocytopenic purpura or acute leukemia or can point to acquired hemophilia. Bruising that only occurs over the hands and forearms suggests the presence of senile purpura.

Each surgical procedure should be explored in depth. The details of bleeding, including timing (immediate or delayed), need for transfusion, comments by the surgeon concerning the characteristics of the bleeding, and any known anatomic sources of bleeding can shed light on the bleeding diathesis. Immediate bleeding may be more characteristic of a disorder of primary hemostasis, whereas delayed bleeding is more common in patients with deficiencies in humoral clotting factors.

Bleeding in patients with an underlying hemorrhagic condition is typically described as "diffuse oozing," without a readily identifiable bleeding source such as a surgical mishap like a severed vessel. If a woman has bled with some procedures, but not others, she should be asked if she was taking oral contraceptive pills or hormone replacement therapy during the procedures in which she had good hemostasis, because these can increase levels of vWF, leading to normalization of hemostasis. If the patient's nonbleeding episodes correlate with times taking estrogen-containing contraceptives, a diagnosis of vWD could be suspected.

Women should be interviewed thoroughly about their menstrual history. Duration and severity of flow are more important than presence or severity of cramping. Features correlated with a higher likelihood of an underlying bleeding disorder include nighttime "flooding," passing clots larger than a quarter, duration longer than 8 days, and development of iron deficiency.

A family history of bleeding should also be elicited. A family history of bleeding with surgical procedures, bleeding requiring transfusions, and menorrhagia leading to hysterectomy at a young age should be queried. However, a negative family history does not rule out a hereditary bleeding disorder.

Certain medications or herbal and dietary supplements increase the risk of bleeding. The use of these agents may precipitate a hemorrhage in those with milder bleeding disorders. Aspirin and NSAIDs impair primary hemostasis, and their use should be avoided before surgery or evaluation of the hemostatic system. Their inclusion in over-the-counter products seems ubiquitous, and careful attention to cold and flu remedies is warranted.

The physical examination may provide useful clues to the cause of the patient's bleeding. Examining the skin may reveal petechiae, indicating thrombocytopenia, or the characteristic ecchymoses and lax skin seen with senile purpura. Telangiectasias around the lips or on the fingertips may signal the presence of hereditary hemorrhagic telangiectasia.

Splenomegaly can be associated with thrombocytopenia and may indicate underlying portal hypertension. Other stigmata of liver disease, such as spider angiomata, gynecomastia, asterixis, and jaundice, also suggest the patient may have liver coagulopathy. A loud systolic murmur radiating to the carotid arteries may indicate severe aortic stenosis, which can cause acquired vWD, with associated gastrointestinal bleeding from arteriovenous malformations. An enlarged tongue, carpal tunnel syndrome, and periorbital purpura may point to amyloidosis, which can lead to dysfibrinogenemia, factor X deficiency, or vascular fragility.

No available test serves as a screening test of global hemostasis, and none can include or exclude the presence of an underlying bleeding disorder. Screening tests may point to the presence of a factor deficiency or a defect in primary hemostasis, although more precise diagnoses require more detailed testing. See Table 30 for differential diagnoses for combinations of abnormal and normal PT and aPTT values.

KEY POINTS

- Bleeding into muscles and joints is characteristic of disorders of humoral clotting factors, whereas mucosal bleeding is more common in disorders of primary hemostasis.

- Features correlated with a higher likelihood of an underlying bleeding disorder in women being evaluated for menorrhagia include nighttime "flooding," passing clots larger than a quarter, duration longer than 8 days, and development of iron deficiency.

Congenital Bleeding Disorders

Hemophilia A and B

Hemophilia A and B are X-linked recessive disorders of hemostasis. Hemophilia A results from factor VIII deficiency and hemophilia B from factor IX deficiency. These disorders present identically and can only be distinguished by measuring the respective clotting factors. They will produce prolongation of the aPTT with a normal PT, and the aPTT mixing study will fully correct. The clinical symptoms are determined by the baseline factor activity in each patient. Those with severe hemophilia have less than 1% factor VIII or IX activity, and these persons will have severe spontaneous bleeding episodes that are clinically manifested at an early age as well as severe bleeding after surgery or trauma. The bleeding episodes occur predominantly in the ankle, knee, and elbow joints, but retroperitoneal, intramuscular, and intracranial bleeding can also occur. Children can present with bleeding after circumcision or have bleeding with loss of deciduous teeth. Patients with moderate hemophilia have factor levels between 1% and 5%, and those with mild disease have factor levels greater than 5%. These persons can occasionally present in adulthood, because they are less likely to experience spontaneous bleeding episodes, and trauma-induced bleeding may not be recognized as clinically significant. Older patients with hemophilia may have been infected with HIV and/or hepatitis C virus from contaminated factor concentrates made from pooled plasma, but transfusion-related risks of HIV and hepatitis B and C viruses are no longer a concern for younger patients with hemophilia.

Treatment relies on replacing the missing clotting factors with factor concentrates. Patients may take factor concentrates in response to bleeding episodes or on a prophylactic basis. Some patients may develop inhibitors, which are neutralizing alloantibodies against factor VIII (or occasionally IX). A patient may have developed an inhibitor if he or she does not clinically respond well to factor VIII or factor IX infusions. Diagnosis is confirmed by measuring a Bethesda titer, which is a measure of the strength of the inhibitor. Patients with hemophilia benefit from being monitored at a comprehensive hemophilia treatment center; this has been shown to decrease morbidity and mortality and reduce cost.

All daughters of men with hemophilia are carriers of the factor deficiency and have a 50% chance of passing the disorder to their sons. They may also experience an increased bleeding tendency, especially if they have low factor VIII or IX levels owing to extreme lyonization, in which patients have a disproportionately inactivated X chromosome carrying the normal factor VIII or IX gene, leading to lower than expected factor levels.

KEY POINTS

- Hemophilia A (factor VIII deficiency) and B (factor IX deficiency) produce prolongation of the activated partial thromboplastin time (aPTT) with a normal prothrombin time, and the aPTT mixing study will fully correct; diagnosis is made by measuring the baseline factor activity.

- Treatment of patients with hemophilia relies on replacing the missing clotting factors with factor concentrates, which can be given in response to bleeding episodes or on a prophylactic basis.

von Willebrand Disease

vWD is the most common inherited bleeding disorder. As many as 1 in 100 persons have low levels of vWF, and approximately 1% of these experience mucocutaneous bleeding problems. Symptoms are similar to those experienced with platelet disorders and may include nosebleeds in children, easy bruising, bleeding gums, and postsurgical bleeding. Gynecologic problems are especially common. Most women with vWD experience heavy menstrual bleeding, and approximately 10% to 30% of women with menorrhagia may be diagnosed with vWD. Additionally, endometriosis (likely related to backflow of menses), miscarriages (unclear mechanism), and postpartum hemorrhage are more common in women with vWD. Type 1 vWD accounts for 80% of all vWD cases and is inherited in an autosomal codominant fashion. In this condition, vWF antigen and activity levels are 30% or less, and factor VIII levels may be normal or low owing to loss of vWF-provided protection from proteolysis. Results of the Platelet Function Analyzer-100 (PFA-100®) are usually prolonged. The PT is normal and the aPTT may be normal or slightly prolonged, because the factor VIII level may be slightly low. Despite this, the pattern of bleeding is similar to that of a platelet disorder rather than of a defect in humoral clotting factor; patients with hemophilia who have levels of factor VIII activity as low as those seen in patients with vWD are asymptomatic, thus the bleeding is due to defects in primary hemostasis from lack of vWF. Diagnosis may be difficult, because many elements influence vWF levels (**Table 31**).

Women with heavy menstrual bleeding may benefit from estrogen-containing oral contraceptives, which may regulate menstruation and raise vWF levels. Desmopressin causes preformed stores of vWF and factor VIII to be released from endothelial cells and may be given for treatment of menstrual or other bleeding or preoperatively as surgical prophylaxis.

TABLE 31. Elements Influencing von Willebrand Factor Levels

Factor	Effect on vWF Synthesis
ABO blood type	Type O persons have vWF levels 25% lower than average
Hypothyroidism	Decreases
Pregnancy and estrogen	Increases
Stress	Increases
Exercise	Increases
Inflammation	Increases
Smoking	Increases

vWF = von Willebrand factor.

Menorrhagia can be treated effectively with antifibrinolytic agents such as tranexamic acid or ε-aminocaproic acid during menses. Finally, factor concentrates consisting of factor VIII and vWF may be given as treatment for severe bleeding episodes or as perioperative therapy for major surgery. These are plasma derived but have undergone a number of steps to inactivate lipid-coated viruses such as HIV and hepatitis B and C. Patients should avoid taking aspirin or NSAIDs, which can worsen bleeding.

Other types of vWD are rare. The various subtypes of type 2 vWD result from production of an abnormally functioning vWF molecule. Type 3 vWD results from the near lack of vWF, and patients with this form of vWD have factor VIII levels low enough to produce defects in humoral hemostasis (for example, muscle hematomas and hemarthroses).

KEY POINTS

- Diagnosis of von Willebrand disease includes von Willebrand factor antigen and activity levels of 30% or less, factor VIII levels that may be normal or low, prolonged Platelet Function Analyzer-100 results, normal prothrombin time, and normal or slightly prolonged activated partial thromboplastin time.

- Treatment of von Willebrand disease depends upon the clinical severity of bleeding; estrogen-containing oral contraceptives and desmopressin can be given for treatment of menstrual or other minor bleeding or preoperatively for surgical prophylaxis.

Acquired Bleeding Disorders
Coagulopathy of Liver Disease

The liver is responsible for synthesis of all clotting factors as well as all anticoagulant and antifibrinolytic factors. Because of this, patients with severe liver failure will have prolonged PT and aPTT values resulting from decreased levels of coagulation factors. Despite this, patients are not protected against thrombosis, because protein C and S levels and antithrombin levels are low as well. Fibrinogen levels are low, and the fibrinogen may be dysfunctional because of abnormal glycosylation. Patients may also undergo accelerated fibrinolysis. Somewhat paradoxically, factor VIII levels are supranormal because it is produced in extrahepatic endothelial cells, and a hepatically synthesized factor is required for factor VIII clearance. Portal hypertension and associated splenomegaly may lead to a decreased platelet count, and qualitative platelet dysfunction is common in advanced liver disease, which may further exacerbate bleeding. Patients experiencing bleeding may require vitamin K, if deficiency is suspected, or transfusion with cryoprecipitate, fresh frozen plasma, and platelets. Antifibrinolytic agents may be beneficial for mucocutaneous bleeding. H

KEY POINTS

- Laboratory evaluation for coagulopathy of liver disease will show prolonged prothrombin time and activated partial thromboplastin time, low fibrinogen levels and possibly dysfunctional fibrinogen because of abnormal glycosylation, and supranormal factor VIII levels.

- Patients with coagulopathy of liver disease who are experiencing bleeding may require transfusion with cryoprecipitate, fresh frozen plasma, and platelets or vitamin K supplementation if deficiency is suspected.

Acquired Hemophilia

Rarely, older patients without a personal or family history of bleeding may present with acute new-onset bleeding. Such bleeding can be mucocutaneous or intramuscular. The PT is normal, but the aPTT is significantly prolonged, and a 1:1 mixing study of the patient's plasma with normal plasma is unsuccessful at completely correcting the aPTT. This is the classic presentation for acquired hemophilia, in which autoantibodies form against factor VIII. This disorder, although rare, carries high morbidity and mortality and is a frequently missed diagnosis; a high level of suspicion is critical for prompt diagnosis and treatment. It may be associated with an underlying autoimmune condition such as systemic lupus erythematosus or malignancy (either lymphoproliferative or solid tumor) but is more commonly idiopathic. Bleeding episodes should be treated with recombinant activated factor VII, and the patient should undergo immunosuppression to decrease the inhibitor levels. H

KEY POINTS

- Bleeding episodes resulting from acquired factor VIII inhibitor should be treated with recombinant activated factor VII and patients should undergo immunosuppression to eradicate the inhibitor.

Disseminated Intravascular Coagulation

DIC is characterized by abnormal activation of coagulation, generation of thrombin, consumption of clotting factors, and peripheral destruction of platelets. Diagnostic laboratory findings are provided in **Table 32**, although not all of those features may be present. DIC may result from a variety of causes,

TABLE 32. Laboratory Features of Disseminated Intravascular Coagulation (DIC)
Features
Elevated prothrombin time due to consumption of factor VII, which has the shortest half-life of the coagulation factors. Possibly elevated activated partial thromboplastin time if DIC is severe, because of consumption of other coagulation factors.
Low and progressively decreasing fibrinogen levels
Elevated D-Dimer or fibrin degradation products
Low platelets
Microangiopathic hemolytic anemia, which appears as schistocytes on the peripheral blood smear (seen in 50% of patients with DIC)

including sepsis, obstetric emergencies (amniotic fluid embolism, fetal demise, placental abruption), acute leukemias (especially acute promyelocytic leukemia), severe burns, venoms, and shock. No specific therapy for DIC exists, and treatment relies on resolving the underlying cause. Supplemental supportive treatment for patients who are bleeding or who are at risk for bleeding can include administering platelets, fresh frozen plasma to replace clotting factors, or cryoprecipitate to replace fibrinogen. H

KEY POINTS

- Management of disseminated intravascular coagulation focuses on treating the underlying cause.

Transfusion

Cellular Products

Erythrocytes

ABO/Rh System and Compatibility Testing

The ABO blood group system refers to carbohydrate antigens present on erythrocytes that include A or B antigens (blood group A or B, respectively), both (blood group AB), or neither (blood group O). Early in life, persons develop IgM antibodies to the A or B antigens not expressed on their erythrocytes. Thus, persons who have blood group A will have antibodies against B antigens and vice versa (**Table 33**). Anti-A and anti-B IgM antibodies bound to antigen on the erythrocyte cell surface activate complement and lead to life-threatening hemolytic reactions.

The Rh proteins on erythrocytes harbor the Rh antigens D, C, c, E, and e, the D antigen being the most immunogenic. Alloantibodies to Rh antigens develop from alloantigen exposure either through pregnancy or previous transfusion. Testing for D antigen is part of routine compatibility testing. IgG antibodies to Rh antigens can produce severe hemolytic transfusion reactions and hemolytic disease in the newborn if the mother is Rh(D)-negative and has been sensitized and the child is Rh(D)-positive; the use of anti-D immune globulin to

TABLE 33. ABO Compatibility Between Donor and Recipient Erythrocytes and Fresh Frozen Plasma

	Recipient ABO Blood Group			
	A	**B**	**AB**	**O**
Recipient erythrocyte antigen	A	B	A and B	None
Recipient isohemagglutinins[a]	Anti-B	Anti-A	None	Anti-A, Anti-B
Compatible donor erythrocytes	A, O	B, O	Any	O
Compatible donor plasma	A, AB	B, AB	AB	Any

[a]Isohemagglutinins are IgM antibodies directed at ABO blood group antigens.

NOTE: Rh(D)-negative patients should receive Rh(D)-negative erythrocytes; Rh(D)-positive patients can receive Rh(D)-negative or Rh(D)-positive erythrocytes.

prevent sensitization in pregnant women who are Rh(D)-negative has decreased the incidence of the latter.

Compatibility testing consists of typing and screening, in which the ABO and Rh(D) phenotypes of the recipient's erythrocytes are determined, followed by screening of the recipient's serum for the presence of alloantibodies to erythrocyte antigens generated as a result of previous transfusion or pregnancy. The ABO type and Rh(D) status of the donor erythrocytes are then verified and cross-matched by incubating the recipient's serum with donor erythrocytes.

If alloantibodies to erythrocyte antigens are discovered, their specificity must be determined so that donor erythrocytes lacking that antigen can be identified. Patients with a history of alloimmunization should never receive erythrocytes containing that antigen, even if repeat alloantibody screening is negative, because anamnestic responses can occur, resulting in delayed hemolytic transfusion reactions.

Clinical Transfusion Issues

Persons with O-negative blood are considered universal erythrocyte donors. As such, O-negative blood should be given in emergencies when the recipient's blood type is not available. One unit of packed red blood cells is 250 to 300 mL and is expected to increase the hemoglobin level by 1 g/dL (10 g/L) in the absence of bleeding, erythrocyte destruction, or sequestration. Prestorage leukoreduction decreases the amount of contaminating leukocytes in the erythrocyte product and reduces the risk of febrile nonhemolytic transfusion reactions, cytomegalovirus transmission, and class I HLA alloimmunization and subsequent platelet transfusion refractoriness. Universal leukoreduction is mandated in many countries. In the United States, more than 80% of institutions have implemented universal leukoreduction policies. **Table 34** discusses modifications to erythrocyte and other cellular products.

The goal of erythrocyte transfusion is to improve oxygen delivery. Considering the potential risks associated with blood transfusion and compensatory mechanisms that exist to maintain oxygen delivery, physicians should use clinical judgment to determine when a transfusion is necessary based on symptoms, the extent of the anemia, and the presence of cardiopulmonary comorbidity.

TABLE 34. Cellular Transfusion Product Modifications

Modification[a]	Notes
Leukoreduction[b]	Reduces the number of leukocytes present in the transfused erythrocyte or platelet product. Reduces class I HLA alloantibody production and subsequent platelet transfusion refractoriness, febrile nonhemolytic transfusion reactions, and transmission of CMV. Leukoreduction cannot be relied on to prevent transfusion-associated GVHD.
Irradiation	Radiation destroys lymphocytes in erythrocyte and platelet transfusion products. Used to prevent transfusion-associated GVHD, which is mediated by donor lymphocytes. Indicated in patients with severe, inherited T-cell immunodeficiency syndromes or Hodgkin lymphoma or recipients of allogeneic or autologous hematopoietic stem cell transplantation; purine analog-based chemotherapy (fludarabine, cladribine, deoxycoformycin), alemtuzumab, or rabbit antithymocyte globulin therapy; and in immunocompetent patients receiving HLA-matched platelets or transfusions from relatives. Irradiation can weaken the erythrocyte membrane, causing reduced cell viability and potassium leakage.
Washing	Removes the proteins residing in the small amount of plasma of erythrocyte and platelet transfusions and is used in patients with a history of severe/recurrent allergic reactions, IgA deficiency (when IgA-deficient donors are unavailable), or complement-dependent autoimmune hemolytic anemia. Also reduces the amount of potassium transfused for use in patients who are at risk for hyperkalemia.

CMV = cytomegalovirus; GVHD = graft-versus-host disease; HLA = human leukocyte antigen.

[a]Transfusion of CMV-negative blood products for immunocompromised recipients who are CMV seronegative is controversial and not universally performed because modern era leukocyte filters are highly effective at reducing the inoculum of CMV-infected leukocytes.

[b]More than 80% of blood banks in the United States adhere to universal leukoreduction. For those that do not, leukoreduction should be performed for chronically transfused patients, those with a history of a febrile hemolytic transfusion reaction, patients who are potential candidates for or recipients of a solid-organ or hematopoietic stem cell transplant, and immunocompromised recipients who are CMV seronegative.

Strategies to Minimize Blood Transfusion

Randomized studies have shown that a more restrictive approach to erythrocyte transfusion is safe and reduces the need for erythrocyte transfusion in well-defined clinical scenarios. For hemodynamically stable, hospitalized medical and postsurgical patients, a transfusion threshold hemoglobin level of less than 7 to 8 g/dL (70-80 g/L) is recommended based on data demonstrating equivalent or improved outcomes for (1) patients in the ICU when transfused at a hemoglobin level of 7 g/dL (70 g/L) or less; (2) patients after surgical hip fracture repair who have pre-existing cardiovascular disease or risk factors for cardiovascular disease who are transfused at a hemoglobin level of 8 g/dL (80 g/L) or less or for symptomatic anemia; and (3) patients with acute upper gastrointestinal bleeding, no acute coronary syndrome, and no history of peripheral vascular disease or stroke when transfused at a hemoglobin level of 7 g/dL (70 g/L) or less. Evidence in patients with underlying cardiovascular disease is limited, but a transfusion threshold of 8 g/dL (80 g/L) or less or transfusion based on the presence of symptoms (chest pain, heart failure, hypotension, and tachycardia not responsive to intravenous fluids) has been proposed. Data on appropriate transfusion thresholds in acute coronary syndromes are lacking and decisions must be made on a case-by-case basis.

Erythropoiesis-stimulating agents (ESAs; erythropoietin and darbepoetin) are used to promote erythrocyte production and reduce the need for transfusion. However, several studies have shown a detrimental impact with the use of ESAs in select clinical situations, especially when a higher hemoglobin level is targeted. ESAs used to target a higher hemoglobin level increase the risk of cerebral infarction, hypertension, and vascular access thrombosis in patients with anemia of chronic kidney disease. A study in patients with chronic heart failure targeting a hemoglobin level of 13 g/dL (130 g/L) demonstrated a similar increased risk of thromboembolic events. ESAs are associated with an increased risk of venous thrombosis and mortality in patients with cancer. In light of these safety concerns, ESA use must be carefully individualized.

Preoperative autologous blood donation can reduce the need for donor blood and reduces many of the risks associated with blood transfusion (febrile nonhemolytic reactions, hemolytic and allergic reactions, graft-versus-host disease [GVHD], alloimmunization). Other strategies include intraoperative hemodilution or use of intraoperative cell salvage technology, a method for retaining and reusing erythrocytes lost during intraoperative bleeding.

(Continued)

HVC

Platelets

ABO/Rh System, Human Leukocyte Antigen System, and Compatibility Testing

ABO blood group antigens are expressed on platelets, and transfusion of ABO-matched platelets produces a modestly increased platelet count compared with ABO-mismatched platelets. Although ABO-mismatched platelets may be used, anti-A or -B antibodies in the plasma of the platelet product can uncommonly lead to hemolytic transfusion reactions. Rh antigens are not expressed on platelets but are present at trace levels owing to contaminating erythrocytes. As such, alloimmunization after exposure to Rh(D)-positive platelets can infrequently occur in Rh(D)-negative recipients. If Rh(D)-positive platelets must be given to a woman of child-bearing potential who is Rh(D)-negative, anti-D immune globulin should be coadministered to reduce the low risk of alloimmunization.

Class I HLA proteins are expressed on the surface of platelets, and alloantibody generation to these antigens may lead to platelet transfusion refractoriness and necessitate the use of class I HLA-matched platelets in affected patients (see Platelet Transfusion Refractoriness).

Clinical Transfusion Issues

Sources for platelet transfusion include random donor-pooled platelets, which include platelets from four to six combined blood donors, and single-donor platelets obtained through apheresis. Random donor-pooled and apheresis platelets are expected to increase the platelet count by 20,000 to 30,000/µL (20-30 × 10⁹/L). Advantages to the use of single-donor platelets include the ability to select a platelet product for a patient based on HLA type, platelet cross-match compatibility, and ABO blood group. Leukoreduction of platelet products yields the same benefits seen with erythrocyte leukoreduction (see Table 34).

Patients with thrombocytopenia with clinically significant active bleeding or patients without bleeding in whom nonneuraxial surgery is planned should be transfused to a target platelet count of 50,000 to 100,000/µL (50-100 × 10⁹/L) depending on the clinical circumstances. For patients with central nervous system bleeding or undergoing neurosurgery, the target platelet count is greater than 100,000/µL

(100 × 10⁹/L). Platelet transfusions may also be indicated for patients with qualitative platelet function defects and clinically significant bleeding.

Prophylactic platelet transfusion for platelet counts of 10,000/μL (10 × 10⁹/L) or less in patients with thrombocytopenia due to decreased bone marrow production (hematologic malignancies undergoing chemotherapy or hematopoietic stem cell transplantation) decreases the risk of bleeding compared with platelet transfusion at the onset of clinical bleeding and is recommended for hospitalized patients. Patients with active fever or infection or acute promyelocytic leukemia, however, require a higher platelet transfusion threshold.

The AABB (formerly the American Association of Blood Banks) also recommends prophylactic platelet transfusion to platelet count of 20,000/μL (20 × 10⁹/L) or greater in patients having an elective central venous catheter placed and to 50,000/μL (50 × 10⁹/L) or greater for patients undergoing elective diagnostic lumbar puncture.

Platelet Transfusion Refractoriness

Platelet transfusion refractoriness is defined as an increase in the platelet count of less than 10,000/μL (10 × 10⁹/L), measured 10 to 60 minutes after transfusion on at least two separate occasions. Refractoriness to platelet transfusion occurs in 10% to 25% of patients receiving chemotherapy for acute myeloid leukemia and is associated with an increased risk of bleeding and mortality. Nonimmune causes of platelet transfusion refractoriness include sepsis, disseminated intravascular coagulation (DIC), medications that can lead to decreased platelet survival (for example, amphotericin B), and platelet sequestration due to splenomegaly.

Alloimmunization is an important cause of platelet transfusion refractoriness due to production of alloantibodies to class I HLA antigens (and less commonly platelet-specific antigens) on donor platelets. Patients at risk are those who have previously been transfused or exposed to fetal antigens during pregnancy. HLA-matched platelets are used for transfusion if available. If the recipient is heterozygous for an HLA haplotype for which the donor is homozygous, the recipient may not reject the contaminating lymphocytes in the platelet product and is at risk of transfusion-associated GVHD. As such, HLA-matched platelets must be irradiated to prevent this complication, regardless of the state of the recipient's immune system. Other options for the alloimmunized patient include the use of HLA-compatible platelets missing the antigen to which the patient is alloimmunized or platelet crossmatching, a process in which the patient's serum is incubated with donor platelets. Class II HLA antigens present on transfused leukocytes are important in the initial immune response to class I HLA antigens on donor platelets. Thus, the use of leukoreduced blood products significantly decreases the risk of alloimmunization. **H**

- If Rh(D)-positive platelets must be given to a woman of childbearing potential who is Rh(D)-negative, anti-D immune globulin should be coadministered to reduce the risk of alloimmunization.

- Platelet transfusion refractoriness, defined as an increase in platelet count less than 10,000/μL (10 × 10⁹/L) when measured within 1 hour after transfusion, may be caused by alloimmunization or nonimmune factors, including sepsis, hypersplenism, disseminated intravascular coagulation, and some medicines, such as amphotericin B.

- In patients with hematologic malignancies undergoing chemotherapy or hematopoietic stem cell transplantation, prophylactic platelet transfusions for platelet counts less than 10,000/μL (10 × 10⁹/L) decrease the risk of bleeding compared with platelet transfusion at the onset of clinical bleeding.

Plasma Products

Fresh Frozen Plasma

Fresh frozen plasma (FFP) is plasma collected from whole blood through centrifugation or collected through apheresis and stored at -18 °C (0.04 °F) or colder within 6 to 8 hours of donation. FFP contains all of the coagulation factors. One unit of FFP is 200 to 280 mL. The appropriate dose of FFP and administration schedule must take into account the patient's plasma volume, the factor activity goal, and the half-life of the affected factor(s). In general, an effective dose of FFP can range from 10 to 15 mL/kg. When used to treat patients with multiple clotting factor deficiencies and clinically significant active bleeding (advanced liver impairment or DIC), FFP may need to be administered every 8 to 12 hours to achieve adequate hemostasis. Redosing should be guided by monitoring the prothrombin and activated partial thromboplastin times, clotting factor levels, and achievement of hemostasis. FFP use is excessive in the United States and other countries despite published guidelines regarding its use. FFP is ineffective at treating mild coagulopathies characterized by an INR of 1.85 or less. Indications for the use of FFP, as well as other plasma-based products, are outlined in **Table 35**. **H**

Antibodies to A and B antigens may be present in FFP, and ABO-identical or ABO-compatible FFP must be used (see Table 33). Rh(D) compatibility is not necessary. FFP is an acellular product. As such, infections caused by intracellular pathogens like cytomegalovirus are significantly reduced. The risk of other transfusion-associated infections is similar (see Transfusion Complications).

Cryoprecipitate

When FFP is thawed at 4 °C (39.2 °F), a cryoprecipitate remains enriched for factors VIII and XIII, fibrinogen, and

TABLE 35. Plasma-Derived Therapeutic Products

Product	Indication(s) for Use
Fresh frozen plasma	Replacement solution for plasma exchange
	Prevention of coagulopathy from massive transfusion
	Treatment of bleeding associated with multiple acquired clotting factor deficiencies (liver disease, disseminated intravascular coagulation)
	Major warfarin-associated hemorrhage (when a 4-factor prothrombin complex concentrate is not available)
Cryoprecipitate	Congenital or acquired fibrinogen deficiency
	Dysfibrinogenemia
	Factor XIII deficiency
	Treatment of hemophilia A and von Willebrand disease when another more suitable product is not available
Immune globulin	Acquired or congenital hypogammaglobulinemia
	Autoimmune disorders
Albumin	Replacement solution for plasma exchange
	Spontaneous bacterial peritonitis
Prothrombin complex concentrates[a]	Major warfarin-associated hemorrhage
Factor VIII[b]	Hemophilia A, treatment and prevention of bleeding
von Willebrand protein-rich factor VIII[c]	Von Willebrand disease, treatment and prevention of bleeding
Factor IX[b]	Hemophilia B, treatment and prevention of bleeding
Fibrinogen	Congenital fibrinogen deficiency, treatment of bleeding
Thrombin[b]	Small vessel bleeding despite standard surgical techniques or when surgical intervention is not feasible (topical application)
Protein C concentrate	Severe congenital protein C deficiency (prevention and treatment of venous thrombosis and purpura fulminans)
Antithrombin[b]	Hereditary antithrombin deficiency (perisurgical and obstetrical procedure prophylaxis and treatment of established venous thrombosis)
α_1-antitrypsin	Congenital α_1-antitrypsin deficiency (high-risk phenotype, α_1-antitrypsin level <11 µmol/L, ≥18 years of age and airflow obstruction by spirometry)
C1-esterase inhibitor	Hereditary angioedema, acute attacks

[a]4-Factor prothrombin complex concentrate (containing factors II, VII, IX, and X) is preferred over 3-factor prothrombin complex concentrates in which factor VII is missing.

[b]Recombinant product available and preferred as a way of reducing risk of transmissible infections.

[c]Select plasma-derived factor VIII products are rich in von Willebrand protein.

von Willebrand factor (vWF). A unit is 10 to 20 mL. Cryoprecipitate is used to treat fibrinogen deficiency, dysfibrinogenemia, and factor XIII deficiency (see Table 35). Cryoprecipitate can be used as a source of vWF for patients with von Willebrand disease, but vWF-containing factor VIII concentrates are preferred. The widespread availability of plasma-derived and recombinant factor VIII products has largely eliminated the use of cryoprecipitate in the management of hemophilia A.

Other Plasma-Derived Transfusion Products

Inactivated 4-factor prothrombin complex concentrate contains factors II, VII, IX, and X and is indicated for the treatment of major warfarin-associated bleeding in conjunction with vitamin K. If unavailable, FFP can be used in its place or a 3-factor prothrombin complex concentrate (missing factor VII) with a supplemental dose of FFP or recombinant activated factor VII (see Table 35).

KEY POINTS

- Fresh frozen plasma is ineffective for treating mild coagulopathies characterized by an INR of 1.85 or less.   **HVC**

- Inactivated 4-factor prothrombin complex concentrate contains factors II, VII, IX, and X and is indicated in conjunction with vitamin K for the treatment of major warfarin-associated bleeding.

Transfusion Complications

Hemolytic Reactions

Acute Hemolytic Transfusion Reaction

Intravascular acute hemolytic transfusion reactions are characterized by the immediate destruction of donor erythrocytes by recipient antibodies. These reactions are most commonly caused by ABO incompatibilities or, occasionally, alloantibodies to other erythrocyte antigens. Signs and symptoms include fever, chills, dyspnea, red urine, flank pain, kidney injury, DIC, and hypotension/shock. Therapy consists of transfusion discontinuation, intravenous hydration, and appropriate cardiovascular support. Blood should be sent for transfusion reaction evaluation. A direct antiglobulin (Coombs) test is positive if blood is drawn before the destruction of all donor erythrocytes. Extravascular acute hemolytic transfusion reactions are caused by non–complement-fixing alloantibodies and are usually not life threatening. Patients may have fever, chills, jaundice, or worsening anemia but are often asymptomatic. Treatment is supportive.

Delayed Hemolytic Transfusion Reaction

Delayed hemolytic transfusion reactions are typically caused by an anamnestic alloantibody response upon re-exposure to an erythrocyte antigen. The alloantibody is undetectable at the time of initial antibody screening but increases rapidly after erythrocyte transfusion. These reactions occur 2 to 10 days after transfusion, are often extravascular, and produce similar clinical signs and symptoms as an extravascular acute hemolytic transfusion reaction. A repeat antibody screen and direct antiglobulin test will be positive. Treatment is supportive. The rate of onset of delayed hemolytic transfusion reactions is slower than that of intravascular acute reaction and signs and symptoms are not as severe. Intravenous fluid hydration and close monitoring are typically sufficient. **H**

KEY POINTS

- Signs and symptoms of acute hemolytic transfusion reaction include fever, chills, dyspnea, red urine, flank pain, kidney injury, disseminated intravascular coagulation, and hypotension/shock.

- Therapy for acute hemolytic transfusion reaction consists of transfusion discontinuation, intravenous hydration, and appropriate cardiovascular support.

- Delayed hemolytic transfusion reactions occur 2 to 10 days after transfusion, are often extravascular, and present with fever, jaundice, and worsening anemia.

Nonhemolytic Transfusion Reactions

Transfusion-associated Circulatory Overload

Transfusion-associated circulatory overload is a common, underreported adverse event in which hypervolemia develops toward completion or within several hours of a blood product transfusion. Signs and symptoms include dyspnea, hypoxia, tachycardia, headache, and hypertension, and physical examination demonstrates evidence of pulmonary edema or other signs of volume overload. Risk factors include age older than 60 years, chronic kidney disease, heart failure, number of blood products transfused, and volume transfused per hour. Management consists of transfusion discontinuation, diuretic therapy, and supportive care. Prevention includes a slower infusion rate (1 mL/kg/hour) and diuretic therapy between transfusions to maintain euvolemia for those at risk.

Transfusion-related Acute Lung Injury

Transfusion-related acute lung injury (TRALI) is the leading cause of transfusion-related mortality. It is characterized by the development of acute lung injury within 6 hours of transfusion of erythrocytes, platelets, or FFP. TRALI is mediated by initial priming of neutrophils in the recipient's lung parenchyma (endothelial damage, for example) followed by their activation by anti-HLA and antineutrophil antibodies present in donor plasma. Signs and symptoms escalate quickly and include dyspnea, hypoxia, fever, chills, and hypotension. Chest radiograph reveals diffuse bilateral pulmonary infiltrates. Preventive measures include excluding multiparous women from donating plasma-rich blood products, deferring any blood product donation from those implicated in a previous TRALI reaction, and using solvent/detergent-treated plasma. Management includes transfusion discontinuation and supportive care, which frequently includes a brief course of mechanical ventilation.

Febrile Nonhemolytic Transfusion Reaction

Febrile nonhemolytic transfusion reactions are common and occur within several hours of an erythrocyte or platelet transfusion. Febrile nonhemolytic transfusion reactions are mediated by the generation of leukocyte-derived cytokines during erythrocyte and platelet storage. Symptoms include fever, chills, rigors, or dyspnea. Management consists of transfusion discontinuation to exclude a more serious transfusion reaction, acetaminophen for fever, and meperidine for rigors. Leukoreduction of packed red blood cells and platelets before storage significantly reduces the rate of febrile nonhemolytic transfusion reactions. **H**

KEY POINTS

- Signs and symptoms of transfusion-associated circulatory overload include dyspnea, hypoxia, tachycardia, headache, and hypertension, and physical examination demonstrates evidence of volume overload.

- Transfusion-related acute lung injury is characterized by the development of acute lung injury within 6 hours of transfusion of erythrocytes, platelets, or fresh frozen plasma, with signs and symptoms escalating quickly to include dyspnea, hypoxia, fever, chills and hypotension.

- Transfusion discontinuation and supportive care are the primary interventions for all nonhemolytic transfusion reactions.

Allergic Reactions and Anaphylaxis

Rarely, anaphylaxis occurs within seconds to several minutes of transfusion of erythrocytes, platelets, plasma, cryoprecipitate, or other plasma-derived blood product. Patients with IgA deficiency are at higher risk because of the presence of anti-IgA antibodies (see MKSAP 17 Infectious Diseases). Manifestations include the sudden onset of respiratory distress, bronchospasm, angioedema, urticaria, nausea and vomiting, abdominal pain, tachycardia, and hypotension. Management consists of transfusion discontinuation, exclusion of other transfusion reactions, and appropriate management of anaphylaxis (see MKSAP 17 Pulmonary and Critical Care Medicine). Prevention includes the use of donors who are IgA deficient for those with anti-IgA antibodies or washing of erythrocyte and platelet products to reduce the volume of allergen-containing plasma in the product.

Less severe allergic reactions occur because of recipient IgE antibodies with reactivity to allergens in the plasma of the transfused product. Signs and symptoms are largely restricted to urticaria. Management consists of transfusion discontinuation to exclude a more severe allergic reaction and administration of antihistamines. Transfusion can be safely resumed for those with waning urticaria and no signs or symptoms of a more serious reaction. Cellular blood product washing reduces the risk of a reaction and should be considered for those with more severe reactions. **H**

KEY POINTS

- Patients with IgA deficiency are at high risk for an anaphylactic transfusion reaction because of the presence of anti-IgA antibodies.

- Treatment of patients experiencing anaphylaxis from transfusion consists of transfusion discontinuation, exclusion of other transfusion reactions, and appropriate anaphylaxis management.

- Management of allergic reactions consists of transfusion discontinuation to exclude a more severe allergic reaction and administrations of antihistamines.

Transfusion-associated Graft-versus-Host Disease

Transfusion-associated GVHD is a rare but fatal complication of erythrocyte and platelet transfusion in which viable donor lymphocytes generate an immune response to recipient tissues. This typically occurs in recipients who are immunocompromised and unable to destroy the donor lymphocytes or in immunocompetent patients who are heterozygous for an HLA haplotype for which the donor is homozygous. Signs and symptoms occur several days to 1 month after transfusion and include a diffuse maculopapular rash, jaundice, abdominal pain, nausea and vomiting, diarrhea, abnormal liver chemistries, and severe pancytopenia. Irradiation of blood products before transfusion destroys donor lymphocytes and has largely eliminated this complication. **H**

KEY POINTS

- Signs and symptoms of transfusion-associated graft-verus-host disease occur several days to 1 month after transfusion and include a diffuse maculopapular rash, jaundice, abdominal pain, nausea and vomiting, diarrhea, abnormal liver chemistries, and severe pancytopenia.

Infectious Complications

Transmission of bacterial infection from contaminated blood products is an uncommon but potentially life-threatening complication of transfusion. Various gram-positive and gram-negative bacteria have been implicated, including skin, enteric, and environmental organisms (**Table 36**). Platelets must be stored at room temperature and are associated with a higher risk of bacterial contamination. Signs and symptoms occur within minutes to several hours after transfusion and include fever, chills, rigors, tachycardia, and hypotension. In addition to blood cultures from the patient and culture of the

TABLE 36.	Transfusion-Transmitted Infections
Pathogen	**Risk of Transmission (when known)**
Bacterial pathogens	
Staphylococcus aureus	1 in 2500 platelet transfusions
Escherichia coli	
Acinetobacter	
Klebsiella	
Anaplasma (human granulocytic ehrlichiosis)	
Viral pathogens	
Hepatitis A	
Hepatitis B[a]	1 in 280,000 erythrocyte units
Hepatitis C[a]	1 in 1,150,000 erythrocyte units
HIV[a]	1 in 1,500,000 erythrocyte units
HTLV-1/2[a]	1 in 1,900,000 erythrocyte units
West Nile virus[a]	
Dengue fever	
Parasitic pathogens	
Babesiosis	
Malaria	
Leishmaniasis	
Chagas disease[a]	
Prion diseases	
Variant Creutzfeldt-Jakob disease	

HTLV = human T-cell lymphotropic virus type 1/2.

[a]Donated blood is screened for these pathogens. Syphilis is also screened, as is cytomegalovirus on a subset of donated blood to serve as a source for immunocompromised recipients who are cytomegalovirus seronegative.

CONT.

transfused product, an evaluation to exclude other transfusion reactions is important, because signs and symptoms of a transfusion-transmitted bacterial infection can be similar to other serious reactions. Management of suspected bacterial infection includes antibiotic therapy with gram-positive and gram-negative coverage. Preventive measures include surveillance cultures of stored platelet products. Table 36 includes other transfusion-transmissible pathogens. H

KEY POINTS

- Management of a suspected transfusion-associated bacterial infection includes antibiotic therapy with gram-positive and gram-negative coverage.

H Therapeutic Apheresis

Therapeutic apheresis is a procedure in which blood is passed through an extracorporeal device that separates the various blood components. The affected component is either discarded (as in leukapheresis or plasmapheresis) or treated (as in photopheresis), and the unaffected components are returned to the patient. Plasma exchange and erythrocyte exchange entail the removal of plasma or erythrocytes through apheresis followed by infusion of a crystalloid/colloid or plasma solution or donor erythrocytes to replace what was removed. Although simple erythrocyte transfusion and erythrocyte exchange have not been compared rigorously in sickle cell disease, exchange has the advantage of not increasing blood viscosity, avoiding iron overload, and decreasing the concentration of hemoglobin S more effectively. **Table 37** reviews the indications for therapeutic apheresis.

Apheresis complications include potential transfusion reactions if donor erythrocytes, plasma, or albumin is used (see Transfusion Reactions). Hypotension may occur as a result of volume depletion or in combination with flushing and abdominal pain in patients taking ACE inhibitors who are undergoing plasma exchange, especially when albumin is used as the replacement solution. This is thought to be the result of decreased clearance of bradykinin generated during plasma exchange for those taking ACE inhibitors. As such, ACE inhibitors should be withheld for 24 hours before plasma exchange, if appropriate. Other complications may include the development of hypocalcemia resulting from binding of ionized calcium to citrate. Plasma exchange with crystalloid or non–plasma-containing colloid can lead to coagulopathy caused by clotting factor depletion. H

KEY POINTS

- Erythrocyte exchange does not increase blood viscosity, avoids iron overload, and more effectively decreases the concentration of hemoglobin S compared with erythrocyte transfusion.

TABLE 37. Indications for Therapeutic Apheresis[a]
Plasmapheresis/Plasma Exchange
Thrombotic thrombocytopenic purpura
Clopidogrel/ticlopidine-associated thrombotic microangiopathy
Hyperviscosity syndrome (Waldenström macroglobulinemia and multiple myeloma)
Paraproteinemic polyneuropathies
Guillain-Barré syndrome (acute inflammatory demyelinating polyneuropathy)
Chronic inflammatory demyelinating polyradiculoneuropathy
Myasthenia gravis
ANCA-associated rapidly progressive glomerulonephritis
Anti-glomerular basement membrane disease
Recurrent focal segmental glomerulosclerosis
Severe, symptomatic cryoglobulinemia
Antibody-mediated renal allograft rejection
Fulminant Wilson disease
Erythrocyte Exchange
Severe babesiosis[b]
Sickle cell disease with acute cerebral infarct
Sickle cell disease with severe acute chest syndrome[c]
Leukapheresis
Hyperleukocytosis syndrome
Plateletpheresis
Symptomatic extreme thrombocytosis[d]
Extracorporeal Photopheresis
Cardiac allograft rejection, prophylaxis
Erythrodermic cutaneous T-cell lymphoma/Sézary syndrome
Selective Blood Component Removal
LDL cholesterol for familial hypercholesterolemia

[a]This list includes diseases for which apheresis is an accepted part of frontline therapy for a particular indication, either as the sole therapeutic modality or in combination with other therapy. It is not an all-inclusive list.

[b]Erythrocyte exchange for severe malaria is a category II indication (accepted second-line therapy).

[c]Erythrocyte exchange for acute chest syndrome is a category II indication but recommended by many as first-line therapy for those severely affected.

[d]The use of plateletpheresis is a category II indication for patients with life-threatening thrombosis or hemorrhage associated with thrombocytosis (for example, in a patient with essential thrombocytosis).

Data from Szczepiorkowski ZM, Winters JL, Bandarenko N, et al; Apheresis Applications Committee of the American Society for Apheresis. Guidelines on the use of therapeutic apheresis in clinical practice--evidence-based approach from the Apheresis Applications Committee of the American Society for Apheresis. J Clin Apher. 2010;25(3):83-177. [PMID: 20568098]

Thrombotic Disorders
Pathophysiology of Thrombosis and Thrombophilia

The balance of multiple procoagulant and anticoagulant factors, including coagulation proteins, platelets, leukocytes, erythrocytes, and components of the vascular wall, prevents thrombosis development. Procoagulant activity necessary for hemostasis is modulated by the natural anticoagulant system (proteins C and S, antithrombin, tissue factor pathway inhibitor). Fibrinolysis limits thrombus growth and facilitates clot resolution, resulting in reestablishment of intravascular blood flow. Thrombosis occurs when this balance is disturbed. The contributing factors of reduced blood flow (stasis), blood hypercoagulability (thrombophilia), and vascular wall abnormalities have been described as Virchow triad. Thrombosis is typically multifactorial, with genetic and acquired factors contributing.

Thrombophilia

Blood hypercoagulability is referred to as thrombophilia and can be inherited or acquired. Venous thromboembolism (VTE) is often multifactorial, and risk factors potentiate each other, often in more than just additive fashion.

Inherited Thrombophilic Conditions
Thrombophilia Testing

When thrombophilia testing is contemplated, a four-component strategy (the "4Ps") should be considered: Patient selection, Pretest counseling, Proper laboratory test interpretation, and Provision of education and advice. No general consensus exists on who should undergo thrombophilia testing. Identifying a thrombophilia often does not change treatment decisions in a patient with VTE. The evidence-based 2012 anticoagulation treatment guidelines of the American College of Chest Physicians and a 2012 guidance document of the International Society on Thrombosis and Haemostasis recommend against routine thrombophilia testing because identification of inherited abnormalities does not alter the duration of recommended anticoagulation or reliably predict risk of VTE recurrence. However, in patients with VTE assessed to be at intermediate risk for recurrence by traditional predictors, finding a strong thrombophilia (homozygous factor V Leiden [FVL] or II20210; double heterozygous FVL plus II20210; deficiency of protein C, S, or antithrombin; antiphospholipid antibody [APLA] syndrome) may be one motivator for long-term anticoagulation (**Table 38**).

TABLE 38. Risk of Venous Thromboembolism Associated with Various Thrombophilias

Thrombophilia	Risk Relative to Persons Without the Respective Thrombophilia	
	First VTE	**Recurrent VTE**
Thrombophilia not present	Reference group	Reference group
Heterozygous G20210A	3.8 (95% CI, 3.0-4.9)[a]	1.45 (95% CI, 0.96-2.21)[b]
Heterozygous FVL	4.9 (95% CI, 4.1-5.9)[a]	1.56 (95% CI, 1.14-2.12)[b]
Homozygous G20210A	Insufficient data	Insufficient data
Heterozygous FVL + heterozygous G20210A	20 (95% CI, 11.1-36.1)[a]	4.81 (95% CI, 0.50-46.3)[b]
Homozygous FVL	18 (95% CI, 4.1-41)[c]	2.65 (95% CI, 1.18-5.97)[b]
Protein S deficiency	30.6 (95% CI, 26.9-55.3)[d]	Increased, but insufficient data for accurate risk assessment
Protein C deficiency	24.1 (95% CI, 13.7-42.4)[d]	
Antithrombin deficiency	28.2 (95% CI, 13.5-58.6)[d]	
APLA	Increased, but data insufficient and too heterogeneous for accurate risk assessment	Available evidence is of very low quality: Any APLA positive: 1.41 (95% CI, 0.99-2.00)[e] Anticardiolipin positive: 1.53 (95% CI, 0.76-3.11)[e] Lupus anticoagulant positive: 2.83 (95% CI, 0.83-9.64)[e]

APLA = antiphospholipid antibody; FVL = factor V Leiden; VTE = venous thromboembolism.

Data from: [a]Emmerich J, Rosendaal FR, Cattaneo M, et al. Combined effect of factor V Leiden and prothrombin 20210A on the risk of venous thromboembolism--pooled analysis of 8 case-control studies including 2310 cases and 3204 controls. Study Group for Pooled-Analysis in Venous Thromboembolism [erratum in: Thromb Haemost 2001 Dec;86(6):1598]. Thromb Haemost. 2001 Sep;86(3):809-16. [PMID: 11583312] [b]Segal JB, Brotman DJ, Necochea AJ, et al. Predictive value of factor V Leiden and prothrombin G20210A in adults with venous thromboembolism and in family members of those with a mutation: a systematic review. JAMA. 2009 Jun 17;301(23):2472-85. [PMID: 19531787] [c]Juul K, Tybjaerg-Hansen A, Schnohr P, Nordestgaard BG. Factor V Leiden and the risk for venous thromboembolism in the adult Danish population. Ann Intern Med. 2004 Mar 2;140(5):330-7. [PMID: 14996674] [d]Lijfering WM, Brouwer JL, Veeger NJ, et al. Selective testing for thrombophilia in patients with first venous thrombosis: results from a retrospective family cohort study on absolute thrombotic risk for currently known thrombophilic defects in 2479 relatives. Blood. 2009 May 21;113(21):5314-22. [PMID: 19139080] [e]Garcia D, Akl EA, Carr R, Kearon C. Antiphospholipid antibodies and the risk of recurrence after a first episode of venous thromboembolism: a systematic review. Blood. 2013 Aug 1;122(5):817-24. [PMID: 23760616]

CONT.

Guidelines have not addressed whether screening family members of patients in whom a strong thrombophilia has been detected is beneficial. Consultation with a thrombosis specialist in these circumstances is advisable.

Factor V Leiden

FVL is the most common inherited thrombophilia. It results from a point mutation (G1691A) in the factor V gene, which leads to an amino acid substitution that renders factor V resistant to inactivation by activated protein C (APC). FVL accounts for greater than 90% of APC resistance, with other causes being less common factor V mutations and acquired conditions, including APLA syndrome, pregnancy, and cancer. FVL is inherited in an autosomal dominant fashion; its prevalence is 3% to 8% in whites and 1.2% in blacks in the United States. It is rarely found in African and Asian populations. Homozygous FVL occurs in 1 in 500 to 1600 whites. FVL is diagnosed by polymerase chain reaction (PCR) testing of the FVL gene. However, the presence of FVL can be detected through an APC resistance assay that assesses the ability of protein C to inactivate factor Va. This is a very sensitive test that effectively excludes FVL if normal and is the preferred initial screening test, because it is usually less expensive than the genetic test. An abnormal result suggests heterozygous or homozygous FVL, depending on the degree of abnormality, but must be followed up by PCR testing of the FVL gene.

Additional factors that further increase VTE risk include age, smoking, obesity, and estrogen use. A systematic review showed that FVL heterozygosity is only a very mild risk factor for VTE recurrence compared with absence of FVL; FVL homozygosity is a stronger risk factor. It is unknown whether homozygous FVL is a risk factor for arterial thrombosis, but heterozygous FVL is not.

Prothrombin *G20210A* Gene Mutation

The prothrombin *G20210A* gene mutation (PGM) occurs in the noncoding region and is the second most common inherited risk factor for VTE. It is inherited in an autosomal dominant fashion, and persons with the mutation have slightly higher levels of circulating prothrombin (factor II) than those without it; this has been speculated to be the mechanism of the increased VTE risk. The prevalence in the United States is 2% in whites and 0.5% in blacks. Homozygosity for PGM occurs in approximately 1 in 4000 persons of white European descent. It is diagnosed by PCR testing of the prothrombin gene. Obtaining factor II activity levels is not helpful.

Heterozygous PGM confers a three-fold increased risk of first-time VTE. The VTE risk in persons homozygous for the mutation has not been defined. A systematic review showed that heterozygosity compared with absence of the mutation was not associated with an increased risk of VTE recurrence. No clinically meaningful association has been demonstrated between PGM and arterial thromboembolism. However, a mild association has been suggested between PGM and stroke and myocardial infarction risks in certain subpopulations, such as younger patients.

Antithrombin Deficiency

Antithrombin is an enzyme that interrupts the coagulation process, mainly by inhibiting thrombin and activated factors X and IX (factors Xa and IXa). Antithrombin deficiency (ATD) is inherited in an autosomal dominant fashion. Quantitative (type I) and qualitative (type II) defects exist, and the risk for VTE appears to depend on the genetic defect and deficiency subtype, ranging from mildly thrombogenic to more pronounced. Inherited ATD is uncommon. The prevalence in the general population is 1 in 500 to 5000. Deficiencies are typically heterozygous; homozygous deficiencies are typically not compatible with life. Many causes exist for acquired low antithrombin levels (**Table 39**). ATD is diagnosed by assaying antithrombin activity. Acquired causes must be ruled out. Genetic testing is not feasible for routine clinical practice. A thrombosis specialist can conduct further testing to clarify the subtype of ATD to assess thrombosis risk.

ATD is considered a risk factor for VTE, but the risk depends on the subtype. It is unclear whether ATD is a risk factor for arterial thromboembolism. A large family study showed no association between ATD and arterial thrombosis. Antithrombin concentrates may be used as adjunctive therapy with routine pharmacologic VTE prophylaxis or as a supplement when treating acute VTE.

Protein C Deficiency

Protein C is a vitamin K–dependent natural anticoagulant; it is converted during the coagulation process to APC, which inactivates coagulation factors Va and VIIIa. Quantitative

TABLE 39. Conditions Associated with Decreased Coagulation Factor Levels

Coagulation Factor	Condition
Protein C	Acute thrombosis
	Warfarin therapy
	Liver disease
	Protein-losing enteropathy
Protein S	Acute thrombosis
	Warfarin therapy
	Liver disease
	Inflammatory states
	Estrogens (contraceptives, pregnancy, postpartum state, hormone replacement therapy)
	Protein-losing enteropathy
Antithrombin	Acute thrombosis
	Heparin therapy
	Liver disease
	Nephrotic syndrome
	Protein-losing enteropathy

(type I) and qualitative (type II) defects exist, but their clinical appearance is almost identical. Protein C deficiency is inherited in an autosomal dominant fashion. The diagnosis is made by obtaining a protein C activity assay, also referred to as functional protein C. Genetic testing is not feasible for routine clinical practice. See Table 39 for causes of acquired low levels.

The prevalence of inherited protein C deficiency is 1 in 500 to 600. Homozygous or double heterozygous protein C deficiency may develop in fetuses in approximately 1 in 1,000,000 pregnancies. Protein C deficiency is a risk factor for primary VTE, recurrent VTE, and arterial thromboembolism.

Plasma-derived protein C concentrate is indicated in infants with catastrophic thrombotic complications (purpura fulminans) due to severe protein C deficiency at birth.

Protein S Deficiency

Protein S is another natural vitamin K–dependent anticoagulant. It is a cofactor for APC. Protein S deficiency is inherited in an autosomal dominant fashion and is classified into three types, although their clinical manifestations are nearly identical. Evaluation of protein S deficiency includes measurement of protein S activity (also referred to as functional protein S) and free protein S antigen; interpretation of these studies is often challenging and may be facilitated by a thrombosis specialist. Genetic testing is not feasible for routine clinical practice. See Table 39 for causes of acquired low levels.

The prevalence of inherited protein S deficiency is between 1 in 800 and 1 in 3000; however, rates of VTE vary among individuals and families with the deficiency. It is considered a higher risk thrombophilia.

The heterogeneity in the clinical phenotype of patients with protein S deficiency must be taken into consideration when deciding duration of anticoagulant therapy and family counseling. A large family study showed that protein S deficiency is a risk factor for arterial thromboembolism in persons younger than 55 years. No protein S concentrate exists.

Other Inherited Thrombophilic Disorders

A family history of VTE is a risk factor for first-time VTE whether a thrombophilia is detectable in the family or not. This risk is conferred by unknown factors. Having one first-degree relative with a history of VTE increases a person's risk of VTE 2.2-fold; having one or more affected relatives increases the risk 3.9-fold.

Dysfibrinogenemias are rare inherited disorders that can lead to a clotting or bleeding phenotype. An elevated serum homocysteine level is a risk factor for arterial and venous thrombosis. However, lowering levels with vitamins B_6 or B_{12} or folic acid does not influence the risk of a first or recurrent thrombotic event. Polymorphisms in the methylene tetrahydrofolate reductase (*MTHFR*) gene exist that, in the homozygous or double heterozygous state, sometimes lead to increased homocysteine levels. Meta-analyses show that the *MTHFR* polymorphisms in North America, where food is supplemented

with folic acid, are not risk factors for venous or arterial thrombosis or pregnancy complications.

Elevated plasma factor VIII levels are an independent and dose-dependent risk factor for a first episode of VTE. Population-based controlled studies have demonstrated that elevations in factor VIII greater than 150% confer a 4.8-fold greater risk for first-episode VTE than levels less than 100%. Results of studies investigating whether elevated factor VIII levels are also a risk factor for recurrent VTE have been inconclusive. Therefore, decisions on duration and intensity of anticoagulation cannot be made based on factor VIII levels. Consequently, clinical testing for factor VIII levels is not part of a thrombophilia evaluation.

Studies of abnormalities of fibrinolysis (protein and activity levels and genetic polymorphisms) as risk factors for arterial or venous thrombosis have yielded conflicting or indecisive results. Therefore, testing for abnormalities in the fibrinolytic pathway (plasminogen, tissue plasminogen activator, plasminogen activator inhibitor-1, and thrombin-activatable fibrinolysis inhibitor) is not meaningful. Results neither explain the cause of a thrombotic event nor influence decisions on duration of anticoagulant therapy.

KEY POINTS

- Evidence-based guidelines recommend against routine **HVC** thrombophilia testing because identification of inherited abnormalities does not alter the duration of recommended anticoagulation or reliably predict the risk of recurrence.

- Factor V Leiden (FVL) is the most common inherited thrombophilia, diagnosed by polymerase chain reaction test and activated protein C (APC) resistance assay; an abnormal APC assay result suggests heterozygous or homozygous FVL, but must be confirmed by a genetic test.

- Heterozygous prothrombin *G20210A* gene mutation confers a three-fold increased risk for initial venous thromboembolism (VTE) but is not associated with increased risk for VTE recurrence.

Acquired Thrombophilic Conditions

Overview

Several environmental and medical conditions lead to an increased risk for VTE. The most significant risk factors are surgery (OR 21.7), trauma (OR 12.7), hospital or nursing home confinement (OR 8.0), and malignant neoplasm undergoing chemotherapy (OR 6.6); other factors (active malignancy not undergoing chemotherapy, central venous catheter or pacemaker placement, superficial vein thrombosis, neurologic disease with extremity paresis) have an OR between 3.0 and 5.6. Central venous access catheters, estrogen therapy and pregnancy, obesity, inflammatory disorders, chemotherapy, glucocorticoid therapy, and smoking are additional risk factors.

Surgery, Trauma, Hospitalization, Immobility

Hip and knee arthroplasty, cancer surgery, and pelvic and abdominal surgery are associated with a particularly high VTE risk. Although outpatient and minor inpatient surgeries can increase the VTE risk, particularly if additional VTE risk factors are present, the overall risk is very low. Approximately 40% of VTEs are associated with hospitalization, occurring either in the hospital or shortly after discharge, typically within 3 months. Therefore, patient awareness of VTE symptoms and postdischarge VTE prophylaxis in patients at high risk may be important, even if the patient is mobile after discharge. Forty percent or more of hospital VTEs are preventable with VTE prophylaxis.

Cancer

Approximately 20% of all VTEs occur in patients with cancer. The risk for VTE is determined by general risk factors (age, obesity, personal or family history of VTE, coexisting medical conditions, inherited and acquired thrombophilias) and cancer-specific risk factors (cancer type, stage, chemotherapy type, hormonal therapy, surgery, central venous catheters). Active cancer or cancer actively being treated with chemotherapy or radiation therapy increases the VTE risk approximately five- to six-fold, but a history of cancer, or cancer that has undergone curative therapy without evidence of residual disease, does not.

Approximately 6% of patients with unprovoked VTE have an undiagnosed cancer at the time of the VTE, and about 10% of patients with unprovoked VTE will be diagnosed with a cancer in the year following the VTE diagnosis. It is unknown whether extensive screening for cancer in a patient with unprovoked VTE is beneficial and leads to decreased cancer-associated morbidity or improved survival. Cancer should be considered in select patients, such as those with recent weight loss and other unexplained symptoms or abnormalities on routine laboratory testing, such as anemia. Routine extensive screening for underlying cancer in all patients with unprovoked VTE, beyond that recommended for age and gender, is not recommended.

Antiphospholipid Antibody Syndrome

APLAs are acquired autoantibodies against phospholipids and phospholipid-binding proteins such as cardiolipin and β_2-glycoprotein I (β_2-GPI). In vitro, they can prolong clotting tests, but in vivo they increase the risk of venous and arterial thrombosis. Antiphospholipid syndrome (APS) can be a primary disorder with no underlying comorbidity or a secondary disorder associated with autoimmune diseases, malignancy, or drugs.

APLAs (**Figure 14**) may be detected and measured in several ways. Lupus anticoagulants (also termed lupus inhibitors) are APLAs that prolong clotting times (such as the prothrombin time [PT], activated partial thromboplastin time [aPTT], dilute Russell viper venom time). This prolongation is not corrected with a normal plasma mixing study, but corrects

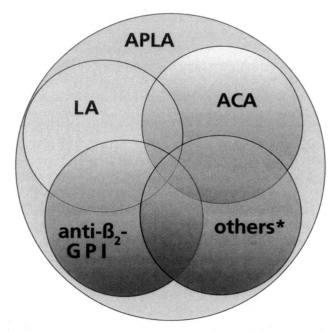

FIGURE 14. APLAs are acquired autoantibodies against phospholipids and phospholipid-binding proteins such as cardiolipin and β_2-GPI; LAs are APLAs that prolong clotting times although patients are actually thrombophilic. Some patients may have one or more APLAs present.

APLA = antiphospholipid antibody; ACA = anticardiolipin antibody; anti-β_2-GPI = anti-β_2-glycoprotein-I antibody; LA = lupus anticoagulant.

*Other antibodies, of unclear clinical significance: antiphosphatidyl-serine, -ethanolamine, and -inositol antibodies.

when excess phospholipids are added. Anticardiolipin antibodies (ACAs) are APLAs that react with cardiolipin or proteins associated with cardiolipin and are also responsible for false-positive tests for syphilis (such as the rapid plasma reagin test) that use cardiolipin in their assays.

The diagnostic criteria for APS include venous or arterial thrombosis or pregnancy loss plus moderate to high antibody titers or a lupus anticoagulant that is positive on repeat testing at least 3 months apart (**Table 40**).

No full consensus exists regarding which APLAs to test for in suspected APS. The Sydney criteria include IgG and IgM ACAs and anti-β_2-GPI antibodies, as well as lupus anticoagulant (see Table 40). The clinical significance of IgA antibodies and antibodies against other phospholipids is unclear. The prevalence of APS is poorly defined, but APLAs are found in nearly 50% of patients with systemic lupus erythematosus, but only 1% to 5% of the general population. Not infrequently, APLAs are transiently positive at the time of an acute thrombotic event, but the clinical significance of these elevations is questionable.

Positivity of all three APLA tests (lupus anticoagulant, ACA, and anti-β_2-GPI antibodies) is associated with the highest risk for thrombosis and pregnancy loss. APS is also implicated in recurrent VTE when anticoagulation is discontinued. However, limited data exist on the degree to which APLAs increase the risk of recurrence, particularly in patients whose index event was provoked. Presence of a

TABLE 40. Diagnostic Criteria for Antiphospholipid Syndrome

Clinical Criteria	Definitions
Vascular events	One or more objectively confirmed symptomatic episodes of arterial, venous, or microvascular thrombosis. Histopathologic specimens must demonstrate thrombosis in the absence of vessel wall inflammation to qualify
Pregnancy morbidity	One or more unexplained fetal deaths at or beyond the 10th week of gestation, with normal fetal morphology; or
	One or more premature births of a morphologically normal neonate before the 34th week of gestation because of eclampsia, severe preeclampsia, or placental insufficiency; or
	Three or more unexplained, consecutive, spontaneous abortions before the 10th week of gestation in the absence of maternal anatomic, chromosomal, or hormonal abnormalities or paternal chromosomal abnormalities
Laboratory Criteria	**Definitions**
Lupus anticoagulant	Positive result for a lupus anticoagulant using a phospholipid-dependent clotting assay (aPTT, dilute Russell viper venom assay, kaolin clotting time, dilute PT) with evidence of phospholipid dependence present on two or more occasions at least 12 weeks apart; or
Anticardiolipin antibody	Medium- or high-titer IgG or IgM anticardiolipin antibody measured using a standardized ELISA on two or more occasions at least 12 weeks apart; or
β_2-Glycoprotein I antibody	High-titer anti-β_2-glycoprotein I IgG or IgM antibody measured using a standardized ELISA on two or more occasions at least 12 weeks apart

aPTT = activated partial thromboplastin time; ELISA = enzyme-linked immunosorbent assay; PT = prothrombin time.

Data from Miyakis S, Lockshin MD, Atsumi T, et al. International consensus statement on an update of the classification criteria for definite antiphospholipid syndrome (APS). J Thromb Haemost. 2006;4(2):295-306. [PMID: 16420554]; and Devreese K, Hoylaerts MF. Laboratory diagnosis of the antiphospholipid syndrome: a plethora of obstacles to overcome. Eur J Haematol. 2009;83(1):1-16. [PMID: 19226362]

lupus anticoagulant is a stronger risk factor for recurrence than ACA and anti-β_2-GPI antibodies; triple positivity confers the highest risk of recurrence. Finally, warfarin therapy is unsuccessful in preventing recurrent thrombosis in 5% to 15% of patients. Occasionally, this is a result of invalidity of the INR for assessing warfarin therapy, because the INR may be inappropriately elevated in some patients because of a lupus anticoagulant, potentially leading to inaccurate measurement of anticoagulation.

Because of the high rate of recurrent VTE, patients with APS and a history of unprovoked VTE should receive anticoagulation therapy indefinitely. A target INR range of 2 to 3 is as effective in preventing recurrent VTE as an INR range of 3 to 4. Whether patients with arterial thrombosis and APS are more effectively treated with antiplatelet or anticoagulant therapy is unknown. Rituximab has been shown to decrease APLA titers in some patients, but whether decreasing or eliminating APLAs leads to a decreased thrombosis risk has not been studied.

Catastrophic APS is a rare, life-threatening condition that results in multiorgan failure from widespread microvascular thrombosis. Anticoagulation, high-dose glucocorticoids and other immunosuppressants, and plasma exchange are the treatment modalities.

Medications

Many medications increase the risk for thrombosis, often in conjunction with acquired hypercoagulable states (such as obesity, smoking, and age) or inherited thrombophilias. The VTE risk with estrogen-progestin contraceptives is highest with the fourth-generation pills (containing the progestin drospirenone) and contraceptive patches and rings, followed by third-generation pills, and then second-generation pills. Somewhat limited data exist regarding the risk of VTE with progestin-only contraceptives. It appears that injectable progestin-only contraceptives do increase the risk of VTE, but oral progestin contraceptives (mini-pill) carry less risk, and progestin-releasing intrauterine devices do not increase risk (see MKSAP 17 General Internal Medicine for more information on contraceptives by generation).

Hormone replacement therapy with estrogen-progestin agents also increases the risk for VTE. Whether so-called "bioidentical hormones," compound hormonal preparations, or phytoestrogens increase the risk for thrombosis is unknown. Chemotherapy, particularly combination therapy, increases the risk for thrombosis in patients with cancer, as do specific drugs such as tamoxifen and anastrozole. Bevacizumab increases the risks for thrombosis and bleeding. Erythropoiesis-stimulating agents confer a mild risk for VTE in patients with cancer, increasing the VTE risk 1.6-fold.

Other Acquired Thrombophilic Conditions

Thrombosis may occur as a complication of systemic or local infection. Head and neck infections may trigger cerebral and sinus vein thrombosis, likely through inflammation of the jugular vein. Inflammatory conditions slightly increase the risk of VTE, as do glucocorticoids. Nephrotic syndrome predisposes to VTE, sometimes owing to urine antithrombin loss but often because of unknown factors. Liver disease can lead to an increased risk of thrombosis because of decreased synthesis of anticoagulants (for example, antithrombin, proteins C and S) and fibrinolytic factors. Myeloproliferative neoplasms (MPNs) (polycythemia vera, essential thrombocythemia, and myelofibrosis) are strong risk factors for thrombosis, more often arterial but also venous. Complete blood count abnormalities may be the first indicator of an MPN, and the presence of the *JAK2 V617F* mutation is a helpful diagnostic tool. Paroxysmal nocturnal hemoglobinuria (PNH) is a rare disorder that predisposes patients to arterial and venous thrombosis with a predilection for splanchnic vein thrombosis.

KEY POINTS

HVC
- Routine extensive screening for underlying cancer in all patients with unprovoked venous thromboembolism is not recommended.

- Because of the high rate of recurrent venous thromboembolism (VTE), patients with antiphospholipid syndrome and a history of unprovoked VTE should undergo anticoagulation indefinitely.

- The risk of venous thromboembolism with estrogen-progestin contraceptives is highest with the fourth-generation pills and contraceptive rings and patches; progestin-releasing intrauterine devices do not increase risk.

- Polycythemia vera, essential thrombocythemia, and myelofibrosis are strong risk factors for arterial and venous thrombosis.

Deep Venous Thrombosis and Pulmonary Embolism

VTE encompasses deep venous thrombosis (DVT) and pulmonary embolism (PE). Superficial thrombophlebitis is not included in this term.

Prevention

VTE prophylaxis should be considered for every hospitalized patient based on individual risk assessment for VTE and bleeding and formal VTE prophylaxis guidelines used in all hospitals (see MKSAP 17 General Internal Medicine). If prophylaxis is indicated, pharmacologic agents are the preferred choice. Mechanical VTE prophylaxis with graded compression stockings or intermittent pneumatic compression devices is not recommended either with or in place of pharmacologic prophylaxis, although intermittent pneumatic compression devices have shown some efficacy in surgical patients and may be an option for nonsurgical patients with a contraindication to pharmacologic therapy. VTE prophylaxis is often only given during a patient's hospitalization. However, for many patients, some degree of VTE risk persists for weeks after discharge, and a heightened level of suspicion that extremity or pulmonary symptoms may be caused by VTE is appropriate, particularly if additional VTE risk factors are present. The benefit of postdischarge prophylaxis (up to 5 weeks) is well established in patients after hip fracture, hip replacement, and major cancer surgery. Prolonged prophylaxis may also be considered in other patients at high risk, such as patients with previous VTE or significant immobility after hospital discharge. The role of inferior vena cava (IVC) filters in patients considered at high risk for PE, such as trauma patients, is unclear.

Diagnosis

The symptoms and signs of VTE, including extremity pain, swelling, warmth, and reddish discoloration in DVT and shortness of breath, chest pain, nonproductive cough, and tachycardia in PE, are notoriously nonspecific, and sensitivity and specificity of these signs and symptoms are low. Because of this, pretest probability models such as the Wells criteria have been developed and validated to assist in clinical decision making when evaluating patients with either potential diagnosis. In patients with low pretest probability for DVT (Wells DVT score ≤1; **Table 41**) or PE (Wells PE score ≤4; **Table 42**), obtaining a D-dimer blood test is suggested; if negative, no further testing is needed, because a VTE has been effectively excluded. However, if the D-dimer assay is positive or the Wells score indicates that DVT or PE is likely (Wells DVT score >1; Wells PE score >4), an imaging study is indicated. When

TABLE 41.	Wells Criteria for Deep Venous Thrombosis	
Variables		**Points**
Leg Symptoms and Findings		
Calf swelling ≥3cm		+1
Swollen unilateral superficial veins (nonvaricose)		+1
Unilateral pitting edema		+1
Swelling of the entire leg		+1
Localized tenderness along the deep venous system		+1
History		
Previously documented DVT		+1
Active cancer or treatment in previous 6 months		+1
Paralysis, paresis, recent cast immobilization of legs		+1
Recently bedridden for ≥3 days; major surgery		+1
Alternative explanation for leg symptoms at least as likely		−2

DVT = deep venous thrombosis

0-1 points = DVT unlikely; obtain D-dimer assay. If negative, no further evaluation; if positive, obtain Doppler ultrasonography.

>1 point = DVT likely; obtain Doppler ultrasonography.

From Wells PS, Anderson DR, Rodger M, et al. Evaluation of D-dimer in the diagnosis of suspected deep-vein thrombosis. N Engl J Med. 2003 Sep 25;349(13):1228. [PMID: 14507948]. Reprinted with permission from Massachusetts Medical Society.

TABLE 42.	Wells Criteria for Pulmonary Embolism	
Variables		**Points**
Symptoms and Signs		
Hemoptysis		1
Heart rate >100/min		1.5
Clinical signs and symptoms of DVT		3
History		
Previously documented DVT or PE		1.5
Active cancer		1
Bedridden ≥3 days or major surgery in previous 4 weeks		1.5
Other		
PE is most likely diagnosis		3

DVT = deep venous thrombosis; PE = pulmonary embolism.

≤4 points = PE unlikely.

4-6 points = moderate possibility of PE.

>6 points = high probability of PE.

Republished with permission of Schattauer, from Wells PS, Anderson DR, Rodger M, et al. Derivation of a simple clinical model to categorize patients probability of pulmonary embolism: increasing the models utility with the SimpliRED D-dimer. Thromb Haemost. 2000 Mar;83(3):418. [PMID: 10744147]

H CONT.

using the D-dimer for pretest probability assessments, a moderately or highly sensitive assay should be used.

Knowledge of superficial versus deep vein anatomy is important when making VTE treatment decisions. The femoral vein (previously termed superficial femoral vein) is the main deep vein in the thigh; because the term "superficial" can lead to confusion, this vein was renamed. The soleal vein is a deep intramuscular distal leg vein. In the arm, the brachial vein is a deep vein and the basilic vein is a superficial vein. Lower extremity DVTs are termed "proximal" if they involve the popliteal or more proximal veins and "distal" if only calf veins are affected.

When imaging is indicated, duplex ultrasonography and CT angiography (CTA) are the diagnostic tests of choice for DVT and PE, respectively. Duplex ultrasonography interpretations are operator dependent; the diagnosis of recurrent DVT can be particularly challenging. PEs are categorized as "massive" if associated with cardiovascular shock or persistent hypotension, "submassive" if associated with right ventricular dysfunction on echocardiography or chest CT or with serum cardiac enzyme elevation (troponin or B-type natriuretic peptide), and "low risk" if cardiac enzyme level and echocardiography are normal. The categories correspond to mortality rates, ranging from greater than 30% to less than 1%. Although chest CTA is a sensitive test for the detection of PE, suboptimal contrast filling of pulmonary arteries, intravascular flow artifacts, and over- and underinterpretation of changes can lead to false-positive and false-negative readings, particularly of subsegmental PEs. When a discrepancy occurs between clinical

pretest probability assessment of PE and CTA imaging findings, review of the CTA by an experienced radiologist and additional testing for VTE (Doppler ultrasonography of the legs, ventilation-perfusion lung scan, D-dimer testing) are indicated to confirm the diagnosis.

Treatment

Outpatient management and early discharge for patients with PE or DVT are safe, feasible, cost-effective management options. Hospital admission is appropriate for patients who are too ill to be managed at home (those needing supplemental oxygen or intravenous pain medications) or for whom social and financial circumstances make this the better option. Outpatient management is safe for up to 50% of patients with PE, even some with mild right heart strain on cardiac echocardiography. Early ambulation rather than bedrest is suggested for patients with DVT and PE.

In patients with acute isolated distal DVT with only mild symptoms and no risk factors for progression (such as immobility or cancer), no anticoagulation is necessary, but serial Doppler ultrasonography approximately 5 to 7 days after initial diagnosis and then 10 to 14 days later is suggested, because approximately 15% of these DVTs progress to proximal veins. Risk factors for extension are a positive D-dimer assay, thrombosis that is extensive or close to the proximal veins, no reversible provoking factor for DVT, active cancer, history of VTE, and inpatient status. Patients with acute isolated distal DVT with severe symptoms or risk factors for extension, and those with proximal DVT, require anticoagulation. For patients with incidentally found asymptomatic proximal DVT or PE, the same initial and long-term anticoagulation is suggested as for comparable patients with symptomatic DVT. Because of radiation exposure with lung scanning, patients with diagnosed DVT and no PE symptoms should not routinely undergo chest CTA.

The role of thrombolytic therapy in the management of DVT is unclear and a matter of clinical investigation. At publication, anticoagulant therapy alone is preferred to pharmacomechanical thrombectomy/thrombolysis for proximal DVT.

Systemic thrombolytic therapy with anticoagulation is suggested for PE with hypotension. The best treatment for patients with submassive PE is unknown, but thrombolytics may be considered in younger patients at low risk for bleeding.

Anticoagulant treatment options in the acute setting are a parenteral anticoagulant (low-molecular-weight heparin [LMWH], fondaparinux, or unfractionated heparin [UFH]) and initiation of warfarin or monotherapy with a new oral anticoagulant (NOAC), including apixaban, dabigatran, edoxaban, and rivaroxaban. When choosing a NOAC, differences between the drugs, dosing regimens, and FDA approval must be considered. Dabigatran and edoxaban were studied in patients with acute VTE only after patients had received at least 5 days of parenteral anticoagulant therapy. In studies of rivaroxaban and apixaban, no such initial bridging therapy was required. Parenteral anticoagulant administration must overlap with

CONT.

warfarin for at least 5 days and until the INR is greater than 2 for 24 hours. In most patients, LMWH or fondaparinux is preferred to UFH, because they have less nonspecific protein binding and lead more rapidly to therapeutic anticoagulation. Intravenous UFH is indicated in severely ill patients with VTE who may require thrombolytic therapy or medical intervention such as central venous catheters or arterial lines, during which temporary dose reduction or anticoagulant interruption may become necessary. Therapy with a NOAC is an option in many patients with acute VTE, unless intravenous UFH is necessary. NOACs should not be used in patients who must be hospitalized, who have an extreme BMI (>40), have kidney disease with a creatinine clearance less than 30 mL/min, or, given the nonreversibility of the NOACs, who are at significantly increased risk for bleeding.

Decisions on anticoagulation therapy duration depend on the recurrent VTE risk without anticoagulation, the bleeding risk with anticoagulants, and the patient's preference. Treatment recommendations are summarized in **Table 43**. Patients with distal leg DVT have a low risk for recurrence. In patients with proximal leg DVT or PE, the cumulative VTE recurrence risk after discontinuation of anticoagulation is (1) 1% after 1 year and 3% after 5 years for VTE provoked by major surgery; (2) 5% after 1 year and 15% after 5 years for VTE provoked by a nonsurgical reversible risk factor; and (3) 10% after 1 year and 30% after 5 years for unprovoked VTE. Risk scoring systems have been developed to predict the risk of recurrence in individual patients (HERDOO-2 score, DASH score, Vienna model), but have not been sufficiently validated for use in routine clinical care. When extended (long-term) anticoagulation therapy is chosen, the risks, benefits, and burden of long-term therapy must be re-evaluated periodically. Aspirin appears to lower the risk of recurrent VTE in some patients with unprovoked VTE treated for a standard length of time with full-dose anticoagulant therapy, but it is much less effective than continued anticoagulant therapy. Therefore, aspirin is not an alternative to anticoagulation. However, in patients with unprovoked VTE who discontinue anticoagulant therapy, daily aspirin therapy is reasonable if it is well tolerated and the patient does not have a high bleeding risk.

The only clear indication for an IVC filter is in patients with acute pelvic or proximal leg DVT who cannot undergo anticoagulation because of active bleeding or a very high bleeding risk. It is unclear whether an IVC filter is beneficial in patients with recurrent leg DVT despite therapeutic anticoagulation. **H**

Long-term Complications

Fifty percent of patients with DVT recover completely, but 33%, 9%, and 7% develop mild, moderate, or severe postthrombotic syndrome (PTS), respectively, most often within 1 to 2 years of the acute DVT. PTS manifests as painful extremities, edema, stasis dermatitis, and skin ulcers.

TABLE 43. Duration of Anticoagulant Therapy for Venous Thromboembolism[a]	
Type of Thrombotic Event	**Duration of Anticoagulant Therapy**
Distal leg DVT	
Provoked or unprovoked, mild symptoms	No anticoagulation suggested, but monitor with serial duplex ultrasonography for 2 weeks
Provoked or unprovoked, moderate-severe symptoms	3 months
Proximal leg DVT or PE	
Provoked (by surgery, trauma, immobility)	3 months
Unprovoked	Extended[b]
Recurrent	Duration of therapy depends on whether VTE events were provoked or unprovoked
Two provoked VTE events	3 months after each event
Second unprovoked VTE	Extended[b]
Upper extremity DVT, proximal	At least 3 months
Cancer-associated DVT or PE	As long as the cancer is active or being treated. LMWH is the preferred anticoagulant.
Chronic thromboembolic pulmonary hypertension	Extended[b]

DVT = deep venous thrombosis; LMWH = low-molecular-weight heparin; PE = pulmonary embolism; VTE = venous thromboembolism.

[a]Decisions regarding duration of anticoagulation must always weigh the risk of VTE recurrence, risk of bleeding, and patient preference.

[b]Indicates long-term anticoagulation therapy with periodic (such as once per year) re-evaluation of the risks, benefits, and burdens of long-term therapy and discussion of new clinical study results and new anticoagulant drugs.

Data from Kearon C, Akl EA, Comerota AJ, et al; American College of Chest Physicians. Antithrombotic therapy for VTE disease: antithrombotic therapy and prevention of thrombosis, 9th ed: American College of Chest Physicians Evidence-Based Clinical Practice Guidelines [erratum in: Chest. 2012 Dec;142(6):1698-1704]. Chest. 2012 Feb;141(2 Suppl):e419S-94S. [PMID: 22315268]

Although compression stockings do not appear to prevent PTS, they may be effective in alleviating symptoms. Venous stents may improve PTS in select patients if significant pelvic vein narrowing is demonstrated. Chronic thromboembolic pulmonary hypertension (CTEPH) is defined as an elevated mean pulmonary artery pressure of greater than 25 mm Hg. Patients with large or recurrent PEs are at risk. Chronic shortness of breath and general malaise are key symptoms. Ventilation-perfusion lung scanning is the appropriate test to evaluate for CTEPH; chest CTA is not a sensitive test. Long-term anticoagulant therapy is indicated if CTEPH is present. See MKSAP 17 Pulmonary and Critical Care Medicine for full discussion.

KEY POINTS

- Venous thromboembolism (VTE) prophylaxis should be considered for every hospitalized patient based on individual risk assessment for VTE and bleeding.

HVC
- A low-probability Wells score with a negative D-dimer blood test rules out venous thromboembolism.

- Anticoagulant therapy alone is preferred for proximal deep venous thrombosis, and thrombolytic therapy with anticoagulation is suggested for pulmonary embolism with hypotension.

- Anticoagulation duration is 3 months for provoked venous thromboembolism (VTE) and extended for unprovoked VTE or following a second unprovoked VTE episode.

HVC
- The only clear indication for an IVC filter is in patients with acute pelvic or proximal leg DVT who cannot be anticoagulated because of active bleeding or a very high risk for bleeding

Other Sites of Thrombosis

Superficial Venous Thrombophlebitis

Superficial venous thrombophlebitis (SVT) may occur unprovoked or in the setting of varicose veins, trauma, phlebotomy, intravenous catheters, underlying hypercoagulable states, cancer, infections, or inflammatory disorders (inflammatory bowel disease, thromboangiitis obliterans [Buerger disease], and Behçet syndrome). Because patients may have concurrent DVT, duplex ultrasonography is indicated when SVT of the great or small saphenous vein is present, if extremity swelling is more pronounced than would be expected from the SVT alone, and if symptoms progress. DVT or PE develops in up to 3.3% of patients with isolated SVT. Nonextensive SVT (less than 5 cm in length and not near the deep venous system) requires only symptomatic therapy consisting of analgesics, anti-inflammatory medications, and warm or cold compresses for symptom relief. Patients with extensive SVT may benefit from a short course of anticoagulant therapy. The only randomized trial in the management of SVT showed that 6 weeks of a prophylactic dose of fondaparinux compared with placebo is beneficial for preventing local thrombosis progression and development of DVT and PE. However, because of a lack of data, optimal length of anticoagulation and drug choice are not known.

KEY POINT

- Nonextensive superficial venous thrombophlebitis requires only symptomatic therapy with analgesics, anti-inflammatory medications, and warm or cold compresses.

Upper Extremity DVT

Upper extremity DVT accounts for 1% to 4% of all DVTs. Approximately 80% are secondary to central venous catheters or cancer, and 20% are primary events. Little direct evidence exists to support any particular duration of anticoagulant therapy after a first unprovoked upper extremity DVT. Management consists of anticoagulation for at least 3 months (see Table 43) for unprovoked or catheter-associated proximal DVT and maintaining catheter placement if the central venous catheter is functional and still needed. Anticoagulation should be continued as long as the catheter remains in place. If the catheter is removed, anticoagulation should be given for 3 months. DVT may also be due to thoracic outlet syndrome (effort thrombosis, Paget-Schroetter syndrome) from external compression of the axillary vein by the clavicle, a cervical rib, or enlarged or aberrantly inserted muscles. No uniform approach exists for treatment of these patients. Upper extremity DVTs carry a risk of PE, but it has not been well quantified.

KEY POINT

- Approximately 80% of upper extremity deep venous thromboembolisms occur secondary to central venous catheters or cancer, with only 20% occurring as primary events.

Budd-Chiari Syndrome

Presentations of hepatic vein thrombosis (Budd-Chiari syndrome) range from asymptomatic and incidentally discovered to fulminant liver failure. Patients can have various degrees of right upper quadrant or diffuse abdominal pain. The cause is often multifactorial. The most common risk factor, present in nearly 50% of patients, is an MPN such as polycythemia vera, essential thrombocythemia, and primary myelofibrosis. The *JAK2* mutation is frequently present in patients with Budd-Chiari syndrome (29%) even if no hematologic abnormalities suggesting an MPN are present. Any of the inherited and acquired thrombophilias can also contribute to the development of Budd-Chiari syndrome, as can estrogens and pregnancy. PNH can be detected in almost 20% of patients with Budd-Chiari syndrome. The diagnosis is made by Doppler ultrasonography, contrast-enhanced CT, or MRI. Thrombolytic therapy can be considered in the acute setting of fulminant

CONT.

thrombosis but must be balanced against the increased risk for bleeding associated with liver failure. Anticoagulation is usually appropriate. The duration may be long term, but depends on a patient's risk for bleeding, which may be significant owing to esophageal varices, coagulopathy from liver synthetic dysfunction, and thrombocytopenia from hypersplenism. **H**

Portal and Mesenteric Vein Thrombosis

Portal vein thrombosis (PVT) is often silent and may only be discovered during evaluation of variceal gastrointestinal bleeding. The most common symptom is nonspecific right upper quadrant abdominal pain of acute or subacute onset. It is associated with inherited and acquired thrombophilias, MPNs, *JAK2* positivity without overt MPN, PNH, intra-abdominal neoplasia, infection, trauma, surgery, and neonatal umbilical vein catheterization. PVT occurs in up to 26% of patients with cirrhosis. It is diagnosed by Doppler ultrasonography, CT, or magnetic resonance venography. Cavernous transformation of the portal vein (collateral vessel formation in the porta hepatis) reflects old PVT. In acute PVT, extension of thrombus into the mesenteric veins may lead to intestinal infarction. Superior mesenteric vein thrombosis typically presents with nonspecific abdominal pain and nausea. Symptoms are vague, often leading to a delay in diagnosis. By the time of diagnosis, small bowel ischemic changes may be present. Gastrointestinal bleeding and peritonitis develop when transmural ischemia has occurred. The causes of superior mesenteric vein thrombosis are similar to those of portal vein thrombosis. Patients with acute portal or mesenteric vein thrombosis typically undergo anticoagulation for at least 3 months. Decisions regarding long-term anticoagulation in these patients, as well as patients with incidentally discovered thrombosis, must balance the often unknown risk of recurrent thrombosis with the risk of bleeding. **H**

Splenic Vein Thrombosis

Pancreatitis and pancreatic malignancies are the main causes of splenic vein thrombosis. Abdominal surgery and trauma, intra-abdominal infection, and thrombophilias are also causative. Symptoms are often subtle, and diagnosis frequently occurs coincidentally during abdominal imaging studies ordered for other reasons. Anticoagulant treatment duration depends on the triggering factors. Incidentally discovered splenic vein thrombosis likely does not require anticoagulation

after appropriate evaluation for an underlying, treatable cause (MPN, PNH) has been concluded. Pancreatitis-associated thrombosis may not require anticoagulation therapy either, particularly because the risk for intra-abdominal bleeding with such therapy may be high.

Cerebral and Sinus Vein Thrombosis

Thrombosis of the cerebral, cortical, and sinus veins is also referred to as cerebral and sinus vein thrombosis (CSVT). The cause is often multifactorial, with risk factors being thrombophilias, estrogen therapy and pregnancy, and infections such as mastoiditis, otitis, sinusitis, and meningitis. A cause for CSVT is identified in 85% of patients. The most frequent but least specific symptom is severe headache of subacute or acute onset, which is present in 90% of patients. Routine noncontrast and contrast head CT and brain MRI scans are often unrevealing, resulting in missed diagnoses; CT venography or magnetic resonance venography are the appropriate studies if CSVT is suspected. Approximately 40% of patients with CSVT have a hemorrhagic infarct, a consequence of the venous occlusion. In the acute setting, even with hemorrhagic infarct, heparin is given followed by oral anticoagulation, unless the hemorrhage is very pronounced. The optimal duration of anticoagulant therapy is unknown. Expert opinion suggests 3 to 6 months if the thrombosis was associated with a transient risk factor, 6 to 12 months if the event was unexplained and no higher risk thrombophilia has been detected, and long term if a higher risk thrombophilia is detected or the event is recurrent. Increased intracranial pressure (pseudotumor cerebri) can be a late complication. CSVT accounts for up to 10% of patients with presumed idiopathic intracranial hypertension. **H**

Retinal Vein Thrombosis

Central retinal vein occlusion (CRVO) leads to sudden, extensive vision loss. A branch retinal vein occlusion (BRVO) causes a painless sectorial decrease in vision resulting in misty or distorted vision. BRVO is more common than CRVO and typically results from pressure on the vein from the overlying arteriosclerotic thickened branch retinal artery. Risk factors for BRVO and CRVO include hypertension, hyperlipidemia, and diabetes mellitus. Management by an ophthalmologist and a thrombosis specialist may be the best approach for optimal treatment of patients with CRVO, because indications for anticoagulant use are not clearly defined (see MKSAP 17 General Internal Medicine section for further information).

Unexplained Arterial Thrombosis

Arterial thrombotic and thromboembolic events in young persons (younger than 50 years) are uncommon unless significant arteriosclerotic risk factors, or atrial fibrillation, are present. A systematic evaluation can be helpful in identifying causes (**Table 44**). Relatively little is known about thrombophilias predisposing to arterial thrombosis. Whether patients found to have a strong thrombophilia should be treated with antiplatelet therapy or anticoagulant therapy is also unknown.

Anticoagulants

The most common anticoagulants used in VTE prevention and treatment are UFH, LMWH, fondaparinux, and warfarin. NOACs apixaban, dabigatran, edoxaban, and rivaroxaban are FDA approved for VTE treatment. The parenteral direct thrombin inhibitors argatroban and lepirudin are reserved for the treatment of heparin-induced thrombocytopenia (HIT), and bivalirudin is used for patients during percutaneous transluminal coronary angioplasty, including patients who also have HIT.

Unfractionated Heparin

UFH potentiates the natural anticoagulant activity of antithrombin and acts as a nonspecific anticoagulant, mostly against thrombin and factor Xa. UFH bioavailability varies greatly because of avid protein binding. It is typically monitored by the aPTT, although anti-factor Xa plasma levels may be used. Whether either monitoring method leads to superior safety or efficacy of heparin therapy is unknown. UFH is mostly cleared by the reticuloendothelial system and, to a lesser degree, by the kidneys. Lower doses may be required for therapeutic anticoagulation in patients with kidney injury and higher doses needed during extensive acute VTE. Weight-based heparin dosing nomograms achieve therapeutic aPTTs faster than other approaches to selecting a UFH dose. The half-life of UFH depends on the dose given; it is 60 minutes with a bolus dose of 100 U/kg. A patient receiving continuous intravenous UFH at therapeutic doses will likely return to the baseline aPTT within 3 to 4 hours after discontinuing heparin. Protamine can be used to reverse anticoagulation with UFH. Long-term use of UFH leads to an increased risk of osteoporosis. **H**

KEY POINTS

- Weight-based heparin dosing nomograms achieve therapeutic activated partial thromboplastin times faster than other approaches to selecting an unfractionated heparin dose.
- Protamine can be used to reverse anticoagulation with unfractionated heparin.

Low-Molecular-Weight Heparin

LMWH is made from UFH through chemical and physical processes that select the smaller polysaccharides; these lower weight molecules have different properties than UFH. Like UFH, LMWH potentiates antithrombin action, although this effect is greater against factor Xa than against thrombin. Because of this, aPTT measurement does not reflect LMWH activity; if it is necessary to assess anticoagulant effect, anti-Xa activity must be measured. LMWH also has greater bioavailability, more predictable pharmacokinetics, and a prolonged half-life when administered subcutaneously. This allows administration once or twice daily based on weight and without routine monitoring. Other differences between LMWH and UFH include less risk for HIT development and decreased osteoporosis risk. Monitoring is generally unnecessary. LMWH should be used cautiously, in reduced doses or not at all, in patients with severe kidney disease (creatinine clearance <30 mL/min). Dosing in obese patients should be based on actual body weight, but anti-Xa activity measured 3 to 4 hours after subcutaneous injection may be helpful in select patients with extreme BMIs (>40) to assess actual anticoagulant effect. LMWH is only partially reversible by protamine. It is unknown whether fresh frozen plasma (FFP), nonactivated prothrombin complex concentrates (PCCs), activated PCCs, or recombinant factor VIIa are beneficial in LMWH-associated major bleeding. Use of these reversal agents is not evidence based. **H**

KEY POINTS

- Low-molecular-weight heparin's predictable pharmacokinetics enable weight-based dosing without laboratory monitoring.
- Low-molecular-weight heparin should be used cautiously, in reduced doses or not at all, in patients with severe kidney disease (creatinine clearance <30 mL/min).

Fondaparinux

Fondaparinux is a synthetic pentasaccharide that acts as an anticoagulant by potentiating antithrombin inhibition of factor Xa. It is administered subcutaneously, reaches its peak plasma level after approximately 3 hours, and, because of a half-life of approximately 17 hours, is dosed once daily. Because fondaparinux does not bind significantly to plasma proteins, it can be given without laboratory monitoring as a fixed dose for VTE prophylaxis and in body-weight-adjusted dosing for VTE treatment. It is cleared by the kidneys, so it should be used with caution in patients with a creatinine clearance of 30 to 50 mL/min. It is contraindicated in patients with a creatinine clearance less than 30 mL/min. No agent is available to reverse anticoagulation with fondaparinux. It is unknown whether FFP, nonactivated PCCs, activated PCCs, or recombinant factor VIIa are beneficial as reversal agents. **H**

TABLE 44.	Structured Approach for the Evaluation of Patients with Unexplained Arterial Thromboembolism

Is Arteriosclerosis the Underlying Problem?

Arteriosclerotic changes demonstrated on imaging studies (CT, contrast arteriogram, or other radiologic imaging studies) or pathology specimens?

Arteriosclerosis risk factors present?

    Cigarette smoking

    High blood pressure

    High LDL cholesterol

    Low HDL cholesterol

    High lipoprotein(a)

    Diabetes mellitus

    Obesity

    Family history of arterial disorders in young relatives (<50 years)

Has the Heart Been Thoroughly Evaluated as an Embolic Source?

Atrial fibrillation evaluated by ECG or ambulatory or event monitor

Cardiomyopathy with possible left ventricular or atrial thrombus

Patent foramen ovale on cardiac echocardiography with bubble study and Valsalva maneuver

Other Causes

Is the patient receiving estrogen therapy (contraceptive pill, ring, or patch; hormone replacement therapy)?

Does the patient use cocaine or anabolic steroids?

Is there evidence for Buerger disease (does patient smoke cigarettes or cannabis)?

Does patient have symptoms suggesting a vasospastic disorder (Raynaud phenomenon)?

Were anatomic abnormalities seen in the artery leading to the ischemic area (web, fibromuscular dysplasia, dissection, vasculitis, external compression)?

Does patient have evidence of a rheumatologic or autoimmune disease (arthritis, purpura, or vasculitis)? Consider laboratory evaluation for vasculitis and immune disorder.

Is there a suggestion of an infectious arteritis?

Could the patient have hyperviscosity or cryoglobulins?

Thrombophilia Evaluation

Hemoglobin and platelet count

Antiphospholipid antibodies

Anticardiolipin IgG and IgM antibodies

Anti-β_2-glycoprotein I IgG and IgM antibodies

Lupus anticoagulant

Protein C activity

Protein S activity and free protein S antigen

Antithrombin III activity

Homocysteine (in younger patients)

Consider factor V Leiden and prothrombin *G20210A* mutation[a]

JAK2 mutation and PNH testing if CBC abnormalities

Do not test for *MTHFR* polymorphisms, PAI-1 or tPA levels or polymorphisms, or fibrinogen or factor VIII activities.

CBC = complete blood count; ECG = electrocardiography; *MTHFR* = methylene tetrahydrofolate reductase; PAI-1 = plasminogen activator inhibitor 1; PNH = paroxysmal nocturnal hemoglobinuria; tPA = tissue plasminogen activator.

[a]The purpose of testing is to detect the homozygous or double heterozygous state.

Adapted with permission of Elsevier Science and Technology Journals, from Moll S. Nonarteriosclerotic arterial occlusive disease. In: Kitchens CS, Konkle BA, Kessler CM, eds. *Consultative Hemostasis and Thrombosis.* 3rd ed. Philadelphia, PA: Saunders; 2013:396; permission conveyed through Copyright Clearance Center, Inc.

- Fondaparinux can be dosed once daily because of a half-life of approximately 17 hours and can be given without laboratory monitoring because it does not bind significantly to plasma proteins.
- Fondaparinux should be used with caution in patients with a creatinine clearance of 30 to 50 mL/min and is contraindicated in those with a creatinine clearance less than 30 mL/min.

Warfarin

Vitamin K antagonists such as warfarin inhibit vitamin K epoxide reductase, an enzyme complex needed for synthesis of coagulation factors II, VII, IX, and X and proteins C and S. Warfarin's effect is measured by the PT, expressed as the INR.

Dosing nomograms should be used when initiating warfarin and at follow-up evaluations. Individual dosage requirements vary between 0.5 and 50 mg/d and depend on the patient's diet, medications, comorbidities, age, and genetic factors. Warfarin is metabolized by the cytochrome P-450 enzyme complex, including the cytochrome P-2C9 (CYP2C9) enzyme. Clinical testing for individual polymorphisms is available but has not been convincingly shown to lead to improved clinical outcomes and is not recommended as part of routine care.

Because warfarin leads to a gradual onset of anticoagulation, and paradoxically leads to hypercoagulability in the first 5 days of initiation owing to its rapid effect of lowering protein C activity levels, it must be administered initially with a rapidly acting parenteral anticoagulant when treating an acute thrombotic event. Both should be administered together for at least 5 days regardless of the INR, because decrease of the shorter half-life coagulation factor VII may lead to an increase in INR that does not reflect protective anticoagulation. During this time, the INR should be checked several times. If the INR increases to greater than 2 during these first 5 days, the parenteral anticoagulant

should be continued and the warfarin dose interrupted or decreased. After this period, and with the INR greater than 2 for 24 hours, the short-acting anticoagulant should be discontinued; thereafter, monitoring can decrease to weekly, then monthly, with a stable, therapeutic INR. In patients with very stable INRs, monitoring can be extended to every 12 weeks. Point-of-care full-blood fingerstick monitors yield reliable results and are available for clinical practices and for appropriately selected patients to self-test their INR at home.

Dietary vitamin K intake influences the INR. Patients should not avoid all foods containing vitamin K, but rather consume a consistent diet. In some patients with fluctuating INRs, daily supplementation with vitamin K (100-150 µg/d) can stabilize the INR. Many medications also influence the metabolism of warfarin, leading to INR elevations or decreases. Preemptive dose adjustments and close monitoring are warranted when interacting medications are started or stopped.

Warfarin's half-life is 20 to 60 hours (mean, 32-40 hours). The bleeding risk associated with a procedure determines whether warfarin must be stopped beforehand and when. Warfarin must be discontinued at least 5 days before major surgery. The patient's thromboembolic risk should determine whether bridging therapy with a parenteral anticoagulant is needed perioperatively (see MKSAP 17 General Internal Medicine). Managing elevated INRs and bleeding in patients taking warfarin depends on the degree of INR elevation and bleeding risk factors or active bleeding (Table 45). PCCs are plasma products from human donors. Four-factor PCC contains all vitamin K–dependent coagulation factors and has been available in the United States since 2013; 3-factor PCCs contain factors II, IX, and X, but relatively little factor VII. Four-factor PCC is capable of restoring individual clotting factor activity in nearly 100% of patients within minutes of administration, whereas 3-factor PCCs must be supplemented with FFP or a low dose of recombinant factor VIIa to more optimally lower the INR (see Transfusion).

TABLE 45. Management Strategy for Elevated INRs and Bleeding in Patients Taking Vitamin K Antagonists			
INR	**Bleeding**	**Risk Factors for Bleeding**[a]	**Intervention**
Supratherapeutic but <5	No	No/yes	Lower or omit next VKA dose(s) Reduce subsequent dose(s)
5-9	No	No	Omit next VKA dose(s) Reduce subsequent dose(s)
	No	Yes	Vitamin K, 1-2.5 mg PO
>9	No	No/yes	Vitamin K, 2.5-5 mg PO
Serious bleed at any INR	Yes	NA	Vitamin K, 10 mg IV + 4f-PCC (or 3f-PCC + FFP or rVIIa)

3f-PCC = 3-factor prothrombin complex concentrate; 4f-PCC = 4-factor PCC; FFP = fresh frozen plasma; IV = intravenous; NA = not applicable; PO = by mouth; rVIIa = recombinant activated factor VII; VKA = vitamin K antagonist.

[a]Coagulopathy, moderate or severe thrombocytopenia, recent major surgery, previous major bleeding episode.

- In some patients taking warfarin with fluctuating INRs, daily supplementation with vitamin K (100-150 µg/d) can stabilize the INR.

- Four-factor prothrombin complex concentrate (PCC) can restore individual clotting factor activity in nearly 100% of patients, whereas 3-factor PCCs must be supplemented with fresh frozen plasma or a low dose of recombinant activated factor VIIa.

New Oral Anticoagulants

The NOACs (apixaban, dabigatran, edoxaban, and rivaroxaban), also referred to as target-specific oral anticoagulants, share several features, including (1) rapid onset of action (maximal anticoagulant plasma levels in 3 or fewer hours after oral intake), (2) no need for routine monitoring of their anticoagulant effect in most patients, (3) no dietary restrictions, (4) relatively few clinically important interactions with medications, (5) short half-lives of about 12 hours when kidney function is normal, (6) contraindications or need for dose modifications in moderate to severe kidney disease, and (7) lack of established reversal agents and strategies for patients with major hemorrhage. These medications are FDA approved and available for specific indications (**Table 46**). NOACs influence routine coagulation tests (PT, aPTT) to various degrees. Additionally, coagulation-based thrombophilia tests (proteins C and S, antithrombin activities, lupus anticoagulant) and coagulation factor levels are influenced by these medications, rendering the obtained results unreliable.

When to discontinue these medications before surgery depends on the expected bleeding risk with the surgery and the patient's kidney function. For standard-risk procedures and in a patient with normal kidney function, discontinuation is typically 24 to 36 hours before surgery; for surgeries and interventions with high risk for bleeding, the NOAC should be discontinued at least 60 hours (2.5 days) beforehand. When kidney function is impaired, the half-lives of the drugs are increased, so the drug must be discontinued sooner before

TABLE 46. Key Features of the New Oral Anticoagulants

	Dabigatran	Rivaroxaban	Apixaban	Edoxaban
Class of anticoagulant	Direct factor IIa inhibitor	Direct factor Xa inhibitor	Direct factor Xa inhibitor	Direct factor Xa inhibitor
T_{max} (h)	2	3	3	1-2
Half-life (h)	12-17	7-11	9-14	9-11
Protein binding	35%	95%	87%	54%
Renal elimination	80%	66% (33% as active metabolite)	25%	35%
FDA-approved indications	Atrial fibrillation VTE treatment	Atrial fibrillation VTE treatment VTE prevention	Atrial fibrillation VTE treatment VTE prevention	Atrial fibrillation VTE treatment
Dosing				
Atrial fibrillation	CrCl >30 mL/min: 150 mg twice daily CrCl 15-30 mL/min: 75 mg twice daily CrCl ≤15 mL/min: do not use	CrCl >50 mL/min: 20 mg once daily CrCl 15-50 mL/min: 15 mg once daily CrCl ≤15 mL/min: do not use	5 mg twice daily 2.5 mg twice daily if ≥2 criteria present: ≥80 years of age Weight ≤60 kg (132 lb) Creatinine ≥1.5 mg/dL (133 µmol/L)	60 mg once daily CrCl 15-50 mL/min: 30 mg once daily CrCl >95 mL/min: do not use
VTE prevention	NA	10 mg once daily	2.5 mg twice daily	NA
VTE treatment	CrCl >30 mL/min: 150 mg twice daily CrCl <30 mL/min: do not use	CrCl >30 mL/min: 15 mg twice daily × 3 wks, then 20 mg once daily CrCl ≤30 mL/min: do not use	VTE treatment: 10 mg twice daily × 1 wk, then 5 mg twice daily Reduction in VTE recurrence: 2.5 mg twice daily	60 mg once daily 30 mg once daily with the following criteria: CrCl 30-50 mL/min Weight ≤60 kg (132 lb) Concomitant p-glycoprotein inhibitor use

CrCl = creatinine clearance; h = hour; NA = not applicable; T_{max} = time to maximum concentration; VTE = venous thromboembolism.

surgery. If major bleeding occurs with any of the NOACs, therapy with oral charcoal is appropriate for patients who ingested the medication within approximately 2 hours of presentation. Further management is supportive. Dabigatran is dialyzable; apixaban, edoxaban, and rivaroxaban, because of their higher plasma protein–binding, are not. Because of a lack of data, it is unknown whether treatment with activated or nonactivated PCCs, recombinant factor VIIa, or FFP is clinically beneficial, or whether antifibrinolytic therapy with tranexamic acid or ε-aminocaproic acid has any beneficial reversal effect.

In clinical treatment trials of acute VTE, some NOACs (rivaroxaban, apixaban) were used immediately upon diagnosis of acute VTE, whereas others (dabigatran, edoxaban) were started after initial therapy with parenteral anticoagulants. Few patients with cancer, extreme body weight, very old age, multiple comorbidities, or APS were included in the VTE treatment trials of the NOACs. Therefore, they should be used with caution, if at all, in these special populations.

KEY POINT

- Apixaban, dabigatran, edoxaban, and rivaroxaban share several features, including rapid onset of action, no need for routine monitoring, no dietary restrictions, short half-lives, contraindications or need for dose modifications in moderate to severe chronic kidney disease, and lack of reversal agents.

Hematologic Issues in Pregnancy

Gestational Anemia

Pregnancy results in significant changes in metabolism, fluid balance, and circulation, all of which impact the hemoglobin value. Starting in the sixth week of gestation, maternal plasma volume begins to increase, but no increase in erythrocyte mass occurs in response. The result is a dilutional anemia evident by the seventh or eighth week of pregnancy, with a hemoglobin value that should not be less than 11 g/dL (110 g/L) in the first trimester or 10 g/dL (100 g/L) in the second or third trimesters. Hemoglobin values less than these should prompt a search for other causes of anemia, of which iron deficiency is the overwhelming culprit.

Iron and folate deficiencies commonly occur during pregnancy independent of fluid shifts induced by the gravid state (see Erythrocyte Disorders).

KEY POINT

- Hemoglobin values less than 11 g/dL (110 g/L) in the first trimester or less than 10 g/dL (100 g/L) in the second and third trimesters of pregnancy should prompt a search for causes of anemia other than the expected gestational anemia.

Sickle Cell Disease

Care of pregnant patients with sickle cell disease (SCD) should be multidisciplinary and ideally involves a hematologist specifically trained in hemoglobinopathies and a maternal-fetal medicine specialist.

Women with SCD considering pregnancy should take prenatal vitamins without iron because of the predisposition to iron overload from frequent blood transfusions; however, folic acid supplementation should be continued throughout pregnancy. Other medications taken for SCD should be reviewed for possible contraindications in pregnancy. Hydroxyurea should be discontinued even though adverse effects in human fetuses have not been demonstrated. Other therapies, such as ACE inhibitors or iron chelation, are contraindicated in pregnancy. Pneumococcal and yearly influenza vaccines are safe to administer during pregnancy (see General Internal Medicine for further information on vaccination recommendations).

Compared with women without SCD, those with SCD are at increased risk for maternal pregnancy complications. Although maternal mortality risk has improved with better care, it remains nine-fold higher than in women without SCD (0.16% in SCD vs. 0.01% in non-SCD).

A recent study showed a significantly increased relative risk of venous thromboembolism (VTE) (pregnancy-related VTE was 0.09% in normal controls, 0.15% in sickle cell trait, and 2.9% in SCD), but no guidelines provide clear indications for prophylactic anticoagulation. Other complications include preeclampsia, eclampsia, infection, cardiomyopathy, intrauterine fetal demise, and intrauterine growth restriction. Vaso-occlusive crises are overall increased during pregnancy, and 28% of women have vaso-occlusive pain episodes at the time of delivery (mostly in women with hemoglobin SS subtype). Development of vaso-occlusive episodes appears to be a predictor for increased maternal morbidity and mortality. Preventing dehydration, for example from pregnancy-induced vomiting, may decrease the incidence of vaso-occlusive crises. If vaso-occlusive crises occur, NSAIDs for pain control are considered safe before 30 weeks' gestation. Opiate analgesics are safe to use in pregnant patients with SCD, but increased narcotic tolerance must be considered during peripartum anesthesia. Chronic opioid use during pregnancy can lead to fetal narcotic withdrawal syndrome.

Although prophylactic transfusions during pregnancy can reduce pain crises, neither transfusion nor exchange transfusion has been shown to reduce pregnancy-related morbidity or mortality, and increased risk for alloantibody production in this population must be considered.

Because pregnant women with SCD have a higher risk of morbidity and mortality, they should be closely monitored for SCD-related complications and promptly treated.

KEY POINTS

- Hydroxyurea, ACE inhibitors, and iron chelation therapy should be discontinued during pregnancy.
- Although prophylactic transfusions during pregnancy can reduce pain crises in patients with sickle cell disease, neither transfusion nor exchange transfusion has been shown to reduce pregnancy-related morbidity or mortality, and increased risk for alloantibody production in this population must be considered.

Thrombocytopenia in Pregnancy

Thrombocytopenia in pregnancy is common, occurring in approximately 7% to 12% of pregnant women. Most cases of thrombocytopenia in pregnancy are mild and have no adverse outcomes for the mother or fetus, although occasionally a low platelet count may signal a more complex, potentially life-threatening condition. Therefore, it is critical to distinguish between different causes of thrombocytopenia in pregnancy.

Gestational Thrombocytopenia

Gestational thrombocytopenia is the cause of a low platelet count in 75% of pregnant women with thrombocytopenia. It generally occurs in the latter half of pregnancy and causes no complications of maternal or fetal health. The patient should have no history of thrombocytopenia outside of pregnancy, and the platelet count should never be less than 50,000/μL (50 × 10⁹/L). No laboratory studies can confirm the diagnosis. It requires no treatment, but careful monitoring is necessary, especially in the final month of pregnancy to ensure the platelet count remains greater than 50,000/μL (50 × 10⁹/L). The mechanism is thought to be the result of a mild consumptive process, but unlike true disseminated intravascular coagulation, the prothrombin and activated partial thromboplastin times are normal, and fibrinogen levels are not depressed. The peripheral blood smear should show an absence of schistocytes, thus proving the thrombocytopenia is not due to a microangiopathic process.

KEY POINT

- In patients with gestational thrombocytopenia, the platelet count should never decrease to less than 50,000/μL (50 × 10⁹/L), and no schistocytes should appear on peripheral blood smear.

Immune Thrombocytopenic Purpura

If a patient has a history of immune thrombocytopenic purpura (ITP), any thrombocytopenia that occurs during pregnancy is assumed to be due to ITP. Additionally, a platelet count that decreases to less than 50,000/μL (50 × 10⁹/L) with normal coagulation values and an absence of schistocytes on peripheral blood smear is considered consistent with a diagnosis of ITP. Management in the first 8 months of pregnancy

should be the same as for any nonpregnant patient, which includes avoiding therapy unless the patient is bleeding or has a platelet count less than 30,000/μL (30 × 10⁹/L). In the final month, a target platelet count of 50,000/μL (50 × 10⁹/L) is desirable, which allows for an emergent cesarean section to be performed safely if needed. If immunosuppressive therapy is required, glucocorticoids such as prednisone are considered relatively safe in pregnancy, although they can increase blood pressure and plasma glucose level, cause weight gain, and may contribute to adverse pregnancy outcomes. Glucocorticoids given to the mother have no effect on fetal platelet counts. Intravenous immune globulin is another first-line therapeutic option for patients with ITP because it is also considered safe for use in pregnancy. Splenectomy should be deferred, if possible. See Platelet Disorders chapter for more information about ITP.

KEY POINT

- Therapy for immune thrombocytopenic purpura during pregnancy is generally not necessary unless the platelet count decreases to less than 30,000/μL (30 × 10⁹/L); however, a platelet count of 50,000/μL (50 × 10⁹/L) is desirable in the final month of pregnancy so a cesarean section can be performed safely if necessary.

Microangiopathy of Pregnancy

The HELLP (Hemolysis, Elevated Liver enzymes, and Low Platelets) syndrome, preeclampsia, and acute fatty liver of pregnancy are part of a spectrum of disorders called the "thrombotic microangiopathy of pregnancy." Symptoms and laboratory features for each overlap (**Table 47**), but making the distinction among the disorders may not be critical, because the most effective therapy for each is emergent delivery of the fetus. If microangiopathic hemolytic anemia and thrombocytopenia worsen following delivery, thrombotic thrombocytopenic purpura should be suspected and plasma exchange therapy initiated. **H**

KEY POINT

- The most effective therapy for HELLP (Hemolysis, Elevated Liver enzymes, and Low Platelets) syndrome, preeclampsia, and acute fatty liver of pregnancy is emergent delivery of the fetus.

Thrombophilia and Venous Thromboembolism in Pregnancy

Epidemiology, Pathophysiology, and Risk Factors **H**

Pregnant women have an approximately five-fold increased risk of thromboembolism compared with nonpregnant women. Eighty percent of events are venous, and the remaining 20% are arterial. Approximately 50% of VTEs occur antepartum. The incidence of VTE declines quickly in the 6 weeks following delivery, and returns to baseline 4 months postpartum. However, the postpartum period is often

TABLE 17. Clinical and Laboratory Features of the Thrombotic Microangiopathies of Pregnancy

Feature	Preeclampsia	HELLP	AFLP	TTP
Hypertension	+++	+++	+	+
Proteinuria	+++	++	+/−	+/−
Abdominal pain	+/−	++	++	+/−
Jaundice	+/−	+/−	++	+/−
Neurologic findings	+	+	+	++
Thrombocytopenia	+	+++	+	+++
Hemolysis	+/−	+++	+	+++
Kidney disease	+/−	+	++	+
Disseminated intravascular coagulation	+/−	++	+++	+/−
Elevated liver chemistry tests	+	+++	+++	+/−
Hypoglycemia	+/−	+/−	+++	+/−

AFLP = acute fatty liver of pregnancy; HELLP = Hemolysis, Elevated Liver enzymes, and Low Platelets; TTP = thrombotic thrombocytopenic purpura.

+++ = always present

++ = usually present

+ = likely to be present

+/− = may or may not be present

CONT.

considered to be the 6 weeks after delivery. VTE complicates one to two of 1000 pregnancies. Deep venous thrombosis of the leg is left-sided in 80% of patients, probably because of stenosis of the left common iliac vein from the overlying right common iliac artery and the lumbar vertebral body posteriorly (May-Thurner syndrome) accentuated by the pregnant uterus. Other contributors to hypercoagulability during pregnancy are a decrease in protein S and increase in fibrinogen, factors VII and VIII, von Willebrand factor, and other procoagulant levels.

The strongest risk factor for pregnancy-associated VTE is a history of VTE. Risk factors for pregnancy-associated VTE are typically the same as those in nonpregnant women, including obesity, advanced age, comorbid conditions such as heart disease, and thrombophilias. Delivery by cesarean section carries up to a 3.6-fold increased risk for postpartum VTE. An association has been suggested between inherited thrombophilias and adverse pregnancy outcomes, such as recurrent early pregnancy loss (<10 weeks), one or more losses after 10 weeks' gestation, intrauterine growth restriction, preeclampsia, and eclampsia, but this association is controversial.

KEY POINT

- Pregnancy is associated with an approximately five-fold increased risk for thromboembolism, with the highest risk for venous thromboembolism occurring in the first 6 weeks postpartum.

Prevention

Despite the increased risk for thrombosis associated with pregnancy, anticoagulation is not indicated for women at average risk in the antepartum or postpartum periods. However, prophylactic anticoagulation should be considered in select women with increased risk for VTE. Unfortunately, adequate data are not available to definitively determine which patients should receive anticoagulant prophylaxis or at what doses. Expert recommendations exist to help guide clinical decision making. Consultation with a thrombosis expert or maternal-fetal medicine specialist is suggested. In patients with a very high risk of VTE, prophylaxis should be started as soon as pregnancy is documented, because VTE risk is relatively evenly distributed throughout pregnancy. Because the postpartum period carries the highest VTE risk, women at high risk should also receive postpartum anticoagulation for 6 weeks.

Diagnosis

When symptoms and signs suggest new deep venous thrombosis, duplex compression ultrasonography of the extremity is the recommended initial diagnostic test. If results are normal or unclear, pelvic magnetic resonance venography may be appropriate. For suspected pulmonary embolism, Doppler ultrasonography of the legs should be performed whether leg symptoms are present or not. If ultrasonography is normal, chest radiography is the next test, followed by a ventilation-perfusion lung scan if normal. If chest radiography is abnormal, CT pulmonary arteriography is appropriate. D-dimer testing is not useful in pregnant women, because it is always positive and lacks predictive value.

Treatment

For pregnant women with acute VTE, full-dose, weight-adjusted, low-molecular-weight heparin (LMWH), rather than unfractionated heparin (UFH), is the treatment of choice.

CONT.

Anticoagulants should be continued for at least 6 weeks post-partum, for a minimum therapy duration of 3 months. It is unclear whether periodic anti-Xa level determination and LMWH dose adjustment based on the results is beneficial. In the final month of pregnancy, a switch from LMWH to UFH can be considered because of UFH's shorter half-life. This allows an epidural catheter for anesthesia to be placed when the activated partial thromboplastin time for UFH is normal, whereas a 24-hour period is necessary after the last LMWH dose before placing a catheter. In addition, UFH can be completely reversed with protamine if major bleeding occurs, whereas LMWH is only partially reversible. An alternative is continued LMWH and labor induction. Patients should stop LMWH at least 24 hours before epidural anesthesia. LMWH and warfarin are acceptable to take while breastfeeding but fondaparinux and the new oral anticoagulants are not. **H**

KEY POINTS

- During pregnancy, weight-based, low-molecular-weight heparin is the treatment of choice for venous thromboembolism.

- Anticoagulation therapy for venous thromboembolism should be continued for at least 6 weeks postpartum, for a therapy duration of at least 3 months.

Issues in Oncology

Introduction

Medical oncology is currently at a threshold between the old and the new. Conventional approaches to histologic diagnosis and clinical staging are being supplemented and sometimes replaced by molecular profiling. New treatment paradigms, including targeted therapy, immunotherapy, and the use of immunoconjugates, are emerging to supplant the long-standing treatment strategies of surgery, radiation therapy, and chemotherapy.

Although the primary site of the tumor and its histology may eventually be of secondary importance to the molecular characteristics of the tumor, clinical evaluation remains fundamental to the management of patients with cancer. Before patients can be treated, staging and an individualized clinical assessment must be done, and mutually determined goals of therapy must be established. Additionally, determining the goals of therapy requires an understanding of the unique terminology used in cancer care, particularly when interpreting the results of clinical trials and discussing with patients whether certain therapeutic options should be considered.

Staging

Once cancer is diagnosed, clinicians must order appropriate tests to identify disease extent. This workup constitutes staging. Although newer methods for describing the extent of disease exist and several tumor-specific systems are used (such

as for certain lymphomas and small cell lung cancer), most solid tumor malignancies are described using the "TNM" classification, in which "T" describes the primary tumor and is designated as T1-4, and the numerals increase with increasing tumor size or extent of local invasion; "N" represents the degree of locoregional lymph node involvement and is designated by N0-3, with N0 indicating no involvement and N1 or greater representing increasing lymph node involvement; and "M" represents the absence or presence of nodal metastasis and is designated by M0 or M1. Differing T, N, and M classifications may then be grouped into disease-specific stages (such as stage I or stage II) to characterize the extent of certain cancers in individual patients and potentially provide prognostic information and help guide appropriate therapy.

The patterns of disease spread as well as the selection of appropriate tests and imaging modalities vary depending on cancer type. Therefore, a proper cancer workup requires knowledge of the individual disease entity so that the necessary tests can be obtained. Tests with a very low yield should not be ordered in the absence of specific directing symptoms. For example, imaging is appropriate in the staging of patients with lung cancer because bone and brain metastases are common in the early course of this disease. However, patients with presumed locoregional colorectal cancer rarely present with bone and brain metastases; consequently, routine imaging as part of staging is not necessary. Thoughtfully performed staging is generally the most accurate prognostic indicator and largely dictates the therapeutic strategy for patients with cancer.

KEY POINTS

- Most solid tumor malignancies are staged according to the "TNM" classification, in which "T" reflects tumor size or extent of local invasion (T1-4); "N" represents the degree of locoregional lymph node involvement (N0-N3), and "M" represents the absence or presence of nodal metastasis (M0-M1).

- During staging of patients with cancer, tests with a very low yield should not be ordered in the absence of specific directing symptoms. **HVC**

Performance Status

A primary consideration in managing patients with cancer is an individual's performance status, which indicates a patient's well-being and ability to perform daily activities. Two measures of performance status are widely used: the Karnofsky score and the Zubrod score (also called the Eastern Cooperative Oncology Group/World Health Organization Performance Scale) (**Table 48**).

Patients with an excellent performance status typically have a better overall prognosis and the ability to tolerate more aggressive therapies compared with those with a poor performance status. Less toxic regimens or no chemotherapy may be warranted in patients with a poor performance status and in those for whom supportive, comfort-oriented care may be most appropriate. Patients who are otherwise medically well

TABLE 48. Oncology Performance Status Systems

ECOG/WHO Performance Scale[a]

| 0 - Fully active; no restrictions on activities |
| 1 - Unable to do strenuous activities, but able to carry out light housework and sedentary activities |
| 2 - Able to walk and manage self-care, but unable to work; out of bed more than 50% of waking hours |
| 3 - Confined to a bed or a chair more than 50% of waking hours; capable of limited self-care |
| 4 - Completely disabled. Totally confined to a bed or chair; unable to do any self-care |
| 5 - Death |

Karnofsky Performance Scale

| 100 - Normal; no symptoms or evidence of disease |
| 90 - Minor symptoms, but able to carry on normal activities |
| 80 - Some symptoms; normal activity requires effort |
| 70 - Unable to carry on normal activities, but able to care for self |
| 60 - Needs frequent care for most needs; some occasional assistance with self-care |
| 50 - Needs considerable assistance with self-care and frequent medical care |
| 40 - Disabled; needs special care and assistance |
| 30 - Severely disabled; hospitalized |
| 20 - Very ill; significant supportive care is needed |
| 10 - Actively dying |
| 0 - Death |

ECOG/WHO = Eastern Cooperative Oncology Group/World Health Organization.

[a]Also called the Zubrod Score.

but in whom a poor performance status score has acutely developed based on tumor-related symptoms and whose performance status would be expected to improve with tumor regression should be considered for aggressive therapy, with recognition of the higher risks involved.

Virtually all clinical oncology trials enroll only patients with good performance status. Therefore, the applicability of the results of these trials to patients with a poorer performance status is limited. Chronologic age is rarely, if ever, a major contraindication to aggressive therapy. Patients in their 80s who are otherwise healthy may be able to tolerate more aggressive therapy, whereas younger patients with multiple medical comorbidities, such as liver or kidney conditions that affect the ability to tolerate treatment, may be unable to receive aggressive therapy.

KEY POINTS

- The term *performance status* is used to indicate a patient's well-being and ability to perform daily activities.

HVC
- Less toxic regimens or no chemotherapy may be warranted in patients with cancer and a poor performance status and for whom supportive, comfort-oriented care may be most appropriate.

- Chronologic age is rarely, if ever, a major contraindication to aggressive cancer therapy.

Goals of Therapy

Establishing clear and realistic treatment goals is essential in the care of patients with cancer. When considering goals, it is important for physicians to discuss with patients that virtually all therapies are associated with risks and side effects. In medically fit patients with locoregional disease, cure is often the stated goal. As the cancer stage increases, the likelihood of cure becomes more remote. For most patients with unresectable, metastatic solid tumors, cure is not a realistic goal, and alternative goals need to be established. In patients who are unfit for aggressive therapy because of medical comorbidities and poor performance status, who have been intolerant to treatment, or who have experienced disease progression despite use of standard therapies, a focus on comfort-oriented management may be most appropriate. Acknowledging that a patient's disease is incurable often leads to appropriate and adequate use of analgesics and other comfort-oriented measures, whereas establishing unrealistic measures for outcomes may impede adequate symptom management. Goals of care other than cure may include lengthening of overall survival time, control of disease growth, amelioration or prevention of disease-related symptoms, and maintaining a level of quality of life acceptable to the patient. Clinicians should reassure patients who express fear of cancer-related pain that their pain will be controlled. Palliative care consultation is appropriate at any point in the treatment process to assist patients in establishing goals of care and help develop comprehensive management strategies.

HVC
- In patients with incurable cancer, acknowledging that disease is incurable often leads to appropriate and adequate use of analgesics and other comfort-oriented measures, whereas establishing unrealistic measures for outcomes may impede adequate symptom management.

Understanding Cancer Terminology

Several terms and concepts are important in understanding the potential benefits and harms of specific therapeutic interventions as they are commonly reported.

The *mitotic rate* is a measure of how fast cancer cells are dividing and growing. To find the mitotic rate, the pathologist determines the number of cancer cells that are in mitosis per mm^2 in a histologic section of the tumor. Mitotic rate is used to help find the stage of melanoma and other types of cancer. Higher mitotic rates are linked with lower survival rates.

The term *overall survival* refers to the time from initiation of therapy until death. This period is frequently quoted as the *median survival time* for a population of patients in a published study. Such medians are not necessarily applicable to any one individual as some patients may live considerably shorter and some considerably longer than the median survival time. Because it is difficult to extrapolate data from studies regarding overall or median survival, physicians should take care when discussing such information with their patients to avoid setting unrealistic expectations. In addition, it should be noted that as a result of increased screening and improved imaging techniques, primary cancer diagnoses and recurrences are being identified earlier in the course of the patient's disease. This "lead time bias" in more recent reports may make comparisons with older data problematic. Improvements in overall survival by a new treatment are thus best determined from randomized controlled trials and should not be inferred from comparisons with historical controls.

Progression-free survival, or more accurately, *progression-free interval*, refers to the time from initiation of therapy until the time therapy is no longer controlling tumor growth. This term is frequently misunderstood to indicate improved overall survival, just as improvements in overall survival are often misunderstood to indicate improvements in the cure rate.

An additional metric of clinical activity is the *overall response rate*, which refers to the percentage of patients involved in a clinical trial whose tumor undergoes a prespecified degree of shrinkage on imaging studies such as CT scan or MRI. Although tumor shrinkage is both encouraging and a clear indicator of an agent's antitumor activity, it does not tend to correlate well with long-term outcome such as overall survival, and its true benefit to the patient is not always clear. If, however, a patient is symptomatic due to tumor bulk, then shrinking of that tumor may provide good palliation of symptoms.

It is imperative that clinicians understand the practical meaning of these measures as they relate to various treatment options and are able to convey their significance to their patients to facilitate informed discussions and development of realistic treatment goals.

- The term *overall survival* refers to the time from initiation of therapy until death and is frequently quoted as the *median survival time* for a population of patients in a published study.
- *Progression-free survival*, or more accurately, *progression-free interval*, refers to the time from initiation of therapy until the time therapy is no longer controlling tumor growth and does not intrinsically indicate improved overall survival.
- *Overall response rate* refers to the percentage of patients involved in a clinical trial whose tumor undergoes a prespecified degree of shrinkage on imaging studies.

Treatment Approaches

Cancer treatments traditionally have comprised of local treatment for the primary tumor with either surgery or radiation therapy and systemic treatment with chemotherapy. New approaches based on molecular characteristics of the tumor, or personalized medicine, have recently been becoming part of clinical practice.

Traditional Cancer Therapies

The primary treatment of locoregional solid tumor malignancies is surgical resection. A general goal is usually resection of all known gross disease with clear surgical margins, which is potentially curative.

Following surgery, TNM classification, and staging, further therapeutic interventions may be warranted. Chemotherapy or radiation therapy is often used in conjunction with surgery to potentially increase the cure rate. When these therapies are given after definitive surgery with curative intent, they are referred to as *adjuvant* therapy, and when they are given before planned definitive surgery with curative intent, they are referred to as *neoadjuvant* therapy. Adjuvant or neoadjuvant chemotherapy or chemoradiotherapy is incorporated into management strategies for most solid tumors and is given for eradication of micrometastatic disease. Whether local or distant recurrence is more likely and whether radiation therapy, chemotherapy, or a combination of the two is most appropriate depends on the tumor type.

Unfortunately, adequate technology to accurately identify which patients will truly benefit from adjuvant or neoadjuvant therapies does not yet exist, although progress has been made in this area. For example, *predictive assays* are highly desirable as they can identify who is at risk for recurrence and who will benefit from treatment. In breast cancer, a commercially available assay analyzes 21 genes within an individual tumor to demonstrate the patient's likelihood for recurrence and benefit from adjuvant chemotherapy; a value of less than 18 indicates a low recurrence score (RS), a value of 18 to 30 indicates an intermediate RS, and a value of greater than 30 indicates a high RS. This tool is useful in discriminating between patients who should or should not receive treatment, and, as such, is a predictive test. However, similar assays in patients with colorectal cancer have been unable to discriminate between which patients will or will not benefit from therapy despite identifying which patients are at higher risk for recurrence; these are called *prognostic assays*. Although prognostic assays may lead to increased emotional comfort in patients and clinicians, they add expense and do not provide information that is useful in therapeutic decision making.

For a small number of cancers, *conversion therapy* may be administered before surgery in patients with surgically unresectable disease that might become resectable with a favorable response to chemotherapy, radiation, or both. This therapy is intended to shrink visible metastatic disease away from critical vascular structures to facilitate resection. The incidence of truly unresectable disease converted to resectable disease is, unfortunately, relatively low.

KEY POINTS

- The primary treatment for locoregional solid tumor malignancies is surgical resection, which is often combined with chemotherapy or radiation to potentially increase the cure rate.

- Adjuvant therapy is given after and neoadjuvant therapy is given before definitive surgery with curative intent to eradicate micrometastatic disease in patients with cancer.

- *Predictive assays* can identify who is at risk for cancer recurrence and who will benefit from treatment, whereas *prognostic assays* can identify who is at risk for recurrence but not who will benefit from treatment.

Personalized Medicine

Traditional cancer chemotherapy has involved cytotoxic agents with minimal selectivity for tumor cells over normal cells. More recently, increased understanding of tumor growth and survival mechanisms has led to development of the so-called targeted agents. These agents are designed to have more selective toxicity on tumor cells based on specific tumor biology; however, many still confer substantial toxicities, the risk for which should not be understated in therapeutic decisions.

The goal of personalized medicine is to direct therapeutic approaches that are optimally beneficial to an individual patient through a better understanding of the molecular makeup of the individual and the tumor. One aspect of personalized medicine is identification of specific tumor markers that can help clinicians decide whether to include or exclude certain therapies in individual patients. For example, the anti–epidermal growth factor receptor monoclonal antibodies cetuximab and panitumumab are active against metastatic colorectal cancer, but only in patients whose tumors do not have mutations in the K-*ras* or N-*ras* genes. Performing genotypic analysis of all patients with metastatic colorectal tumors to exclude use of these agents in patients with colorectal cancer in whom *ras* mutations have been identified (50% of all patients with colorectal cancer) has become standard practice. Identification of this *exclusionary* marker does not make available any new treatment options to patients with colorectal cancer because these therapies were available before the utility of *ras* genotyping was understood; however, identification of the *ras* mutations in these patients will preclude the use of agents that will not be beneficial and may even cause unnecessary harm, toxicity, and expense.

Conversely, approximately 20% to 25% of breast cancer tumors and a similar percentage of gastroesophageal tumors demonstrate *HER2* growth factor receptor overexpression on the cell surface. Although *HER2* overexpression has been identified as a poor prognostic factor, the development of the anti-*HER2* therapies, such as the monoclonal antibody trastuzumab, has led to availability of specific therapies that are used only against tumors with demonstrated *HER2* overexpression. Thus, the presence of *HER2* constitutes an *inclusionary* marker that has made available a previously unavailable therapeutic strategy.

Other examples include the use of the tyrosine kinase inhibitor imatinib against a growth factor–activating mutation in gastrointestinal stromal tumors; the small molecule inhibitor vemurafenib that acts against a mutation in the *BRAF* gene, which is present in 40% of patients with melanoma; and erlotinib, another tyrosine kinase inhibitor active against an activating mutation present in some patients with non–small cell lung cancer. In these scenarios, pretesting for the presence of tumor mutations dictates appropriate therapy.

Other technologies are evolving. Antibodies that target overexpression of specific factors on tumor cells are being conjugated to radiotherapeutic agents or toxins; these agents have demonstrated clinical activity and are routinely used to treat many malignancies. Active immunotherapeutic strategies have also been developed over the past several years, including the monoclonal antibody ipilimumab, which has demonstrated benefit in patients with metastatic melanoma by blocking innate immune regulatory mechanisms and allowing the immune system to more effectively attack tumors. Development of other immunostimulatory strategies is currently in progress and appears promising.

KEY POINT

- The goal of personalized medicine is to direct therapeutic approaches that are optimally beneficial to an individual patient through a better understanding of the molecular makeup of the individual and the tumor.

Breast Cancer

Introduction

In the United States, breast cancer is the most common cancer among women, excluding skin cancer, and is the second leading cause of cancer-related death in women, exceeded only by lung cancer. The lifetime risk of developing invasive breast cancer is about one in eight. In 2013, approximately 232,340 new cases of invasive breast cancer; 64,640 new cases of ductal carcinoma in situ; and 39,620 breast cancer–related deaths were estimated to have occurred. Breast cancer incidence in men is less than 1% that of women.

Epidemiology and Risk Factors

Breast cancer incidence increases with age. Ninety-five percent of new cases occur in women aged 40 years or older, with a median age at diagnosis of 61 years. Breast cancer incidence rates in the United States are highest in non-Hispanic white women and second highest in black women. Other risk factors for breast cancer are listed in **Table 49**.

Women with a strong family history of breast cancer should be referred to a qualified genetic counselor for possible genetic testing for breast cancer susceptibility genes such as *BRCA1* and *BRCA2*. The most common features suggestive of a familial breast cancer syndrome are detailed in the highlights of the National Comprehensive Cancer Network guidelines in **Table 50** on page 76. The United States Preventive Services Task Force guidelines for *BRCA1/2* testing are listed in **Table 51** on page 76.

KEY POINTS

- Breast cancer incidence increases with age, with 95% of cases developing in women older than 40 years, and incidence is highest in non-Hispanic white women and second highest in black women.

- Women with a strong family history of breast cancer should be referred to a qualified genetic counselor for possible genetic testing for breast cancer susceptibility genes such as *BRCA1/2*.

Chemoprevention and Other Risk Reduction Strategies

Breast cancer screening is discussed in MKSAP 17 General Internal Medicine.

The Gail Model Risk Assessment Tool (www.cancer.gov/bcrisktool/) can be used to estimate any woman's 5-year and lifetime breast cancer risk. Women older than 35 years with a 5-year breast cancer risk of 1.7% or higher or with lobular carcinoma in situ are candidates for breast cancer prophylaxis with antiestrogen treatments such as tamoxifen prior to menopause and, in addition, raloxifene or exemestane after menopause (**Table 52**, on page 77). Atypical ductal hyperplasia is associated with a high risk of breast cancer independent of the Gail Model risk.

The American Cancer Society (ACS) recommends screening certain high-risk women with breast MRI and annual mammography. These recommendations are listed in **Table 53** on page 77.

Women with *BRCA1/2* mutations should undergo breast cancer screening with MRI beginning at age 25 years and mammography beginning at age 30 years. Ovarian cancer screening with semiannual pelvic examinations, pelvic ultrasonography, and serum CA-125 measurement should begin at age 30 years. However, the effectiveness of ovarian cancer screening is not known, and surgical prophylaxis as detailed below is strongly recommended for *BRCA1/2* mutation carriers. Ovarian cancer screening is not recommended in women at average risk of ovarian cancer.

In women who are *BRCA1/2* carriers with one prior diagnosis of breast cancer, tamoxifen decreases the risk of contralateral breast cancer by 40% to 60%. Surgical prophylaxis options for carriers of *BRCA1/2* mutations include prophylactic bilateral mastectomy, which decreases the risk of breast cancer by greater than 90%, and prophylactic bilateral salpingo-oophorectomy (BSO), which decreases the risk of ovarian cancer by 80%, whether done before or after menopause. If done before menopause, prophylactic BSO also decreases the risk of breast cancer by 50%. Prophylactic BSO is recommended in women who carry deleterious *BRCA1/2* mutations between ages 35 and 40 years, once childbearing is complete. A recent registry study recommends risk-reducing BSO by age 35 years in women with *BRCA1* mutations because of a 4% risk of ovarian cancer between ages 35 and 40 years. Women with *BRCA2* mutations in this study did not develop ovarian cancer until after age 40 years.

KEY POINTS

- Women older than 35 years with a 5-year breast cancer risk of 1.7% or higher or with lobular carcinoma in situ or atypical ductal hyperplasia are candidates for breast cancer prophylaxis with tamoxifen prior to menopause and with tamoxifen, raloxifene, or exemestane after menopause.

- Women with *BRCA1/2* mutations should undergo breast cancer screening with MRI beginning at age 25 years and mammography beginning at age 30 years.

- Surgical prophylaxis options for *BRCA1/2* mutation carriers include prophylactic bilateral mastectomy (90% decreased risk of breast cancer) and prophylactic bilateral salpingo-oophorectomy (80% decreased risk of ovarian cancer).

TABLE 49. Breast Cancer Risk Factors

Breast Cancer Risk Factor Category	Breast Cancer Risk Factors	Increase in Breast Cancer Risk or Lifetime Breast Cancer Risk
Reproductive factors	Early menarche, late menopause, first full-term pregnancy after age 30 years, or nulliparous	RR 1.2-3.5
Lifestyle	Obesity (BMI ≥30), lack of regular exercise, vitamin D deficiency, alcohol intake	RR 1.2-1.6 Obesity: RR 1.6 for BMI >30.7 versus BMI <22.9 in postmenopausal women[a] Regular exercise: RR decreased by 25% in physically active women compared with the least active women[b] Vitamin D deficiency: Postmenopausal breast cancer risk decreased by 12% for each 5 ng/mL (12.5 nmol/L) increase in 25(OH)D levels between 27 and 35 ng/mL[c] (67.4 and 87.4 nmol/L) Alcohol: mildly increased risk (RR 1.05) with 2 to 3 drinks per week. RR 1.41 for women consuming 2 to 5 drinks per day[d]
Treatment related: radiation	Prior chest wall radiation in patients younger than age 30 years (e.g., mantle radiation for Hodgkin lymphoma)	RR 5.0, with highest risk for younger age at radiation therapy; risk remains increased for at least 40 years after radiation therapy, with 30% to 50% lifetime risk of breast cancer[e]
Treatment related: HRT	Combination estrogen and progesterone HRT after menopause	RR 1.2-1.4; increased risk begins after 3 years of therapy[a]
Breast density[f]	Increased breast density	Risk increases with each category of breast density; for ≥75% density, RR is 4.7 compared with <10% density[g]
Atypical breast lesions	Atypical ductal or lobular hyperplasia, LCIS	RR 3.8-5.3 for atypical hyperplasia[h] and RR 5.4-8.0 for LCIS[i]; 30% to 35% lifetime risk of breast cancer (bilateral risk)[h,i]
Family history of breast cancer and familial breast cancer syndromes	*BRCA1/2* mutation represents the most common familial breast cancer syndrome (5% to 10% of all breast cancer tumors); others are rare	*BRCA1/2* mutations (RR 3.0 to 7.0) confer a 50% to 87% lifetime risk of breast cancer and a 20% to 45% lifetime risk of ovarian cancer

25(OH)D = 25-hydroxyvitamin D; HRT = hormone replacement therapy; LCIS = lobular carcinoma in situ; RR = relative risk.

[a]Data from Clemons M, Goss P. Estrogen and the risk of breast cancer. N Engl J Med. 2001 Jan 25;344 (4):276-85. Erratum in: N Engl J Med. 2001 Jun 7;344(23):1804. [PMID: 11172156]

[b]Data from Lynch BM, Neilson HK, Friedenreich CM. Physical activity and breast cancer prevention. Recent Results Cancer Res. 2011;186:13-42. [PMID: 21113759]

[c]Data from Bauer SR, Hankinson SE, Bertone-Johnson ER, Ding EL. Plasma vitamin D levels, menopause, and risk of breast cancer: dose-response meta-analysis of prospective studies. Medicine (Baltimore). 2013 May;92(3):123-31. [PMID: 23625163]

[d]Data from Bagnardi V, Rota M, Botteri E, et al. Light alcohol drinking and cancer: a meta-analysis. Ann Oncol. 2013 Feb;24(2):301-8. [PMID: 22910838] and Smith-Warner SA, Spiegelman D, Yaun SS, et al. Alcohol and breast cancer in women: a pooled analysis of cohort studies. JAMA. 1998 Feb 18;279(7):535-40. [PMID: 9480365]

[e]Data from Swerdlow AJ, Cooke R, Bates A, et al. Breast cancer risk after supradiaphragmatic radiotherapy for Hodgkin's lymphoma in England and Wales: a National Cohort Study. J Clin Oncol. 2012 Aug 1;30(22):2745-52. [PMID: 22734026]

[f]Breast density refers to the amount of radiologically dense breast tissue appearing on a mammogram.

[g]Data from Boyd NF, Guo H, Martin LJ, et al. Mammographic density and the risk and detection of breast cancer. N Engl J Med. 2007 Jan 18;356(3):227-36. [PMID: 17229950]

[h]Data from Degnim AC, Visscher DW, Berman HK, et al. Stratification of breast cancer risk in women with atypia: a Mayo cohort study. J Clin Oncol. 2007 Jul 1;25(19):2671-7. [PMID: 17563394] and Marshall LM, Hunter DJ, Connolly JL, et al. Risk of breast cancer associated with atypical hyperplasia of lobular and ductal types. Cancer Epidemiol Biomarkers Prev. 1997 May;6(5):297-301. [PMID: 9149887]

[i]Data from Bodian CA, Perzin KH, Lattes R. Lobular neoplasia. Long term risk of breast cancer and relation to other factors. Cancer. 1996 Sep 1;78(5):1024-34. [PMID: 8780540]

TABLE 50.	Highlights of NCCN Criteria for Breast and/or Ovarian Cancer Syndrome Genetic Testing[a]
Individual with a family history of a known deleterious *BRCA1/2* mutation
Individual with breast cancer diagnosed before age 45 years
Individual with breast cancer diagnosed before age 50 years if family history includes very few female first- or second-degree relatives or if one relative is diagnosed with breast cancer at any age
Individual with breast cancer diagnosed at any age if one or more relatives is diagnosed with epithelial ovarian cancer
Breast cancer in women of Ashkenazi (Eastern European) Jewish ancestry
Men with breast cancer diagnosed at any age
Individual with more than three family members[b] with breast cancer, ovarian cancer, pancreatic cancer, and/or aggressive prostate cancer
Individual with triple-negative breast cancer[c] diagnosed before age 60 years
Individual with epithelial ovarian cancer diagnosed at any age

BCRA1/2 = breast cancer susceptibility 1 or breast cancer susceptibility 2 genes; NCCN = National Comprehensive Cancer Network.

[a]Full testing guidelines can be accessed at www.nccn.org/professionals/physician_gls/f_guidelines.asp.

[b]First-, second-, or third-degree relatives.

[c]Negative for estrogen receptors, progesterone receptors, and *HER2* amplification.

TABLE 51.	U.S. Preventive Services Task Force Recommendations[a] for Breast and/or Ovarian Cancer Syndrome Genetic Testing[b]
Women of Non–Ashkenazi Jewish Heritage:
Two first-degree relatives with breast cancer, one of whom received the diagnosis at age 50 years or younger
A combination of three or more first- or second-degree relatives with breast cancer regardless of age at diagnosis
A combination of both breast and ovarian cancer among first- and second-degree relatives
A first-degree relative with bilateral breast cancer
A combination of two or more first- or second-degree relatives with ovarian cancer regardless of age at diagnosis
A first- or second-degree relative with both breast and ovarian cancer at any age
A history of breast cancer in a male relative
Women of Ashkenazi Jewish Heritage:
Any first-degree relative (or two second-degree relatives on the same side of the family) with breast or ovarian cancer

[a]Full testing recommendations can be accessed at: www.uspreventiveservicestaskforce.org/Page/Document/RecommendationStatementFinal/brca-related-cancer-risk-assessment-genetic-counseling-and-genetic-testing.

[b]Applies to patients without a personal history of breast or ovarian cancer and without a known deleterious breast cancer susceptibility gene 1 (*BRCA1*) or breast cancer susceptibility gene 2 (*BRCA2*) mutation present in their family. Both maternal and paternal family histories are important.

Staging and Prognosis of Early-Stage Breast Cancer

Breast cancer staging and prognosis is detailed in **Table 54**.

Stage I and II disease are classified as early breast cancer. According to the American Society of Clinical Oncology guidelines, imaging studies to identify occult metastatic disease are not needed for staging of early breast cancer unless worrisome signs or symptoms are present. The risk of distant metastases at diagnosis in these patients is very low. Clinical features associated with a more favorable prognosis include hormone receptor–positive cancer, small tumor size, low tumor grade, negative lymph nodes, and lack of *HER2* overexpression or extensive lymphovascular invasion. Based on these clinical characteristics, the benefit of adjuvant therapy in terms of recurrence and survival can be estimated using risk calculators such as www.adjuvantonline.com.

Women with hormone receptor–positive breast cancer (about 75% of cases) respond to antiestrogen therapy and have the best prognosis. *HER2* overexpression or gene amplification is present in approximately 20% of patients with breast cancer and predicts response to anti-*HER2* agents. Tumors negative for estrogen receptor, progesterone receptor, and *HER2* overexpression are called triple-negative tumors and are a particularly aggressive subtype.

TABLE 52. Chemoprophylaxis Agents for Breast Cancer Risk Reduction

Considerations	Medications		
	Tamoxifen	**Raloxifene**	**Exemestane**
Mechanism of action	SERM	SERM	Aromatase inhibitor: prevents conversion of androgens to estrogens
Dose (all are 5 years in duration)	20 mg/d orally	60 mg/d orally	25 mg/d orally
Breast cancer risk reduction	49%	Less effective than tamoxifen: retains 76% of the effectiveness of tamoxifen	65%
Important toxicities	Vasomotor symptoms, cataracts, vascular events (stroke, TIA, DVT and PE), and endometrial cancer and uterine sarcoma in postmenopausal women	Vasomotor symptoms, cataracts, vascular events (25% lower risk of vascular events than tamoxifen)	Vasomotor symptoms, arthralgia, headaches, and insomnia
Indicated for use in premenopausal women	Yes	Not studied; should not be used unless part of a clinical trial	Not effective in premenopausal women
Other	Contraindicated in women with prior thromboembolic events	Contraindicated in women with prior thromboembolic events	At 3-year follow-up, no increase in osteoporosis, fractures, endometrial cancer, vascular events, or cardiac disease

DVT = deep venous thrombosis; PE = pulmonary embolism; SERM = selective estrogen receptor modulator; TIA = transient ischemic attack.

TABLE 53. American Cancer Society Recommendations for MRI Breast Cancer Screening

Women with *BRCA1/2* mutations

Women who are a first-degree relative of a *BRCA1/2* carrier, but are untested[a]

Women with a strong family history of breast cancer with a lifetime breast cancer risk of ≥20% to 25% as calculated by models[b] largely dependent on family history

Women who had radiation to the chest wall between ages 10 and 30 years (e.g., mantle radiation therapy for Hodgkin lymphoma)

Women with a history of other rare familial breast cancer syndromes

BRCA1/2 – breast cancer susceptibility 1 or breast cancer susceptibility 2 genes.

[a]Testing for the *BRCA1* or *BRCA2* mutation that is present in the family is strongly recommended, but some patients decide to defer testing. In this situation where their carrier status is unknown, breast MRI screening is recommended. If they are later tested and do not carry the mutation, MRI screening should be stopped.

[b]Models that can be used to estimate lifetime risk of breast cancer to determine if MRI screening is appropriate (please note that the Gail Model is not recommended for this use):

- BRCAPRO: www4.utsouthwestern.edu/breasthealth/cagene/default.asp
- Claus model: Claus EB, Risch N, Thompson WD. The calculation of breast cancer risk for women with a first degree family history of ovarian cancer. Breast Cancer Res Treat. 1993 Nov;28(2):115-20. [PMID: 8173064]
- Tyrer-Cuzick (also called IBIS Breast Cancer Risk Evaluation Tool): www.ems-trials.org/riskevaluator

---

TABLE 54. Breast Cancer Stage and Survival

Stage	Tumor Size and Nodes	5-Year Relative Survival
I	≤2 cm, negative lymph nodes	95%
IIA	≤2 cm if 1 to 3 positive lymph nodes; 2.1-5 cm if negative lymph nodes	85%
IIB	2.1-5 cm with 1 to 3 positive lymph nodes; or >5 cm tumor with negative lymph nodes	70%
III	Any tumor size with ≥4 positive axillary lymph nodes; positive infraclavicular or supraclavicular nodes, and/or positive ipsilateral internal mammary nodes (clinically detected, or on sentinel node biopsy if ≥4 positive axillary nodes); tumors >5 cm with ≥1 positive nodes; or tumor extension to chest wall or skin	52%
IV	Distant metastases	18%

- Clinical features associated with a more favorable prognosis of early-stage breast cancer include hormone receptor–positive cancer, small tumor size, low tumor grade, and negative lymph nodes.

HVC
- Imaging studies to identify occult metastatic disease are not needed in patients with stage I and II breast cancer unless worrisome symptoms or the following poor prognostic features are present: hormone receptor-negative cancer, *HER2* overexpression, large tumor size, high tumor grade, positive lymph nodes, and the presence of extensive lymphovascular invasion.

Primary Breast Cancer Therapy

Ductal Carcinoma in Situ

Ductal carcinoma in situ (DCIS), classified as stage 0 breast cancer, usually presents as calcifications on mammography but can occasionally present as a palpable mass.

Given that DCIS is a cancer that is not life-threatening while it remains noninvasive, whether DCIS is being overdiagnosed and overtreated in many women is controversial. The ultimate goal would be to identify, potentially through molecular techniques, the patients in whom risk of progressing to invasive cancer is low enough that they could safely be monitored and forego surgical and radiation treatment (see Issues in Oncology). However, currently, it is not possible to accurately determine which patients are at such minimal risk.

The goal of treatment of DCIS is to prevent progression to invasive cancer. Excision alone without radiation is associated with a 30% risk of local recurrence at 10 years, with half of these recurrences consisting of invasive cancers. Risk factors for recurrence include young age, high tumor grade, the presence of comedo-type necrosis (necrosis in the center of the involved spaces), margin width, and tumor size.

DCIS can be treated with breast-conserving therapy, which consists of wide excision (lumpectomy) followed by breast radiation, or mastectomy. Mastectomy may be necessary if the DCIS is more extensive or if clear margins cannot be obtained by a wide excision. Sentinel lymph node biopsy is recommended if there is microinvasion (≤1 mm foci of invasion) or if a mastectomy is done in those in whom invasion is found on final pathologic results.

Approximately 80% of DCIS is estrogen receptor positive. In patients with estrogen receptor–positive DCIS, adjuvant tamoxifen decreases the risk of local recurrence of both DCIS and invasive cancer by 20% to 25% and of contralateral breast cancer by 50%. Because tamoxifen in DCIS confers no apparent benefit for survival, a discussion about treatment decisions should focus on potential toxicities and patients' needs and preferences. With treatment, patients with DCIS have a 15-year cause-specific survival rate of 97%.

- Ductal carcinoma in situ (DCIS) can be treated with breast-conserving therapy or mastectomy if the disease is more extensive or if clear margins cannot be obtained by a wide excision.

- In patients with estrogen receptor–positive DCIS, adjuvant tamoxifen decreases the risk of local recurrence of both DCIS and invasive cancer by 20% to 25% and of contralateral breast cancer by 50%, but it does not confer a survival advantage.

Invasive Breast Cancer

Breast-conserving therapy (wide excision followed by breast radiation) and mastectomy are the two surgical options used to treat invasive breast cancer. Breast-conserving therapy is an effective option in patients with tumors measuring 5 cm or less involving a single quadrant of the breast and with clear margins after excision. Mastectomy is recommended for tumors involving the skin, chest wall, or more than one quadrant of the breast, and for inflammatory breast cancer. Patients with tumors measuring 5 cm or greater who would otherwise be candidates for breast-conserving therapy may receive chemotherapy or antiestrogen treatment before surgery to decrease tumor size to facilitate breast conservation. Mastectomy may be appropriate for patients in whom radiation is contraindicated and is an option for women with familial breast cancer syndromes (including *BRCA1/2* mutations) owing to the increased risk of subsequent ipsilateral and contralateral breast cancers.

At the time of definitive breast surgery, lymph nodes in the ipsilateral axilla are routinely sampled to complete breast cancer staging and guide treatment decisions. In patients with no palpable lymph nodes and no abnormal nodes seen on ultrasound (if an ultrasound is done), a sentinel lymph node biopsy is usually done. The sentinel lymph node procedure uses radioactive colloid and/or blue dye injected near the area of the tumor or in the subareolar area to identify and then remove the lymph node or a few lymph nodes to which breast cancer would initially spread. If the sentinel lymph node biopsy is negative, or if there are less than three positive sentinel nodes in a woman who is to receive whole breast radiation and adjuvant therapy, axillary lymph node dissection is not required. In patients with clinically involved lymph nodes or with three or more involved sentinel lymph nodes, axillary lymph node dissection is done to remove additional lymph nodes. The sentinel lymph node procedure is associated with a much lower risk of lymphedema, sensory loss, and shoulder abduction defects than is axillary lymph node dissection.

Primary breast radiation usually consists of whole breast radiation with a boost given to the lumpectomy bed. Chest wall radiation after mastectomy is recommended in patients with tumors measuring greater than 5 cm, positive tumor margins, skin or chest wall involvement, inflammatory breast cancer, or four or more positive axillary lymph nodes. Depending on other risk factors, it may be recommended in women with one to three positive axillary lymph nodes. Postmastectomy radiation in these patients decreases the risk for local recurrence and systemic metastases.

For women aged 70 years and older with tumors measuring less than 2 cm, no clinically involved lymph nodes, and estrogen receptor–positive breast cancer, wide excision without sentinel lymph node biopsy or whole breast radiation followed by antiestrogen therapy alone is an acceptable treatment option. Whole breast radiation in this setting does decrease the risk for local recurrence, but does not increase breast cancer–specific or overall survival.

Men with breast cancer have the same surgical options as women; however, owing to smaller breast size and more frequent involvement of the areola, many men are not candidates for breast-conserving therapy, and most are treated with mastectomy. Sentinel lymph node sampling is appropriate in men with clinically lymph node–negative breast cancer, and the indications for postmastectomy radiation are the same for men as for women with breast cancer.

KEY POINTS

- Breast-conserving therapy is effective for patients with invasive breast cancer with tumors 5 cm or less involving a single quadrant of the breast and clear margins after excision.

- Mastectomy is recommended for patients with invasive breast cancer with tumors involving the skin, chest wall, or more than one quadrant of the breast and for inflammatory breast cancer.

- Chest wall radiation therapy after mastectomy is recommended in patients with invasive breast cancer with tumors greater than 5 cm, positive tumor margins, skin or chest wall involvement, inflammatory breast cancer, and for many patients with any positive axillary lymph nodes.

Adjuvant Systemic Therapy for Nonmetastatic Breast Cancer

Adjuvant systemic therapy is used to eradicate occult microscopic foci of breast cancer to prevent or delay systemic recurrence for stages I to III breast cancer, stages in which the cancer is not metastatic and is potentially curable. The type of adjuvant therapy recommended depends on tumor characteristics such as stage and tumor biology as well as patient status and preferences.

Adjuvant Endocrine Therapy

Most patients with hormone receptor–positive breast cancer receive adjuvant antiestrogen therapy which includes aromatase inhibitors, tamoxifen, and ovarian suppression in premenopausal women. Hormonal therapies reduce the overall risk of local and distant recurrence by 40% to 50% and the risk of contralateral cancer by 50% to 65%.

For premenopausal women, tamoxifen, a selective estrogen receptor modulator, is routinely recommended. Recent results from two large international studies, the ATLAS (Adjuvant Tamoxifen: Longer Against Shorter) and aTTom (Adjuvant Tamoxifen Treatment Offers More) trials, are showing superior results with 10 rather than 5 years of tamoxifen adjuvant therapy, changing the standard of care for premenopausal women. Premenopausal women who previously completed 5 years of tamoxifen also benefit further from taking an aromatase inhibitor for 5 years once they become postmenopausal. Ovarian ablation or suppression decreases the risk of breast cancer recurrence by 25% and is sometimes used in premenopausal women with contraindications to tamoxifen. Clinical trials are investigating whether ovarian suppression may provide additional benefit to patients receiving adjuvant antiestrogen therapy and/or chemotherapy.

For women who are postmenopausal at breast cancer diagnosis or who become postmenopausal after the first 2 to 3 years of tamoxifen therapy, treatment should include an aromatase inhibitor. A meta-analysis of postmenopausal women with early breast cancer who took adjuvant tamoxifen for 5 years or an adjuvant aromatase inhibitor for 5 years reported a decreased rate of breast cancer recurrence (12% versus 15% at 5 years, rate ratio 0.77) in the aromatase inhibitor arm. Current antiestrogen adjuvant therapy options for postmenopausal women include 2 years of tamoxifen therapy followed by 3 to 5 years of an aromatase inhibitor, or 5 years of an aromatase inhibitor. Women who cannot tolerate more than 2 to 3 years of an aromatase inhibitor can switch to tamoxifen to complete 5 years of antiestrogen therapy.

The three approved aromatase inhibitors, anastrazole, letrozole, and exemestane, have comparable efficacy. Aromatase inhibitors prevent peripheral conversion of androgens to estrogens in postmenopausal women. They should not be used in premenopausal women as they are inactive in women with intact ovarian function. The main side effects of aromatase inhibitors are arthralgia and bone pain; vaginal dryness; sexual dysfunction; and higher risks of osteoporosis, fractures, cardiovascular risk, and hyperlipidemia. Compared with tamoxifen, the aromatase inhibitors confer a lower risk of venous thrombosis and endometrial cancer. Patients taking aromatase inhibitors should have their bone density monitored, and if the T score falls below -2.5, bisphosphonate treatment can be initiated.

Tamoxifen increases the risk of endometrial cancer and venous thromboembolic events in women over age 55 years. Other toxicities include hot flushes, vaginal discharge, and sexual dysfunction. Yearly pelvic examinations are recommended, and abnormal vaginal bleeding should be reported to their physicians.

Men with hormone receptor–positive breast cancer (85% of male breast cancers) are treated adjuvantly with tamoxifen. Data supporting the use of aromatase inhibitors in men are insufficient.

- In women with hormone receptor–positive breast cancer, antiestrogen therapy reduces the overall risk of local and distant recurrence by 40% to 50% and the risk of contralateral breast cancer by 50% to 65%.

- Women with hormone receptor–positive breast cancer experienced superior benefit when they took adjuvant tamoxifen for 10, rather than 5, years.

- Treatment of women who are postmenopausal at breast cancer diagnosis or who become postmenopausal after the first 2 to 3 years of tamoxifen therapy should include an aromatase inhibitor.

Adjuvant Chemotherapy

Adjuvant chemotherapy is usually recommended for patients with high-risk breast cancer features, such as hormone receptor–negative status, HER2 amplification, high-grade tumor, extensive lymphovascular invasion, and positive lymph nodes. For all women with hormone receptor–positive and lymph node–negative cancer and for postmenopausal women with one to three positive lymph nodes, commercially available molecular prognostic profiles can help determine the benefit of adjuvant chemotherapy. The most commonly used molecular prognostic profile in the United States is the 21-gene recurrence score (see Issues in Oncology).

Patients with hormone receptor–negative breast cancer generally have a greater benefit from adjuvant chemotherapy, with a proportional reduction in risk of recurrence and breast cancer–related death of more than 50% compared with a risk reduction of 25% in patients with hormone receptor–positive breast cancer. The decision to use adjuvant chemotherapy is individualized to the patient and involves assessment of the degree of benefit in decreasing risk of distant recurrence, potential toxicities, comorbidities, and patient preferences.

Adjuvant chemotherapy usually consists of two or three agents given sequentially or concurrently for 3 to 6 months. Commonly used agents include the anthracyclines (doxorubicin or epirubicin), cyclophosphamide, and the taxanes (paclitaxel or docetaxel). Common side effects of these regimens include bone marrow suppression with anemia and neutropenia, alopecia, hypersensitivity reactions, neuropathy, nausea, and premature menopause and infertility when given to premenopausal women (see Effects of Cancer Therapy and Survivorship). Rare but serious toxicities include cardiomyopathy from anthracyclines, interstitial pneumonitis from cyclophosphamide or the taxanes, and myelodysplasia and acute leukemia from the anthracyclines and/or cyclophosphamide. The risk of cardiomyopathy after four cycles of anthracycline therapy is

1.5%. The risk of acute leukemia after regimens with cyclophosphamide and doxorubicin is 0.5%.

For women with HER2-positive breast tumors measuring 0.5 cm or larger and/or positive lymph nodes, adjuvant chemotherapy combined with trastuzumab is recommended. Trastuzumab is a monoclonal antibody directed against the HER2 receptor. When added to adjuvant chemotherapy, trastuzumab decreases the risk of breast cancer recurrence by 53% and the risk of breast cancer–related death by 34%. Adjuvant trastuzumab is given for 1 year. Trastuzumab toxicities include infusion reactions and cardiomyopathy. The risk of cardiomyopathy is higher in patients receiving anthracycline-containing regimens (2% to 4%) compared with non–anthracycline-containing regimens (0.4%) and is higher in older women or those with preexisting cardiac risk factors. Cardiac function should be evaluated at baseline with echocardiography or multigated acquisition scan and every 3 months during adjuvant trastuzumab therapy (see Effects of Cancer Therapy and Survivorship). Other anti-HER2 agents are being studied in adjuvant clinical trials.

Nearly half of all breast cancers are diagnosed in women older than age 65 years, yet many adjuvant chemotherapy trials have not included older women owing to comorbidities or upper-age-limit eligibility. Consequently, evidence-based guidelines for women in this age group are lacking. Studies support treating healthy older women the same as younger women with early-stage breast cancer. Older women have a higher risk for cardiotoxicity, which should be considered when clinicians formulate treatment recommendations.

The indications for adjuvant chemotherapy in men with breast cancer and the regimens used are the same as those for women with early-stage breast cancer.

- Patients with hormone receptor–negative breast cancer generally have a greater benefit from adjuvant chemotherapy, with a proportional reduction in risk of recurrence compared with patients with hormone receptor–positive breast cancer.

- Patients with HER2-positive breast tumors measuring 0.5 cm, or larger and/or positive lymph nodes, should receive a combination of adjuvant chemotherapy and trastuzumab; the addition of trastuzumab decreases the risk of breast cancer recurrence by 53% and the risk of breast cancer–related death by 34%.

Locally Advanced and Inflammatory Breast Cancer

Locally advanced breast cancer (stages IIIA-IIIC) is characterized by tumors measuring greater than 5 cm with lymph node involvement, skin or chest wall involvement, and/or extensive axillary lymph node involvement. This type of cancer is treated with initial chemotherapy (neoadjuvant chemotherapy), followed by surgery, and then radiation. Patients with tumors measuring greater than 5 cm without other locally advanced features such as skin or chest wall involvement can often have breast-conserving surgery after chemotherapy. Tumors with chest wall or skin invasion (T4 cancers) require mastectomy after chemotherapy; surgical staging of the axilla is also required. Postmastectomy or postlumpectomy radiation is recommended for these locally advanced breast cancers, which often also require radiation of draining lymph nodes. Locally advanced cancer is associated with a high risk of distant and local recurrence.

Inflammatory breast cancer is an aggressive and rapidly progressive type of cancer characterized by erythema and edema of the skin of the breast called "peau d'orange" for its resemblance to the skin of an orange (**Figure 15**).

In the United States, inflammatory breast cancer constitutes 1% to 2% of cases of breast cancer. The inflammatory appearance mimicking mastitis is caused by tumor emboli in the dermal lymphatics, which are often seen on skin biopsy but are not required for the diagnosis; an underlying breast mass may also be palpable. The diagnosis is established based on the clinical appearance of the breast. Tumors of inflammatory breast cancer are usually high grade, most are hormone receptor negative, and many have *HER2* amplification. At diagnosis, nearly all patients have axillary lymph node involvement and approximately one third have distant metastases. Because of the high risk for metastases in patients with inflammatory cancer, staging with CT and bone scanning is recommended.

Inflammatory breast cancer is treated with neoadjuvant chemotherapy, followed by mastectomy with axillary node dissection, and then postmastectomy chest wall radiation therapy. Despite multimodality treatment, prognosis is still worse for patients with inflammatory breast cancer than for those with other types of locally advanced breast cancer, with a 5-year relative survival rate of approximately 40%.

KEY POINTS

- Inflammatory breast cancer is characterized by erythema and edema of the skin of the breast, which can resemble the skin of an orange ("peau d'orange"); the diagnosis is established based on the clinical appearance of the breast.
- Because of the high risk for metastases in patients with inflammatory breast cancer, staging with CT and bone scanning is recommended.
- Inflammatory breast cancer is treated with neoadjuvant chemotherapy, followed by surgery, and then radiation.

Breast Cancer Follow-up and Survivorship

After completing surgery, radiation therapy, and chemotherapy, patients with early-stage breast cancer should receive follow-up monitoring every 3 to 6 months for 2 years, every 6 months during years 2 through 5, and then annually. Monitoring should include annual mammography, whereas screening MRI of the breast is reserved for patients who have a high risk for subsequent breast cancer from *BRCA1/2* mutations, a strong family history of breast cancer, or other indications as based on the ACS guidelines (see Table 53).

Surveillance blood tests and other imaging studies are not recommended, as these have not been shown to improve survival. Investigative laboratory tests and imaging studies should be reserved for patients with worrisome symptoms or findings on examination. Most hormone receptor–negative breast cancer recurrences develop within 5 years of diagnosis. However, in patients with hormone receptor–positive breast cancer, half of the recurrences arise 5 years or more after diagnosis.

Quality-of-life issues should be monitored in survivors of breast cancer. Vasomotor symptoms are common in younger women owing to chemotherapy-induced early menopause and antiestrogen treatment in patients with hormone receptor–positive breast cancer. Hot flushes may be improved with selective serotonin reuptake inhibitors such as escitalopram, or with serotonin-norepinephrine reuptake inhibitors such as venlafaxine. However, in patients taking tamoxifen, it is important to avoid the use of strong and moderately strong CYP2D6 inhibitors, such as bupropion, fluoxetine, and paroxetine, as these drugs can inhibit tamoxifen activation. Testing patients for CYP2D6 polymorphisms is not currently recommended. Gabapentin at bedtime can help decrease night sweats. Aromatase

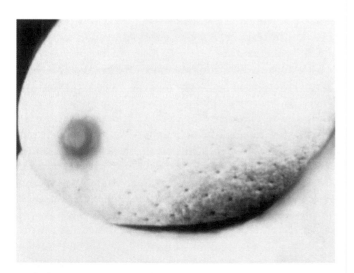

FIGURE 15. Inflammatory breast cancer often has this characteristic "p'eau d'orange" (orange peel) appearance of the skin, due to tumor emboli in the dermal lymphatics. Erythema is often present as well.

inhibitor–induced arthralgia can be treated with NSAIDs, a break in treatment, or changing to another aromatase inhibitor or to tamoxifen. Regular exercise can ameliorate aromatase-inhibitor arthralgia. Other common problems facing survivors of breast cancer include sexual dysfunction, fatigue, insomnia, and cognitive dysfunction, including impaired memory, decreased concentration, and word-finding difficulty. Patients can experience a treatment-related decrease in bone density caused by chemotherapy-induced early menopause or aromatase inhibitors. Bone density should be monitored every 1 to 2 years during, as well as initially after, aromatase inhibitor treatment and should be monitored in patients with chemotherapy-induced premature menopause. Additionally, patients should be monitored for decreased arm mobility and lymphedema, with prompt referral to physical therapy if such symptoms occur. Patients who wish to preserve fertility after breast cancer treatment should be referred to fertility specialists before starting chemotherapy. Clinicians should reassure patients that becoming pregnant following breast cancer diagnosis and treatment does not increase the risk of breast cancer recurrence nor does it decrease survival. Premenopausal women with breast cancer who do not wish to become pregnant should use a nonhormonal method of birth control.

An established fertility preservation option for a woman with a partner is in vitro fertilization with embryo freezing. Newer options, often done as part of clinical trials, include freezing of unfertilized eggs and ovarian cryopreservation with future reimplantation. Embryo preservation also gives parents with *BRCA1/2* mutations the option of preimplantation genetic diagnosis (if desired by the parents, embryos without the mutation can be selected for implantation).

KEY POINTS

HVC
- After completion of treatment, follow-up monitoring in patients with early-stage breast cancer should occur every 3 to 6 months for 2 years, every 6 months during years 2 through 5, and then annually, with annual mammography for all survivors, and MRI of the breast reserved for those at high risk for recurrence.

HVC
- Surveillance blood tests and other imaging tests should not be routinely performed and are reserved for patients with symptoms or findings of disease.

- Therapy-related hot flushes in breast cancer survivors may be improved with selective serotonin reuptake inhibitors or serotonin-norepinephrine reuptake inhibitors, with avoidance of strong and moderately strong CYP2D6 inhibitors, which can inhibit tamoxifen activation.

- Breast cancer survivors should undergo monitoring for decreased arm mobility and lymphedema, with prompt referral to physical therapy in the presence of such symptoms.

Metastatic Breast Cancer

Recurrent breast cancer with distant metastases is not curable. The average overall survival from the start of systemic chemotherapy to death is 2 years, although patients with hormone-sensitive breast cancer are often treated for years with antiestrogen therapy before chemotherapy is begun. The goals of treatment in this setting are to improve survival, palliate symptoms, and minimize treatment toxicity. Clinical trials of new treatments, including new molecularly targeted therapies, should be considered for patients with metastatic breast cancer whenever possible. It is important to discuss goals of care with patients and involve palliative care teams when appropriate.

Patients with a history of early-stage breast cancer who develop findings suspicious for metastatic disease should undergo biopsy of the suspected metastatic lesions if possible to confirm the diagnosis and facilitate repeat assessment of hormone receptor status and *HER2* overexpression. Most patients with recurrence outside the central nervous system can undergo imaging-guided needle biopsies in locations such as the spine. Discordance between the status of these molecular markers in the primary tumor and the metastatic site occurs in 10% to 15% of patients with breast cancer for both estrogen receptor status and *HER2* amplification, usually resulting in a change in treatment.

Systemic treatment is the mainstay of therapy for patients with metastatic breast cancer; surgery and radiation have ancillary roles. Radiation is used to treat painful bone metastases. Surgery can stabilize impending pathologic fractures. Either may be used to treat oncologic emergencies, such as spinal cord compression and brain metastases. Patients who present with de novo metastatic disease currently do not undergo resection of the primary breast cancer, although randomized trials are currently studying whether this approach may confer survival benefits in patients in whom the systemic disease is responding to therapy.

Initial treatment for metastatic breast cancer depends on hormone receptor and *HER2* status, disease sites, and patient comorbidities and preferences. For hormone receptor-positive cancer, antiestrogen therapy usually is given initially. Antiestrogen therapy works best in patients with bone and soft tissue metastases and in those with a longer disease-free interval since the initial breast cancer diagnosis. Antiestrogen treatments for metastatic breast cancer include aromatase inhibitors, tamoxifen, ovarian suppression in premenopausal women, fulvestrant (an estrogen receptor down-regulator), megestrol acetate, and estradiol. A newer approach combines antiestrogen treatment with molecularly targeted therapy affecting downstream pathways. The combination of exemestane and the mammalian target of rapamycin (mTOR) inhibitor, everolimus, is effective in patients in whom resistance to aromatase inhibitor therapy has developed.

Patients with hormone receptor–negative cancer, those with impending visceral crisis due to extensive metastases, or those who do not respond to antiestrogen therapy are treated with chemotherapy. Generally, single-agent chemotherapy is given, although combination therapy is appropriate in patients with extensive visceral metastases in whom a higher response rate is needed. Chemotherapeutic agents can be used sequentially in patients with good performance status who wish to continue palliative treatment.

Patients with *HER2*-amplified metastatic breast cancer are treated with monoclonal antibodies against the *HER2* receptor. These drugs can be used as single agents, in multiple anti-*HER2* drug combinations, given with antiestrogen therapy in hormone receptor–positive cancer, or combined with nonanthracycline-based chemotherapies. A more recent approach uses an antibody drug conjugate of trastuzumab linked to the antimitotic agent ado-trastuzumab emtansine. Trastuzumab delivers the potent chemotherapeutic agent directly to the cancer cells that overexpress *HER2*.

Patients with breast cancer with lytic bone metastases are treated with bisphosphonates to decrease bone pain and skeletal-related events such as bone fractures and reduce the need for palliative radiation therapy. These agents can cause transient aches as well as fever, kidney injury, hypocalcemia, and osteonecrosis of the jaw. Denosumab, a monoclonal antibody against the receptor activator of nuclear factor κB ligand (RANKL), is an alternative option for reducing the morbidity related to metastatic bone lesions. Denosumab can also cause hypocalcemia and osteonecrosis of the jaw. Patients who take bisphosphonates or denosumab should receive a baseline dental evaluation, schedule regular dental appointments during treatment, maintain good oral hygiene, and report any jaw pain or areas of poor gingival healing. Coordination with an oral surgeon is needed to minimize risk before any invasive dental procedures are performed.

KEY POINTS

- Recurrent breast cancer with distant metastases is not curable, and the goals of treatment in such patients are to improve survival, palliate symptoms, and minimize treatment toxicity.
- Patients with a history of early-stage breast cancer who develop findings suspicious for metastatic disease should undergo biopsy of a suspected metastatic lesion, if possible, to confirm the diagnosis and facilitate repeat assessment of hormone receptor status and *HER2* overexpression.
- Recurrent metastatic hormone receptor–positive breast cancer is usually treated with initial antiestrogen therapy, which works best in patients with bone and soft tissue metastases and in those with a longer disease-free interval since the initial breast cancer diagnosis.

Ovarian Cancer

Epidemiology and Risk Factors

Ovarian cancer is the leading cause of gynecologic cancer-related deaths, with an estimated 22,240 new cases and 14,230 deaths in the United States in 2013. The lifetime risk for developing ovarian cancer is 1.4%, and the median age at diagnosis is 63 years. Epithelial cancer accounts for 95% of ovarian cancer and is the type discussed in this section.

The most important risk factor for ovarian cancer is family history. Ten percent to 15% of ovarian cancer is hereditary, mostly due to *BRCA1/2* mutations. The lifetime risk of ovarian cancer in hereditary syndromes is detailed in **Table 55**. Current guidelines recommend *BRCA1/2* testing for all women with ovarian cancer (see Breast Cancer).

Factors that decrease the risk of ovarian cancer include previous pregnancy, prior oral contraceptive pill (OCP) use, and tubal ligation or hysterectomy. OCP use for 15 years or

TABLE 55. Lifetime Risk of Ovarian Cancer	
Family History or Mutation Status	**Lifetime Risk of Ovarian Cancer**
Average population risk (no family history of ovarian cancer or related cancers)	1.4%
Family history of ovarian cancer with negative testing for a familial ovarian cancer syndrome	Previously listed as 5%, but now uncertain if risk is increased above population baseline if genetic testing is negative
BRCA1 mutation	35% to 46%
BRCA2 mutation	13% to 23%
Lynch syndrome[a] (also called HNPCC)	3% to 14%

BRCA1 = breast cancer susceptibility 1 gene; *BRCA2* = breast cancer susceptibility 2 gene; HNPCC = hereditary nonpolyposis colon cancer.

[a]Also has increased risks of colon cancer, other gastrointestinal cancers, endometrial cancer, and urinary tract cancers.

more decreases the risk of ovarian cancer by 50%, with the protective effect lasting approximately 30 years after OCP cessation, but even shorter use results in some protection. Endometriosis, polycystic ovary syndrome, infertility, intrauterine device use, and cigarette smoking all increase the risk. Ovulation induction for treatment of infertility does not increase ovarian cancer risk.

KEY POINTS

- All women with ovarian cancer are eligible for *BRCA1/2* testing.

- Oral contraceptive pill (OCP) use for 15 years or more decreases the risk of ovarian cancer by 50%, with the protective effect lasting 30 years after OCP cessation, but even shorter use results in some protection.

Screening and Risk-Reduction Strategies

Women at average risk of ovarian cancer should not undergo screening. The predictive value of serum CA-125 testing and ultrasonography are each less than 3% and lead to a high rate of false-positive results and unnecessary surgeries. Prospective randomized studies have shown no difference in the stage of ovarian cancer at detection or in the rate of ovarian cancer–related deaths when annual serum CA-125 assays and transvaginal ultrasounds are used. Despite a lack of data showing that screening in high-risk patients is effective, most guidelines recommend women with hereditary ovarian cancer syndromes undergo ovarian cancer screening beginning at age 30 years (or 5 to 10 years younger than the age at which ovarian cancer was diagnosed in the youngest relative) with pelvic examinations, serum CA-125 measurement, and transvaginal ultrasonography performed every 6 months.

In women who carry deleterious *BRCA1/2* mutations, prophylactic bilateral salpingo-oophorectomy (BSO) is recommended between ages 35 and 40 years, once childbearing is complete. A recent registry study recommends risk-reducing BSO by age 35 years in women with *BRCA1* mutations because of a 4% risk of ovarian cancer between ages 35 and 40 years. Women with *BRCA2* mutations in this study did not develop ovarian cancers until after age 40 years.

KEY POINTS

HVC
- Women at average risk for ovarian cancer should not receive ovarian cancer screening; the predictive values of serum CA-125 testing and ultrasonography are each less than 3% and lead to a high rate of false-positive results and unnecessary surgeries.

- Prophylactic bilateral salpingo-oophorectomy reduces ovarian cancer risk by 80%, with a residual 1% to 3% risk of primary peritoneal cancer in women with hereditary syndromes.

Diagnosis

Although ovarian cancer is sometimes diagnosed early when an ovarian mass is felt on examination or seen on imaging, ovarian cancer is usually advanced at diagnosis owing to the absence of effective screening tests and usual lack of symptoms in patients with early-stage disease. Severe or persistent symptoms such as abdominal or pelvic pain, bloating, early satiety, or anorexia should raise suspicion for ovarian cancer, particularly in postmenopausal women. Dyspnea due to pleural effusion or symptoms of bowel obstruction may be presenting symptoms.

Ultrasound findings suggestive of a malignant ovarian mass include a solid component that is often nodular or papillary and the presence of ascites and/or peritoneal masses. If ovarian cancer is suspected, CT or MRI of the abdomen and pelvis and chest imaging are usually done to assess disease extent.

Serum CA-125 levels are elevated in most women with advanced ovarian cancer, but this finding is less sensitive for detecting earlier-stage disease. In addition, the finding of elevated serum CA-125 levels is not specific and levels can be elevated in other malignancies; in several benign gynecologic conditions common in premenopausal women; and in liver failure, colitis, peritonitis, diverticulitis, and heart failure. The decision to proceed to surgery should depend more on imaging findings than on biomarkers such as the serum CA-125 level. If ovarian cancer is diagnosed, it is helpful to measure preoperative serum CA-125 levels to determine whether this marker will be useful for assessing treatment response.

In patients with an adnexal mass without ascites, diagnosis is usually established by surgical exploration, as there is survival benefit from intact removal of the adnexal mass in early-stage disease. In patients with advanced disease, diagnosis may be made by cytologic evaluation of ascites or pleural fluid, or by image-guided biopsy of peritoneal masses.

KEY POINTS

- Severe or persistent symptoms such as abdominal or pelvic pain, bloating, early satiety, or anorexia should raise suspicion for ovarian cancer, particularly in postmenopausal women.

- Ultrasound findings suggestive of a malignant ovarian mass include a solid component that is often nodular or papillary and the presence of ascites and/or peritoneal masses.

- Ovarian cancer diagnosis is usually established by surgical exploration, cytologic evaluation of ascites or pleural fluid, or by image-guided biopsy of peritoneal masses in patients with more advanced cancer.

Treatment

Ovarian cancer staging, treatment, and prognosis are detailed in **Table 56**. Stage I ovarian cancer without high-risk features is treated with surgery alone. Patients with stage I ovarian cancer with high-grade or clear cell histology, cyst rupture, or positive peritoneal cytologic results should receive adjuvant chemotherapy after surgery. Patients with stages II, III, and IV ovarian cancer and initially resectable disease can undergo surgery first followed by postoperative chemotherapy. If disease is not resectable initially, neoadjuvant chemotherapy is given, usually for two to three cycles, followed by resection in patients with an adequate response to chemotherapy; chemotherapy is completed after surgery.

Optimal surgical debulking (residual masses <1 cm), ideally performed by a gynecologic oncologist, improves survival. Surgery involves total abdominal hysterectomy and BSO; staging by examination of the abdomen and pelvis, including peritoneal washings and lymph node evaluation; and tumor debulking by removal of all neoplastic tissue that can be safely excised.

For stage II and optimally debulked stage III cancer, intraperitoneal chemotherapy through an indwelling peritoneal catheter should be considered. It results in a 16-month improvement in overall survival in patients with stage III disease compared with intravenous chemotherapy regimens, but is associated with more toxicity. Physicians and patients should discuss the risks and benefits of this approach.

KEY POINTS

- Surgical treatment of ovarian cancer should be done by a gynecologic oncologist and involves total abdominal hysterectomy and bilateral salpingo-oophorectomy; staging by examination of the abdomen and pelvis, including peritoneal washings and lymph node evaluation; and optimal tumor debulking.

- Intraperitoneal chemotherapy results in a 16-month improvement in overall survival in patients with stage II and optimally debulked stage III ovarian cancer compared with intravenous chemotherapy, but it is associated with more toxicity.

Monitoring and Follow-up

Patients with ovarian cancer undergo follow-up monitoring every 2 to 4 months for the first 2 years following completion of surgery and first-line chemotherapy, with subsequent monitoring every 3 to 6 months through 5 years after treatment, and then annually. Follow-up visits include a thorough history, physical examination, and pelvic examination. Guidelines differ on whether to monitor serum

TABLE 56. International Federation of Gynecology and Obstetrics Ovarian Cancer Staging, Treatment, and Survival			
Stage	**Definition**	**Treatment**	**5-Year Overall Survival**
Stage I disease (favorable)	Cancer in one or both ovaries, not high grade or clear cell, negative peritoneal washings, no rupture	Surgery alone	>90%
Stage I disease (unfavorable); stage II disease	Unfavorable stage I disease: Confined to ovaries but with high-grade or clear cell histology, rupture, or positive peritoneal washings Stage II disease: spread beyond ovaries but confined to pelvis	Surgery followed by chemotherapy	Stage I: 75% to 80% Stage II: 60% to 70%
Optimally debulked stage III disease	Spread to abdomen, with residual tumor masses <1 cm after debulking surgery	Surgery followed by intravenous or intraperitoneal chemotherapy	Intravenous chemotherapy: 40% Intraperitoneal chemotherapy: 50%
Suboptimally debulked stage III disease or stage IV disease	Stage III (suboptimal) disease: spread to abdomen with residual masses >1 cm after debulking surgery Stage IV disease: spread beyond abdomen	Surgery (usually done even for stage IV disease) and chemotherapy, with order of treatment depending on initial tumor resectability	Stage III: 20% to 30% Stage IV: 10% to 15%

CA-125 levels, although a recent trial suggested that such monitoring might result in earlier initiation of treatment for recurrence, but no difference in overall survival. Imaging studies and other blood tests are reserved for addressing specific clinical concerns. If not given on initial diagnosis, a referral for genetic counseling should be provided at initial follow-up.

KEY POINT

HVC • Follow-up for patients who have completed treatment for ovarian cancer includes a periodic history, physical examination, and pelvic examination for 5 years after treatment; routine monitoring of CA-125 levels, other laboratory testing, and imaging studies does not improve survival and should be reserved for addressing specific clinical concerns.

Management of Recurrent Ovarian Cancer

More than 70% of women with advanced ovarian cancer will experience a relapse after first-line chemotherapy, and recurrent ovarian cancer is not curable. The goal of treatment of recurrent ovarian cancer is to improve cancer-related symptoms and extend survival. Discussion and shared decision making about goals of care and referral to a palliative care team are appropriate in the management of patients with recurrent disease.

Secondary cytoreductive surgery is best considered for patients with a progression-free interval of at least 12 months, good performance status, and a local recurrence that can potentially be rendered free of gross disease with surgery.

An elevated serum CA-125 level in a patient with a normal physical examination and CT scan and no disease symptoms constitutes the most common presentation at relapse. Patients with an isolated serum CA-125 recurrence who are not comfortable with surveillance alone can be treated with tamoxifen or an aromatase inhibitor. Initiating cytotoxic treatment confers no known benefit in this setting.

Cytotoxic chemotherapy is indicated for patients with significant disease on CT scan or physical examination or in those with disease progression–related symptoms. Treatment options include single-agent or combination chemotherapy, often involving a platinum agent if the cancer has not developed resistance, as well as anti-angiogenesis inhibitors such as bevacizumab.

Ascites can be managed with periodic paracentesis for symptomatic relief. Patients with bowel obstruction from advanced ovarian cancer are unlikely to benefit from surgery. Chemotherapy benefit in patients with bowel obstruction is often limited, and treatment should focus on comfort and palliation.

KEY POINTS

• The goal of treatment of recurrent ovarian cancer is to improve cancer-related symptoms and extend survival.

• Secondary cytoreductive surgery is best considered for patients with ovarian cancer and a progression-free interval of at least 12 months, good performance status, and a local recurrence that can potentially be rendered free of gross disease with surgery.

Cervical Cancer
Epidemiology and Risk Factors

Over 12,000 new cases of invasive cervical cancer and approximately 4000 cervical cancer–related deaths occur in the United States each year. The mean age at diagnosis is 48 years. Invasive cervical cancer incidence in the United States has decreased by more than 80% since the 1940s, largely owing to Pap smear screening. The incidence and mortality rates are higher in countries lacking screening programs.

Nearly all cases of cervical cancer are precipitated by persistent human papillomavirus (HPV) infection. HPV, most commonly subtypes 16 and 18, is detected in more than 99% of patients with cervical cancer. Both squamous cell carcinoma and adenocarcinoma are associated with HPV infection. The HPV vaccine is ideally given before sexual activity begins: if given to adolescents and young women before they develop HPV infection, it is 90% effective at preventing infection and 97% to 100% effective at preventing cervical intraepithelial neoplasia and invasive cervical cancer.

Cervical Pap smears can detect precancerous lesions that occur several years before the development of invasive disease. See MKSAP 17 General Internal Medicine for cervical cancer screening guidelines and HPV vaccine recommendations.

KEY POINTS

• Nearly all cases of cervical cancer are precipitated by human papillomavirus infection (subtypes 16 and 18).

• The human papillomavirus vaccine, given before infection develops, is 90% effective at preventing infection and 97% to 100% effective at preventing cervical intraepithelial neoplasia and invasive cervical cancer. **HVC**

Diagnosis, Staging, and Treatment

The most common presenting symptoms of cervical cancer are abnormal vaginal discharge, postcoital bleeding, or vaginal bleeding between menstrual cycles or after menopause. Diagnosis of cervical cancer is established by biopsy of the cervix. Colposcopy with directed biopsy is done if there is no visible lesion, with cervical conization done if colposcopy is nondiagnostic. The most common histologies are squamous cell carcinoma (69% of cervical cancers) and adenocarcinoma (25%).

Staging, most often performed using the International Federation of Gynecology and Obstetrics system (**Table 57**), is done clinically and includes a pelvic examination and chest radiograph. CT, MRI, and PET/CT are often useful in planning therapy, although they are not part of the formal staging evaluation.

Primary treatment of cervical cancer based on clinical stage is outlined in Table 57. Chemotherapy given with radiation therapy improves survival in patients with intermediate-risk and high-risk cervical cancer but not in the neoadjuvant or adjuvant setting.

KEY POINTS

- The most common presenting symptoms of cervical cancer are abnormal vaginal discharge, postcoital bleeding, or vaginal bleeding between menstrual cycles or after menopause.
- Chemotherapy given with radiation therapy improves survival in patients with intermediate- and high-risk cervical cancer but not in the neoadjuvant or adjuvant setting.

Prognosis and Surveillance

The most important prognostic factor in cervical cancer is clinical stage followed by involvement of pelvic or paraaortic lymph nodes. The 5-year overall survival rate is 90% to 95% for patients with early-stage clinical disease and negative lymph nodes; the survival rate in patients with positive lymph nodes decreases to 70%. Patients with regionally advanced tumors have a 40% to 50% survival rate at 5 years.

Surveillance of patients with cervical cancer includes clinical evaluation every 3 to 6 months for 2 years, followed by evaluation every 6 months until year 5, and then annually. Surveillance evaluation should include a history, physical examination, and pelvic examination with cervicovaginal cytology. Yearly chest radiography is optional, and other imaging is done only as clinically indicated. In appropriate candidates, localized pelvic recurrence may be cured with pelvic exenteration.

KEY POINTS

- In patients with cervical cancer, surveillance evaluation (a history, physical examination, and pelvic examination with cervicovaginal cytology) should occur every 3 to 6 months for 2 years, followed by evaluation every 6 months until year 5, and then annually.

Gastroenterological Malignancies
Colorectal Cancer

This section discusses staging through follow-up and prognosis of patients with colorectal cancer. Epidemiology, pathophysiology, risk factors, and clinical manifestations will be discussed in MKSAP 17 Gastroenterology and Hepatology. Colorectal cancer screening is discussed in MKSAP 17 General Internal Medicine.

Colorectal cancer is a common malignancy in both men and women in developed countries and is second only to lung cancer as a cause of cancer-related deaths in the United States. Symptoms and signs of bowel disease include bleeding per rectum, melena, persistent cramping or bloating, and chronic diarrhea or constipation and may indicate the presence of a

TABLE 57.	International Federation of Gynecology and Obstetrics Cervical Cancer Staging	
Stage	**Treatment**
I: Carcinoma is strictly confined to the cervix IA: Microscopic disease only	I: Radical hysterectomy or radiation; ovarian preservation can be done if fertility desired IA: Simple hysterectomy, cone biopsy, or removal of cervix alone are options
IIA (nonbulky) and IIB (bulky): Cervical carcinoma invades beyond the uterus, but not to the pelvic wall or lower third of the vagina	IIA: same as for stage I IIB: same as for stage III
III: The tumor extends to the pelvic wall and/or involves the lower third of the vagina and/or causes hydronephrosis or nonfunctioning kidney	III: Radiation with concurrent platinum-based chemotherapy
IV: The carcinoma extends beyond the true pelvis or involves (biopsy proven) the mucosa of the bladder or rectum IVA: spread to adjacent organs IVB: distant metastases	IVA: same as for stage III IVB: palliative chemotherapy, with palliative radiation for local symptoms such as bleeding or pain

benign polyp, another nonmalignant process, or cancer. Such symptoms and signs warrant investigation regardless of age.

Colorectal cancer is a cancer of the large intestine. The most distal 12 to 15 centimeters of the large intestine, the portion below the peritoneal reflection and therefore within the pelvis, is referred to as the rectum; the rest of the organ is referred to as the colon. Metastatic disease from either the colon or the rectum is referred to as colorectal cancer. The need for a permanent colostomy is one of the most common fears in patients in whom colorectal cancer is diagnosed, and usually this fear is unfounded.

KEY POINTS

- The need for a permanent colostomy is one of the most common fears in patients in whom colorectal cancer is diagnosed, and usually this fear is unfounded.

Staging

The preoperative staging workup should include a complete colonoscopy (if technically feasible) and contrast-enhanced CT scans of the chest, abdomen, and pelvis. Preoperative measurement of serum carcinoembryonic antigen (CEA) levels is also routinely done. PET scans have not been demonstrated to improve preoperative staging and should not be used routinely. Patients with local or locoregional rectal cancer require further preoperative staging with endorectal ultrasonography or a pelvic MRI to assess the depth of tumor penetration (T stage), degree of lymph node involvement (N stage), and any metastasis (M stage).

Staging using the TNM cancer staging system is the most accurate predictor of outcome in patients with colorectal cancer (**Table 58**).

KEY POINTS

HVC
- PET scans have not been demonstrated to improve preoperative staging in patients with colorectal cancer and should not be routinely used.

TABLE 58.	Staging of Colorectal Cancer	
Stage	**Description**	**Approximate 5-Year Disease-Free Survival**
I	Tumor does not invade the full thickness of bowel wall (T1, T2); lymph nodes not involved (N0)	90%-95%
II	Tumor invades full thickness of the bowel and may invade into pericolonic or perirectal fat (T3, T4); lymph nodes not involved (N0)	70%-85%
III	One or more lymph nodes involved with cancer (N1, N2); any T stage	25%-70%
IV	Metastatic tumor spread to distant site (M1); any T stage; any N stage	0%-10%

Surgical Management

Colon Cancer

Patients with colon cancer without preoperative evidence of metastatic disease should undergo surgical resection of the primary tumor and the regional lymph nodes. Surgery of the colon should almost never result in a need for permanent colostomy, although a temporary colostomy, usually reversed after a few months, may be needed for emergent surgery due to obstruction or perforation or if the bowel is not evacuated properly before surgery. Surgery involving tumors of the upper two thirds of the rectum also should only very rarely require permanent colostomy, although temporary ostomies may be needed more frequently. Patients with colon cancer confirmed as stage I at surgery require no further treatment. In stage II colon cancer, data do not show a clear survival advantage for administration of adjuvant chemotherapy; consequently, surgery alone is acceptable standard practice for most patients. An exception is patients with stage II colon cancer with characteristics associated with a high risk for recurrence (T4 disease and inadequate lymph node sampling [<12 lymph nodes examined], lymphovascular invasion, poorly differentiated histology, or clinical perforation or obstruction). In these patients, the prognosis is similar to that of patients with stage III disease, and adjuvant chemotherapy may be appropriate.

Rectal Cancer

Patients with rectal tumors that are not full thickness and do not have lymph node involvement (stage I) on pretreatment imaging usually undergo surgery, with a total mesorectal excision being the preferred procedure. The mesorectum is a fatty sheath covering the rectum that contains the regional lymph nodes. A total mesorectal excision entails a sharp dissection of the pelvis outside of the mesorectum to allow removal of the mesorectum fully intact en bloc with the rectum. However, considerable expertise is required to avoid complications with this procedure, which should be performed only by a subspecialized surgeon. If local lymph node metastases or full-thickness tumor penetration is found after surgery in those patients thought to be stage I preoperatively, then postoperative chemotherapy and radiation therapy are indicated. Otherwise, if pathology confirms stage I cancer, no further therapy is needed. In patients with tumors that are too distal to permit an adequate margin of resection without resection of the anal sphincter muscles, an abdominal-peritoneal resection is likely to be required, which results in a permanent colostomy. Patients who have full-thickness rectal tumors (T3-T4) or clearly enlarged lymph nodes on preoperative imaging require combined-modality therapy with neoadjuvant radiation and chemotherapy and adjuvant chemotherapy alone. More recently, an accepted alternative has been chemotherapy first, followed by chemoradiotherapy, and then surgery, with no postoperative treatment ("total neoadjuvant therapy").

- Patients with colon cancer without preoperative evidence of metastatic disease should undergo surgical resection of the primary tumor and the regional lymph nodes.

- Treatment for patients with rectal tumors that are not full thickness and with no lymph node involvement (stage I) on pretreatment imaging is usually surgery alone.

Adjuvant Treatment of Colorectal Cancer

Colon Cancer

The first drug successfully used for adjuvant treatment of colorectal cancer was 5-fluorouracil (5-FU), and this agent, now in its sixth decade of clinical use, remains at the center of current treatment strategies. Newer drugs are most typically used in combination with 5-FU. 5-FU is usually given with the reduced folate leucovorin, which is inactive alone but causes 5-FU to bind more tightly to its target enzyme. Capecitabine is an oral prodrug that is converted to 5-FU in the body. Use of this agent requires a highly reliable, motivated patient who is able to adhere to a complex oral medication schedule. In patients with stage III disease, adjuvant 5-FU–based chemotherapy given for approximately 6 months after surgery has been shown to reduce the risk of cancer recurrence and death; therefore, all patients with stage III disease, regardless of age, should receive adjuvant chemotherapy barring specific medical or psychiatric contraindications. The FOLFOX (leucovorin, 5-FU, and oxaliplatin) regimen and the CAPOX (capecitabine plus oxaliplatin) regimens have been shown to be modestly but statistically significantly more effective than the same regimens without oxaliplatin in patients with stage III disease (but not in those with stage II disease); these two regimens are equally acceptable. Not all drugs that are useful for treating metastatic disease are active in the adjuvant setting. Irinotecan, bevacizumab, and cetuximab have all been shown to be ineffective in improving survival in the adjuvant setting, yet, as discussed below, all are part of standard treatment of metastatic disease. For patients with stage II disease and a high risk for recurrence, treatment with 5-FU/leucovorin or capecitabine may be appropriate. Whether the addition of oxaliplatin in patients with high-risk stage II disease is appropriate has been challenged by recent data, and patient care must be individualized based on the extent of risk factors for recurrence and the patient's overall medical condition. Although no definitive standards exist, a consensus statement from the American Society of Clinical Oncology recommends that all patients with stage II colon cancer consult with a medical oncologist to discuss the risks and benefits of adjuvant treatment.

Rectal Cancer

Radiation therapy is not routinely indicated for completely resected colon cancer. However, because of the anatomic location of rectal cancer and the difficulty in obtaining adequate tumor-free margins, local recurrence rates tend to be higher than those for completely resected colon cancer. Therefore, neoadjuvant chemoradiotherapy is indicated in patients with locally advanced (T3-T4) rectal cancer, in addition to adjuvant therapy. Clinical trials have established that 5-FU given by protracted intravenous infusion or capecitabine is an equally acceptable chemotherapeutic option to be given concurrently with radiation therapy. Data evaluating the addition of oxaliplatin during radiation have been disappointing, and this therapy is not currently recommended. The FOLFOX or CAPOX regimen is typically used after neoadjuvant chemoradiotherapy and surgery for approximately 4 months to complete a total of approximately 6 months of therapy (inclusive of pre- and postoperative treatments). More recently, use of this 4-month combination chemotherapy as an initial treatment, followed by chemoradiation and then surgery, has become an acceptable alternative.

- Adjuvant 5-fluorouracil–based chemotherapy given for approximately 6 months after surgery reduces the risk of cancer recurrence and death in patients with stage III colon cancer.

- For patients with stage II colon cancer and a high risk for recurrence, the prognosis is similar to that for patients with stage III disease, and treatment with 5-fluorouracil/leucovorin or capecitabine may be appropriate.

- Neoadjuvant and adjuvant chemotherapy is indicated in patients with stage III or IV rectal cancer.

Metastatic Disease

Most patients with stage IV colorectal cancer have treatable, but not curable, disease. A long disease-free interval, a limited number of metastases, and metastases confined to a single organ (such as liver or lung) are favorable prognostic factors. A few such patients may have disease amenable to curative surgical resection. Patients with a limited number of liver-only lesions (≤3) have been reported to have long-term disease-free survival rates of 25% to 50% in selected studies. Results are less encouraging as the number of lesions increases. Otherwise, the primary treatment modality is chemotherapy. 5-FU, often modified by the reduced folate leucovorin, is the basis of most chemotherapy regimens used in colorectal cancer. Often, the drugs oxaliplatin or irinotecan are added to these agents. The FOLFOX regimen or the 5-FU, leucovorin, and irinotecan (FOLFIRI) regimen are equally acceptable. Bevacizumab, a monoclonal antibody against vascular endothelial growth factor (VEGF), modestly improves outcome when added to chemotherapy regimens. Recent data support the use of either continued bevacizumab or ziv-aflibercept, another anti-VEGF agent, together with second-line chemotherapy.

All patients with metastatic colorectal cancer should undergo tumor genotyping to identify mutations in the K-*ras and* N-*ras* genes because the anti–epidermal growth factor receptor antibodies, cetuximab and panitumumab, are inactive in the 50% of tumors that harbor mutations. Cetuximab and panitumumab typically cause an acneiform rash, which can be uncomfortable and socially debilitating; however, for reasons that remain unclear, antitumor activity and the development of rash are tightly correlated, and patients who do not experience a substantial skin rash are extremely unlikely to benefit from these agents.

KEY POINTS

- In some patients, metastatic colorectal cancer confined to a single organ may be curable with surgical resection of the primary tumor and metastasis.

- 5-fluorouracil, leucovorin, irinotecan, and oxaliplatin are used to treat patients with metastatic colorectal cancer.

- Bevacizumab, a monoclonal antibody against vascular endothelial growth factor, modestly improves outcome in patients with metastatic colon cancer when added to chemotherapy regimens.

- All patients with metastatic colorectal cancer should undergo tumor genotyping to identify mutations in the K-*ras* and N-*ras* genes because the anti–epidermal growth factor receptor antibodies, cetuximab and panitumumab, are inactive in the 50% of tumors that harbor mutations.

Postoperative Surveillance

The role of postoperative surveillance in patients with colorectal cancer, regardless of whether postoperative therapy has been given, is to identify surgically curable recurrence, such as oligometastatic liver disease or lung metastases, rather than to assess for more disseminated disease. Treatment of small-volume, widely metastatic, but asymptomatic, disease discovered on surveillance has not been associated with improved outcomes and may subject patients to significant treatment toxicity. CT scans of the chest, abdomen, and pelvis are recommended annually for at least the first 3 years postoperatively. PET scanning should not be used for routine surveillance but may be used to further evaluate an equivocal finding on CT scans in some patients. Colonoscopy is typically recommended 1 year after resection, 3 years later, and then every 5 years unless abnormalities are found. The main purpose of colonoscopy is to identify new polyps rather than survey for local recurrence, which is relatively rare. Serum CEA levels are measured every 3 to 6 months for the first 2 years, and then every 6 months, to complete a total of 5 years. The finding of abnormal serum CEA levels, if testing has been repeated and confirmed, warrants additional investigation, as it may indicate recurrent disease. However, therapy should not be started based on serum CEA elevation alone.

KEY POINTS

- Postoperative surveillance of patients with colorectal cancer includes CT scans of the chest, abdomen, and pelvis annually for at least the first 3 years postoperatively and colonoscopy 1 year after resection, 3 years later, and then every 5 years with the goal of identifying surgically curable recurrence.

- Treatment of small-volume, widely metastatic, but **HVC** asymptomatic, disease discovered on surveillance has not been associated with improved outcomes and may subject patients to significant treatment toxicity.

- PET scanning should not be used for routine surveil- **HVC** lance of patients with colorectal cancer but may be used to further evaluate an equivocal finding on CT scans in some patients.

Anal Cancer

Anal cancer is an epidermoid, or squamous cell carcinoma, in contradistinction to rectal cancer, which is an adenocarcinoma. Anal cancers are typically associated with human papillomavirus (HPV) infection and also have increased incidence in patients with HIV infection. Whereas current management of rectal cancer uniformly involves surgical resection, anal cancer is often curable with radiation therapy and concurrent chemotherapy with mitomycin plus 5-FU. This chemotherapeutic regimen was established in the 1970s, and results of studies that have explored newer, alternative agents have not demonstrated improved outcomes. Anal tumors may continue to regress for at least 6 months up to 1 year after completion of chemoradiation therapy. Therefore, treatment failure should not be declared unless unequivocal growth or metastases are documented after completion of radiation therapy. Salvage surgery is performed in patients with local tumor growth after radiation plus chemotherapy; however, this procedure necessarily removes the sphincter muscle, thus requiring a permanent colostomy.

See MKSAP 17 General Internal Medicine for discussion of HPV vaccination.

KEY POINTS

- Anal cancer is often curable with radiation therapy and concurrent chemotherapy with mitomycin plus 5-fluorouracil.

- Because anal tumors may continue to regress for 6 months to 1 year following completion of radiation therapy, treatment failure should not be declared unless unequivocal growth or metastases are documented after completion of radiation therapy.

Pancreatic Cancer

To determine the extent of disease in pancreatic cancer, clinicians use the American Joint Committee on Cancer (AJCC)

TNM cancer staging system. To determine treatment approach, exocrine pancreatic cancer is typically classified based on whether it is surgically resectable, borderline resectable, or either locally advanced or metastatic unresectable disease.

Resectable tumors are confined to the pancreas or just beyond it that correspond to stage IA (tumor limited to the pancreas and ≤2 cm in diameter), IB (tumor limited to the pancreas but >2 cm in diameter), and IIA (tumor extension beyond the pancreas but without involvement of the celiac axis) without involved lymph nodes or evidence of metastatic disease.

Borderline resectable pancreatic cancer is that which extends to nearby blood vessels but that may be removed completely with surgery, such as some stage III tumors (involving the celiac axis or superior mesenteric artery with or without involved lymphadenopathy) without evidence of metastatic disease.

Unresectable cancers cannot be removed entirely by surgery and may include locally advanced disease that has not yet spread to distant organs but still cannot be completely surgically removed (stage IIB [localized tumor or with extension beyond the pancreas but with associated involved lymph nodes] and most stage III cancers).

Metastatic cancer has spread to distant organs and might involve surgery to ameliorate symptoms, but surgery cannot excise the tumor completely or cure the cancer.

Surgical resection is the only potential curative intervention for pancreatic cancer. Patients with a clinical presentation and CT or MRI scans consistent with a resectable pancreatic cancer should undergo definitive resection of the pancreatic mass. Endoscopic or percutaneous needle biopsy should not be attempted prior to definitive surgery, as these procedures have a high false-negative rate in this setting, and would therefore not change management; a suspicious pancreatic mass would require resection whether the needle biopsy showed cancer or not. Although only 15% to 20% of cases are considered resectable at presentation and the overall cure rate in patients undergoing surgical resection is low, patients without evidence of metastatic disease who appear to have resectable disease should undergo resection because it is the only potentially curative option. For patients with locally unresectable disease, neoadjuvant chemoradiation remains controversial.

Postoperative adjuvant therapy with chemotherapy, local radiation, or the combination is also controversial.

For decades, gemcitabine alone was considered an appropriate standard treatment for metastatic pancreatic cancer. More recently, a combination regimen of oxaliplatin, irinotecan, 5-FU, and leucovorin (FOLFIRINOX), has been shown to provide better outcomes; however, this regimen has substantial toxicity and is only a reasonable option in patients who are both medically well (have an excellent performance status) and who are highly motivated. A more

recent trial has shown that the addition of liposomally encapsulated paclitaxel (nab-paclitaxel) to gemcitabine also improves outcome modestly, albeit with some increased toxicity.

KEY POINT

- Patients with pancreatic cancer without evidence of metastatic disease who have technically resectable disease should undergo resection because it is the only potentially curative option.

Gastroesophageal Cancer

This section discusses treatment of patients with gastroesophageal cancer. Epidemiology, risk factors, and clinical manifestations of esophageal cancer are discussed in MKSAP 17 Gastroenterology and Hepatology, Disorders of the Esophagus. The same aspects of gastric cancer are discussed in MKSAP 17 Gastroenterology and Hepatology, Disorders of the Stomach and Duodenum.

Staging of gastroesophageal cancer is based on the TNM cancer staging system. In simple terms, stage I disease is a superficial lesion that has not spread and does not penetrate the full thickness of the esophagus or stomach wall, whereas stage II disease is a full-thickness lesion. Stage III disease is defined by spread to locoregional lymph nodes, and stage IV disease is defined by the presence of distant metastatic disease. Virtually all gastric and gastroesophageal junction cancers are adenocarcinomas, as are approximately 95% of esophageal cancers. About 5% of esophageal cancers are of squamous cell histology, although currently, patients with adenocarcinomas and squamous cell carcinoma receive the same treatments.

Although only 30% to 40% of patients have potentially resectable disease at presentation, patients with local and locoregional disease (AJCC stages I, II, and III) are typically treated surgically. Unfortunately, recurrence rates are high and cure rates with surgical resection remain low. Studies have shown that administration of neoadjuvant chemotherapy improves outcome to a modest, but statistically significant, degree. The addition of preoperative radiation therapy, as well as chemotherapy, is also supported by some—although less robust—clinical data. As such, surgery alone is no longer the preferred approach, and neoadjuvant chemotherapy or chemoradiation therapy is routinely used.

Because of the low cure rates for locoregional therapy for esophageal cancer, chemotherapy has been added to many treatment regimens, and many patients are currently treated with combination chemoradiation therapy following surgery for resectable disease. However, the optimal treatment regimen and the overall effectiveness of different treatment approaches have not yet been established.

Treatment of metastatic (stage IV) gastroesophageal cancer remains unsatisfactory and palliative. Numerous agents have shown modest activity, and combination cisplatin-based regimens are typically used owing to the insufficient activity of single agents.

Up to 20% of gastric cancers and 30% of gastroesophageal junction adenocarcinomas recently have been found to overexpress the *HER2* growth factor receptor, which is a target for the anti-*HER2* monoclonal antibody trastuzumab. Therefore, evaluation of all metastatic gastroesophageal carcinomas for *HER2* is performed, and trastuzumab is added to chemotherapy regimens in patients whose tumors express *HER2*.

KEY POINTS

- Patients with local and locoregional gastroesophageal cancer (American Joint Committee on Cancer stages I, II, and III) are typically treated surgically.

- Treatment of metastatic gastroesophageal cancer is palliative and usually consists of cisplatin-based therapy or cisplatin-based therapy plus trastuzumab in patients with *HER2* tumor expression.

Neuroendocrine Tumors

Neuroendocrine tumors (NETs) are rare in incidence, but because of their often relatively indolent course, the prevalence of NETs in the population is disproportionately higher than the incidence. NETs arising from the endocrine cells of the pancreas are called pancreatic NETs, whereas those arising from all other neuroendocrine tissues of the aerodigestive tract are called carcinoid tumors. Although older literature categorized pancreatic NETs (previously called islet cell tumors) and carcinoids together, these two entities clearly behave differently, with several anticancer agents showing activity against pancreatic NETS but not against carcinoid tumors. Typically, NETs of the gastrointestinal tract are well to moderately differentiated and indolent in growth pattern. However, NETs may be poorly differentiated, in which case they typically exhibit a very aggressive growth pattern and are treated like small cell lung cancer. Most NETs are hormonally nonfunctioning, but about 25% are hormone producing. For example, carcinoid tumors typically produce serotonin, which can cause the classic carcinoid syndrome of diarrhea and facial flushing. Pancreatic NETs, when hormonally active, may produce any of the pancreatic endocrine hormones, including insulin, gastrin, glucagon, somatostatin, or vasoactive intestinal peptide, with resulting hormonal syndromes based on the type of hormone elaborated.

Although patients with hormonally functioning tumors may present with hormonal symptoms, those with nonfunctioning tumors may be asymptomatic and have metastatic disease for many years before diagnosis. The liver is overwhelmingly the most common site of metastasis, and diagnosis is often established through an incidental finding of hepatomegaly.

Because well-differentiated NETs are so indolent, patients often can be effectively managed with expectant observation and serial imaging. Triple-phase contrast-enhanced CT scanning or MRI with gadolinium are the preferred imaging modalities. Indium 111 pentetreotide scanning can be used to establish the presence of somatostatin receptors, which are commonly expressed on these tumors. Tumors that have demonstrated somatostatin receptors and are hormonally symptomatic or show clear growth under observation may be treated with the somatostatin analogues octreotide or lanreotide. Mechanical interventions, such as hepatic arterial embolization, radiofrequency ablation, or surgical debulking, may be used to reduce symptomatic tumor bulk in the liver or to decrease hormone production.

In pancreatic NETs, the small-molecule inhibitors sunitinib (an anti-VEGF agent) and everolimus (an anti–mammalian target of rapamycin [mTOR] agent), and the oral cytotoxic combination of capecitabine and temozolomide, are active. However, these agents have not demonstrated the same activity in carcinoid tumors. Chemotherapy is minimally effective in carcinoid tumors, and no specific agents are FDA approved for this indication.

KEY POINTS

- Most neuroendocrine tumors are hormonally nonfunctioning, but about 25% that manifest are hormone producing.

- Because well-differentiated neuroendocrine tumors are **HVC** so indolent, patients often can be effectively managed with expectant observation and serial imaging using triple-phase contrast-enhanced CT scanning or MRI with gadolinium.

- In pancreatic neuroendocrine tumors, the small-molecule inhibitors sunitinib and everolimus and combination capecitabine and temozolomide are active.

Gastrointestinal Stromal Tumors

Although gastrointestinal stromal tumors (GISTs) were once considered rare, significant improvements in molecular diagnostics and therapy have led to increased recognition of these tumors. GISTs are the most common tumor of mesenchymal origin, or sarcoma, of the gastrointestinal tract, representing 1% to 3% of all gastrointestinal tumors, and are derived from the precursors of the intestinal cells of Cajal. Almost all GISTs have an activating mutation in the c-*kit* proto-oncogene, leading to constitutive activation of the KIT receptor tyrosine kinase. CD-117, the immunohistochemical marker for the KIT protein, is the hallmark of most GISTs. GISTs may also present with mutations in the platelet-derived growth factor-α receptor.

Localized GISTs typically appear as isolated, discrete masses anywhere along the digestive tract. Localized GISTs are managed with surgical resection. For patients undergoing a potentially curative resection of a localized GIST, tumors with favorable risk factors require no further treatment, whereas patients with higher-risk tumors are treated with an extended course of the small-molecule receptor tyrosine kinase inhibitor imatinib, which blocks c-*kit* tyrosine kinase phosphorylation. In such patients, recurrence-free survival and overall survival are superior in patients who receive 3 years of imatinib therapy versus 1 year of therapy.

Metastatic disease is extremely refractory to standard cytotoxic chemotherapy agents; however, imatinib is remarkably effective in this setting, and lifelong treatment with this drug typically is recommended until disease progresses or treatment toxicity becomes unacceptable. However, despite its outstanding efficacy, imatinib is not curative. More recently, other agents such as sunitinib and dasatinib have shown activity in the treatment of GISTs that have become refractory to imatinib.

KEY POINTS

- Patients with localized gastrointestinal stromal tumors are managed with surgical resection.

- Following surgery, patients with localized gastrointestinal stromal tumors and tumors with favorable risk factors require no further treatment, whereas those with higher-risk tumors are treated with an extended course of imatinib.

- Patients with metastatic gastrointestinal stromal tumors are treated with lifelong imatinib until disease progresses or treatment toxicity is no longer tolerable.

Lung Cancer

This section will focus on treatment and follow-up of patients with lung cancer. See MKSAP 17 Pulmonary and Critical Care Medicine for discussion of epidemiology, risk factors, screening, diagnosis, and staging.

The initial step in developing a therapeutic plan for lung cancer is to obtain a tissue diagnosis to determine whether the tumor is non–small cell lung cancer (NSCLC) or small cell lung cancer (SCLC) and to exclude metastatic disease from another site. It is important to obtain an adequate biopsy sample (with at least a core biopsy) to allow for additional molecular studies that may be helpful in guiding therapy in some patients.

NSCLC constitutes 80% to 90% of cases, SCLC is responsible for approximately 10% of cases, and the management of these two forms of lung cancer differs significantly. Unfortunately, most patients with lung cancer have advanced, and often incurable, disease at diagnosis, reflecting the relatively asymptomatic nature of early-stage disease. Nonetheless, lung cancer research efforts have led the way in improving therapy through molecular targeting, resulting in

multiple targeted therapies that are now readily available to patients and have dramatically affected treatment efficacy and tolerability.

KEY POINTS

- The initial step in developing a therapeutic plan for lung cancer is to obtain a tissue diagnosis to determine whether the tumor is non–small cell lung cancer or small cell lung cancer and to exclude metastatic disease from another site.

- Most patients with lung cancer have advanced, and often incurable, disease at diagnosis, reflecting the relatively asymptomatic nature of early-stage disease.

Non-Small Cell Lung Cancer

Diagnosis and Staging

The clinical manifestations and diagnosis of lung tumors are discussed in MKSAP 17 Pulmonary and Critical Care Medicine.

NSCLC includes several different histologic types, including squamous cell carcinoma, adenocarcinoma, large cell carcinoma, and other less commonly occurring tumors. It may also be characterized by various paraneoplastic syndromes, including hypercalcemia due to secretion of parathyroid hormone-related protein, hypertrophic pulmonary osteoarthropathy, and inflammatory myopathies. Adenocarcinoma is the most common subtype, accounting for about 50% of cases. Correct assignment of subtype, especially adenocarcinoma versus squamous cell carcinoma, is important to allow for proper treatment in patients with metastatic disease. Additionally, adenocarcinoma can be associated with genetic mutations that help predict the response to tyrosine kinase inhibitors.

The histologic subtypes of NSCLC are all staged similarly; selection of therapy is based primarily on disease stage. Stage I disease is characterized by a solitary tumor without regional (peribronchial or hilar) or mediastinal lymph node involvement. Stage IA disease consists of tumors measuring less than 3 cm, whereas stage IB disease consists of tumors measuring greater than 3 cm but less than 5 cm. Patients with stage II disease have tumors greater than 5 cm; regional lymph node involvement; tumor invasion into local structures, such as the pleura or chest wall; or tumors that are located near the carina. Most patients with stage III disease have mediastinal lymph node involvement. Patients with stage IV disease have metastatic disease or an ipsilateral malignant pleural effusion.

KEY POINTS

- Non–small cell lung cancer may be characterized by various paraneoplastic syndromes, including hypercalcemia due to secretion of parathyroid hormone–related protein, hypertrophic pulmonary osteoarthropathy, and inflammatory myopathies. *(Continued)*

- Correct assignment of subtype, especially adenocarcinoma versus squamous cell carcinoma, is important to allow for proper treatment in patients with metastatic disease.

Treatment

Lung cancer treatment varies significantly based on cancer stage, as noted below. A vital component of treatment, regardless of stage, is smoking cessation. Continued smoking has been shown to increase the risk of complications associated with treatment as well as reducing the potential efficacy of treatment. Furthermore, it is associated with higher risks of secondary cancers in patients with lung cancer.

Surgery with curative intent is recommended for patients with stage I or II NSCLC. Because many patients with lung cancer have concomitant chronic obstructive pulmonary disease, evaluating baseline pulmonary function with measurement of D_{LCO} and spirometry in all potential surgical candidates is necessary. Depending on results of baseline pulmonary function testing, further evaluation to assess predicted postoperative pulmonary function and exercise capacity may be indicated. Some patients are considered to have unresectable disease based on poor pulmonary function or the presence of extensive medical comorbidities rather than disease stage. In these patients or those of advanced age, stereotactic ablative radiation therapy may be an alternative treatment option, as phase II trials have found it can result in tumor control rates similar to surgery. Patients with stage III disease with mediastinal lymph node involvement and those with metastatic disease or an ipsilateral malignant pleural effusion (stage IV) are not typically treated with surgery.

Although adjuvant chemotherapy is not usually recommended following surgery for stage I disease, it may be beneficial in patients with high-risk tumors (poorly differentiated histology, vascular invasion, need for wedge resections, tumors greater than 4 cm, visceral pleural involvement, and incomplete lymph node sampling). Adjuvant chemotherapy has a proven role in patients with resected stage II and resected stage III disease. Cisplatin-based combination therapy has demonstrated a clear survival advantage in these settings.

Adjuvant radiotherapy has been shown to decrease the risk of locoregional recurrence, although its effect on overall survival in patients with stage I and II NSCLC has not been established. Consequently, radiotherapy is not typically given to patients with negative tumor resection margins but may be considered for those with an incompletely resected tumor.

For most patients with stage III NSCLC, combined chemoradiation therapy given with curative intent is the preferred treatment approach. There is no single standard chemotherapy regimen used, but treatment with cisplatin-

or carboplatin-based chemotherapy can be given. Adjuvant chemotherapy does not improve survival following definitive chemoradiation. In highly selected patients with stage III disease, surgery may be considered an appropriate therapeutic option. For patients with T3N1 disease, surgery can be done as initial therapy, although the procedure should include mediastinal lymph node dissection. If mediastinal lymph nodes are negative, adjuvant chemotherapy should be given. In patients with positive mediastinal lymph nodes, sequential chemotherapy and radiation is recommended. For patients with limited mediastinal lymph node involvement, chemotherapy or chemoradiation can be given initially, followed by surgery in patients without disease progression. However, no data indicate that this approach is superior to definitive chemoradiation therapy. Following surgery, patients with positive margins or multistage mediastinal lymph node involvement who were treated with chemotherapy only before surgery should be offered adjuvant radiotherapy.

Metastatic disease (stage IV) is not curable, and treatment in these patients is, by definition, palliative. Proper assessment of performance status using a validated measure is vital, as the benefit of chemotherapy in this patient population is confined to those with an adequate performance status (see Issues in Oncology for discussion of performance status scales). In addition, it is important to address issues surrounding goals of care and provision of palliative care in patients with metastatic NSCLC (see Issues in Oncology for discussion of palliative care goals and benefits).

Selected patients with a single site of metastasis can be treated with resection of the metastatic lesion and aggressive treatment of the primary tumor. However, most patients who present with metastatic disease have multiple sites of metastasis and are treated with systemic therapy. Recommended treatments for patients with metastatic disease are based on the pattern of metastatic spread and the results of histologic and molecular assessment. Recent evidence has indicated that squamous cell carcinoma and adenocarcinoma each respond differently to certain chemotherapeutic agents. Additionally, mutations in the epidermal growth factor receptor (EGFR), translocation of the *ALK* and *EML-4* genes, or mutation of the *ROS1* gene have been identified in a few non–squamous cell lung cancers, usually adenocarcinomas. Patients with EGFR mutations have been found to derive significant benefit from treatment with erlotinib, whereas those with *ALK* translocations and *ROS1* mutations derive similar benefit from crizotinib; these agents are recommended as initial therapy in these patients when mutation status is known before treatment is initiated. In patients who must start treatment before mutation test results are available, these agents can be used later in treatment.

Patients without an activating mutation are treated with chemotherapy. Platinum-containing doublet regimens are widely used in the first-line treatment of metastatic NSCLC and are typically combined with pemetrexed for patients with adenocarcinoma or gemcitabine for squamous cell tumors. For patients in whom the histologic subtype is uncertain, paclitaxel or docetaxel can be used. Bevacizumab, a monoclonal antibody directed against vascular endothelial growth factor, can be combined with chemotherapy for patients with non–squamous cell histology. Patients receiving platinum-based chemotherapy are typically treated for an initial four to six cycles because more than six cycles has not been shown to be beneficial.

Following the initial course of therapy, management options include observation and maintenance chemotherapy. Maintenance therapy is typically given until the patient experiences disease progression or an unacceptable level of toxicity. In such cases, the platinum-containing drug is stopped, and patients continue to receive the same drug that was used in combination with the platinum-based agent (continuation maintenance) or a different drug (switch maintenance). Bevacizumab should be continued along with maintenance therapy in patients receiving this agent, as it has been shown to improve progression-free survival. Patients with an activating mutation detected after initial platinum-based chemotherapy is started should receive the appropriate tyrosine kinase inhibitor as maintenance therapy if it was not used sooner. Maintenance chemotherapy results in improved progression-free survival and is therefore considered an accepted treatment option in patients with responsive or stable disease following four to six cycles of a platinum-based treatment. If disease progression occurs while on or after first-line chemotherapy, patients are often treated with single-agent chemotherapy consisting of docetaxel or pemetrexed (for non–squamous cell cancers). However, response rates in patients receiving second-line therapy are low, and median survival is relatively short following progression after first-line treatment. Patients with an EGFR mutation or *ALK* translocation can be treated with erlotinib or crizotinib, respectively, as maintenance therapy if they were initially treated with chemotherapy. It is especially important to address goals of care and symptom management in patients whose disease progresses after they receive first-line chemotherapy.

Following curative-intent treatment for NSCLC, patients should undergo follow-up monitoring with a periodic history, physical examination, and CT of the chest. Follow-up monitoring is important in the detection of recurrence and new primary lung cancers, which occur at a rate of approximately 3% per year. In addition, smoking cessation counseling is important in the care of lung cancer survivors.

Despite these treatment interventions, the 5-year survival rate for patients with NSCLC is only 10% to 15%. This low survival rate is largely attributable to the finding that 70% of patients present with stage III or IV disease. However, 5-year survival rates for patients with stage IA disease is only 73%, decreasing to 36% for those with stage IIB disease, and lower for those with stage III disease.

- Surgery is recommended for patients with stage I or stage II non–small cell lung cancer.
- Adjuvant chemotherapy is appropriate for patients with resected stage II and stage III non–small cell lung cancer.
- For patients with stage III non–small cell lung cancer, the preferred treatment is combined chemotherapy and radiation.
- Metastatic non–small cell lung cancer (stage IV) is not curable and treatment is palliative; the benefit of systemic therapy in this patient population is confined to those with adequate performance status. **HVC**
- Patients with metastatic non–small cell lung cancer and adequate performance status should be treated with systemic therapy selected based on the pattern of metastatic spread and the results of histologic and molecular assessment. **HVC**

Small Cell Lung Cancer

Diagnosis and Staging

SCLC is a neuroendocrine tumor that is seen almost exclusively in smokers. Large cell neuroendocrine carcinoma is a form of lung cancer that is distinct from small cell carcinoma histologically but behaves and is treated similarly to SCLC. SCLC is characterized by rapid growth, with most patients presenting with locally advanced or metastatic disease. Like NSCLC, SCLC can be associated with several paraneoplastic syndromes, including hyponatremia due to the syndrome of inappropriate antidiuretic hormone secretion, hypertrophic pulmonary osteoarthropathy, inflammatory myopathies, Cushing syndrome caused by ectopic adrenocorticotropic hormone deficiency, and other various hematologic and neurologic syndromes. SCLC is also associated with superior vena cava syndrome (see Oncologic Urgencies and Emergencies).

Staging of SCLC involves a two-stage system that was first used in early clinical trials conducted by the Veterans Administration Lung Study Group. Limited-stage disease is defined as cancer confined to a single hemithorax, which could include ipsilateral supraclavicular lymph node disease, and requires that all disease be encompassed by a single radiation portal. Extensive disease refers to disease that extends beyond a single hemithorax. Typically performed staging studies include CT of the chest, abdomen, and pelvis; whole-body bone scintigraphy; and MRI of the brain. The most recent update of lung cancer staging has recommended that SCLC be staged with the TNM system used for staging NSCLC; however, because most patients with SCLC present with locally advanced or metastatic disease, the use of the TNM staging system does not alter treatment decisions in most patients.

- Limited-stage small cell lung cancer is defined as cancer confined to a single hemithorax, which could include ipsilateral supraclavicular lymph node disease, and requires that all disease be encompassed by a single radiation portal.
- Extensive-stage small cell lung cancer refers to disease that extends beyond a single hemithorax.

Treatment

The role of surgery in the management of patients with SCLC is limited to those with very early-stage disease (<10% of patients). Although no firm criteria can be used to identify patients for surgery, eligible patients should optimally have single, small primary tumors without associated lymph node involvement (T1-2 and N0). Patients require extensive preoperative evaluation to exclude occult disease, including invasive staging of the mediastinum with endobronchial ultrasonography or mediastinoscopy. Although no prospective data are available to guide clinical decision making, retrospective data indicate 5-year survival rates of 15% to 48% following resection depending on disease stage. Patients treated with surgery typically receive adjuvant chemotherapy, as currently available data indicate that surgery alone is suboptimal.

Limited-stage SCLC that is too advanced for surgical resection is potentially curable, but treatment outcomes are poor, with 5-year survival rates of only 10% to 15%. The mainstay of treatment is combined chemotherapy and radiation therapy. The addition of radiation to chemotherapy in patients with limited-stage disease has been shown to improve survival compared with chemotherapy alone, which is associated with a high risk of local recurrence. Radiation is typically started with cycle 1 or cycle 2 of chemotherapy. Cisplatin or carboplatin can be used in combination with etoposide. Patients who experience a complete response or a significant partial response to primary chemoradiation should be offered treatment with prophylactic cranial irradiation to reduce the incidence of brain metastases and improve overall survival.

Extensive-stage SCLC is treated with chemotherapy usually consisting of cisplatin or carboplatin combined with etoposide or irinotecan and given for four to six cycles. Although response rates to chemotherapy are high, overall treatment outcomes remain poor. Nonetheless, survival in patients with extensive-stage SCLC who receive chemotherapy is superior to those who do not receive chemotherapy. As with limited-stage disease, cisplatin or carboplatin is used as initial therapy, but carboplatin is most commonly used owing to its more favorable side effect profile. Patients with extensive-stage disease who respond to initial chemotherapy also should be offered prophylactic cranial irradiation.

Unfortunately, even in the setting of significant tumor response, patients with extensive-stage SCLC will likely experience recurrent disease. The median survival following relapse of extensive disease is 4 months, but patients can still benefit from treatment depending on the timing and extent of the relapse and response to initial therapy. Patients with a good performance status who had a good response to initial therapy and whose disease progresses more than 90 days after initial treatment are most likely to benefit from second-line chemotherapy. Conversely, patients who experience relapse less than 90 days after completion of first-line chemotherapy, whose disease progresses while being treated with first-line chemotherapy, or who have a poor performance status are less likely to benefit from second-line chemotherapy. Although second-line chemotherapy can be offered, best supportive care is often more appropriate for these patients. In particular, patients with a poor performance status should not be treated with additional chemotherapy. Except in patients with extensive-stage SCLC who have experienced a late relapse following first-line therapy, combination chemotherapy is not used in the second-line setting because it provides no benefit compared with single-agent chemotherapy, and single-agent chemotherapy confers a reduced risk for side effects.

- Patients with small cell lung cancer who are considered eligible for surgery optimally have single, small primary tumors without associated lymph node involvement (T1-2 and N0) and require invasive staging of the mediastinum with endobronchial ultrasonography or mediastinoscopy to exclude occult disease.
- The mainstay of treatment for patients with limited-stage small cell lung cancer that is too advanced for surgical resection is combined chemotherapy and radiation therapy.
- Extensive-stage small cell lung cancer is treated with chemotherapy usually consisting of a platinum-containing doublet.

Head and Neck Cancer

Cancers arising in the oral cavity, nasopharynx, oropharynx, hypopharynx, larynx, paranasal sinuses, thyroid, and salivary glands are grouped together as head and neck cancer. Squamous cell carcinoma, which arises from the mucosa, constitutes 90% to 95% of cases of head and neck cancer and will be the focus of this chapter. Thyroid cancer is discussed in MKSAP 17 Endocrinology and Metabolism.

Risk Factors

Head and neck cancer constitutes approximately 3% of cancer diagnoses in the United States and is more common among men than women. Tobacco and alcohol use are well-described and potent risk factors that also can cause global mucosal alterations, markedly increasing the risk for second primary cancers involving other head and neck subsites. More recently, human papillomavirus (HPV) infection has emerged as an important risk factor for head and neck cancer, particularly for oropharyngeal cancer. HPV-associated oropharyngeal cancer has dramatically increased in incidence in North America over the past 30 to 40 years, accounting for 70% to 80% of oropharyngeal cancers diagnosed in the United States. This is mostly related to oral sexual contact. While not yet definitively proved, it is hoped that use of the HPV vaccine will be able to reduce the incidence of HPV-associated oropharyngeal cancers.

HPV-associated tumors differ markedly from conventional squamous cell carcinoma of the head and neck. These tumors occur almost exclusively within the oropharynx, develop in younger individuals, and are associated with a significantly improved prognosis, even when diagnosed at an advanced stage. However, despite the improved prognosis of patients with HPV-associated oropharyngeal cancer, HPV status does not currently factor into treatment decisions. Other risk factors for head and neck cancer include Epstein-Barr virus infection, HIV infection, various occupational exposures, and betel nut chewing. Persons with occupations placing them at risk for head and neck cancer include painters, wood workers, textile workers, farmers, and construction workers.

KEY POINTS

- Tobacco, alcohol, and human papillomavirus infection are important risk factors in the development of head and neck cancer.

- Human papillomavirus tumors differ markedly from squamous cell carcinoma of the head and neck as they occur almost exclusively within the oropharynx, develop in younger individuals, and are associated with a significantly improved prognosis.

Clinical Manifestations

Head and neck cancer is characterized by various presenting symptoms, many of which are nonspecific and therefore important for physicians to recognize to avoid unnecessary delays in diagnosis. An isolated neck mass is a common presentation prompting further evaluation. Other symptoms and signs suggestive of head and neck cancer are less obvious and include hearing loss (often unilateral), tinnitus, ear pain, non-healing oral ulcers, loosening of teeth, ill-fitting dentures, throat pain, dysphagia, hoarseness, bleeding, and unilateral nasal obstruction. Weight loss also occurs in patients with more advanced disease at diagnosis.

KEY POINTS

- An isolated neck mass is a common symptom in head and neck cancer and should prompt further evaluation.

Evaluation and Staging

Patients with suspected head and neck cancer require prompt referral to an otolaryngologist. The basis of diagnosis is the history and physical examination, which includes flexible fiberoptic laryngoscopy to facilitate direct visualization of the mucosa of the entire pharynx and larynx. Examination under anesthesia with diagnostic panendoscopy (laryngoscopy, bronchoscopy, and esophagoscopy) is done to obtain a biopsy, better characterize the anatomic extent of disease, and identify second primary cancers. Imaging studies, particularly CT and MRI, are important in evaluating the primary site and regional lymph nodes. PET and PET/CT are especially effective in detecting metastatic disease, and they can also help to clarify the results of MRI and CT imaging.

Staging of head and neck cancer follows the TNM staging system (**Table 59**). Although tumors arising from different anatomic locations are staged differently with regard to T stage, staging of cervical lymph node metastases is similar for all the different anatomic sites. Generally, patients with stage I and II disease have clinically negative lymph nodes, whereas patients with stage III to IVb disease have varying degrees of lymph node involvement. Stage IVc disease is typically limited to patients with distant metastatic disease. Patients with stages I and II disease are generally considered to have localized disease, whereas those with stages III and IVa disease are considered to have locally advanced disease. Although it occurs infrequently, metastatic disease must be excluded, particularly in patients with locally advanced head and neck cancer.

KEY POINTS

- The basis of diagnosis of head and neck cancer is the history and physical examination, which includes flexible fiberoptic laryngoscopy to facilitate direct visualization of the mucosa of the entire pharynx and larynx.

- In patients with head and neck cancer, imaging studies, including CT and MRI, are important in evaluating the primary site and lymph nodes, and PET and PET/CT detect metastatic disease and clarify results of CT and MRI.

Treatment

Treatment of clinical early-stage (typically stage I and II) head and neck cancer consists of surgical resection or definitive radiotherapy. One exception to this is nasopharyngeal cancer, which is treated with radiation alone for stage I disease and combined chemotherapy and radiation for stage II and higher (nonmetastatic) disease. Recurrence rates are generally similar for patients treated surgically or with radiation, and the selected modality most commonly is chosen based on expected morbidity and functional outcomes. For patients treated with surgery, the use of adjuvant radiation or combined chemotherapy and radiation is recommended based on findings at surgery. Factors indicating a need for adjuvant therapy include (Text continued on page 100)

TABLE 59. AJCC TNM Staging System for Head and Neck Cancer

Stage	Anatomic Sites						
	Nasopharynx	Lip and Oral Cavity	Oropharynx	Hypopharynx	Supraglottis	Glottis	Subglottis
Primary Tumor (T)							
T1	Confined to nasopharynx, or extends to oropharynx and/or nasal cavity without parapharyngeal extension[a]	≤2 cm	≤2 cm	≤2 cm and limited to 1 subsite of hypopharynx	Limited to 1 subsite of supraglottis with normal vocal cord mobility	Limited to vocal cord(s) with normal mobility; T1a: 1 vocal cord; T1b: both vocal cords	Limited to subglottis
T2	Parapharyngeal extension[a]	≥2-4 cm	≥2-4 cm	≥2-4 cm and/or invades >1 subsite of hypopharynx or an adjacent site and without fixation of hemilarynx	>1 area of invasion in adjacent subsite of supraglottis or glottis or region outside supraglottis without fixation of the larynx	Extends to supraglottis and/or subglottis, and/or with impaired vocal cord mobility	Extends to vocal cord(s) with normal or impaired mobility
T3	Involves bony structures of skull base and/or paranasal sinuses	>4 cm	>4 cm or extension to lingual surface of epiglottis	>4 cm or fixation of hemilarynx or extension to esophagus	Limited to larynx with vocal cord fixation and/or invades any of the following: postcricoid area, pre-epiglottic space, paraglottic space, and/or inner cortex of thyroid cartilage	Limited to larynx with vocal cord fixation and/or invasion of paraglottic space, and/or inner cortex of thyroid cartilage	Limited to larynx with vocal cord fixation
T4a	T4 (no subcategories): Intracranial extension and/or involvement of cranial nerves, hypopharynx, orbit, or with extension to infratemporal fossa/masticator space	Moderately advanced local disease[b]. Lip: invades through cortical bone, inferior alveolar nerve, floor of mouth, or skin of face; Oral cavity: invades adjacent structures only	Moderately advanced local disease: invades larynx, extrinsic muscle of tongue, medial pterygoid, hard palate, or mandible[c]	Moderately advanced local disease: invades thyroid/cricoid cartilage, hyoid bone, thyroid gland, or central compartment soft tissue[d]	Moderately advanced local disease: invades through thyroid cartilage and/or invades tissues beyond larynx	Moderately advanced local disease: invades through outer cortex of thyroid cartilage and/or invades tissues beyond larynx	Moderately advanced local disease: invades cricoid or thyroid cartilage and/or invades tissues beyond larynx
T4b	n/a	Very advanced local disease: invades masticator space, pterygoid plates, or skull base and/or encases internal carotid artery	Very advanced local disease: invades lateral pterygoid muscle, pterygoid plates, lateral nasopharynx, or skull base or encases carotid artery	Very advanced local disease: invades prevertebral fascia, encases carotid artery, or involves mediastinal structures	Very advanced local disease: invades prevertebral space, encases carotid artery, or invades mediastinal structures	Very advanced local disease: invades prevertebral space, encases carotid artery, or invades mediastinal structures	Very advanced local disease: invades prevertebral space, encases carotid artery, or invades mediastinal structures

(Continued on the next page)

TABLE 59.	AJCC TNM Staging System for Head and Neck Cancer *(Continued)*						
Stage	**Anatomic Sites**						
	Nasopharynx	**Lip and Oral Cavity**	**Oropharynx**	**Hypopharynx**	**Supraglottis**	**Glottis**	**Subglottis**
Regional Lymph Nodes (N)[e]							
N1	Unilateral metastasis in cervical lymph node(s), ≤6 cm, above supra-clavicular fossa, and/or unilateral or bilateral, retropharyngeal lymph nodes, ≤6 cm[f]		Single ipsilateral node ≤3 cm				
N2a	N2 (not divided into sub-categories): Bilateral metastasis in cervical lymph node(s), ≤6 cm, above supra-clavicular fossa[f]		Single ipsilateral node >3 cm and ≤6 cm				
N2b	n/a		Multiple ipsilateral nodes, none >6 cm				
N2c	n/a		Bilateral or contralateral nodes, none >6 cm				
N3	Metastasis in a lymph node(s)[f] >6 cm (N3a) and/or to supraclavicular fossa (N3b)[f,g]		One or more nodes >6 cm				
Distant Metastasis (M)							
M0	No distant metastasis		No distant metastasis				
M1	Distant metastasis		Distant metastasis				
Anatomic Stage/Prognostic Groups							
Stage I	T1N0M0		T1N0M0				
Stage II	T2N0M0 or T1-2N1M0		T2N0M0				
Stage III	T1-2N2M0 or T3N0-2M0		T3N0M0 or T1-3N1M0				
Stage IVA	T4N0-2M0		T4aN0-2M0 or T1-3N2M0				
Stage IVB	Any T,N3,M0		Any T, N3, M0 or T4b, any N, M0				
Stage IVC	Any T, any N, M1		Any T, any N, M1				

AJCC = American Joint Committee on Cancer; n/a = not applicable.

[a]Parapharyngeal extension denotes posterolateral infiltration of tumor.

[b]Superficial erosion alone of bone/tooth socket by gingival primary is not sufficient to classify a tumor as T4.

[c]Mucosal extension to lingual surface of epiglottis from primary tumors of the base of the tongue and vallecula does not constitute invasion of larynx.

[d]Central compartment soft tissue includes prelaryngeal strap muscles and subcutaneous fat.

[e]For hypopharynx, metastases at level VII are considered regional lymph node metastases.

[f]Midline nodes are considered ipsilateral nodes.

[g]Supraclavicular zone or fossa is relevant to the staging of nasopharyngeal carcinoma and is the triangular region originally described by Ho. It is defined by three points: (1) the superior margin of the sternal end of the clavicle, (2) the superior margin of the lateral end of the clavicle, (3) the point where the neck meets the shoulder. Note that this would include caudal portions of levels IV and VB. All cases with lymph nodes (whole or part) in the fossa are considered N3b.

With kind permission from Springer Science+Business Media: Edge SB, Byrd DR, Compton CC, Fritz AG, Greene F, Trotti A, eds. AJCC Cancer Staging Manual. 7th Ed. New York, NY: Springer; 2010.

close or positive surgical margins, the presence of lymphovascular or perineural invasion, and identification of T3 or T4 disease. The expected 5-year survival rate for patients with early-stage disease is 70% to 90%, although patients with tobacco- or alcohol-related cancer have a substantial risk of developing a second primary cancer.

Initial treatment of locally advanced disease consists of surgery or combined-modality therapy, depending on the expected morbidity and functional outcomes associated with these treatments. In general, surgery is preferred for oral cavity cancers because these tumors are usually easily accessible and can be resected with good functional outcomes using modern reconstruction techniques. Locally advanced tumors arising from other anatomic sites are more commonly treated with combined-modality therapy to preserve organ function. Concurrent chemotherapy and radiation is the accepted standard of care, with sequential chemotherapy and radiation or radiation alone for patients who cannot tolerate combined-modality therapy. The most commonly used agent is high-dose cisplatin. Cetuximab, a monoclonal antibody directed against the epidermal growth factor receptor, is also an accepted standard of care in this setting. In patients treated with combined chemotherapy and radiation, surgery for removal of the primary tumor is reserved for identification of residual cancer at the time of posttreatment assessment. Posttreatment neck dissection in patients treated with chemoradiotherapy is used only in those with residual disease in the cervical lymph nodes following treatment as assessed by PET/CT (or MRI in patients in whom contrast is contraindicated). The expected 5-year survival for patients with locally advanced disease is approximately 40% to 60%.

Patients treated with primary surgery for locally advanced disease almost always require adjuvant radiation or combined chemotherapy. Although many patients can receive radiation alone, patients with positive surgical margins or those with extracapsular extension of metastatic disease with lymph node involvement are at especially high risk of recurrence and should receive combined chemotherapy and radiation. Neck dissection is recommended based on T stage and lymph node status at diagnosis.

Chemotherapy is used in patients with metastatic disease, and treatment outcomes are generally poor, with a median survival of typically less than 1 year. Various agents are active against metastatic head and neck cancer and are chosen based on prior treatment history, timing of recurrence, and performance status. Cetuximab has also been shown to be effective in this setting as a single agent or combined with chemotherapy. Given the poor prognosis of patients with metastatic disease, early discussions about goals of care and symptom management are essential.

The treatment of head and neck cancer can result in significant functional impairment and disfigurement, dramatically affecting quality of life. Optimal management of patients with head and neck cancer requires a multidisciplinary treatment team consisting of not only physicians, but also nurses, speech and swallowing therapists, and nutritionists. Surgery can result in permanently altered speech and swallowing and disfigurement. Radiation or combined-modality therapy often causes xerostomia, thickening of saliva, mucositis, dysphagia, odynophagia, and malnutrition. Insertion of a percutaneous gastrostomy tube prior to treatment is recommended for some patients, particularly those with significant dysphagia or malnutrition at diagnosis. Late complications can include trismus, peripheral neuropathy, kidney failure, chronic pain, hypothyroidism, tooth decay, and second cancers.

KEY POINTS

- Treatment of clinical early-stage (typically stage I and II) head and neck cancer consists of surgical resection or definitive radiotherapy depending on expected morbidity and functional outcomes.

- Initial treatment of locally advanced head and neck cancer consists of surgery (most likely with adjuvant radiation or combined chemotherapy) or combined-modality therapy.

- Patients treated with primary surgery for locally advanced head and neck cancer almost always require adjuvant radiation or combined chemotherapy.

- Chemotherapy is used in patients with metastatic head and neck cancer, and treatment outcomes are generally poor, with a median survival of typically less than 1 year.

Posttreatment Surveillance

Posttreatment surveillance of patients with head and neck cancer is particularly important, especially in patients with tobacco- or alcohol-related cancers owing to the increased risk for second primary cancers. Surveillance in these patients is directed at both assessment of cancer recurrence and identification of potential second cancers. Conversely, patients with HPV-associated oropharyngeal cancer experience a much lower rate of second primary cancers.

The primary means of surveillance monitoring of patients with head and neck cancer is direct examination, most commonly by flexible fiberoptic laryngoscopy combined with conventional physical examination. Use of imaging, other than to establish a posttreatment baseline assessment, is recommended only as signs or symptoms warrant. Posttreatment surveillance should be done every 1 to 3 months for the first year, every 2 to 6 months for the second year, every 4 to 8 months for years 3 through 5, and yearly thereafter. Tobacco and alcohol cessation counseling is a vital component of posttreatment care because continued cigarette smoking or alcohol use is associated with decreased head and neck cancer–specific survival. Other recommendations include assessment of thyroid function every 6 to 12 months for patients treated with neck radiation and periodic dental evaluation for those treated with oral cavity radiotherapy. Speech, hearing, and swallowing evaluations are also performed as needed. Low-dose CT surveillance should be considered for patients with a history of alcohol- or tobacco-related cancer because of the documented survival benefit associated with its use in this setting.

- The primary means of surveillance monitoring of patients with head and neck cancer is direct examination, most commonly by flexible fiberoptic laryngoscopy combined with conventional physical examination.
- Tobacco and alcohol cessation counseling is a vital component of posttreatment care of patients with head and neck cancer because continued cigarette smoking or alcohol use is associated with decreased head and neck cancer–specific survival

Genitourinary Cancer

Prostate Cancer

Epidemiology and Risk Factors

Prostate cancer is the second most common cancer in the United States, with an estimated 238,590 cases diagnosed in 2013. The mortality rate of prostate cancer is disproportionally low to its high incidence. The incidence of prostate cancer varies significantly throughout the world, although these data are confounded significantly by the use of prostate-specific antigen (PSA) screening (see MKSAP 17 General Internal Medicine for a discussion of current issues relating to PSA screening).

Risk factors for developing prostate cancer are numerous and include ethnicity, certain genetic and dietary factors, and age, the most important risk factor. Currently available data indicate markedly increasing prostate cancer prevalence with advancing age. Black men have a significantly higher age-adjusted incidence of prostate cancer than white or Hispanic men and receive a diagnosis at an earlier age, with a higher serum PSA level and Gleason score, and they have more advanced disease at diagnosis.

- Risk factors for developing prostate cancer are numerous and include ethnicity, certain genetic and dietary factors, and age, which is the most important risk factor.

Diagnosis and Staging

An estimated 80% of newly diagnosed cases of prostate cancer in the United States are based on initial identification of an elevated serum PSA level. However, digital rectal examination (DRE) remains an important component of diagnosis because 20% of men diagnosed with prostate cancer undergo biopsy after identification of a palpable nodule on DRE. In addition to identification of actual nodules on DRE, prostate asymmetry or focal induration should prompt referral for biopsy, regardless of the serum PSA level. Prostate biopsy is performed by urologists, commonly using transrectal ultrasonography for guidance. Twelve specimens are taken, with six samples taken from each lobe. A negative biopsy, although reassuring, does not exclude prostate cancer, and in a man with an elevated PSA level or abnormal findings on DRE, close follow-up with possible repeat biopsy is warranted.

Mostly all cases of prostate cancer are adenocarcinomas (approximately 95%), which will be the focus of this section. Other histologies include transitional cell carcinoma, small cell carcinoma, and lymphoma. Important components of the pathology report include the Gleason score, the location and extent of cancer, and the presence of perineural invasion and extraprostatic extension. The Gleason score is a scoring system in which architectural features of prostate cancer cells are graded, with 1 representing the most well-differentiated histology and 5 representing the least well-differentiated histology. Two scores, representing the two most prevalent differentiation patterns identified in a biopsy specimen, are added together to derive a composite score (for example, $3 + 4 = 7$). The most prevalent differentiation pattern identified is listed first. The Gleason score has been correlated closely with the prevalence of nonorgan-confined disease and outcomes after definitive local therapy.

Staging of prostate cancer follows the TNM system. The most common stage at diagnosis is T1c, referring to clinically silent prostate cancer diagnosed on the basis of an elevated serum PSA level. Clinical staging is based on information obtained from the prostate biopsy, DRE, and, in some patients, imaging studies. Use of these data, along with the serum PSA level and Gleason score, facilitates risk stratification into five different risk categories (**Table 60**). This information is instrumental in guiding decisions on the need for imaging evaluation and local therapy. Imaging studies to assess for possible metastatic disease or regional lymph node involvement are only indicated for men with poor-risk features (typically men with intermediate, high, or very high–risk cancer).

- A negative biopsy, although reassuring, does not exclude prostate cancer; patients with an elevated serum prostate-specific antigen level or abnormal findings on digital rectal examination require close follow-up with possible repeat biopsy.
- In patients with prostate cancer, imaging studies to assess for possible metastatic disease or regional lymph node involvement are only indicated for men with poor-risk features (typically men with intermediate, high, or very high–risk cancer).

HVC

Treatment

Management options in men with clinically localized prostate cancer include observation, active surveillance, radiation therapy, brachytherapy, and radical prostatectomy. Active

TABLE 60. Prostate Cancer Risk Stratification

Risk Category	Definition
Very Low	Stage T1c, serum PSA <10 ng/mL (10 µg/L), Gleason score ≤6, fewer than 3 biopsy cores positive, ≤50% cancer in each core, PSA density <0.15 ng/mL/g
Low	T1-T2a, Gleason score ≤6, PSA <10 ng/mL (10 µg/L)
Intermediate	T2b-T2c OR Gleason score 7 OR PSA 10-20 ng/mL (10-20 µg/L)
High	T3a OR Gleason score 8-10 OR PSA >20 ng/mL (20 µg/L)
Very High	T3b-T4, primary Gleason pattern 5, >4 cores with Gleason score 8-10

PSA = prostate-specific antigen.

Adapted with permission from the NCCN Clinical Practice Guidelines in Oncology (NCCN Guidelines®) for Prostate Cancer V.1.2015. © National Comprehensive Cancer Network, Inc 2014. All rights reserved. Accessed January 16, 2015. To view the most recent and complete version of the guideline, go online to NCCN.org. NATIONAL COMPREHENSIVE CANCER NETWORK®, NCCN®, NCCN GUIDELINES®, and all other NCCN Content are trademarks owned by the National Comprehensive Cancer Network, Inc.

surveillance is the postponement of definitive local therapy coupled with surveillance using serum PSA measurement, DRE, and repeat prostate biopsy. It is only appropriate for men with very low–risk or low-risk prostate cancer with a life expectancy of at least 10 years. Men undergoing active surveillance receive referral for definitive local therapy if there is any evidence of disease progression. As of this writing, no randomized trials have compared the use of active surveillance with initial, definitive local therapy.

Options for local therapy include external-beam radiotherapy, brachytherapy, and radical prostatectomy. At the present time, there are no data supporting the use of proton beam radiotherapy in the treatment of prostate cancer. Unfortunately, no randomized trials to date have compared treatment outcomes or incidence of complications among these modalities. Furthermore, comparison of different studies is complicated by selection bias. However, some conclusions can be drawn. For men with low-risk, clinically localized prostate cancer, all three modalities offer excellent disease control. Radiation is often associated with symptoms of urinary irritation (urgency, frequency, dysuria), with brachytherapy causing these symptoms more commonly than external-beam radiotherapy. Radical prostatectomy is more commonly associated with urinary incontinence, with approximately 60% to 70% of patients having urinary leakage 2 months following surgery. Problems with sexual function are frequent in men treated with both radiation and surgery, although these complications occur more commonly following surgery. Bowel complications are associated with radiation therapy and include increased urgency, increased frequency, and diarrhea; however, these complications occur in only approximately 10% to 20% of men. Prostate cancer treatment–related complications occur most commonly in

the first few months after treatment, and they improve or resolve over time in most men.

Men with intermediate and high-risk disease, who were treated with surgery, should be treated with adjuvant androgen deprivation therapy (ADT) with a gonadotropin-releasing hormone (GnRH) if found to have lymph node metastasis. For men treated with external beam radiation, those with high-risk disease should be treated with ADT with a GnRH agonist for 2 to 3 years, while those with intermediate risk disease only require treatment for 4-6 months. For all men who have completed local therapy, follow-up monitoring for relapse and treatment-related complications is vital. Follow-up monitoring consists of a history and physical examination with serum PSA measurement. After radical prostatectomy, the serum PSA level should be undetectable; a PSA of 0.2 ng/mL (0.2 µg/L) or greater indicates active prostate cancer. However, after radiation therapy, the serum PSA level declines to a nadir but does not typically become undetectable; a PSA rise of 2 ng/mL (2 µg/L) or more above the nadir is considered a recurrence following radiotherapy.

Patients with a biochemical recurrence (a rising serum PSA level and no evidence of local disease progression) are treated with ADT, but the optimal timing of therapy remains to be defined. Studies have indicated that early initiation of therapy, before identification of clinical evidence of metastasis, is associated with decreased prostate cancer mortality rates but no improvement in overall survival. ADT consists of inhibiting androgen synthesis by using a GnRH agonist or blocking the androgen receptor with an antiandrogen agent. Bilateral orchiectomy is a reasonable alternative to GnRH agonist therapy, particularly in the very elderly. Initial treatment consists of a GnRH agonist alone or a GnRH agonist with an antiandrogen agent (a so-called complete androgen blockade). ADT is associated with a response rate of 80% to 90%. As of this writing, no evidence supports one approach over the other, and consensus guidelines indicate that either is appropriate. ADT is associated with significant side effects, including fatigue, loss of muscle mass, osteoporosis, dyslipidemia, hyperglycemia, and sexual dysfunction. Although intermittent androgen deprivation has been studied as a means of limiting ADT-associated morbidity, insufficient evidence exists indicating an improvement in morbidity without sacrificing efficacy; therefore, this approach is not recommended as a routine standard of care.

KEY POINTS

- Active surveillance, with the use of serum prostate-specific antigen measurement, digital rectal examination, and repeat prostate biopsy, is appropriate only for men with very low–risk or low-risk prostate cancer who have a life expectancy of at least 10 years. **HVC**

- Options for local therapy of patients with prostate cancer include external-beam radiotherapy, brachytherapy, and radical prostatectomy; proton beam radiotherapy is not recommended.

(Continued)

- Any identifiable level of prostate specific antigen (PSA) following surgery indicates active prostate cancer, whereas a progressive increase in the serum PSA level is required to demonstrate recurrence following radiotherapy.

Metastatic Prostate Cancer

Metastatic disease invariably develops in men with a biochemical recurrence. The most common site of metastasis is bone, and men with osseous metastatic disease are at risk for pain and fracture. Treatments available to target bone metastases include external-beam radiotherapy and bone-targeted radiopharmaceutical agents. Radiation is most appropriate for men with pain limited to one or a few metastatic sites. For men with multifocal bone pain due to metastatic disease, treatment with a radiopharmaceutical agent is indicated. Radium-223 has recently been approved by the FDA for this indication, and it has been shown to relieve symptoms and improve overall survival. Another important treatment for men with osseous metastatic disease is osteoclast inhibition. This form of therapy, using zoledronic acid or denosumab, reduces the incidence of skeletal-related events such as fracture or pain and mitigates bone loss due to ADT.

Whether they are being treated for biochemical recurrence or overt metastatic disease, men who receive ADT eventually experience disease progression. Prostate cancer that progresses despite ADT is considered castrate resistant. Disease in men who are treated with only a GnRH agonist may respond to the addition of an antiandrogen agent in this setting. In addition, castrate-resistant disease may be responsive to secondary endocrine therapies, including ketoconazole, megestrol, glucocorticoids, and estrogens. In addition, two newer therapies that target pathways of androgen biosynthesis have recently been approved by the FDA for treatment of castrate-resistant prostate cancer: abiraterone and enzalutamide. Both of these agents have been shown to improve overall survival in placebo controlled trials. Sipuleucel-T, an autologous dendritic cell–based therapeutic vaccine, has also been shown to improve survival in men with asymptomatic or minimally symptomatic castrate-resistant metastatic prostate cancer. Patients whose disease does not respond to these therapies or in whom disease progresses after an initial response eventually require chemotherapy. Docetaxel plus prednisone is the most commonly used first-line regimen. This combination has been found to improve survival compared with mitoxantrone, which was the standard of care previously. Cabazitaxel is a newer taxane that also has demonstrated efficacy in the treatment of metastatic castrate-resistant prostate cancer. Although chemotherapy is effective in patients with advanced prostate cancer, the median survival of such patients is less than 2 years. Given this prognosis, the use of chemotherapy in the setting of metastatic castrate-resistant prostate cancer should be discussed within the context of goals of care and palliative care.

- In patients with prostate cancer, zoledronic acid and denosumab reduce the incidence of skeletal-related events such as fracture or pain and mitigate bone loss due to androgen deprivation therapy.
- Painful bone metastases in patients with prostate cancer can be treated with external-beam radiotherapy and bone-targeted radiopharmaceutical agents.
- Patients with a biochemical recurrence of prostate cancer (a rising serum prostate-specific antigen level and no evidence of local disease progression) are treated with androgen deprivation therapy.

Testicular Cancer

Although the most common cancer among male adolescents and men aged 15 to 35 years, testicular cancer is rare among cancers, accounting for only 1% of all adult cancers in the United States. Testicular cancer management represents a true success story among solid tumors because it has been one of the most curable cancers since the late 1970s. The 5-year survival rate for all patients with testicular germ cell tumors is approximately 95%. Mostly all testicular cancers are germ cell tumors, which will be discussed in this section. Germ cell tumors can be pure seminomas or nonseminomas.

For most men, testicular cancer symptoms are attributable to local disease and include testicular swelling, identification of a testicular mass, or, occasionally, a dull pain in the lower abdomen, perianal region, or scrotum. Occasionally, men will present with symptoms caused by metastatic disease. Physical examination typically reveals a firm, often painless, testicular mass.

After a palpable mass is identified, testicular ultrasonography is performed to confirm the presence of a solid mass, following which radical inguinal orchiectomy is usually performed. Needle biopsy is contraindicated, as this can result in an increased recurrence rate. In conjunction with histologic sampling, it is important to measure serum tumor marker levels, which include β-human chorionic gonadotropin, lactate dehydrogenase, and α-fetoprotein. The serum α-fetoprotein level is never elevated in patients with pure seminomas, and β-human chorionic gonadotropin is only elevated in approximately 20% of patients with pure seminomas. Nonseminomatous germ cell tumors can contain elements of seminoma, but those elements are mixed with tumors with nonseminomatous histologies, which include yolk sac tumor, choriocarcinoma, and embryonal carcinoma. This distinction is important for determining the correct treatment. Once a diagnosis is made, a clinical stage is determined by tumor marker assessment and CT to identify metastatic disease and assess retroperitoneal lymph nodes.

Treatment depends on stage, histology, and, in patients with advanced disease, risk assessment based on disease extent and tumor marker levels. Because many testicular cancer treatments can affect future fertility, obtaining a sperm count and discussing sperm banking should occur before treatment is initiated unless treatment needs to start emergently. For patients with seminoma confined to the testis (stage I), orchiectomy is usually curative. Options following surgery include active surveillance, single-agent carboplatin, and radiation to para-aortic lymph nodes. Active surveillance consists of regular tumor marker and imaging assessments with the purpose of evaluating for evidence of recurrence. Patients with stage II seminomas receive adjuvant radiotherapy or cisplatin-based chemotherapy depending on the extent of lymphadenopathy. Conversely, in patients with stage I nonseminomatous germ cell tumors, depending on pathologic risk factors, post-surgical therapy can include active surveillance, one cycle of cisplatin-based chemotherapy, or retroperitoneal lymph node dissection (RPLND). High-risk patients usually receive RPLND or chemotherapy. Patients with stage II disease receive RPLND if retroperitoneal lymph nodes are small, with possible adjuvant chemotherapy depending on the extent of disease identified at surgery. For patients with bulky retroperitoneal lymphadenopathy identified on CT, cisplatin-based chemotherapy is recommended. Treatment of advanced disease depends on both histology and risk assessment based on clinical extent of disease and tumor marker levels. All patients with advanced disease receive chemotherapy, most commonly bleomycin, etoposide, and cisplatin, given for three to four cycles. Following treatment, patients are observed closely with periodic history, physical examination, and imaging and tumor marker assessments. For patients with residual radiographic abnormalities following treatment, surgery is sometimes recommended. Patients with relapsed or refractory disease are treated with salvage chemotherapy, and sometimes, autologous hematopoietic stem cell transplantation.

Survivorship issues are particularly important in men with testicular germ cell tumors because of the risk for various treatment-related complications, such as infertility from chemotherapy or RPLND, and the risk for second cancers, including some solid tumors and acute leukemia. There is an increased risk for metabolic syndrome (insulin resistance, hypertension, dyslipidemia, abdominal obesity) after chemotherapy or radiation treatment. Other potential complications include pulmonary toxicity, kidney failure, peripheral neuropathy, ototoxicity, Raynaud phenomenon, and cardiovascular disease.

KEY POINTS

- For most patients with testicular cancer, symptoms are attributable to local disease and include testicular swelling, a testicular mass, or occasionally, a dull pain in the lower abdomen, perianal region, or scrotum.

- After a palpable testicular mass is identified, patients undergo testicular ultrasonography to confirm the presence of a solid mass, following which radical inguinal orchiectomy is usually performed.

- For patients with seminoma confined to the testis (stage 1), orchiectomy is usually curative.

Renal Cell Carcinoma

Renal cell carcinomas arise in the renal cortex and are the most common type of tumors affecting the kidney. The next most common tumor, transitional cell carcinoma of the renal pelvis, is not considered a renal cell carcinoma and is treated similarly to bladder cancer. Patients with renal cell carcinoma are often asymptomatic until they have advanced disease, but possible symptoms include hematuria, an abdominal mass, abdominal pain, and unexplained weight loss. However, the classic triad of flank pain, hematuria, and a palpable abdominal mass occurs in only approximately 9% of patients. Incidental identification of asymptomatic renal mass lesions has been occurring with increasing frequency owing to the large number of abdominal ultrasounds and CT scans done for other reasons.

Renal cell carcinoma has been associated with various paraneoplastic syndromes, including erythrocytosis, AA amyloidosis, polymyalgia rheumatica, and hepatic dysfunction. For patients with symptoms suggestive of renal cell carcinoma, radiographic evaluation with abdominal ultrasonography or CT is recommended. Identification of a solid mass or complex cyst requires further intervention. Small lesions should be biopsied if possible. Larger lesions can be removed without biopsy if imaging findings are consistent with malignancy. Additionally, CT to evaluate the local disease extent and assess for metastatic disease is also recommended.

Patients with nonmetastatic disease undergo radical or partial nephrectomy. For patients who are not surgical candidates, active surveillance or ablative treatment can be considered for those with small tumors. No established adjuvant therapy for renal cell carcinoma is available, although studies using targeted agents are ongoing; consequently, patients with localized renal cell carcinoma are observed following surgery regardless of the local extent of disease. Selected patients with metastatic disease at presentation undergo cytoreductive nephrectomy, which has been associated with improved survival in some studies. Patients with lung-only metastasis and good performance status benefit most. Common sites of metastasis in renal cell carcinoma are the lung, liver, bone, and renal fossa.

Previously, metastatic renal cell carcinoma treatment was disappointing because responses to cytotoxic chemotherapy were limited and survival was often short. Although interleukin-2 can result in long-term remission in about 10% of patients, this agent is expensive, not widely available, and is associated with significant toxicity. However, because of rapidly expanding knowledge about the molecular pathogenesis of renal cell carcinoma, multiple targeted therapies are now available, and many of these agents have been shown to have significant activity against renal cell carcinoma. These agents are categorized as vascular endothelial growth factor (VEGF) inhibitors and mammalian target of rapamycin (mTOR) inhibitors. VEGF inhibitors include bevacizumab and various VEGF tyrosine kinase inhibitors, such as sunitinib, sorafenib, pazopanib, and axitinib. The mTOR inhibitors include temsirolimus and everolimus. Unfortunately, no studies comparing any of these agents have been published to date. Most patients receive a VEGF tyrosine kinase inhibitor in the first-line setting. Those with high-risk disease, which is determined by performance status, elevated serum lactate dehydrogenase level, elevated serum calcium level, and anemia, are often treated with an mTOR inhibitor, although sunitinib is also active against high-risk disease. Agents with demonstrated activity in second-line treatment include axitinib, sorafenib, and everolimus. Bevacizumab, a monoclonal antibody directed against VEGF, can also be used with interferon alfa in first-line treatment or as a single agent in second-line or later treatment.

KEY POINTS

- The classic triad of flank pain, hematuria, and a palpable abdominal mass occurs only in approximately 9% of patients with renal cell carcinoma.

- For patients with suspected renal cell carcinoma, radiographic evaluation with abdominal ultrasonography or CT is recommended, with histologic sampling done on identification of a kidney lesion that is characterized by a mass or a complex cyst.

- Patients with nonmetastatic renal cell carcinoma undergo radical or partial nephrectomy.

- The response of metastatic renal cell carcinoma to traditional cytotoxic chemotherapy is limited and associated with short survival; however, multiple targeted therapies, including vascular endothelial growth factor inhibitors, have significant activity against renal cell carcinoma and may improve survival in select patients.

Bladder Cancer

Bladder cancer is the most commonly diagnosed cancer of the urinary tract. In the United States, almost all bladder cancer is transitional cell carcinoma, which will be the focus of this section. The incidence of bladder cancer has increased by more than 50% during the past 20 to 30 years. Risk factors include advanced age, white ethnicity, various occupational exposures, and cigarette smoking; smoking is the most important risk factor and encompasses current and former smokers and individuals exposed to second-hand smoke. Individuals at occupational risk include metal workers, painters, miners, textile workers, and leather workers, among others.

The most common presenting symptom is painless hematuria, although some patients experience other urinary symptoms, such as frequency, urgency, or dysuria. Identification of new-onset hematuria in patients older than 40 years mandates urologic evaluation with cystoscopy. Biopsy or resection can be performed during initial cystoscopy, depending on the status of the lesion. Most bladder cancer is superficial and does not invade into muscle. These lesions often can be treated locally with transurethral resection of the bladder tumor. Following resection, additional treatment with intravesical bacillus Calmette-Guérin or chemotherapy is usually given, with the amount of treatment determined by risk assessment. The risk of recurrence and of new primary tumors is high following a diagnosis of superficial bladder cancer; consequently, careful surveillance is essential following initial treatment.

Cystectomy is recommended only for patients with frequent, high-grade recurrences occurring within a short period. Conversely, patients with muscle-invasive disease often are treated with radical cystectomy, although bladder-sparing approaches can be considered in some patients. Neoadjuvant cisplatin-based chemotherapy is also recommended, as it can improve survival in patients with muscle-invasive disease; however, the role of adjuvant chemotherapy is much less clear.

Treatment outcomes for patients with metastatic bladder cancer are disappointing. Although cisplatin-based regimens have been shown to improve survival, cures are uncommon, and median survival is only about 15 months.

KEY POINTS

- Identification of new-onset hematuria in patients older than 40 years mandates urologic evaluation with cystoscopy.

- Most bladder cancer is superficial, does not invade into muscle, and can usually be treated locally with transurethral resection of the bladder tumor.

- Patients with muscle-invasive bladder cancer often are treated with radical cystectomy, although bladder-sparing approaches can be considered in some patients.

Lymphoid Malignancies
Epidemiology and Risk Factors

Transient palpable lymphadenopathy is a common physical finding, particularly among young patients, and is virtually always benign, with less than 1% of cases persisting and later found to be lymphoma. Local or systemic infection with bacteria or viruses, drug reactions, and autoimmune disease can all be characterized by transient lymphadenopathy.

Lymphoma is the most common subtype of the hematologic malignancies and is heralded by lymphadenopathy. The fifth most common malignancy, lymphoma constitutes 5% of all cancers and 3% of cancer-related deaths in the United States. In 2013, the American Cancer Society estimated there would be 79,030 new cases of lymphoma diagnosed in the Unites States, 88% of which would be non-Hodgkin lymphoma (NHL) and 12% of which would be Hodgkin lymphoma. The incidence of lymphoma has doubled over the past 30 years; however, Surveillance Epidemiology and End Result statistics (SEER) reported a drastic improvement in 5-year relative survival rates for both non-Hodgkin (47% in 1975-1977 versus 71% in 2002-2008) and Hodgkin lymphoma (72% in 1975-1977 versus 87% in 2002-2008).

NHL occurs more often in men, and the incidence increases with age. Hodgkin lymphoma has a bimodal age distribution, occurring between ages 15 and 45 years and after age 55 years. The cause of some subtypes of lymphoma remains unknown. One exception is mucosa-associated lymphoid tissue (MALT) lymphoma, which is caused by an underlying infection with *Helicobacter pylori*. Other infections, including Epstein-Barr virus, HIV, human T-cell lymphotrophic virus type-1 (HTLV-1), and hepatitis B and C viruses, can also directly drive transformation of lymphoid tissue to lymphoma or contribute indirectly to transformation by causing immunodeficiency, which is also a risk factor for lymphoma. For example, patients who receive immunosuppressive drugs such as cyclosporine or tacrolimus following transplantation may develop lymphoproliferative disorders that evolve to high-grade B-cell NHL.

In addition to chronic inflammation caused by infectious agents, genetic factors and occupational risk factors predisposing to lymphoma include exposure to herbicides, chlorinated organic compounds, and other fertilizing material used in farming. Hodgkin lymphoma survivors have an increased lifetime risk of acquiring NHL, presumably because of the lifelong T-cell defect associated with Hodgkin lymphoma.

KEY POINTS

- The cause of some lymphoma subtypes is underlying infection, including *Helicobacter pylori*, Epstein-Barr virus, HIV, human T-cell lymphotrophic virus type-1, and hepatitis B and C virus infections.

- In addition to chronic inflammation caused by infectious agents, genetic factors and occupational risk factors predisposing to lymphoma include exposure to herbicides, chlorinated organic compounds, and other fertilizing material used in farming.

Evaluation and Diagnosis

Initial workup of patients with lymphadenopathy includes a detailed history of recent travel, insect bites, sexual encounters, injection drug use, blood product transfusions, and all new medications. Fever, night sweats, or unexpected weight loss should be documented. A comprehensive physical examination determines the number of sites, size (small versus large), and consistency (firm and fixed versus soft and moveable) of lymphadenopathy. In addition, careful assessment for enlarged Waldeyer tonsillar ring nodes and hepatic and splenic enlargement is warranted. Patients with soft, small, freely moveable lymph nodes that are limited to one or two adjacent sites and who have no other significant history or physical examination findings can be followed with serial examinations over 6 to 8 weeks and require no other laboratory studies or imaging. Persistent or enlarging lymphadenopathy, particularly when associated with systemic symptoms, may require

further assessment, including a chest radiograph, complete blood count with differential, and a serum chemistry panel.

To establish a diagnosis of lymphoma, it is optimal to perform an excisional biopsy to preserve lymph node architecture. Core needle biopsy can be used for deep lymph nodes in place of excision, but fine-needle aspiration should be avoided. The biopsy specimen is used for histopathologic, cytogenetic, fluorescence in situ hybridization (FISH), and immunophenotypic analysis and gene expression profiling. Routine blood tests should include a complete blood count with differential, erythrocyte sedimentation rate, and chemistry panel, including serum urate levels. Serum levels of lactate dehydrogenase, β_2-microglobulin, and immune globulins should also be assessed to assist in diagnosis and establish prognosis. Screening for viral infections, including hepatitis B and C viruses, HIV, HTLV-1, human herpesvirus-8, Epstein-Barr virus, and when indicated in gastric lymphoma, *H. pylori* infection, is appropriate to identify possible causative drivers of lymphoma.

After a histologic diagnosis of lymphoma is made, a total-body PET/CT scan and an iliac crest bone marrow biopsy are done to complete staging. Patients with aggressive lymphoma with involvement of the testes, sinuses, bone marrow, and ocular sites require a lumbar puncture owing to an increased risk for central nervous system involvement.

KEY POINTS

- Patients with small, soft, freely moveable lymph nodes **HVC**
  that are limited to one or two adjacent sites and who
  have no other significant history or physical examination findings can be followed with serial examinations
  and require no laboratory studies or imaging.

- Persistent or enlarging lymphadenopathy, particularly
  when associated with systemic symptoms, may require
  further assessment, including a chest radiograph, a
  complete blood count with differential, a serum chemistry panel, and assessment for viral infections.

- Excisional biopsy and core biopsy for deep lymphadenopathy are appropriate for diagnosing lymphoma;
  however, fine-needle aspiration should not be used.

Classification, Staging, and Prognosis of Malignant Lymphoma

NHL consists of more than 20 lymphoma subtypes defined by cell surface antigen expression and other morphologic features, including unique molecular profiles. NHL falls into two categories based on a B-cell immunophenotype or a T-cell or natural killer (NK)–cell lineage immunophenotype. B-cell lymphomas account for 85% of all cases of NHL, with T-cell (13%) and NK-cell (2%) lymphomas constituting the remainder. Classification of NHL and Hodgkin lymphoma is summarized in the 2008 World Health Organization 2008 classification system.

Staging of lymphoma consists of structural disease assessment using physical examination, CT imaging, and biopsy of potential disease sites and disease activity assessment using PET scanning to quantify the standard uptake value (SUV). SUV activity is an indicator of glucose uptake and metabolism, with more aggressive, quickly growing lymphomas using more glucose and thus associated with a higher SUV score. The Ann Arbor staging criteria can be used for determining disease extent for most forms of lymphoma (**Figure 16**).

Lymphomas are classified into three prognostic groups: indolent, aggressive, and highly aggressive. Traditional methods of staging used for other cancers are inadequate for prognosis and treatment planning for NHL. Because of this, the International Prognostic Index (IPI) was developed which generates a score based on patient age, performance status, serum lactate dehydrogenase level, disease stage, and degree of extranodal involvement. The IPI score correlates with progression-free and overall survival after standard therapy, and separate IPI scoring systems have been developed for diffuse large B-cell lymphoma (DLBCL) (revised IPI), mantle cell lymphoma (MIPI), and follicular lymphoma (FLIPI); however, new therapies, plus treatment with rituximab, have lessened the predictive value of these indices.

Indolent lymphomas may not require therapy for decades but are difficult to cure. Conversely, aggressive lymphomas, and particularly, highly aggressive lymphomas such as Burkitt lymphoma, require immediate therapy and often can be cured. Newer modalities of prognostic testing are available, including next-generation sequencing that assesses major portions of tumor genomes to identify mutations predictive of outcome to available therapies. Consequently, classic staging and IPI scores will likely become less relevant over time.

KEY POINTS

- The Ann Arbor staging criteria can be used for determining extent of disease for most forms of lymphoma.

- Use of International Prognostic Index (IPI) scores can help determine the prognosis of patients with diffuse large B-cell lymphoma (revised IPI), mantle cell lymphoma (MIPI), and follicular lymphoma (FLIPI), although new therapies, in addition to treatment with rituximab, have lessened the predictive value of these indices.

Overview and Treatment of Indolent Lymphomas

Follicular Lymphoma

Follicular lymphoma constitutes 20% of all cases of NHL in the United States and Europe and 70% of all cases of indolent

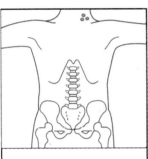

Stage I

- Involvement of single lymph node region; or
- Involvement of single extralymphatic site (stage IE)

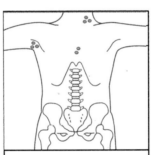

Stage II

- Involvement of ≥2 lymph node regions on same side of diaphragm
- May include localized extralymphatic involvement on same side of diaphragm (stage IIE)

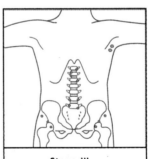

Stage III

- Involvement of lymph node regions on both sides of diaphragm
- May include involvement of spleen (stage IIIS) or localized extranodal disease (stage IIIE) or both (IIIE+S)

For Hodgkin lymphoma:

III1

- Disease limited to upper abdomen — spleen, splenic hilar, celiac, or portahepatic nodes

III2

- Disease limited to lower abdomen — periaortic, pelvic or inguinal nodes

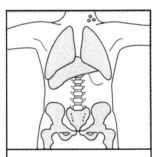

Stage IV

- Disseminated (multifocal) extralymphatic disease involving one or more organs (e.g., liver, bone, marrow, lung, skin), +/- associated lymph node involvement; or
- Isolated extralymphatic disease with distant (nonregional) lymph node involvement

FIGURE 16. Ann Arbor Staging System for Hodgkin and non-Hodgkin lymphoma.

Reprinted with permission from DeVita, VT, Lawrence TS, Rosenberg SA. *DeVita, Hellman, and Rosenberg's Cancer: Principles & Practice of Oncology.* 9th Ed. Philadelphia, PA: Lippincott Williams & Wilkins; 2011.

NHL, ranking second in incidence to DLBCL (30%). Follicular lymphoma is characterized by the presence of surface B-cell markers (CD10, 19, 20, and 22) and small cells on morphologic analysis. Incidence increases with increasing age (median age at presentation, 60 years). Invariably, patients present with advanced-stage disease, including bone marrow involvement (stage IV). However, unlike patients with large cell lymphoma, patients with follicular lymphoma have an indolent clinical course (that is, disease is slow to progress), with most patients having lymphadenopathy but no other symptoms at presentation, and some patients not requiring therapy for decades. Diagnosis is confirmed by biopsy of a palpable lymph node and cytogenetic analysis identifying a translocation [t(14:18)] that causes an overexpression of the *BCL2* oncogene.

An international prognostic score specific for follicular lymphoma (FLIPI) has been created that provides prognostic information and helps to guide therapeutic choices. Routinely, therapy is withheld until patients become symptomatic because it is generally not curative, and early initiation of therapy does not change long-term prognosis. Disease causing localized symptoms can be treated effectively with involved-field radiation therapy combined with rituximab. Symptomatic systemic disease requires multiagent therapy that traditionally includes rituximab plus cyclophosphamide, doxorubicin, vincristine, and prednisone (R-CHOP); rituximab plus cyclophosphamide, vincristine, and prednisone (R-CVP); or rituximab and bendamustine. Radioimmunoconjugates that consist of an anti-CD20 antibody directed against CD20-expressing lymphoma and that deliver targeted cytotoxic radiation by being conjugated with a radioisotope (tositumomab and ibritumomab) have been used effectively to induce long-term remissions. Autologous and allogeneic hematopoietic stem cell transplantation (HSCT) is used in younger patients with advanced symptomatic follicular lymphoma whose disease is responsive to standard chemotherapy. Allogeneic transplantation remains the only curative therapy but is associated with a significant risk for morbidity and mortality. New therapeutic approaches include maintenance rituximab for 2 years after completion of rituximab and chemotherapy. Combining rituximab with immune modulators such as lenalidomide may also be effective and may eliminate the need for cytotoxic chemotherapy. Salvage therapy with ibrutinib, a Bruton tyrosine kinase inhibitor, has recently been shown to be highly effective.

KEY POINTS

- The clinical course of patients with follicular lymphoma is usually indolent, with most patients having lymphadenopathy but no symptoms at presentation, and some patients requiring no therapy for decades.

- Allogeneic hematopoietic stem cell transplantation remains the only curative therapy for follicular lymphoma but is associated with a significant risk for morbidity and mortality.

Mucosa-associated Lymphoid Tissue Lymphoma

MALT lines the entire gastrointestinal tract, providing for immune surveillance and initiating immunologic responses to pathogens. Chronic antigen stimulation can lead to clonal expansion of MALT and progress to malignant transformation manifesting as lymphoma. The lymphoma originates in B cells in the marginal zone of MALT and expresses the CD20 surface antigen. The clinical course of MALT lymphoma is usually indolent, and presentation is usually localized. Gastric MALT lymphoma occurs most commonly, but MALT lymphoma can occur throughout the gastrointestinal tract and can also be characterized as extranodal marginal-zone lymphoma when involving a tissue independent of a lymph node. Constituting 50% of all cases of gastric lymphomas, gastric MALT lymphomas usually are localized (stage I and II) and almost always (70% to 98%) are caused by chronic inflammation of an ulcer bed resulting from infection with *H. pylori* diagnosed by upper endoscopy and biopsy. Strikingly, complete remissions are achieved in greater than 70% of patients with limited disease without chemotherapy after completion of antimicrobial therapy directed against *H. pylori* infection and concomitant proton pump inhibitor treatment.

For MALT lymphoma that is not localized to the stomach, or rarely, that is localized to the stomach but does not respond to eradication of *H. pylori* infection, surgical removal, involved-field radiation therapy, and, when indicated, anti-CD20–directed therapy with R-CVP may be effective. Isolated splenic MALT lymphoma is characterized by asymptomatic splenomegaly, circulating lymphocytosis, and a low level of monoclonal serum proteins. Complete responses can occur following splenectomy.

Patients with chronic autoimmune disease, such as Sjögren syndrome or Hashimoto thyroiditis, can present with MALT lymphoma of the salivary glands and thyroid, respectively. Other less frequent sites of presentation include the orbits, lungs, and bladder, all usually associated with a form of chronic inflammation. The large cell variant of MALT lymphoma requires the aggressive chemotherapy used to treat DLBCL.

KEY POINTS

- In patients with mucosa-associated lymphoid tissue lymphoma, complete remission is achieved in most patients with limited disease without chemotherapy after completion of antimicrobial therapy directed against *Helicobacter pylori* infection and concomitant proton pump inhibitor therapy. **HVC**

- For mucosa-associated lymphoid tissue lymphoma that is not localized to the stomach or is not responsive to *Helicobacter pylori* infection eradication, treatment includes surgical removal, involved-field radiation therapy, and, when indicated, anti-CD20–directed therapy with rituximab combined with multiagent chemotherapy.

Chronic Lymphocytic Leukemia

B-cell chronic lymphocytic leukemia (CLL) is the most common form of adult leukemia, accounting for 10% of hematologic malignancies. Patients with CLL present at a median age of 70 years, and, with newer therapies, median survival for affected patients is approaching that of age-matched controls. Patients are usually asymptomatic at presentation, with CLL identified by a relative lymphocytosis on a routine complete blood count. Although common in western countries, CLL occurs uncommonly in Japan and China and usually is characterized by a T-cell phenotype. Younger patients develop CLL less frequently, and, when they do, they usually have more aggressive disease. No definitive causative factors are associated with CLL, although it is more common among first-degree relatives.

Diagnosis is confirmed by flow cytometry indicating co-expression of cell surface antigens CD5 and CD23. Several staging criteria from the Rai or Binet staging systems are used. Early-stage disease (stage 0) is limited to patients with elevated lymphocyte counts, mid-stage disease (stage I and II) is associated with lymphadenopathy and splenomegaly, and late-stage disease (stage III and IV) is characterized by suppression of normal hematopoiesis (anemia and thrombocytopenia).

Prognosis is determined by gene mutation status (immune globulin variable heavy-chain mutation) and FISH or array-based karyotyping. In patients with CLL, a deletion of chromosome 17p is concerning because it is associated with a short median survival (<3 years). Whether to initiate therapy depends on several factors, including disease stage, patient age and comorbidities, lymphocyte doubling time, and other prognostic markers. Asymptomatic patients with low-stage disease (stage 0 to II) can be observed without therapy, often for decades. When therapy is indicated, the goal in most patients is palliation. Combination therapy with rituximab and multiagent chemotherapy (fludarabine, cyclophosphamide, and prednisone or rituximab and bendamustine) has been the most effective treatment regimen. Curative therapy (allogeneic HSCT) is reserved for younger patients with aggressive symptomatic disease.

Concomitant autoimmune disease, including immune thrombocytopenia and hemolytic anemia, is common among patients with CLL. Regardless of therapy, patients with CLL have a chronic immunodeficiency that may be characterized by recurrent sinus and pulmonary infections and low serum IgG levels requiring replacement therapy. Surveillance for viral infections and early initiation of antimicrobial agents for presumed bacterial infections are essential. Consideration for live virus vaccines including herpes zoster should be made early in the course of disease before a more profound immunodeficiency develops. Patients are at increased risk for second malignancies and transformation from CLL to a large cell lymphoma (Richter transformation) requiring aggressive multiagent chemotherapy with R-CHOP.

Hairy Cell Leukemia

Hairy cell leukemia is a rare disorder with only 2000 new cases diagnosed annually in the United States and Europe. The incidence is higher in men (5 to 1) and older patients. This disorder is characterized by an accumulation of malignant B cells in the bone marrow and spleen that manifests as pancytopenia and progressive splenomegaly without lymphadenopathy. Typically, an attempt at bone marrow aspiration is unsuccessful (a "dry tap") owing to reticulin fibrosis and packing of the marrow with B cells that have the classic appearance of thread-like projections emanating from the cell surface ("hairy" cells) (Figure 17). Diagnosis is established by bone marrow biopsy results and confirmed by expression of specific cell surface antigens. Treatment with a purine analog such as cladribine plus rituximab for resistant disease results in complete and durable remission in most patients.

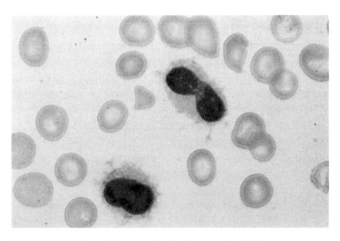

FIGURE 17. Hairy cell leukemia depicted by a peripheral blood smear showing atypical lymphocytes with thread-like cytoplasmic projections from the cell surface.

- Hairy cell leukemia is characterized by an accumulation of malignant B cells in the bone marrow and spleen that manifests as pancytopenia and progressive splenomegaly without lymphadenopathy.

- Treatment of hairy cell leukemia with purine analogs plus rituximab for resistant disease results in complete and durable remission for most patients.

Overview and Treatment of Aggressive Lymphomas

Diffuse Large B-Cell Lymphoma

DLBCL is the most common form of lymphoma, and when considered together along with the other less common form, diffuse large T-cell lymphoma, represents 30% of all lymphoma cases. Most patients with DLBCL present with advanced (stage III and IV) disease, fever, night sweats, or weight loss (B symptoms), and experience rapid disease progression without therapy. The way in which the T-cell variant presents depends on the course and subtype of disease.

The IPI is used to assist in determining prognosis before therapy and considers age, serum lactate dehydrogenase level, number of extranodal sites, disease stage, and performance status. Standard therapy for all patients with DLBCL, regardless of stage or prognosis, is R-CHOP. Studies evaluating more aggressive initial therapy for advanced disease in patients with high IPI scores including rituximab plus hyperfractionated cyclophosphamide, vincristine, doxorubicin, and dexamethasone (R-hyper-CVAD), as well as the addition of novel agents, including immune modulators such as lenalidomide, are ongoing. Involved-field radiation therapy is added for patients with bulky disease, with expected cure rates ranging from less than 20% for those with advanced disease and high IPI scores to more than 80% for those with localized disease and low IPI scores. Autologous HSCT is used as salvage therapy in patients with recurrent, chemotherapy-sensitive disease who experienced a disease-free interval of longer than 1 year from initial therapy. The use of allogeneic transplantation in patients with DLBCL remains investigational. Patients with the T-cell variant of large cell lymphoma are treated with CHOP, but outcomes for these patients vary significantly.

The most aggressive forms of large cell lymphoma are Burkitt lymphoma and lymphoblastic lymphoma. Onset of disease is acute, and patients usually present with life-threatening metabolic and structural abnormalities. Treatment is the same as that used to treat acute lymphoblastic leukemia (R-hyper-CVAD for CD20-positive disease), and it is associated with high response rates (80%) and is curative in nearly 50% of patients.

- Most patients with diffuse large B-cell lymphoma present with advanced (stage III and IV) disease, have B symptoms (fever, night sweats, or weight loss), and will experience rapid disease progression without therapy.

- Standard therapy for all patients with diffuse large B-cell lymphoma, regardless of stage or prognosis, is rituximab plus cyclophosphamide, doxorubicin, vincristine, and prednisone (R-CHOP).

Mantle Cell Lymphoma

Overexpression of cyclin D1, a cell-cycle gene regulator, is associated with a chromosomal translocation [t(11:14)] and can result in mantle cell lymphoma, a rare form of NHL that has a varied clinical course depending on the extent of disease. Usually, patients present with advanced disease characterized by lymphadenopathy, weight loss, and sometimes fever, and have diffuse sites of involvement, including the gastrointestinal tract, bone marrow, and bloodstream. Previously, most patients with mantle cell lymphoma treated with R-CHOP experienced brief remissions and limited median survival (<3 years). Newer approaches using more intensive chemotherapy such as R-hyper-CVAD and including autologous HSCT have increased median survival rates and, occasionally, resulted in durable complete remissions. Allogeneic HSCT, although associated with a significant risk of morbidity and mortality, can produce long-term remissions, even in patients with relapsed disease. Newer FDA approved agents active against relapsed disease include bortezomib, a proteasome inhibitor; temsirolimus; and ibrutinib.

Fifteen percent of patients with mantle cell lymphoma present with localized and indolent disease. This group is younger (<65 years), has normal serum lactate dehydrogenase and serum β_2-microglobulin levels, and has no B symptoms. Median survival in these patients exceeds 6 years, and initiation of therapy can be delayed until symptoms develop. The variable course of mantle cell lymphoma led to the development of a graded prognostic score (MIPI) to guide therapy.

- Most patients with mantle cell lymphoma present with advanced disease characterized by lymphadenopathy, weight loss, and occasionally fever, and have diffuse sites of involvement, including the gastrointestinal tract, bone marrow, and bloodstream.

- Allogeneic hematopoietic stem cell transplantation, although associated with a significant risk of morbidity and mortality, can produce long-term remissions in patients with mantle cell lymphoma, even in those with relapsed disease.

Hodgkin Lymphoma

Hodgkin lymphoma encompasses four classic histologic subtypes (nodular sclerosing, mixed cellularity, lymphocyte predominant, and lymphocyte depleted) and one nonclassic subtype (nodular lymphocyte-predominant subtype expressing the CD20 cell surface antigen). Hodgkin lymphoma is distinctive among lymphomas because it commonly presents locally, is associated with firm lymphadenopathy, and allows for therapy to be more readily limited in intensity and duration based on stage and risk factors compared with other types of lymphoma. The presentation is consistent among subtypes and is characterized by palpable, firm lymph nodes, and, in some patients, B symptoms. Other physical examination findings include splenomegaly (30%) and hepatomegaly (5%).

Hodgkin lymphoma is curable in most patients, even those with advanced disease. Therapy is not based on histology in classic Hodgkin lymphoma but rather on stage. The staging evaluation consists of PET scanning and a bone marrow biopsy after lymph node biopsy results confirm a diagnosis.

Stage I and II disease in patients without B symptoms (limited to lymph nodes and the same side of the diaphragm) can be treated effectively with radiation alone or radiation combined with a short course of chemotherapy. Patients with advanced disease (stage III and IV) or those with B symptoms, regardless of stage, usually require a full course of chemotherapy. The combination of doxorubicin, bleomycin, vinblastine, and dacarbazine remains the standard of care for all stages of classic Hodgkin lymphoma when chemotherapy is indicated. Rituximab is added to this combination in patients with CD20-positive disease (nodular lymphocyte–predominant subtype).

The goal of treatment is to administer the least amount of chemotherapy sufficient to achieve a durable remission (cure) while avoiding early and late (chronic) therapy-related toxicity. Therapy-related toxicities include bleomycin-induced pneumonitis, doxorubicin-induced cardiac dysfunction, vincristine-induced neuropathy, and late second malignancies and myelodysplasia. Early repeat PET scanning provides important prognostic information in patients with Hodgkin lymphoma, but not in those with NHL. Patients with Hodgkin lymphoma who have a normal PET scan after two to three cycles of chemotherapy, regardless of residual lymphadenopathy, have more than a 90% likelihood of long-term disease response compared with those with residual PET activity, who have less than a 15% likelihood of being cured with standard therapy. Multiple prognostic risk scores are available to assist in determining long-term prognosis, but PET findings in response to two to three cycles of chemotherapy may be more predictive.

Multiple effective salvage therapies are available for patients with recurrent and resistant Hodgkin lymphoma. Patients with recurrent chemotherapy-sensitive disease are usually candidates for autologous HSCT, whereas those with disease resistant to salvage chemotherapy may achieve long-term remissions with allogeneic HSCT. Brentuximab, an anti-CD30 monoclonal antibody, is also effective as salvage therapy. Patients with Hodgkin lymphoma, including those cured by therapy, may have long-term deficits in T-cell function and should be monitored for late reactivation of viruses.

KEY POINTS

- Hodgkin lymphoma is curable in most patients, even those with advanced disease.

- Patients with stage I and II Hodgkin lymphoma without B symptoms can be treated effectively with radiation alone or radiation combined with a short course of chemotherapy, whereas those with stage III and IV disease or with B symptoms, regardless of stage, usually require a full course of chemotherapy.

- Patients with recurrent chemotherapy-sensitive Hodgkin lymphoma usually are candidates for autologous hematopoietic stem cell transplantation, whereas those with disease resistant to salvage chemotherapy may achieve long-term remissions with allogeneic hematopoietic stem cell transplantation.

Cutaneous T-Cell Non-Hodgkin Lymphoma

The more common forms of cutaneous T-cell NHL are lymphomas expressing T-cell surface antigens (CD4) that infiltrate skin and initially cause rash (mycosis fungoides), and occasionally, circulate in the blood (Sézary syndrome). The large CD4-expressing malignant T cells have classic cerebriform-appearing nuclei and clonal T-cell receptor gene rearrangements. Presentation begins with small areas of pruritic erythema. Disease progression manifests with raised plaques, diffuse skin erythema, and skin ulcers. In the final stages of disease progression, organ infiltration and evolving immunodeficiency cause recurrent bacterial infections, sepsis, and death.

Therapy is guided by disease stage. Early-stage disease (stages I and II) is limited to the skin only and is associated with a median survival of more than 20 years. Early-stage disease is treated effectively with topical glucocorticoids and, when needed, additional retinoids such as bexarotene as well as psoralen and ultraviolet A (PUVA) therapy that can be combined with interferon alfa. Advanced-stage disease (stages III and IV) is characterized by extensive skin and organ involvement and is associated with a median survival of 4 years. Advanced-stage disease requires more aggressive therapy, including electron-beam radiation therapy; photopheresis; chemotherapy including methotrexate, gemcitabine, and CHOP; purine analogs such as pentostatin; histone deacetylase inhibitors such as romidepsin and vorinostat; and monoclonal antibodies such as alemtuzumab. Allogeneic HSCT may be curative in young patients with an appropriate donor.

- Early-stage cutaneous T-cell non-Hodgkin lymphoma is treated with topical glucocorticoids, retinoids (when needed), and psoralen and ultraviolet light with interferon alfa.

- Advanced-stage cutaneous T-cell non-Hodgkin lymphoma is treated with chemotherapy, purine analogs, histone deacetylase inhibitors, and monoclonal antibodies.

- Allogeneic hematopoietic stem cell transplantation may be curative in young patients with an appropriate donor.

Cancer of Unknown Primary Site

Introduction

In the United States, approximately 35,000 patients receive a diagnosis of cancer of unknown primary site (CUP) annually. Continued improvements in diagnostic imaging have resulted in decreased frequency of CUP diagnosis.

Diagnosis and Evaluation

CUP is a diagnosis of exclusion established in patients with a solid metastatic tumor after a detailed medical history and physical examination have been done and imaging studies or other diagnostic studies have not identified a primary tumor site.

Diagnostic efforts should focus on identifying whether a patient is among the approximately 20% of patients with CUP who have a more favorable prognosis and who can benefit from a specific treatment strategy. A biopsy obtained from the site that can be sampled in the safest, least invasive manner is performed, and specimens are evaluated by immunohistochemical stains consistent with the tumor's pattern of presentation to attempt to establish a diagnosis of a more treatable subtype of CUP. The clinical evaluation should not involve an exhaustive search for a primary site because detection of an asymptomatic and occult primary tumor does not improve outcome. Physicians should discuss with patients and their families that focusing on identification of the primary tumor can distract from the more important issue of managing the metastatic cancer. Efforts to identify primary tumors should focus only on those tumors that are suggested by the clinical presentation or could be managed with a specific, effective therapy. For example, upper endoscopy and colonoscopy are warranted in patients with evidence or symptoms of gastrointestinal bleeding but should not be done routinely. Men should undergo a testicular examination, a prostate examination, and serum prostate-specific antigen measurement. Women should undergo breast examination, mammography, and a full gynecologic examination.

Measurement of serum tumor marker levels, such as carcinoembryonic antigen, CA-19-9, CA-15-3, and CA-125, is rarely helpful and virtually never diagnostic. Although PET scans may sometimes suggest the location of a primary tumor, these findings are rarely definitive and do not improve long-term outcome.

Although several companies currently offer molecular analyses such as gene expression profiling or microRNA profiling to attempt to identify the site of tumor origin in patients with CUP, these approaches have yet to be validated in randomized prospective trials and are not considered standard practice.

- The clinical evaluation in patients with cancer of unknown primary site should not involve an exhaustive search for a primary tumor because finding an asymptomatic and occult primary site does not improve outcome. **HVC**

- In patients with cancer of unknown primary site, measurement of serum tumor marker levels, such as carcinoembryonic antigen, CA-19-9, CA-15-3, and CA-125, is rarely helpful and virtually never diagnostic. **HVC**

- Although PET scans may sometimes suggest the location of a primary tumor, these findings are rarely definitive and do not improve long-term outcome in patients with cancer of unknown primary site. **HVC**

Prognostic Subgroups of CUP

If a primary tumor site is identified, the patient no longer has CUP and should receive treatment that is appropriate for the new diagnosis. For those patients who retain a CUP diagnosis, evaluation is focused on identifying the prognostic subgroups into which their disease is categorized.

Favorable Subgroups

Isolated Regional Lymphadenopathy

Patients with CUP who have lymphadenopathy in a single lymph node or single lymph node region belong to a potentially more treatable subgroup of patients with CUP.

Women with adenocarcinoma limited to lymph nodes in one or both axillae have locoregional breast cancer until proved otherwise and should undergo MRI of the breasts. If a primary tumor is identified on MRI imaging, the patient should be managed as appropriate for her breast cancer. However, even patients with negative MRI findings should be treated for presumptive stage II breast cancer and undergo mastectomy and appropriate axillary lymph node management. Although a primary breast cancer tumor is identified on pathologic inspection of resected breast specimens in 50% women with CUP and axillary lymphadenopathy, the management and prognosis of these patients are similar to that of women with breast cancer whether or not a primary breast cancer tumor is identified.

Patients with isolated cervical lymphadenopathy should undergo triple endoscopic examination (upper endoscopy, bronchoscopy, and laryngoscopy) to identify a head and neck primary tumor site. However, even patients in whom a primary tumor site is not identified should receive chemotherapy and radiation therapy for head and neck cancer, which yields a high response rate and can be curative in some patients, especially those with squamous cell histology and nonbulky cervical lymphadenopathy. Patients with adenocarcinoma or supraclavicular lymphadenopathy have a worse prognosis; however, treatment recommendations for adenocarcinoma and squamous cell histology in these patients are similar in the absence of identification of other disease sites.

Patients with isolated inguinal lymphadenopathy should undergo a thorough anorectal, perineal, and genital examination. In the absence of identification of a primary site, resection or locoregional radiation therapy may result in a favorable outcome. Resection or localized radiotherapy may also be used to manage other isolated solitary or regional enlarged lymph nodes.

Peritoneal Carcinomatosis in Women

Women with CUP characterized by ascites and abdominal carcinomatosis are regarded as having ovarian cancer until proved otherwise and are managed with cytoreductive surgery and ovarian cancer chemotherapy regimens.

Poorly Differentiated Nonadenocarcinoma

Certain groups of patients with poorly differentiated CUP that cannot be identified as adenocarcinoma may benefit from specific chemotherapeutic approaches. Young men with poorly differentiated carcinoma that is relatively symmetrical around the midline and is characterized by bulky retroperitoneal or mediastinal lymphadenopathy may have an unrecognized germ cell tumor. These patients require measurement of serum α-fetoprotein and β-human chorionic gonadotropin levels, a testicular examination, and testicular ultrasonography. Management consists of platinum-containing germ cell tumor regimens and germ cell treatment paradigms.

Poorly differentiated neuroendocrine tumors constitute another nonadenocarcinoma CUP subgroup that may benefit from specific chemotherapeutic strategies. Metastases predominantly to the liver and to bone are common. Therapy with platinum-based chemotherapy using a regimen similar to that used to treat small cell lung cancer often results in responses, and occasionally, complete clinical responses. Note that only high-grade, poorly differentiated neuroendocrine tumors are sensitive to platinum-based regimens; well-differentiated neuroendocrine tumors do not respond to this approach.

Nonfavorable Subgroups

There are no accepted standard treatment regimens for patients with nonfavorable CUP (those patients with CUP who do not fit into one of the favorable subgroups); therapy tends to be empiric, and the prognosis is often poor. The use of gastrointestinal cancer regimens for CUP that is mostly below the diaphragm and lung cancer regimens for CUP that is mostly above the diaphragm is reasonable. Accurate assessments of performance status, as well as liver, kidney, and bone marrow function, are important when developing treatment strategies. Patients who are medically fit (Eastern Cooperative Oncology Group performance status of 0 or 1; see Table 48) are most likely to benefit from and tolerate aggressive chemotherapy compared with those who are debilitated or have multiple comorbidities and for whom supportive therapy may be appropriate.

Melanoma

Epidemiology, diagnosis, and staging of melanoma are discussed in MKSAP 17 Dermatology.

Treatment

Wide local excision is the standard of care for patients with nonmetastatic melanoma. Recommended margins are 0.5 cm for in situ lesions, 1 cm for melanomas with less than 1 mm of invasion, and 2 cm for melanomas with deeper invasion.

Sentinel lymph node biopsy should be done for melanomas 1 mm thick or greater and should be considered for thin melanomas less than 1 mm thick if high-risk features are present, such as tumor ulceration or a mitotic rate of 1/mm² or more. If the sentinel lymph node is positive or if lymph nodes are involved clinically, complete lymphadenectomy (removal of the remaining nodes in the involved nodal basin) is recommended.

Patients with melanomas that are 4 mm thick or greater or who have lymph node involvement have a 25% to 75% risk of dying from melanoma; adjuvant chemotherapy is not beneficial in these patients. Adjuvant immunotherapy with interferon alfa improves relapse-free survival, but its impact on overall survival is not clear. This agent is associated with significant toxicity, including fever, myalgia, fatigue, myelosuppression, depression, autoimmune disease, hepatotoxicity, cardiac ischemia, arrhythmias, and cardiomyopathy. Adjuvant interferon alfa is an option for patients with positive regional lymph nodes or skin metastases or for those with more advanced lymph node–negative melanoma (2-4 mm with ulceration or >4 mm) with no history of depression or autoimmune disease. Observation is also an acceptable option for these patients.

Patients with metastatic melanoma have a median survival of 11 months, and their disease is relatively chemotherapy resistant. In patients with metastatic disease limited to one or a few sites that is potentially resectable, surgical resection can result in prolonged survival. Immunotherapy or targeted therapy is preferred over chemotherapy. Chemotherapy can be used if patients are not candidates for these other therapies, or after their disease progresses while receiving other treatments. The most active chemotherapeutic agent for metastatic melanoma is dacarbazine, which results in a response rate of 19% to 25%.

Immunotherapy options for metastatic melanoma include interleukin-2 and ipilimumab. Immunotherapy is recommended as initial treatment in patients with metastatic disease that is considered lower-risk, typically defined as patients with minimal or no symptoms from their metastases; normal serum lactate dehydrogenase level; and metastases limited to skin, lymph nodes, or lung. Immunotherapy is also recommended in patients without a targetable mutation, even in the presence of more advanced or symptomatic disease. High-dose interleukin-2 is an option for patients with good performance status and is associated with a 15% response rate and a 5% to 6% rate of complete remission, with 50% of the responses lasting several years.

The monoclonal antibody ipilimumab is an immune check-point blocker that results in a 20% to 30% response rate with durable remissions; 60% of responders in clinical trials maintained a response for at least 2 years. Overall survival was improved to 10 months versus 6.4 months in the non-ipilimumab arm. This agent works by blocking cytotoxic T-lymphocyte antigen-4, leading to T-cell potentiation and an antitumor immune reaction. It is associated with clinically significant autoimmune toxicities, including colitis with risk of perforation, rash, hypophysitis, thyroiditis, hepatitis, and nephritis. These side effects are managed with vigilant follow-up and early use of glucocorticoids. Combined treatment with ipilimumab and nivolumab (an antibody against the programmed death 1 [PD-1] receptor) has led to rapid responses in a high percentage of patients with advanced melanoma in clinical trials. The anti–PD-1 monoclonal antibody pembrolizumab has shown substantial activity, including in patients previously treated with ipilimumab, and has been FDA approved for patients with metastatic melanoma whose disease progresses after other therapies.

All patients with metastatic melanoma should have their tumor assessed for the presence of a driver V600 *BRAF* mutation. For patients with V600 *BRAF* mutation, targeted therapy is recommended initially over immunotherapy for patients with poor performance status and/or more advanced disease. *BRAF* gene mutations are present in 50% to 70% of patients with melanoma. Vemurafenib is a selective *BRAF* inhibitor resulting in a response rate of more than 60% in patients with metastatic melanomas with a V600 *BRAF* mutation, with rapid tumor regression, a median response duration of 5 months, and overall survival of 13.6 months versus 9.7 months in patients receiving dacarbazine. Common side effects include rash, arthralgia, diarrhea, and secondary cutaneous squamous cell carcinoma.

KEY POINTS

- Wide local excision is the standard of care for patients with nonmetastatic melanoma.

- In a clinical trial for patients with metastatic melanoma, ipilimumab, a monoclonal antibody, resulted in a 20% to 30% response rate, with 60% of responders maintaining a response for at least 2 years and improved overall survival of 10 months versus 6.4 months in the non-ipilimumab arm.

- For patients with metastatic melanoma and a V600 *BRAF* mutation, targeted therapy is recommended initially over immunotherapy for patients with poor performance status and/or more advanced disease.

Prognosis and Follow-up

Patients with melanomas less than 1 mm thick with negative lymph nodes and no adverse risk factors have a 95% 5-year survival rate. Patients with 1-mm melanomas with negative lymph nodes have a 5-year survival rate between 50% and 85% (average rate, 70%). Melanomas in patients with positive lymph nodes are associated with a 5-year survival rate of 25% to 70% (average rate, 45%).

Patients with a history of melanoma should undergo annual skin examinations for life, perform monthly skin self-examinations, and undergo physical examination with complete history every 3 to 12 months for 5 years and then annually.

The goal of surveillance is to identify potentially curable recurrences and to monitor for second primary melanomas. Routine blood tests are not recommended. Although guidelines suggest discussing screening chest radiography, CT scanning, or PET/CT scanning with patients who have had higher-risk melanomas (positive lymph nodes, size >4 mm or >2 mm with ulceration), the value of imaging studies in asymptomatic patients is questionable, and many studies therefore recommend against their use.

KEY POINTS

- Patients with a history of melanoma should undergo annual skin examinations for life, perform monthly skin self-examinations, and undergo physical examination with complete history every 3 to 12 months for 5 years and then annually.

HVC
- In the follow-up care of patients with melanoma, routine blood tests are not recommended, and the value of screening chest radiography, CT scanning, or PET/CT scanning is questionable.

Oncologic Urgencies and Emergencies

Structural Urgencies and Emergencies

Superior Vena Cava Syndrome

Superior vena cava (SVC) syndrome is caused by acute obstruction of blood flow to the right atrium from the upper torso, can result in symptoms of progressive dyspnea and cough, and may be associated with swelling of the face and neck. SVC syndrome is usually insidious in onset and may less frequently be characterized by swelling of the upper extremities, chest pain, and pain on swallowing. Other physical findings include venous distention in the neck and chest, cyanosis, and facial plethora.

The most common cause of SVC syndrome is lung cancer (both small cell and non–small cell lung cancer), accounting for 65% of all cases. Other malignancies less commonly associated with SVC syndrome include diffuse large B-cell lymphoma, lymphoblastic lymphoma, acute lymphoblastic leukemia, Hodgkin lymphoma, and germ cell tumors. Mediastinal widening and pleural effusions are common radiographic findings; however, up to 16% of patients have a normal chest radiograph. Tissue biopsy is essential for establishing a histologic diagnosis and guiding therapy for the specific cancer type. Mediastinoscopy is commonly used to obtain tissue in patients with SVC syndrome, and is associated with a procedure-related complication rate of 5%. Percutaneous transthoracic CT-guided needle biopsy is another acceptable approach.

Symptoms can be treated with diuretics and glucocorticoids, if needed, pending results of a tissue diagnosis. Cancer type–specific therapy, including chemotherapy, radiation therapy, or a combination of the two, is usually rapidly effective (typically within 2 weeks) in ameliorating SVC-related symptoms. Anticoagulation may be required if complete patency of the SVC is not established. Salvage approaches have included endovascular stent placement, thrombolytic therapy, and embolectomy, with limited reports of success.

KEY POINTS

- Superior vena cava syndrome can be caused by various malignancies, with small cell lung cancer and non–small cell lung cancer the most common.
- Symptomatic treatment of superior vena cava syndrome is appropriate until a tissue diagnosis is established to guide cancer type–specific therapy, which is usually rapidly effective.

Neoplastic Disease-Induced Acute Central Nervous System Emergencies

Increased Intracranial Pressure

Mass effect within the brain causes progressive increased intracranial pressure (ICP), which, if left untreated, can lead to diffuse brain injury, permanent disability, and death. Although some primary brain tumors (such as glial tumors or lymphoma) may cause increased ICP, metastatic disease is a more common cause. Tumors originating from lung cancer and cutaneous melanoma are the most common malignancy-related causes of increased ICP and are also associated with intracerebral hemorrhage, particularly melanoma. Other less common causes of malignancy-related increased ICP include lymphoma and germ cell tumors.

Headache is typically the first presenting symptom followed by vomiting, altered mental status, focal neurologic deficits, and loss of consciousness as ICP increases. Because progression can be rapid, emergent assessment with CT of the head or MRI of the brain is essential to avoid the late adverse consequences of ICP leading to permanent neurologic dysfunction and death. When increased ICP is suspected in association with an intracerebral mass, lumbar puncture is contraindicated because the procedure can precipitate brainstem herniation. Conversely, diffuse central nervous system (CNS) involvement by a malignancy such as leukemia or carcinomatosis without a defined mass is not a contraindication for a diagnostic lumbar puncture.

Immediate treatment is essential. Glucocorticoids are the initial therapy of choice. Oral administration may be appropriate for patients without severe symptoms or associated clinical findings, although patients with impaired mentation, uncontrolled seizures, or those in whom oral intake of medication cannot be assured should receive intravenous treatment. Dexamethasone, 8 to 10 mg every 6 hours, is recommended for both oral and intravenous administration. Higher-dose dexamethasone (100 mg/d) does not improve responses and is associated with more adverse effects than the recommended dose. In patients with severe symptoms

CONT.

or complications associated with increased ICP, osmotic diuresis with mannitol in addition to glucocorticoids should be considered.

An isolated brain mass in a young patient, particularly in the setting of HIV infection, is suspicious for CNS lymphoma. When primary CNS lymphoma is suspected early in the course of increased ICP, it is appropriate to obtain a tissue biopsy before initiating glucocorticoids to preserve tumor cell viability for diagnostic purposes. In addition to tumor masses, malignant cells (leukemia, lymphoma, and melanoma) can cause obstructing hydrocephalus that usually requires surgical decompression. When ICP is controlled, elective surgical excision followed by focal stereotactic or whole-brain radiation therapy of isolated brain metastases should be considered. Multiple brain metastases are usually treated with radiation therapy and chemotherapy or tumor-specific targeted therapies such as ipilimumab for melanoma.

Cerebral syndrome, a consequence of capillary leakage from vascular beds, can cause edema and mimic brain metastasis. Cranial nerve palsy can be a consequence of viral infections or paraneoplastic syndrome or due to direct invasion of the cranial nerves in the subarachnoid space caused by leptomeningeal carcinomatosis. Other nonmalignant causes of pain and motor dysfunction include degenerative spine disease due to disk and bone spur impingement on nerve roots. Trauma or metastatic disease can cause cauda equina syndrome, which can be confused with spinal cord compression.

Spinal Cord Compression

Up to 10% of patients with cancer will experience neck or back pain followed by progressive neurologic dysfunction due to malignancy-induced compression of the spinal cord. The most common causes of spinal cord compression include cancer of the lung, breast, and prostate, and multiple myeloma. Because any malignancy can cause spinal cord compression, the symptoms of neck or back pain should be evaluated immediately in patients with cancer to avoid the potentially devastating consequences of progressive neurologic deterioration that can become permanent within hours to days.

Expansion of one or multiple vertebral body metastases with extension into the epidural space causes ischemic injury to the spinal cord and resultant neurologic dysfunction. Pain is uniformly the initial symptom followed by a sense of heaviness in the legs, progressing to leg muscle weakness manifesting as difficulty climbing stairs and rising from a sitting position. If untreated, bowel and bladder dysfunction and lower extremity paresis occur. Physical findings can vary, particularly early in the course of compression, with pain on palpation over the involved vertebral body, hyperreflexia, and diffuse lower extremity weakness being the most common findings.

Emergent MRI or CT of the entire spine should be performed to confirm the diagnosis and identify other potential asymptomatic metastatic sites. To avoid permanent neurologic deficits in patients with cancer and back pain, high-dose

intravenous glucocorticoids (dexamethasone, 20 mg) should be administered immediately on presentation followed by maintenance glucocorticoids until definitive therapy is administered on confirmation of spinal cord compression. Early intervention can completely reverse the adverse consequences of spinal cord compression, with standard definitive therapy consisting of surgical decompression or radiation therapy supplemented by chemotherapy in chemotherapy-responsive malignancies such as lymphoma. **H**

KEY POINTS

- Headache is typically the first presenting symptom of increased intracranial pressure (ICP) followed by vomiting, altered mental status, focal neurologic deficits, and loss of consciousness as ICP increases.

- Lumbar puncture is contraindicated when increased ICP is suspected to be caused by an intracerebral mass because the procedure may precipitate brainstem herniation leading to permanent neurologic dysfunction and death.

- Patients with cancer with unremitting neck or back pain should receive immediate medical evaluation, spinal imaging, and intravenous glucocorticoid therapy.

Malignant Pleural and Pericardial Effusions

The initial presentation in patients with cancer can include pleural or pericardial fluid, but more often this finding reflects advancing and incurable disease. Lung cancer, breast cancer, melanoma, and lymphoma are among the more common causes of malignant pleural and pericardial effusions, but any malignancy can cause these findings.

The usual presentation of pleural effusion is dyspnea on exertion, but chest pain, cough, and dyspnea at rest are also common. Patients with cancer and dyspnea should have a chest radiograph or chest CT to confirm the presence and extent of the effusion. Initial thoracentesis may be both diagnostic (with cytologic examination of the pleural fluid) and therapeutic. Thoracoscopy can be useful both for drainage and to allow for pleural biopsy which may be helpful in diagnosis.

In patients with pleural effusion, up to 20 mL/kg of body weight of fluid can be drained from a pleural cavity for symptomatic relief, but to avoid re-expansion pulmonary edema, no more than 1500 mL should be drained at one time. Unfortunately, malignancy-induced pleural effusions recur in 70% of patients. Periodic repeated thoracenteses may be effective with slowly recurring effusions whereas more rapidly recurring effusions may be managed with traditional thoracostomy tube placement or placement of an indwelling pleural catheter, which is a smaller drainage tube that can be managed as an outpatient. If spontaneous obliteration of the pleural space does not occur following prolonged drainage, infusion of agents to cause pleurodesis, including tetracycline, bleomycin, or talc, is effective in treating recurrent malignant effusions.

CONT.

Unlike pleural effusion, pericardial effusion may cause little to no symptoms initially and is usually identified as an enlarged heart on chest radiograph or low voltages on electrocardiogram. Patients with significant accumulation of pericardial fluid may present initially with dyspnea, orthopnea, and chest pain, and later with hemodynamic instability if cardiac tamponade develops. Prompt echocardiography is essential for confirming a diagnosis and facilitating intervention in patients with suspected malignant pericardial effusion.

Immediate subxiphoid cardiocentesis allows for drainage and enables proper cardiac chamber filling. Drainage is usually followed by surgical creation of a pericardial window or partial pericardiectomy. Chemotherapy, cancer-specific targeted therapies, or radiation therapy may be appropriate for patients with responsive disease.

KEY POINTS

- The usual presentation of pleural effusion is dyspnea on exertion, but chest pain, cough, and dyspnea at rest are also common; conversely, pericardial effusion initially presents asymptomatically and is usually identified as an enlarged heart on chest radiograph or low voltages on electrocardiogram.

- In patients with pleural effusion, no more than 1500 mL of fluid should be drained at one time to prevent re-expansion pulmonary edema.

- Recurrent malignant pleural effusions after prolonged drainage should be treated with agents that cause pleurodesis such as tetracycline, bleomycin, or talc.

- Echocardiography is essential to establish an early diagnosis of pericardial effusion to avoid progression to cardiac tamponade.

Metabolic Urgencies and Emergencies

Tumor Lysis Syndrome

Malignancies associated with rapid cell turnover can release large quantities of electrolytes and procoagulants into the circulation, causing the potentially life-threatening complication of tumor lysis syndrome. Spontaneous tumor lysis syndrome occurs commonly in patients with leukemia and Burkitt lymphoma and after treatment of bulky large B-cell lymphoma or advanced chronic lymphocytic leukemia. Rapid cell breakdown results in hyperkalemia, hyperphosphatemia, hyperuricemia, hypocalcemia, and disseminated intravascular coagulation. Hyperuricemia can lead to urate nephropathy and acute kidney injury.

Prevention of tumor lysis syndrome is optimal. Large-volume intravenous hydration with normal saline plus administration of allopurinol to limit hyperuricemia is usually effective. Because of its rapid onset of action and ability to lower urate levels quickly that may be renoprotective, rasburicase should be administered before initiation of chemotherapy in patients with underlying kidney disease or those with

signs of kidney disease, including an elevated serum creatinine level and a low urine output. Hemodialysis may be needed to address fluid overload, uremia, severe hyperkalemia, or hyperphosphatemia.

KEY POINTS

- Spontaneous tumor lysis syndrome occurs commonly in patients with leukemia and Burkitt lymphoma and after treatment of bulky large B-cell lymphoma or advanced chronic lymphocytic leukemia.

- Prevention and treatment of tumor lysis syndrome include large-volume intravenous hydration with normal saline and treatment with allopurinol or rasburicase when kidney disease is present.

Hypercalcemia
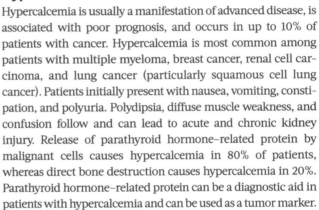

Hypercalcemia is usually a manifestation of advanced disease, is associated with poor prognosis, and occurs in up to 10% of patients with cancer. Hypercalcemia is most common among patients with multiple myeloma, breast cancer, renal cell carcinoma, and lung cancer (particularly squamous cell lung cancer). Patients initially present with nausea, vomiting, constipation, and polyuria. Polydipsia, diffuse muscle weakness, and confusion follow and can lead to acute and chronic kidney injury. Release of parathyroid hormone–related protein by malignant cells causes hypercalcemia in 80% of patients, whereas direct bone destruction causes hypercalcemia in 20%. Parathyroid hormone–related protein can be a diagnostic aid in patients with hypercalcemia and can be used as a tumor marker.

Immediate hydration with large-volume normal saline infusion followed by forced diuresis using furosemide restores intravascular volume and decreases serum calcium levels. In patients with malignancies that initially responded to glucocorticoids, including multiple myeloma, additional glucocorticoid therapy is warranted. Bisphosphonates are the most common medications used to maintain normal serum calcium levels, but can result in hypocalcemia. Osteonecrosis of the jaw and kidney disease can occur with repeated administration of these agents. Receptor activator of nuclear factor κB ligand (RANKL) inhibitors, such as denosumab, are also effective for achieving normocalcemia, are not associated with kidney injury, and are easier to administer and monitor than bisphosphonates. However, there is less clinical experience with these agents and they are significantly more expensive than bisphosphonates. Treatment with chemotherapy or disease-specific targeted agents is appropriate for long-term control of hypercalcemia.

KEY POINTS

- Hypercalcemia is most common among patients with multiple myeloma, breast cancer, renal cell carcinoma, and lung cancer, and can include nausea, vomiting, constipation, and polyuria on presentation followed by polydipsia, diffuse muscle weakness, and confusion.

(Continued)

- Aggressive intravenous hydration followed by forced diuresis is the initial management of patients with hypercalcemia followed by infusion of bisphosphonates or receptor activator of nuclear factor κB ligand (RANKL) inhibitors for long-term control.

Effects of Cancer Therapy and Survivorship

Introduction

Adverse events are common with administration of all forms of antineoplastic therapy; these effects can be acute and chronic and can negatively affect treatment efficacy, quality of life, and survivorship. Transient suppression of hematopoiesis is among the most common acute toxicities, manifesting with anemia, neutropenia, and thrombocytopenia. Newer agents, particularly cancer-specific targeted therapies, cause unique, and sometimes profound, toxicities, requiring expertise and vigilance to avoid vital organ dysfunction. Cardiac, pulmonary, neurocognitive, and reproductive late adverse effects, as well as secondary malignancies, are becoming more common as the number of cancer survivors increases (**Table 61**).

Acute Effects of Cancer Therapy

Hematopoietic Toxicity

Varying degrees of suppression of erythrocyte, leukocyte, and platelet production is common with most forms of antineoplastic therapy. Mild suppression usually reverses spontaneously or after temporary dose reduction or treatment discontinuation. Profound suppression can be life threatening and specific to the hematopoietic lineage.

TABLE 61. Cancer Treatment-Related Toxicities

Chemotherapy Toxicities	Representative Chemotherapeutic Agents
Myelosuppression	Most cytotoxic drugs
Emesis	Cisplatin, doxorubicin, cyclophosphamide
Diarrhea	5-FU, capecitabine, irinotecan
Alopecia	Doxorubicin, paclitaxel, cyclophosphamide
Stomatitis	Doxorubicin, methotrexate
Vesicant (blistering)	Doxorubicin, mitomycin
Peripheral neuropathy	Paclitaxel, docetaxel, cisplatin, vincristine
Pulmonary toxicity	Bleomycin, mitomycin
Kidney toxicity	Cisplatin, ifosfamide
Cardiac toxicity	Doxorubicin
Gonadal toxicity	Alkylating agents (e.g., cyclophosphamide)
Carcinogenicity	Alkylating agents, etoposide, and doxorubicin (AML), cyclophosphamide (bladder cancer), tamoxifen (endometrial cancer)
Hormonal Agent Toxicities	
Osteopenia	Anastrozole, letrozole, exemestane
Thrombosis	Tamoxifen
Biologicals and Targeted Therapy Toxicities	
Infusion reactions	Rituximab, trastuzumab, bevacizumab
Rash	Cetuximab, erlotinib
Fatigue	Sorafenib, sunitinib
Thrombosis/bleeding	Bevacizumab
Reactivation of viral diseases	Rituximab (hepatitis B), alemtuzumab (cytomegalovirus)
Reversible posterior leukoencephalopathy	Rituximab
Immune-related enterocolitis	Ipilimumab
Cardiac toxicity	Trastuzumab
Skin cancers	Vemurafenib

5-FU = 5-fluorouracil; AML = acute myeloid leukemia.

Neutropenia and Fever

Patients with a neutrophil count below 1000/μL (1×10^9/L) are at significantly increased risk of infection. However, antibiotic prophylaxis for prevention of infection during chemotherapy-induced neutropenia is not routinely given except in selected patients with profound neutropenia (defined as ≤100/μL [0.1×10^9/L] neutrophils) expected to last 7 days or longer.

In patients with neutropenia who develop fever or other clinical signs of infection, immediate treatment is necessary to prevent a potentially life-threatening infection as rapid deterioration can occur over 12 to 24 hours, potentially resulting in sepsis, shock, and death. Empiric broad-spectrum antimicrobial treatment is therefore provided before a diagnostic evaluation is completed, even if a likely source of infection is not obvious.

Patients with neutropenic fever are often classified as low- or high-risk. Individuals without significant comorbidities and in whom the duration of neutropenia is expected to be brief (<7 days) are usually considered to be at low risk for complications from neutropenia. Selected low-risk patients with stable vital signs and an unremarkable physical examination may be eligible for outpatient oral therapy at experienced centers with close monitoring capability. Treatment is usually with a fluoroquinolone in combination with an oral β-lactam antibiotic until the neutrophil count recovers. High-risk patients are those with an expected long duration (≥7 days) of neutropenia or the presence of advanced malignant disease or other comorbidities. These individuals are usually treated as inpatients with empiric parenteral broad-spectrum antimicrobial agents selected to also cover any suspected source of infection while further diagnostic evaluation is pursued. Appropriate antibiotic regimens include monotherapy with an antipseudomonal β-lactam agent (ceftazidime, cefepime, meropenem, imipenem, or piperacillin-tazobactam) or combination therapy with activity against both gram-positive and gram-negative organisms. Antifungal agents are usually used initially only in patients who are hemodynamically unstable, or are added in patients who are persistently febrile on broad-spectrum antibiotic treatment without an identifiable source of infection.

Hematopoietic growth factors, including granulocyte colony-stimulating factor and granulocyte-macrophage colony-stimulating factor, can decrease the severity and duration of neutropenia. They are FDA approved for prophylactic use with administration of myelosuppressive chemotherapy, although due to expense and modest effect on clinical outcomes, they are not used routinely. Their use is typically limited to patients receiving regimens expected to cause neutropenia in more than 20% of treated patients and/or profound neutropenia, and in selected patients at high risk of neutropenia-associated infection. The effectiveness of hematopoietic growth factors when used therapeutically to shorten the duration of established neutropenia or in combination with antibiotics in patients with neutropenic fever has not been established; therefore, they are usually used only in patients with profound neutropenia (≤100/μL [0.1×10^9/L] neutrophils) expected to be of long duration or associated with severe sepsis and hemodynamic instability.

KEY POINTS

- Patients presenting with fever and neutropenia (absolute neutrophil count less than 1000/μL [1×10^9/L]) require immediate medical attention and prompt initiation of antimicrobial agents.
- Hematopoietic growth factors, including granulocyte colony-stimulating factor and granulocyte-macrophage colony-stimulating factor, can decrease the severity and duration of neutropenia but due to expense and only modest effect on outcomes, they should be reserved for patients at high risk for neutropenia-associated infection.

HVC

Thrombocytopenia and Anemia

Thrombocytopenia can be life threatening when platelet levels fall below 10,000/μL (10×10^9/L), which is the usual threshold for transfusion. Use of platelet growth factors such as thrombopoietin is not considered standard practice for patients with chemotherapy-induced thrombocytopenia.

Anemia in symptomatic patients is treated with transfusions. General use of erythropoietin is discouraged owing to adverse events such as thrombosis and a decrease in overall survival.

KEY POINT

- Platelet growth factors such as thrombopoietin are not considered standard therapeutic practice for patients with chemotherapy-induced thrombocytopenia and are reserved for those with immune-mediated thrombocytopenia.

HVC

Disorders of Pulmonary Function

Acute and debilitating chronic pulmonary dysfunction can occur after chemotherapy and radiation therapy involving the lung fields. Bleomycin is the most common cause of pulmonary dysfunction associated with cytotoxic chemotherapy and can cause the most severe side effects. Usually, bleomycin pulmonary toxicity occurs after a patient has exceeded a cumulative dose threshold (400 U); however, acute presentations after one dose have also been reported. Onset of bleomycin toxicity can be insidious and is characterized initially by a dry cough. Serial pulmonary function tests can be helpful to monitor for decreases in DLco or forced expiratory volumes, but these tests are not always predictive. Early discontinuation of bleomycin is essential to avoid progressive dyspnea from evolving into bleomycin-induced pneumonitis, pulmonary fibrosis, and even death. Treatment of bleomycin-induced pneumonitis with glucocorticoids can limit its progression, but permanent residual pulmonary dysfunction usually occurs. High fractions of inspired oxygen should be avoided in all patients who received bleomycin previously to avoid late toxicity.

Involved-field radiation therapy, particularly when combined with chemotherapy, can cause pneumonitis that is effectively treated with glucocorticoids. A slow taper of the glucocorticoid dose is essential to avoid glucocorticoid-withdrawal exacerbations of pneumonitis.

KEY POINT

- In patients receiving cytotoxic chemotherapy, early discontinuation of bleomycin is essential to avoid progressive dyspnea due to evolving bleomycin-induced pneumonitis, pulmonary fibrosis, and death.

⊞ Disorders of Genitourinary and Kidney Function

Kidney failure due to renal tubular dysfunction can occur following administration of cisplatin and ifosfamide; consequently, serum electrolyte levels and kidney function must be carefully monitored. High-dose methotrexate used to treat osteosarcoma and lymphoma can also cause renal tubular injury, which can be avoided with aggressive intravenous hydration, forced diuresis, urine alkalization, and administration of leucovorin. Transient kidney disease caused by newer targeted therapies, such as sunitinib and vemurafenib, can be reversed with drug dosage reductions or cessation. Radiation therapy to the kidneys can cause acute and chronic kidney dysfunction.

Hemorrhagic cystitis can occur after any dose of cyclophosphamide or ifosfamide. Aggressive intravenous hydration with forced diuresis can limit renal tubular and bladder damage. The uroprotective agent, mesna, has greatly reduced the incidence of hemorrhagic cystitis. ⊞

KEY POINT

- In patients with cancer undergoing treatment with potentially nephrotoxic drugs, serial assessments of serum electrolyte levels and kidney function are required to avoid permanent kidney damage.

⊞ Immune-Related Toxicities

A new class of antineoplastic therapeutic agents directed against T-cell checkpoint receptors, such as ipilimumab or PD-1 and PD-L1 inhibitors, can cause numerous, potentially permanent and life-threatening, immune-related organ toxicities. These agents have caused autoimmune, hepatic, gastrointestinal, pulmonary, endocrine (hypothalamus, thyroid, and adrenal), and neurologic T-cell–induced damage that usually reverses with glucocorticoids. ⊞

Effects on Bone Health

Aromatase inhibitors, commonly used to treat breast cancer, can cause debilitating osteopenia resulting in pathologic fractures that can be avoided with calcium and vitamin D supplements and, when indicated, by use of serial bone density scans and bisphosphonate therapy.

KEY POINT

- Aromatase inhibitors can cause debilitating osteopenia resulting in pathologic fractures that can be avoided with calcium and vitamin D supplements and, when indicated, by use of serial bone density scans and bisphosphonate therapy.

Late Effects of Cancer Therapy

Secondary Malignancies

Patients with a history of cancer may have an increased lifetime risk for development of secondary malignancies owing to exposure to chemotherapy and radiation (treatment-related neoplasms), genetic susceptibilities (cancer genetic syndromes), shared causative exposures, and the cancerization field effect (for example, an increased risk for a second aerodigestive tract cancer in smokers with a previous cancer of this type). Hematopoietic clonal disorders, including myelodysplasia, leukemia, and lymphoma, can occur decades after completion of therapy. Typical agents associated with therapy-related myelodysplasia include alkylators, anthracyclines, and topoisomerase II inhibitors. Likewise, leukemia and lymphoma can develop as a late consequence of exposure to chemotherapy and radiation. Similarly, radiation-induced solid tumors, such as breast cancer after mantle radiation for Hodgkin lymphoma, are not uncommon, especially in women treated early in life. Thus, the overall cancer rate in cancer survivors is higher than that in the general population.

KEY POINTS

- Myelodysplasia can occur years to decades after patients with cancer receive chemotherapy.
- Radiation-induced solid tumors, such as breast cancer, are not uncommon in women treated early in life with mantle radiation therapy for Hodgkin lymphoma.

Disorders of Cardiac Function ⊞

Various antineoplastic agents can cause acute and chronic cardiac dysfunction. Anthracyclines such as doxorubicin are the most common cause of chemotherapy dose-dependent-induced cardiomyocyte damage, leading to late and irreversible chronic heart failure. Cardiac dysfunction can be avoided by limiting the cumulative dose and discontinuing anthracyclines in patients in whom a decrement of left ventricular function is observed during therapy. However despite these precautions, a 1.5% late risk of cardiac dysfunction after exposure to anthracyclines still exists. Cessation of therapy and aggressive medical management with diuresis and afterload reduction may lead to complete recovery of cardiac function, but sometimes, heart failure is permanent. Acute and reversible cardiac dysfunction can occur after treatment with trastuzumab, a monoclonal antibody directed against

CONT.

the *HER2/neu* receptor, the effects of which are not dose dependent. Involved-field radiation therapy encompassing the heart can cause premature coronary artery stenosis and left ventricular dysfunction. **H**

KEY POINT

- Cardiac dysfunction can often be avoided by limiting the cumulative dose and discontinuing anthracyclines in patients in whom a decrement of left ventricular function is observed during cancer therapy; however, even with precautions, a late risk of heart failure in cancer survivors still exists.

Sexual Function

Sexual dysfunction is common and underreported among patients receiving cancer therapy. Hormonal therapy and radiation of pelvic structures can impair sexual function in both sexes. Anxiety and depression may also play a role. Women may experience vaginal dryness leading to dyspareunia, and hormonal changes can result in loss of libido, arousal, and orgasm. Men develop erectile dysfunction but may also have loss of libido and ability to ejaculate. Physicians should directly inquire to determine if sexual dysfunction is ongoing during and after therapy. Social, emotional, hormonal, and anatomic causes can all be involved in sexual dysfunction. Phosphodiesterase-5 enzyme inhibitors such as sildenafil for erectile dysfunction and topical low-dose estrogen or nonhormonal lubricants for vaginal dryness and discomfort are effective treatments and, when given, should be combined with counseling.

KEY POINT

- Along with counseling, phosphodiesterase-5 enzyme inhibitors such as sildenafil for erectile dysfunction and low-dose estrogen or nonhormonal lubricants for vaginal dryness and discomfort can effectively treat cancer treatment–related sexual dysfunction.

Survivorship

General Principles

More than 14 million cancer survivors are dealing with the toll of treatment and its aftermath in the United States. Consequently, interest in developing guidelines and strategies to care for the immediate and late adverse consequences of cancer has recently increased. The process of both living with cancer as well as living beyond cancer is termed survivorship, and recommendations for survivorship care from the Institute of Medicine include the following:

1. prevention of new and recurrent cancer and of other late effects;

2. surveillance for cancer spread, recurrence, or second malignancies, including screening recommendations for new cancers;

3. intervention for consequences of cancer and its treatment, including medical problems such as lymphedema; neurocognitive changes; sexual dysfunction; symptoms such as pain and fatigue; psychological distress; and financial concerns about employment, insurance, and disability; and

4. coordination of care between specialists and internists to ensure that survivors' health needs are met.

Survivorship Care Plan

A "Survivorship Care Plan" (SCP) should be generated by a patient's oncologist and provided to the patient and the patient's internist when active cancer management is being transitioned to posttreatment care. The objective of the SCP is to summarize critical information needed for the patient's long-term care, including cancer type; treatments received, and their potential consequences; results of diagnostic tests; recommendations for timing and type of follow-up evaluation; and recommendations for preventive practices and health maintenance and well-being. Although several different models for survivorship health care delivery have been developed, it is important for the care providers to establish a clear plan to definitively delineate management responsibility among providers.

For more information on survivorship planning, see the Institute of Medicine's Web site at http://iom.edu/Reports/2005/From-Cancer-Patient-to-Cancer-Survivor-Lost-in-Transition.aspx.

Screening for Second Cancers and Lifestyle Modifications

Because cancer risk is higher among cancer survivors, with a risk as high as 30%, for example, in patients who have had head and neck cancer or lung cancer, diligent adherence to screening guidelines is imperative. Additionally, an emphasis on lifestyle modifications to reduce cancer risk is extremely important and includes smoking cessation, exercise, and weight loss.

Cognitive Function after Cancer Therapy

Cancer survivors often report cognitive dysfunction, particularly impairment of multitasking and executive functions. These problems occur most frequently after chemotherapy ("chemo brain"), endocrine therapy, and brain radiation. Recent studies support patients' reports of impairment in verbal ability, memory, and visuospatial and executive functions. A recent study showed that such symptoms occurred in about 20% of breast cancer survivors. Symptoms seem to improve with time.

Validation of patients' concerns and reassurance that symptoms usually improve over time may be beneficial. Interventions include management of contributing factors such as pain, anxiety, depression, and fatigue, and discontinuation of medications that might contribute to cognitive impairment. Nonpharmacologic interventions may include coping behaviors such as use of reminder notes and avoidance of multitasking. Pharmacologic interventions, such as modafinil, are under study.

Other Issues for Survivors

Fear of recurrence, sleep disorders, anxiety and depression, fatigue, and chronic pain may be part of the survivor experience and require medical management. Vaccination recommendations may differ for cancer survivors. Patients who are immunosuppressed from leukemia or lymphoma or from treatment such as allogeneic hematopoietic stem cell transplantation should not receive live herpes zoster; oral polio; attenuated live influenza; or measles, mumps, and rubella vaccines.

KEY POINTS

- A survivorship care plan and clear delineation of responsibility for follow-up care should be formulated at the completion of cancer therapy and provided to the patient and internist.

- Patients reporting impaired cognitive function after cancer treatment can benefit from validation of their symptoms and being told that their symptoms will likely improve with time.

- Patients with immunosuppression caused by their malignancy or its treatment should not receive live vaccines.

Bibliography

Hematopoietic Stem Cells and Their Disorders

Experts in Chronic Myeloid Leukemia. The price of drugs for chronic myeloid leukemia (CML) is a reflection of the unsustainable prices of cancer drugs: from the perspective of a large group of CML experts. Blood. 2013 May 30;121(22):4439-42. [PMID: 23620577]

Greenberg PL, Tuechler H, Schanz J, et al. Revised international prognostic scoring system for myelodysplastic syndromes. Blood. 2012 Sep 20;120(12):2454-65. [PMID: 22740453]

Hsieh MM, Everhart JE, Byrd-Holt D, Tisdale JF, Rodgers GP. Prevalence of neutropenia in the U.S. population: age, sex, smoking status, and ethnic differences. Ann Intern Med. 2007 Apr 3;146(7):486-92. [PMID: 17404350]

Kantarjian H, O'Brien S, Jabbour E, et al. Improved survival in chronic myeloid leukemia since the introduction of imatinib therapy: a single-institution historical experience. Blood. 2012 Mar 1;119(9):1981-7. [PMID: 22228624]

Lo-Coco F, Awisati G, Vignetti M, et al; Gruppo Italiano Malattie Ematologiche dell'Adulto; German-Austrian Acute Myeloid Leukemia Study Group; Study Alliance Leukemia. Retinoic acid and arsenic trioxide for acute promyelocytic leukemia. N Engl J Med. 2013 Jul 11;369(2):111-21. [PMID: 23841729]

Passamonti F, Thiele J, Girodon F, et al. A prognostic model to predict survival in 867 World Health Organization-defined essential thrombocythemia at diagnosis: a study by the International Working Group on Myelofibrosis Research and Treatment. Blood. 2012 Aug 9;120(6):1197-201. [PMID: 22740446]

Tichelli A, Schrezenmeier H, Socié G, et al. A randomized controlled study in patients with newly diagnosed severe aplastic anemia receiving antithymocyte globulin (ATG), cyclosporine, with or without G-CSF: a study of the SAA Working Party of the European Group for Blood and Marrow Transplantation. Blood. 2011 Apr 28;117(17):4434-41. [PMID: 21233311]

Vardiman JW, Thiele J, Arber DA, et al. The 2008 revision of the World Health Organization (WHO) classification of myeloid neoplasms and acute leukemia: rationale and important changes. Blood. 2009 Jul 30;114(5):937-51. [PMID: 19357394]

Multiple Myeloma and Related Disorders

Cavo M, Rajkumar SV, Palumbo A, et al; International Myeloma Working Group. International Myeloma Working Group consensus approach to the treatment of multiple myeloma patients who are candidates for autologous stem cell transplantation. Blood. 2011 Jun 9;117(23):6063-73. [PMID: 21447828]

Dimopoulos MA, Gertz MA, Kastritis E, et al. Update on treatment recommendations from the Fourth International Workshop on Waldenstrom's Macroglobulinemia. J Clin Oncol. 2009 Jan 1;27(1):120-6. [PMID: 19047284]

Kumar S, Dispenzieri A, Lacy MQ, et al. Revised prognostic staging system for light chain amyloidosis incorporating cardiac biomarkers and serum free light chain measurements. J Clin Oncol. 2012 Mar 20;30(9):989-95. [PMID: 22331953]

Kyle RA, Durie BG, Rajkumar SV, et al; International Myeloma Working Group. Monoclonal gammopathy of undetermined significance (MGUS) and smoldering (asymptomatic) multiple myeloma: IMWG consensus perspectives risk factors for progression and guidelines for monitoring and management. Leukemia. 2010 Jun;24(6):1121-7. [PMID: 20410922]

Leung N, Bridoux F, Hutchison CA, et al; International Kidney and Monoclonal Gammopathy Working Group. Monoclonal gammopathy of renal significance: when MGUS is no longer undetermined or insignificant. Blood. 2012 Nov 22;120(22):4292-5. [PMID: 23047823]

McCarthy PL, Owzar K, Hofmeister CC, et al. Lenalidomide after stem-cell transplantation for multiple myeloma. N Engl J Med. 2012 May 10;366(19):1770-81. [PMID: 22571201]

Palumbo A, Rajkumar SV, San Miguel JF, et al. International Myeloma Working Group consensus statement for the management, treatment, and supportive care of patients with myeloma not eligible for standard autologous stem-cell transplantation. J Clin Oncol. 2014 Feb 20;32(6):587-600. [PMID: 24419113]

Rummel MJ, Niederle N, Maschmeyer G, et al; Stugy group indolent Lymphomas (StiL). Bendamustine plus rituximab versus CHOP plus rituximab as first-line treatment for patients with indolent and mantle-cell lymphomas: an open-label, multicentre, randomised, phase 3 non-inferiority trial [erratum in Lancet. 2013 Apr 6;381(9873):1184]. Lancet. 2013 Apr 6;381(9873):1203-10. [PMID: 23433739]

San Miguel J, Weisel K, Moreau P, et al. Pomalidomide plus low-dose dexamethasone versus high-dose dexamethasone alone for patients with relapsed and refractory multiple myeloma (MM-003): a randomised, open-label, phase 3 trial. Lancet Oncol. 2013 Oct;14(11):1055-66. [PMID: 24007748]

Terpos E, Morgan G, Dimopoulos MA, et al. International Myeloma Working Group recommendations for the treatment of multiple myeloma-related bone disease. J Clin Oncol. 2013 Jun 20;31(18):2347-57. [PMID: 23690408]

Erythrocyte Disorders

Ballas SK, Kesen MR, Goldberg MF, et al. Beyond the definitions of the phenotypic complications of sickle cell disease: an update on management. ScientificWorldJournal. 2012;2012:949535. [PMID: 22924029]

Berentsen S, Tjønnfjord GE. Diagnosis and treatment of cold agglutinin mediated autoimmune hemolytic anemia. Blood Rev. 2012 May;26(3):107-15. [PMID: 22330255]

Bolton-Maggs PH, Langer JC, Iolascon A, Tittensor P, King MJ; General Haematology Task Force of the British Committee for Standards in Haematology. Guidelines for the diagnosis and management of hereditary spherocytosis-2011 update. Br J Haematol. 2012 Jan;156(1):37-49. [PMID: 22055020]

Goodnough LT, Nemeth E, Ganz T. Detection, evaluation, and management of iron-restricted erythropoiesis. Blood. 2010 Dec 2;116(23):4754-61. [PMID: 20826717]

Higgs DR, Engel JD, Stamatoyannopoulos G. Thalassaemia. Lancet. 2012 Jan 28;379(9813):373-83. [PMID: 21908035]

Howard J, Malfroy M, Llewelyn C, et al. The Transfusion Alternatives Preoperatively in Sickle Cell Disease (TAPS) study: a randomised, controlled, multicentre clinical trial. Lancet. 2013 Mar 16;381(9870):930-8. [PMID: 23352054]

Kliger AS, Foley RN, Goldfarb DS, et al. KDOQI US Commentary on the 2012 KDIGO Clinical Practice Guideline for Anemia in CKD. Am J Kidney Dis. 2013 Nov;62(5):849-59. [PMID: 23891356]

Michel M. Classification and therapeutic approaches in autoimmune hemolytic anemia: an update. Expert Rev Hematol. 2011 Dec;4(6):607-18. [PMID: 22077525]

Rachmilewitz EA, Giardina PJ. How I treat thalassemia. Blood. 2011 Sep 29;118(13):3479-88. [PMID: 21813448]

Stabler SP. Clinical practice. Vitamin B12 deficiency. N Engl J Med. 2013 Jan 10;368(2):149-60. [PMID: 23301732]

Iron Overload Syndromes

Crownover BK, Covey CJ. Hereditary hemochromatosis. Am Fam Physician. 2013 Feb 1;87(3):183-90. [PMID: 23418762]

Platelet Disorders

Cuker A, Gimotty PA, Crowther MA, Warkentin TE. Predictive value of the 4Ts scoring system for heparin-induced thrombocytopenia: a systematic review and meta-analysis. Blood. 2012 Nov 15;120(20):4160-7. [PMID: 22990018]

George JN, Al-Nouri ZL. Diagnostic and therapeutic challenges in the thrombotic thrombocytopenic purpura and hemolytic uremic syndromes. Hematology Am Soc Hematol Educ Program. 2012;2012:604-9. [PMID: 23233641]

Neunert C, Lim W, Crowther M, Cohen A, Solberg L Jr, Crowther MA; American Society of Hematology. The American Society of Hematology 2011 evidence-based practice guideline for immune thrombocytopenia. Blood. 2011 Apr 21;117(16):4190-207. [PMID: 21325604]

Bleeding Disorders

Berntorp E. Von Willebrand disease. Pediatr Blood Cancer. 2013;60(Suppl 1):S34-6. [PMID: 23109385]

Carcao MD. The diagnosis and management of congenital hemophilia. Semin Thromb Hemost. 2012 Oct;38(7):727-34. [PMID: 23011791]

Mannucci PM, Tripodi A. Liver disease, coagulopathies and transfusion therapy. Blood Transfus. 2013 Jan;11(1):32-6. [PMID: 23058863]

Sborov DW, Rodgers GM. How I manage patients with acquired haemophilia A. Br J Haematol. 2013 Apr;161(2):157-65. [PMID: 23373521]

Transfusion

Carson JL, Grossman BJ, Kleinman S, et al; Clinical Transfusion Medicine Committee of the AABB. Red blood cell transfusion: a clinical practice guideline from the AABB. Ann Intern Med. 2012 Jul 3;157(1):49-58. [PMID: 22751760]

Carson JL, Terrin ML, Noveck H, et al; FOCUS Investigators. Liberal or restrictive transfusion in high-risk patients after hip surgery. N Engl J Med. 2011 Dec 29;365(26):2453-62. [PMID: 22168590]

Hébert PC, Wells G, Blajchman MA, et al. A multicenter, randomized, controlled clinical trial of transfusion requirements in critical care. Transfusion Requirements in Critical Care Investigators, Canadian Critical Care Trials Group [erratum in N Engl J Med. 1999 Apr 1;340(13):1056]. N Engl J Med. 1999 Feb 11;340(6):409-17. [PMID: 9971864]

Palmer SC, Navaneethan SD, Craig JC, et al. Meta-analysis: erythropoiesis-stimulating agents in patients with chronic kidney disease. Ann Intern Med. 2010 Jul 6;153(1):23-33. [PMID: 20439566]

Roback JD, Caldwell S, Carson J, et al; American Association for the Study of Liver; American Academy of Pediatrics; United States Army; American Society of Anesthesiology; American Society of Hematology. Evidence-based practice guidelines for plasma transfusion. Transfusion. 2010 Jun;50(6):1227-39. [PMID: 20345562]

Stanworth SJ, Estcourt LJ, Powter G, et al; TOPPS Investigators. A no-prophylaxis platelet-transfusion strategy for hematologic cancers. N Engl J Med. 2013 May 9;368(19):1771-80. [PMID: 23656642]

Szczepiorkowski ZM, Winters JL, Bandarenko N, et al; Apheresis Applications Committee of the American Society for Apheresis. Guidelines on the use of therapeutic apheresis in clinical practice--evidence-based approach from the Apheresis Applications Committee of the American Society for Apheresis. J Clin Apher. 2010;25(3):83-177. [PMID: 20568098]

Tonia T, Mettler A, Robert N, et al. Erythropoietin or darbepoetin for patients with cancer. Cochrane Database Syst Rev. 2012 Dec 12;12:CD003407. [PMID: 23235597]

Villanueva C, Colomo A, Bosch A, et al. Transfusion strategies for acute upper gastrointestinal bleeding [erratum in N Engl J Med. 2013 Jun 13;368(24):2341]. N Engl J Med. 2013 Jan 3;368(1):11-21. [PMID: 23281973]

Thrombotic Disorders

Ageno W, Gallus AS, Wittkowsky A, Crowther M, Hylek EM, Palareti G; American College of Chest Physicians. Oral anticoagulant therapy: antithrombotic therapy and prevention of thrombosis, 9th ed: American College of Chest Physicians Evidence-Based Clinical Practice Guidelines. Chest. 2012 Feb;141 (2 Suppl):e44S-88S. [PMID: 22315269]

Baglin T, Gray E, Greaves M, et al; British Committee for Standards in Haematology. Clinical guidelines for testing for heritable thrombophilia. Br J Haematol. 2010 Apr;149(2):209-20. [PMID: 20128794]

Garcia DA, Baglin TP, Weitz JI, et al. Parenteral anticoagulants: antithrombotic therapy and prevention of thrombosis, 9th ed: American College of Chest

Physicians Evidence-Based Clinical Practice Guidelines [erratum in Chest. 2012 May;141(5):1369]. Chest. 2012 Feb;141(2 Suppl):e24S-43S. [PMID: 22315264]

Kearon C, Akl EA, Comerota AJ, et al; American College of Chest Physicians. Antithrombotic therapy for VTE disease: antithrombotic therapy and prevention of thrombosis, 9th ed: American College of Chest Physicians Evidence-Based Clinical Practice Guidelines [erratum in Chest. 2012 Dec;142(6):1698-1704]. Chest. 2012 Feb;141(2 Suppl):e419S-94S. [PMID: 22315268]

Miyakis S, Lockshin MD, Atsumi T, et al. International consensus statement on an update of the classification criteria for definite antiphospholipid syndrome (APS). J Thromb Haemost. 2006 Feb;4(2):295-306. [PMID: 16420554]

Segal JB, Brotman DJ, Necochea AJ, et al. Predictive value of factor V Leiden and prothrombin G20210A in adults with venous thromboembolism and in family members of those with a mutation: a systematic review. JAMA. 2009 Jun 17;301(23):2472-85. [PMID: 19531787]

Hematologic Issues in Pregnancy

Andemariam B, Browning SL. Current management of sickle cell disease in pregnancy. Clin Lab Med. 2013 Jun;33(2):293-310. [PMID: 23702119]

Bates SM, Greer IA, Middeldorp S, Veenstra DL, Prabulos AM, Vandvik PO; American College of Chest Physicians. VTE, thrombophilia, antithrombotic therapy, and pregnancy: antithrombotic therapy and prevention of thrombosis, 9th ed: American College of Chest Physicians Evidence-Based Clinical Practice Guidelines. Chest. 2012 Feb;141(2 Suppl):e691S-736S. [PMID: 22315276]

D'Angelo A, Fattorini A, Crippa L. Thrombotic microangiopathy in pregnancy. Thromb Res. 2009;123(Suppl 2):S56-62. [PMID: 19217478]

James A; Committee on Practice Bulletins—Obstetrics. Practice bulletin no. 123: thromboembolism in pregnancy. Obstet Gynecol. 2011 Sep;118(3):718-29. [PMID: 21860313]

Kamel H, Navi BB, Sriram N, Hovsepian DA, Devereux RB, Elkind MS. Risk of a thrombotic event after the 6-week postpartum period. N Engl J Med. 2014 Apr 3;370(14):1307-15. [PMID: 24524551]

Myers B. Diagnosis and management of maternal thrombocytopenia in pregnancy. Br J Haematol. 2012 Jul;158(1):3-15. [PMID: 22551110]

Porter B, Key NS, Jauk VC, Adam S, Biggio J, Tita A. Impact of sickle hemoglobinopathies on pregnancy-related venous thromboembolism. Am J Perinatol. 2014 Oct;31(9):805-9. [PMID: 24338132]

Sifakis S, Pharmakides G. Anemia in pregnancy. Ann N Y Acad Sci. 2000; 900:125-36. [PMID: 10818399]

Breast Cancer

Albain KS, Barlow WE, Shak S, et al; Breast Cancer Intergroup of North America. Prognostic and predictive value of the 21-gene recurrence score assay in postmenopausal women with node-positive, oestrogen-receptor-positive breast cancer on chemotherapy: a retrospective analysis of a randomised trial. Lancet Oncol. 2010 Jan;11(1):55-65. [PMID: 20005174]

Amir E, Miller N, Geddie W, et al. Prospective study evaluating the impact of tissue confirmation of metastatic disease in patients with breast cancer. J Clin Oncol. 2012 Feb 20;30(6):587-92. [PMID: 22124102]

Baselga J, Campone M, Piccart M, et al. Everolimus in postmenopausal hormone-receptor-positive advanced breast cancer. N Engl J Med. 2012 Feb 9;366(6):520-9. [PMID: 22149876]

Burstein HJ, Temin S, Anderson H, et al. Adjuvant endocrine therapy for women with hormone receptor-positive breast cancer: american society of clinical oncology clinical practice guideline focused update. J Clin Oncol. 2014 Jul 20;32(21):2255-69. [PMID: 24868023]

Chen S, Parmigiani G. Meta-analysis of BRCA1 and BRCA2 penetrance. J Clin Oncol. 2007 Apr 10;25(11):1329-33. [PMID: 17416853]

Davies C, Pan H, Godwin J, et al; Adjuvant Tamoxifen: Longer Against Shorter (ATLAS) Collaborative Group. Long-term effects of continuing adjuvant tamoxifen to 10 years versus stopping at 5 years after diagnosis of oestrogen receptor-positive breast cancer: ATLAS, a randomised trial. Lancet. 2013 Mar 9;381(9869):805-16. Erratum in: Lancet. 2013 Mar 9;381(9869):804. [PMID: 23219286]

Early Breast Cancer Trialists' Collaborative Group (EBCTCG). Effects of chemotherapy and hormonal therapy for early breast cancer on recurrence and 15-year survival: an overview of the randomised trials. Lancet. 2005 May 14-20;365(9472):1687-717. [PMID: 15894097]

Fisher B, Costantino JP, Wickerham DL, et al. Tamoxifen for prevention of breast cancer: report of the National Surgical Adjuvant Breast and Bowel Project P-1 Study. J Natl Cancer Inst. 1998 Sep 16;90(18):1371-88. [PMID: 9747868]

Giuliano AE, Hunt KK, Ballman KV, et al. Axillary dissection vs no axillary dissection in women with invasive breast cancer and sentinel node metastasis: a randomized clinical trial. JAMA. 2011 Feb 9;305(6):569-75. [PMID: 21304082]

Goss PE, Ingle JN, Alés-Martínez JE, et al; NCIC CTG MAP.3 Study Investigators. Exemestane for breast-cancer prevention in postmenopausal women. N Engl J Med. 2011 Jun 23;364(25):2381-91. Erratum in: N Engl J Med. 2011 Oct 6;365(14):1361. [PMID: 21639806]

Hughes KS, Schnaper LA, Bellon JR, et al. Lumpectomy plus tamoxifen with or without irradiation in women age 70 years or older with early breast cancer: long-term follow-up of CALGB 9343. J Clin Oncol. 2013 Jul 1;31(19):2382-7. [PMID: 23690420]

Khatcheressian JL, Hurley P, Bantug E, et al; American Society of Clinical Oncology. Breast cancer follow-up and management after primary treatment: American Society of Clinical Oncology clinical practice guideline update. J Clin Oncol. 2013 Mar 1;31(7):961-5. [PMID: 23129741]

Paik S, Tang G, Shak S, et al. Gene expression and benefit of chemotherapy in women with node-negative, estrogen receptor-positive breast cancer. J Clin Oncol. 2006 Aug 10;24(23):3726-34. [PMID: 16720680]

Saslow D, Boetes C, Burke W, et al; American Cancer Society Breast Cancer Advisory Group. American Cancer Society guidelines for breast screening with MRI as an adjunct to mammography. CA Cancer J Clin. 2007 Mar-Apr;57(2):75-89. Erratum in: CA Cancer J Clin. 2007 May-Jun;57(3):185. [PMID: 17392385]

Vogel VG, Costantino JP, Wickerham DL, et al; National Surgical Adjuvant Breast and Bowel Project (NSABP). Effects of tamoxifen vs raloxifene on the risk of developing invasive breast cancer and other disease outcomes: the NSABP Study of Tamoxifen and Raloxifene (STAR) P-2 trial. JAMA. 2006 Jun 21;295(23):2727-41. Erratum in: JAMA. 2006 Dec 27;296(24):2926. JAMA. 2007 Sep 5;298(9):973. [PMID: 16754727]

Ovarian Cancer

Armstrong DK, Bundy B, Wenzel L, et al; Gynecologic Oncology Group. Intraperitoneal cisplatin and paclitaxel in ovarian cancer. N Engl J Med. 2006 Jan 5;354(1):34-43. [PMID: 16394300]

Bristow RE, Tomacruz RS, Armstrong DK, Trimble EL, Montz FJ. Survival effect of maximal cytoreductive surgery for advanced ovarian carcinoma during the platinum era: a meta-analysis. J Clin Oncol. 2002 Mar 1;20(5):1248-59. [PMID: 11870167]

Buys SS, Partridge E, Black A, et al; PLCO Project Team. Effect of screening on ovarian cancer mortality: the Prostate, Lung, Colorectal and Ovarian (PLCO) Cancer Screening Randomized Controlled Trial. JAMA. 2011 Jun 8;305(22):2295-303. [PMID: 21642681]

Collaborative Group on Epidemiological Studies of Ovarian Cancer, Beral V, Doll R, Hermon C, Peto R, Reeves G. Ovarian cancer and oral contraceptives: collaborative reanalysis of data from 45 epidemiological studies including 23,257 women with ovarian cancer and 87,303 controls. Lancet. 2008 Jan 26;371(9609):303-14. [PMID 18294997]

Rustin GJ, van der Burg ME, Griffin CL, et al; MRC OV05; EORTC 55955 investigators. Early versus delayed treatment of relapsed ovarian cancer (MRC OV05/EORTC 55955): a randomised trial. Lancet. 2010 Oct 2;376(9747):1155-63. [PMID: 20888993]

Vergote I, Tropé CG, Amant F, et al; European Organization for Research and Treatment of Cancer-Gynaecological Cancer Group; NCIC Clinical Trials Group. Neoadjuvant chemotherapy or primary surgery in stage IIIC or IV ovarian cancer. N Engl J Med. 2010 Sep 2;363(10):943-53. [PMID: 20818904]

Cervical Cancer

Burstein HJ, Temin S, Anderson H, et al. Adjuvant endocrine therapy for women with hormone receptor-positive breast cancer: american society of clinical oncology clinical practice guideline focused update. J Clin Oncol. 2014 July 20:32(21);2255-69. [PMID: 24868023]

Chemoradiotherapy for Cervical Cancer Meta-Analysis Collaboration. Reducing uncertainties about the effects of chemoradiotherapy for cervical cancer: a systematic review and meta-analysis of individual patient data from 18 randomized trials. J Clin Oncol. 2008 Dec 10;26(35):5802-12. [PMID: 19001332]

Schiffman M, Castle PE, Jeronimo J, Rodriguez AC, Wacholder S. Human papillomavirus and cervical cancer. Lancet. 2007 Sep 8;370(9590):890-907. [PMID: 17826171]

Gastroenterological Malignancies

Bang YJ, Van Cutsem E, Feyereislova A, et al; ToGA Trial Investigators. Trastuzumab in combination with chemotherapy versus chemotherapy alone for treatment of HER2-positive advanced gastric or gastro-oesophageal junction cancer (ToGA): a phase 3, open-label, randomised controlled trial.

Lancet. 2010 Aug 28;376(9742):687-97. Erratum in: Lancet. 2010 Oct 16;376(9749):1302. [PMID: 20728210]

Conroy T, Desseigne F, Ychou M, et al; Groupe Tumeurs Digestives of Unicancer; PRODIGE Intergroup. FOLFIRINOX versus gemcitabine for metastatic pancreatic cancer. N Engl J Med. 2011 May 12;364(19):1817-25. [PMID: 21561347]

Garcia-Aguilar J, Holt A. Optimal management of small rectal cancers: TAE, TEM, or TME? Surg Oncol Clin N Am. 2010 Oct;19(4):743-60. [PMID: 20883951]

Haller DG, Tabernero J, Maroun J, et al. Capecitabine plus oxaliplatin compared with fluorouracil and folinic acid as adjuvant therapy for stage III colon cancer. J Clinl Oncol. 2011 Apr 10;29(11):1465-71. [PMID: 21383294]

James RD, Glynne-Jones R, Meadows HM, et al. Mitomycin or cisplatin chemoradiation with or without maintenance chemotherapy for treatment of squamous-cell carcinoma of the anus (ACT II): a randomised, phase 3, open-label, 2 × 2 factorial trial. Lancet Oncol. 2013 May;14(6):516-24. [PMID: 23578724]

Joensuu H, Eriksson M, Sundby Hall K, et al. One vs three years of adjuvant imatinib for operable gastrointestinal stromal tumor: a randomized trial. JAMA. 2012 Mar 28;307(12):1265-72. [PMID: 22453568]

Johnston FM, Mavros MN, Herman JM, Pawlik TM. Local therapies for hepatic metastases. J Natl Compr Canc Netw. 2013 Feb 1;11(2):153-60. [PMID: 23411382]

Kulke MH, Siu LL, Tepper JE, et al. Future directions in the treatment of neuroendocrine tumors: consensus report of the National Cancer Institute Neuroendocrine Tumor clinical trials planning meeting. J Clin Oncol. 2011 Mar 1;29(7):934-43. [PMID: 21263089]

Meyerhardt JA, Mangu PB, Flynn PJ, et al; American Society of Clinical Oncology. Follow-up care, surveillance protocol, and secondary prevention measures for survivors of colorectal cancer: American Society of Clinical Oncology clinical practice guideline endorsement. J Clin Oncol. 2013 Dec 10;31(35):4465-70. [PMID: 24220554]

NCCN Guidelines for Treatment of Cancer: Colon/Rectal Cancer. National Comprehensive Cancer Network Web site. www.nccn.org/professionals/physician_gls/f_guidelines.asp#colon. Updated October 3, 2014. Accessed January 22, 2015.

Peeters M, Douillard JY, Van Cutsem E, et al. Mutant KRAS codon 12 and 13 alleles in patients with metastatic colorectal cancer: assessment as prognostic and predictive biomarkers of response to panitumumab. J Clin Oncol. 2013 Feb 20;31(6):759-65. [PMID: 23182985]

Lung Cancer

Agra Y, Pelayo M, Sacristan M, Sacristán A, Serra C, Bonfill X. Chemotherapy versus best supportive care for extensive small cell lung cancer. Cochrane Database Syst Rev. 2003;(4):CD001990. Update in: Cochrane Database Syst Rev. 2009;(4):CD001990. [PMID: 14583943]

Azzoli CG, Baker S Jr, Temin S; American Society of Clinical Oncology. American Society of Clinical Oncology Clinical Practice Guideline update on chemotherapy for stage IV non-small-cell lung cancer. J Clin Oncol. 2009 Dec 20;27(36):6251-66. [PMID: 19917871]

Douillard JY, Rosell R, De Lena M, Riggi M, Hurteloup P, Mahe MA; Adjuvant Navelbine International Trialist Association. Impact of postoperative radiation therapy on survival in patients with complete resection and stage I, II, or IIIA non-small-cell lung cancer treated with adjuvant chemotherapy: the adjuvant Navelbine International Trialist Association (ANITA) Randomized Trial. Int J Radiat Oncol Biol Phys. 2008 Nov 1;72(3):695-701. [PMID: 18439766]

Lung. In: Edge S, Byrd DR, Compton CC, Fritz AG, Greene FL, Trotti A, eds. AJCC Cancer Staging Manual. 7th ed. New York, NY: Springer; 2010:253.

Meert AP, Paesmans M, Berghmans T, et al. Prophylactic cranial irradiation in small cell lung cancer: a systematic review of the literature with meta-analysis. BMC Cancer. 2001;1:5. [PMID: 11432756]

Nair BS, Bhanderi V, Jafri SH. Current and emerging pharmacotherapies for the treatment of relapsed small cell lung cancer. Clin Med Insights Oncol. 2011;5:223-34. [PMID: 21836818]

Pelosof LC, Gerber DE. Paraneoplastic syndromes: an approach to diagnosis and treatment. Mayo Clin Proc. 2010 Sep;85(9):838-54. Erratum in: Mayo Clin Proc. 2011 Apr;86(4):364. [PMID: 20810794]

Pignon JP, Arriagada R, Ihde DC, et al. A meta-analysis of thoracic radiotherapy for small-cell lung cancer. N Engl J Med. 1992 Dec 3;327(23):1618-24. [PMID: 1331787]

Pisters KM, Evans WK, Azzoli CG, et al; Cancer Care Ontario; American Society of Clinical Oncology. Cancer Care Ontario and American Society of Clinical Oncology adjuvant chemotherapy and adjuvant radiation therapy for stages I-IIIA resectable non small-cell lung cancer guideline. J Clin Oncol. 2007 Dec 1;25(34):5506-18. [PMID: 17954710]

Rosell R, Carcereny E, Gervais R; Spanish Lung Cancer Group in collaboration with Groupe Français de Pneumo-Cancérologie and Associazione Italiana Oncologia Toracica. Erlotinib versus standard chemotherapy as first-line treatment for European patients with advanced EGFR mutation-positive non-small-cell lung cancer (EURTAC): a multicentre, open-label, randomised phase 3 trial. Lancet Oncol. 2012 Mar;13(3):239-46. [PMID: 22285168]

Shaw AT, Kim DW, Nakagawa K, et al. Crizotinib versus chemotherapy in advanced ALK-positive lung cancer. N Engl J Med. 2013 June 20;368(25): 2385-94. [PMID: 23724913]

Siegel R, Naishadham D, Jemal A. Cancer Statistics, 2013. CA Cancer J Clin. 2013 Jan;63(1):11-30. [PMID: 23335087]

Soria JC, Mauguen A, Reck M, et al; meta-analysis of bevacizumab in advanced NSCLC collaborative group. Systematic review and meta-analysis of randomised, phase II/III trials adding bevacizumab to platinum-based chemotherapy as first-line treatment in patients with advanced non-small-cell lung cancer. Ann Oncol. 2013 Jan;24(1):20-30. Erratum in: Ann Oncol. 2013 Apr;24(4):1133. [PMID: 23180113]

Temel JS, Greer JA, Muzikansky A, et al. Early palliative care for patients with metastatic non-small-cell lung cancer. N Engl J Med. 2010 Aug 19;363(8): 733-42. [PMID: 20818875]

Vallières E, Shepherd FA, Crowley J, et al; International Association for the Study of Lung Cancer International Staging Committee and Participating Institutions. The IASLC Lung Cancer Staging Project: proposals regarding the relevance of TNM in the pathologic staging of small cell lung cancer in the forthcoming (seventh) edition of the TNM classification for lung cancer. J Thorac Oncol. 2009 Sep;4(9):1049-59. [PMID: 19652623]

Head and Neck Cancer

Adelstein DJ, Li Y, Adams GL, et al. An intergroup phase III comparison of standard radiation therapy and two schedules of concurrent chemoradiotherapy in patients with unresectable squamous cell head and neck cancer. J Clin Oncol. 2003 Jan 1;21(1):92-8. [PMID: 12506176]

Bonner JA, Harari PM, Giralt J, et al. Radiotherapy plus cetuximab for squamous-cell carcinoma of the head and neck. N Engl J Med. 2006 Feb 9;354(6):567-78. [PMID: 16467544]

Cooper JS, Zhang Q, Pajak TF, et al. Long-term follow-up of the RTOG 9501/intergroup phase III trial: postoperative concurrent radiation therapy and chemotherapy in high-risk squamous cell carcinoma of the head and neck. Int J Radiat Oncol Biol Phys. 2012 Dec 1;84(5):1198-205. [PMID: 22749632]

Chaturvedi AK, Engels EA, Pfeiffer RM, et al. Human papillomavirus and rising oropharyngeal cancer incidence in the United States. J Clin Oncol. 2011 Nov 10;29(32):4294-301. [PMID: 21969503]

Fortin A, Wang CS, Vigneault E. Influence of smoking and alcohol drinking behaviors on treatment outcomes of patients with squamous cell carcinomas of the head and neck. Int J Radiat Oncol Biol Phys. 2009 Jul 15;74 (4):1062-9. [PMID: 19036528]

Porceddu SV, Pryor DI, Burmeister E, et al. Results of a prospective study of positron emission tomography-directed management of residual nodal abnormalities in node-positive head and neck cancer after definitive radiotherapy with or without systemic therapy. Head Neck. 2011 Dec;33 (12):1675-82. [PMID: 22076976]

Siegel R, Naishadham D, Jemal A. Cancer statistics, 2013. CA Cancer J Clin. 2013 Jan;63(1):11-30. [PMID: 23335087]

Genitourinary Cancer

de Bono JS, Logothetis CJ, Molina A, et al; COU-AA-301 Investigators. Abiraterone and increased survival in metastatic prostate cancer. N Engl J Med. 2011 May 26;364(21):1995-2005. [PMID: 21612468]

Delongchamps NB, Singh A, Haas GP. The role of prevalence in the diagnosis of prostate cancer. Cancer Control. 2006 Jul;13(3):158-68. [PMID: 16885911]

Fizazi K, Carducci M, Smith M, et al. Denosumab versus zoledronic acid for treatment of bone metastases in men with castration-resistant prostate cancer: a randomised, double-blind study. Lancet. 2011 Mar 5;377(9768):813-22. [PMID: 21353695]

Loblaw DA, Virgo KS, Nam R, et al; American Society of Clinical Oncology. Initial hormonal management of androgen-sensitive metastatic, recurrent, or progressive prostate cancer: 2006 update of an American Society of Clinical Oncology practice guideline. J Clin Oncol. 2007 Apr 20;25(12):1596-605. [PMID: 17404365]

Motzer RJ, Hutson TE, Tomczak P, et al. Overall survival and updated results for sunitinib compared with interferon alfa in patients with metastatic renal cell carcinoma. J Clin Oncol. 2009 Aug 1;27(22):3584-90. [PMID: 19487381]

Parker C, Nilsson S, Heinrich D, et al. Updated analysis of the phase III, double-blind, randomized, multinational study of radium-223 chloride in castra-

tion-resistant prostate cancer (CRPC) patients with bone metastases (ALSYMPCA). American Society of Clinical Oncology Web site. http://meetinglibrary.asco.org/content/95649-114. Published 2012. Accessed October 3, 2014.

Ryan CJ, Smith MR, De Bono, JS, et al. Interim analysis (IA) results of COU-AA-302, a randomized, phase III study of abiraterone acetate (AA) in chemotherapy-naive patients (pts) with metastatic castration-resistant prostate cancer (mCRPC). American Society of Clinical Oncology Web site. http://meetinglibrary.asco.org/content/95300-114. Published 2012. Accessed October 3, 2014.

Sanda MG, Dunn RL, Michalski J, et al. Quality of life and satisfaction with outcome among prostate-cancer survivors. N Engl J Med. 2008 Mar 20;358(12):1250-61. [PMID: 18354103]

Scher HI, Fizazi K, Saad F, et al; AFFIRM Investigators. Increased survival with enzalutamide in prostate cancer after chemotherapy. N Engl J Med. 2012 Sep 27;367(13):1187-97. [PMID: 22894553]

Siegel R, Naishadham D, Jemal A. Cancer Statistics, 2013. CA Cancer J Clin. 2013 Jan;63(1):11-30. [PMID: 23335087]

van den Belt-Dusebout AW, de Wit R, Gietema JA, et al. Treatment-specific risks of second malignancies and cardiovascular disease in 5-year survivors of testicular cancer. J Clin Oncol. 2007 Oct 1;25(28):4370-8. [PMID: 17906202]

von der Maase H, Sengelov L, Roberts JT, et al. Long-term survival results of a randomized trial comparing gemcitabine plus cisplatin, with methotrexate, vinblastine, doxorubicin, plus cisplatin in patients with bladder cancer. J Clin Oncol. 2005 Jul 20;23(21):4602-8. [PMID: 16034041]

Lymphoid Malignancies

Amador-Ortiz C, Chen L, Hassan A, et al. Combined core needle biopsy and fine-needle aspiration with ancillary studies correlate highly with traditional techniques in the diagnosis of nodal-based lymphoma. Am J Clin Pathol. 2011 Apr;135(4):516-24. [PMID: 21411774]

Ferreri AJ, Govi S, Ponzoni M. The role of Helicobacter pylori eradication in the treatment of diffuse large B-cell and marginal zone lymphomas of the stomach. Curr Opin Oncol. 2013 Sep;25(5):470-9. [PMID: 23942292]

Hoster E, Dreyling M, Klapper W, et al; German Low Grade Lymphoma Study Group (GLSG); European Mantle Cell Lymphoma Network. A new prognostic index (MIPI) for patients with advanced-stage mantle cell lymphoma. Blood. 2008 Jan 15;111(2):558-65. Erratum in: Blood. 2008 Jun 15;111(12): 5761. [PMID: 17962512]

Kostakoglu L, Goldsmith SJ, Leonard JP, et al. FDG-PET after 1 cycle of therapy predicts outcome in diffuse large cell lymphoma and classic Hodgkin disease. Cancer. 2006 Dec 1;107(11):2678-87. [PMID 17063502]

Lenz G, Staudt LM. Aggressive lymphomas. N Engl J Med. 2010 Apr 15;362(15): 1417-29. [PMID: 20393178]

Li ZM, Ghielmini M, Moccia AA. Managing newly diagnosed follicular lymphoma: state of the art and future perspectives. Expert Rev Anticancer Ther. 2013 Mar;13(3):313-25. [PMID: 23477518]

Martelli M, Ferreri AJ, Agostinelli C, Di Rocco A, Pfreundschuh M, Pileri SA. Diffuse large B-cell lymphoma. Crit Rev Oncol Hematol. 2013 Aug;87(2): 146-71. [PMID: 23375551]

Molyneux EM, Rochford R, Griffin B, et al. Burkitt's lymphoma. Lancet. 2012 Mar 31;379(9822):1234-44. [PMID: 22333947]

Prince HM, Whittaker S, Hoppe RT. How I treat mycosis fungoides and Sézary syndrome. Blood. 2009 Nov 12;114(20):4337-53. [PMID: 19696197]

Rancea M, Monsef I, von Tresckow B, Engert A, Skoetz N. High-dose chemotherapy followed by autologous stem cell transplantation for patients with relapsed/refractory Hodgkin lymphoma. Cochrane Database Syst Rev. 2013 Jun 20;6:CD009411. [PMID: 23784872]

Sehn LH, Berry B, Chhanabhai M, et al. The revised International Prognostic Index (R-IPI) is a better predictor of outcome than the standard IPI for patients with diffuse large B-cell lymphoma treated with R-CHOP. Blood. 2007 Mar 1;109(5):1857-61. [PMID: 17105812]

van Besien K, Keralavarma B, Devine S, Stock W. Allogeneic and autologous transplantation for chronic lymphocytic leukemia. Leukemia. 2001 Sep;15(9):1317-25. [PMID: 11516091]

Cancer of Unknown Primary Site

Petrakis D, Pentheroudakis G, Voulgaris E, Pavlidis N. Prognostication in cancer of unknown primary (CUP): development of a prognostic algorithm in 311 cases and review of the literature. Cancer Treat Rev. 2013 Nov;39(7): 701-8. [PMID: 23566573]

Varadhachary GR. Carcinoma of unknown orimary: focused evaluation. J Natl Compr Canc Netw. 2011 Dec;9(12):1406-12. [PMID: 22157558]

Melanoma

Chapman PB, Hauschild A, Robert C, et al; BRIM-3 Study Group. Improved survival with vemurafenib in melanoma with BRAF V600E mutation. N Engl J Med. 2011 Jun 30;364(26):2507-16. [PMID: 21639808]

Eggermont AM, Suciu S, Testori A, et al. Long-term results of the randomized phase III trial EORTC 18991 of adjuvant therapy with pegylated interferon alfa-2b versus observation in resected stage III melanoma. J Clin Oncol. 2012 Nov 1;30(31):3810-8. [PMID: 23008300]

Francken AB, Bastiaanet E, Hoekstra HJ. Follow-up in patients with localised primary cutaneous melanoma. Lancet Oncol. 2005 Aug;6(8):608-21. [PMID: 16054572]

Hodi FS, O'Day SJ, McDermott DF, et al. Improved survival with ipilimumab in patients with metastatic melanoma. N Engl J Med. 2010 Aug 19;363(8):711-23. Erratum in: N Engl J Med. 2010 Sep 23;363(13):1290. [PMID: 20525992]

Soong SJ, Ding S, Coit D, et al; AJCC Melanoma Task Force. Predicting survival outcome of localized melanoma: an electronic prediction tool based on the AJCC Melanoma Database. Ann Surg Oncol. 2010 Aug;17(8):2006-14. [PMID: 20379784]

Wong SL, Balch CM, Hurley P, et al; American Society of Clinical Oncology; Society of Surgical Oncology. Sentinel lymph node biopsy for melanoma: American Society of Clinical Oncology and Society of Surgical Oncology joint clinical practice guideline. J Clin Oncol. 2012 Aug 10;30(23):2912-8. [PMID: 22778321]

Oncologic Urgencies and Emergencies

Burazor I, Imazio M, Markel G, Adler Y. Malignant pericardial effusion. Cardiology. 2013;124(4):224-32. [PMID: 23571453]

Patil CG, Pricola K, Garg SK, Bryant A, Black KL. Whole brain radiation therapy (WBRT) alone versus WBRT and radiosurgery for the treatment of brain metastases. Cochrane Database Syst Rev. 2010 Jun 16;(6):CD006121. Update in: Cochrane Syst Rev. 2012;9:CD006121. [PMID: 20556764]

Rampello E, Fricia T, Malaguarnera M. The management of tumor lysis syndrome. Nat Clin Pract Oncol. 2006 Aug;3(8):438-47. [PMID: 16894389]

Taylor JW, Schiff D. Metastatic epidural spinal cord compression. Semin Neurol. 2010 Jul;30(3):245-53. [PMID: 20577931]

Effects of Cancer Therapy and Survivorship

Galardy PJ, Hochberg J, Perkins SL, Harrison L, Goldman S, Cairo MS. Rasburicase in the prevention of laboratory/clinical tumour lysis syndrome in children with advanced mature B-NHL: a Children's Oncology Group Report. Br J Haematol. 2013 Nov;163(3):365-72. [PMID: 24032600]

Hewitt M, Greenfield S, Stovall E, eds. *From Cancer Patient to Cancer Survivor: Lost in Translation.* Washington, DC: The National Academies Press; 2006.

Lopez-Olivo MA, Pratt G, Palla SL, Salahudeen A. Rasburicase in tumor lysis syndrome of the adult: a systematic review and meta-analysis. Am J Kidney Dis. 2013 Sep;62(3):481-92. [PMID: 23684124]

Paul M, Yahav D, Faser A, Leibovici L. Empirical antibiotic monotherapy for febrile neutropenia: systematic review and meta-analysis of randomized controlled trials. J Antimicrob Chemother. 2006 Feb;57(2):176-89. [PMID: 16344285]

Hematology and Oncology Self-Assessment Test

This self-assessment test contains one-best-answer multiple-choice questions. Please read these directions carefully before answering the questions. Answers, critiques, and bibliographies immediately follow these multiple-choice questions. The American College of Physicians is accredited by the Accreditation Council for Continuing Medical Education (ACCME) to provide continuing medical education for physicians.

The American College of Physicians designates MKSAP 17 **Hematology and Oncology** for a maximum of **22** *AMA PRA Category 1 Credits*™. Physicians should claim only the credit commensurate with the extent of their participation in the activity.

Earn "Instantaneous" CME Credits Online

Print subscribers can enter their answers online to earn Continuing Medical Education (CME) credits instantaneously. You can submit your answers using online answer sheets that are provided at mksap.acponline.org, where a record of your MKSAP 17 credits will be available. To earn CME credits, you need to answer all of the questions in a test and earn a score of at least 50% correct (number of correct answers divided by the total number of questions). Take any of the following approaches:

➢ Use the printed answer sheet at the back of this book to record your answers. Go to mksap.acponline.org, access the appropriate online answer sheet, transcribe your answers, and submit your test for instantaneous CME credits. There is no additional fee for this service.

➢ Go to mksap.acponline.org, access the appropriate online answer sheet, directly enter your answers, and submit your test for instantaneous CME credits. There is no additional fee for this service.

➢ Pay a $15 processing fee per answer sheet and submit the printed answer sheet at the back of this book by mail or fax, as instructed on the answer sheet. Make sure you calculate your score and fax the answer sheet to 215-351-2799 or mail the answer sheet to Member and Customer Service, American College of Physicians, 190 N. Independence Mall West, Philadelphia, PA 19106-1572, using the courtesy envelope provided in your MKSAP 17 slipcase. You will need your 10-digit order number and 8-digit ACP ID number, which are printed on your packing slip. Please allow 4 to 6 weeks for your score report to be emailed back to you. Be sure to include your email address for a response.

If you do not have a 10-digit order number and 8-digit ACP ID number or if you need help creating a user name and password to access the MKSAP 17 online answer sheets, go to mksap.acponline.org or email custserv@acponline.org.

CME credit is available from the publication date of July 31, 2015, until July 31, 2018. You may submit your answer sheets at any time during this period.

Hematology Questions

Item 1

A 45-year-old woman is evaluated in the emergency department for a 1-day history of abdominal pain and fever. She also reports unexpected, heavy menstrual bleeding of 1 day's duration and easy bruising of 2 days' duration. Medical and family histories are unremarkable, and she takes no medications.

On physical examination, the patient is oriented to person and place, but not time. Temperature is 38.1 °C (100.6 °F), blood pressure is 170/98 mm Hg, pulse rate is 110/min, and respiration rate is 20/min. Other than confusion, neurologic examination is normal. Subconjunctival hemorrhages are present. Cardiopulmonary examination is normal. Abdominal examination reveals tenderness to palpation without guarding or rebound. Pelvic examination shows blood in the vaginal vault with no cervical motion tenderness or adnexal masses.

Laboratory studies:

Hematocrit	26%
Leukocyte count	10,300/µL (10.3 × 10⁹/L)
Platelet count	24,000/µL (24 × 10⁹/L)
Reticulocyte count	8.3% of erythrocytes
Bilirubin, total	2.3 mg/dL (39.3 µmol/L)
Creatinine	3.2 mg/dL (283 µmol/L)
Lactate dehydrogenase	1500 U/L

Which of the following is the most appropriate diagnostic test to perform next?

(A) ADAMTS-13 activity level
(B) Osmotic fragility test
(C) Peripheral blood smear
(D) Stool Shiga toxin assay

Item 2

A 75-year-old man arrives at the emergency department after passing three large-volume, melenic stools over a 2-hour period. Medical history is significant for atrial fibrillation and hypertension. Medications are warfarin, metoprolol, and lisinopril.

On physical examination, he is diaphoretic and the skin is cool to the touch. Temperature is 36.8 °C (98.2 °F), blood pressure is 82/64 mm Hg, pulse rate is 142/min and irregular, and respiration rate is 20/min. Oxygen saturation is 95% breathing ambient air. Cardiac examination reveals tachycardia. Pulmonary examination is normal. Peripheral pulses are thready. Rectal examination reveals melenic stool that is guaiac positive.

Laboratory studies:

Hemoglobin	8.2 g/dL (82 g/L); 12.8 g/dL (128 g/L) 3 months ago
Leukocyte count	8600/µL (8.6 × 10⁹/L)
Platelet count	183,000/µL (183 × 10⁹/L)
INR	7.4

In addition to intravenous vitamin K and fluid resuscitation, which of the following is the most appropriate treatment?

(A) 4-Factor prothrombin complex concentrate
(B) Activated factor VII
(C) Cryoprecipitate
(D) Fresh frozen plasma

Item 3

A 37-year-old woman is evaluated for a 6-month history of progressive shortness of breath. Although she remains physically active, she becomes dyspneic when walking up multiple flights of stairs or running to catch a bus. Medical history is significant for a diagnosis of a pulmonary embolism 2 years ago, which was associated with oral contraceptive use. She was initially treated with low-molecular-weight heparin followed by therapeutic warfarin for 3 months. She is a nonsmoker. Medical history is otherwise unremarkable, and she takes no medications.

On physical examination, she is afebrile, blood pressure is 128/76 mm Hg at rest, pulse rate is 72/min, and respiration rate is 15/min. Oxygen saturation is 98% breathing ambient air. Pulmonary examination reveals clear lungs. Cardiac examination is significant for a fixed, split S₂, a holosystolic murmur at the left sternal border that increases on inspiration, and a heave. Trace lower extremity bilateral edema is present. The remainder of the examination is noncontributory.

Walking up stairs at the office at a moderate pace, she becomes short of breath after two flights of stairs, oxygen saturation decreases to 92%, and pulse rate increases to 145/min.

A chest radiograph is normal, showing no parenchymal abnormalities. Transthoracic echocardiography shows right atrial and ventricular dilation and moderate tricuspid regurgitation but no other valvular abnormalities.

Which of the following is the most appropriate diagnostic test to perform next?

(A) Pulmonary CT angiography
(B) Serum D-dimer test
(C) Venous Doppler ultrasonography of the legs
(D) Ventilation-perfusion (V/Q) lung scan

Item 4

A 48-year-old woman is evaluated for fatigue and intermittent abdominal discomfort of 2 months' duration and occasional dark urine. Medical and family histories are unremarkable. Her only medication is an oral contraceptive pill.

On physical examination, temperature is 37.2 °C (99.0 °F), blood pressure is 125/74 mm Hg, pulse rate is 68/min, and respiration rate is 13/min. Pallor is observed, and abdominal tenderness is present on palpation. No icterus, bruising, or splenomegaly is noted.

Laboratory studies:

Hemoglobin	7.2 g/dL (72 g/L)
Leukocyte count	3000/µL (3 × 10⁹/L) with a normal differential
Platelet count	125,000/µL (125 × 10⁹/L)
Reticulocyte count	8% of erythrocytes
Bilirubin, total	Normal
Direct antiglobulin (Coombs) test	Negative

A bone marrow biopsy shows 20% cellularity. Flow cytometry reveals erythrocytes lacking CD55 and CD59. Abdominal ultrasonography shows portal vein thrombosis.

Which of the following is the most likely diagnosis?

(A) Aplastic anemia

(B) Myelodysplastic syndrome

(C) Myeloproliferative neoplasm

(D) Paroxysmal nocturnal hemoglobinuria

Item 5

A 36-year-old woman is evaluated in the emergency department for a 1-month history of intermittent abdominal pain, a 1-week history of abdominal swelling, and a 4.5-kg (10 lb) weight gain. She rarely drinks alcohol. Her only medication is an oral combination contraceptive pill.

On physical examination, temperature is 36.4 °C (97.5 °F), blood pressure is 115/76 mm Hg, pulse rate is 92/min, and respiration rate is 16/min. Tender hepatomegaly and tense ascites are noted on abdominal palpation. No jaundice or spider telangiectasias are observed.

Laboratory studies show a hemoglobin level of 11.5 g/dL (115 g/L), leukocyte count of 12,000/µL (12 × 10⁹/L), and platelet count of 335,000/µL (335 × 10⁹/L). A viral hepatitis screening panel and pregnancy test are both negative.

Abdominal Doppler flow ultrasonography shows hepatic vein thrombosis and elevated estimated portal pressures.

Which of the following diagnostic tests is most likely to explain the cause of this patient's condition?

(A) Antiphospholipid antibody

(B) Factor V Leiden

(C) *JAK2 V617F* activating mutation

(D) Prothrombin gene mutation (G20210A)

Item 6

A 24-year-old man is evaluated in the emergency department for prolonged and severe bleeding 3 days after undergoing hemorrhoidectomy. He reports continually bleeding and soaking through four bath towels. Medical history is significant for prolonged bleeding following wisdom tooth removal. Family history is notable for a brother who experienced heavy bleeding with tooth extraction and a maternal grandfather who died of an intracerebral hemorrhage at age 32 years. He takes no medications.

On physical examination, the patient appears pale. Temperature is 36.7 °C (98.1 °F), blood pressure is 90/55 mm Hg, pulse rate is 110/min, and respiration rate is 20/min. Continued rectal bleeding is observed, with no clear source on anoscopy.

Laboratory studies:

Hematocrit	17%
Leukocyte count	12,000/µL (12 × 10⁹/L)
Platelet count	380,000/µL (380 × 10⁹/L)
Activated partial thrombo-plastin time (aPTT)	45 s
Prothrombin time	12.2 s
aPTT following 1:1 mixing study with normal plasma	32 s

Which of the following is the most appropriate diagnostic test to perform next?

(A) Bleeding time

(B) Factor VIII level

(C) Factor XI level

(D) Lupus anticoagulant

Item 7

A 52-year-old man is evaluated for orthopnea and dyspnea on exertion of 4 weeks' duration. Twelve weeks ago, he developed chronic abdominal pain, diarrhea, and weight loss. Two weeks ago, he developed new-onset eczema and nonhealing, painful sores inside his mouth. Medical history is otherwise unremarkable, and he takes no medications.

On physical examination, the patient appears ill and uncomfortable. Temperature is 36.4 °C (97.5 °F), blood pressure is 138/88 mm Hg, pulse rate is 88/min, and respiration rate is 18/min. He has diffuse erythroderma and multiple oral aphthous ulcers. On cardiac examination, prominent jugular venous distention, an S₄ gallop, and a grade 2/6 holosystolic murmur are noted. On pulmonary examination, crackles are auscultated. Palpation of the abdomen elicits generalized tenderness without guarding. Lower extremity edema is present to the knee.

Laboratory studies:

Hemoglobin	13.5 g/dL (135 g/L)
Leukocyte count	18,000/µL (18 × 10⁹/L) with 50% lymphocytes, 10% eosinophils, and 40% neutrophils
Platelet count	155,000/µL (155 × 10⁹/L)
Troponin I	Negative

Electrocardiography shows low QRS voltage in all leads without evidence of ischemic changes. Echocardiography shows restrictive left ventricular filling, increased echogenicity of the endomyocardium, and moderate mitral regurgitation.

A peripheral blood smear demonstrates mature eosinophils. Secondary causes of eosinophilia have been excluded.

Which of the following is the most likely diagnosis?

(A) Acute eosinophilic leukemia

(B) Chronic myeloid leukemia

(C) Hypereosinophilic syndrome

(D) Systemic mastocytosis

Item 8

A 35-year-old woman is evaluated for worsening thrombocytopenia; she is pregnant at 36 weeks' gestation. Medical history is significant for immune thrombocytopenic purpura. Previous platelet counts during this pregnancy have been 80,000 to 100,000/µL (80-100 × 10⁹/L). Her only medication is a prenatal vitamin.

On physical examination, temperature is 37.0 °C (98.6 °F), blood pressure is 165/110 mm Hg, pulse rate is 95/min, and respiration rate is 18/min. Abdominal examination reveals mild right upper quadrant discomfort on palpation. Reflexes are normal, and no clonus is observed. She has lower extremity edema to the level of the knees bilaterally.

Laboratory studies:

Hemoglobin	10.5 g/dL (105 g/L)
Platelet count	21,000/μL (21 × 10⁹/L)
Alanine aminotransferase	480 U/L
Aspartate aminotransferase	600 U/L
Creatinine	1.2 mg/dL (106.1 μmol/L)
Urinalysis	3+ protein

A peripheral blood smear is shown.

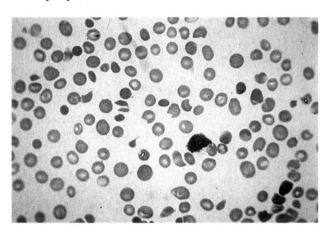

Which of the following is the most appropriate management of this patient's thrombocytopenia?

(A) Emergent delivery

(B) Intravenous immune globulin

(C) Plasma exchange

(D) Prednisone

Item 9

A 44-year-old man is evaluated in follow-up for an episode of unprovoked left proximal leg deep venous thrombosis 3 months ago. Following initial anticoagulation with low-molecular-weight heparin, he began treatment with warfarin. INR testing done every 3 to 4 weeks has shown a stable therapeutic INR. He has mild left leg discomfort after a long day of standing, but it does not limit his activity level. He tolerates warfarin well. Family history is unremarkable, and he takes no other medications.

On physical examination, vital signs are normal. He has mild edema of the left leg below the knee, with post-thrombotic pigmentation. The remainder of the examination is unremarkable.

Which of the following is the most appropriate management?

(A) Continue anticoagulation indefinitely

(B) Discontinue warfarin in another 3 months

(C) Discontinue warfarin now

(D) Discontinue warfarin and perform thrombophilia testing

Item 10

A 28-year-old woman is evaluated for a 1-week history of progressive dyspnea and fatigue. She was diagnosed with Hodgkin lymphoma 2 months ago and is receiving chemotherapy with doxorubicin, bleomycin, vinblastine, and dacarbazine (ABVD). She takes no other medications.

On physical examination, temperature is 36.8 °C (98.2 °F), blood pressure is 134/82 mm Hg, pulse rate is 105/min, and respiration rate is 16/min. Oxygen saturation is 98% breathing ambient air. Conjunctival pallor is noted but no scleral icterus. The lungs are clear to auscultation, and the cardiac examination is normal. The remainder of the examination is unremarkable.

Laboratory studies:

Hemoglobin	6.8 g/dL (68 g/L)
Leukocyte count	1300/μL (1.3 × 10⁹/L)
Platelet count	83,000/μL (83 × 10⁹/L)
Cytomegalovirus IgG antibody	Positive

A peripheral blood smear shows pancytopenia but is otherwise unremarkable.

Which of the following is the most appropriate erythrocyte transfusion product for this patient?

(A) Leukoreduced

(B) Leukoreduced, cytomegalovirus-negative

(C) Leukoreduced, irradiated

(D) Leukoreduced, washed

Item 11

A 70-year-old man is admitted to the hospital for fatigue and malaise of 3 weeks' duration and easy bruising and fever of 1 week's duration. Medical and family histories are unremarkable. He takes no medications.

On physical examination, temperature is 38.1 °C (100.5 °F), blood pressure is 128/83 mm Hg, pulse rate is 115/min, and respiration rate is 13/min; BMI is 28. Conjunctivae are pale. Splenomegaly is noted and lower extremity petechiae are observed.

Laboratory studies show a hemoglobin level of 7.3 g/dL (73 g/L), a leukocyte count of 20,000/μL (20 × 10⁹/L), and a platelet count of 14,000/μL (14 × 10⁹/L). Bone marrow examination reveals 35% lymphoblasts. A peripheral blood smear demonstrates immature cells identified as lymphoid blasts by flow cytometry. Cytogenetic testing using fluorescence in situ hybridization is positive for t(9;22).

In addition to dexamethasone, which of the following is the most appropriate treatment?

(A) Asparaginase

(B) Dasatinib

(C) Daunorubicin

(D) Vincristine

Item 12

A 38-year-old man is evaluated in the hospital for increasing right leg pain and swelling. He experienced a right femur fracture 2 days ago and underwent surgical repair. Medical history is unremarkable, but family history reveals his mother experienced a pulmonary embolism at age 66 years while receiving breast cancer treatment, and a maternal uncle had a "leg clot" at age 82 years. Medications are as-needed oxycodone and prophylactic-dose enoxaparin.

On physical examination, vital signs are normal. The right leg shows increased circumference of 2 cm at the midcalf compared with the left. The surgical site is clean and dry.

Laboratory studies show normal activated partial thromboplastin and prothrombin times.

Doppler ultrasonography shows a right proximal leg deep venous thrombosis.

Which of the following is the most appropriate thrombophilia testing for this patient?

(A) Antiphospholipid antibodies

(B) Factor V Leiden

(C) Prothrombin gene mutation

(D) No thrombophilia testing

Item 13

A 23-year-old man is admitted to the hospital with an acute vaso-occlusive pain episode. He reports pain in his back and legs with no respiratory or abdominal symptoms and rates his pain 10/10. Medical history is significant for homozygous sickle cell anemia (Hb SS). He has vaso-occlusive pain episodes approximately every 2 months. He typically receives erythrocyte transfusions for symptomatic anemia one to three times per year. Medications are folic acid and hydroxyurea.

On physical examination, temperature is 37.2 °C (99.0 °F), blood pressure is 115/70 mm Hg, pulse rate is 96/min, and respiration rate is 20/min. Oxygen saturation is 96% breathing ambient air. Scleral icterus is observed. A grade 2/6 early systolic murmur is heard at the base of the heart. Lungs are clear. No hepatosplenomegaly or tenderness is noted on abdominal examination.

Laboratory studies show a hemoglobin level of 7 g/dL (70 g/L), a mean corpuscular volume of 110 fL, and a serum creatinine level of 0.4 mg/dL (35.4 µmol/L).

A chest radiograph is normal.

Hydration and incentive spirometry are initiated.

Which of the following analgesic regimens is most appropriate for this patient?

(A) As-needed ketoprofen and morphine

(B) As-needed morphine

(C) Scheduled meperidine

(D) Scheduled morphine

Item 14

A 25-year-old woman is evaluated for a 3-hour history of pleuritic chest pain and mild shortness of breath. She is pregnant at 16 weeks' gestation. Her symptoms began acutely; she reports no other symptoms or previous problems during the pregnancy. Medical and family history is unremarkable. Her only medication is a prenatal vitamin.

On physical examination, she is afebrile, blood pressure is 125/88 mm Hg, heart rate is 80/min, and respiration rate is 15/min. Oxygen saturation is 97% breathing ambient

air. Lungs are clear, and cardiac examination is normal. She has a distended, pregnant abdomen. Trace bipedal edema is noted, and the left midcalf circumference is 1.5 cm larger than the right. The remainder of the physical examination is unremarkable.

A chest radiograph is normal.

Which of the following is the most appropriate diagnostic test to perform next?

(A) CT pulmonary angiography

(B) D-dimer test

(C) Lower extremity venous duplex ultrasonography

(D) Ventilation-perfusion lung scan

Item 15

A 42-year-old woman is evaluated for thrombocytopenia. She was admitted to the hospital 1 week ago for newly diagnosed acute myeloid leukemia. She has been receiving leukoreduced, irradiated erythrocyte and platelet transfusions since admission. Yesterday, her platelet count was 8000/µL (8×10^9/L). A platelet count checked 30 minutes after a random, donor-pooled platelet transfusion was 11,000/µL (11×10^9/L). This morning, her platelet count was 6000/µL (6×10^9/L). Thirty minutes after a random, donor-pooled platelet transfusion, the platelet count is 9000/µL (9×10^9/L). She has had four uncomplicated pregnancies and deliveries. Medications are daunorubicin, cytarabine, cefepime, posaconazole, valacyclovir, and ondansetron.

On physical examination, vital signs are normal. No splenomegaly is present. Ecchymoses are seen at previous venipuncture sites. She has scattered petechiae over the lower extremities. The remainder of the examination is normal.

Peripheral blood smear reveals no schistocytes or platelet clumps.

Which of the following is the most appropriate management?

(A) Transfuse ABO-matched platelets

(B) Transfuse HLA-matched platelets

(C) Transfuse washed platelets

(D) Observation

Item 16

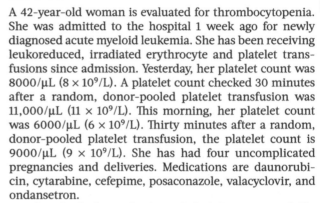

A 56-year-old man is evaluated in the hospital for acute onset right lower extremity pain and swelling. He was admitted to the hospital 2 days ago with hematemesis and underwent emergent upper endoscopy with band ligation of extensive esophageal varices. He received 2 units of packed red blood cells. Medical history is significant for alcoholic cirrhosis. He stopped drinking alcohol 18 months ago. His only outpatient medication is propranolol.

On physical examination, he is alert and oriented. He is afebrile, blood pressure is 128/76 mm Hg, pulse rate is 82/min, and respiration rate is 16/min. Splenomegaly is present. The right calf is 4 cm in circumference larger than the left. The remainder of the physical examination is non-contributory.

Laboratory studies:

Activated partial thrombo-plastin time	39.3 s
Hemoglobin	10.3 g/dL (103 g/L)
Platelet count	78,000/μL (78 × 10⁹/L)
Prothrombin time	16.3 s

A lower extremity Doppler ultrasonography reveals a right leg proximal deep venous thrombosis (DVT).

Which of the following is the most appropriate management of this patient's DVT?

(A) Argatroban

(B) Inferior vena cava filter placement

(C) Intravenous heparin

(D) Rivaroxaban

Item 17

A 30-year-old woman is evaluated in follow-up for anemia diagnosed during a recent evaluation for symptoms of fatigue. She reports no shortness of breath, dizziness, or chest pain. Medical history is notable only for heavy menses. Family history is remarkable for anemia in her mother. Her only medication is an iron supplement. She is white.

On physical examination, the patient appears well. Temperature is 36.9 °C (98.4 °F), blood pressure is 100/60 mm Hg, pulse rate is 80/min, and respiration rate is 12/min. BMI is 25. No lymphadenopathy or organomegaly is identified, and the remainder of her physical examination is unremarkable.

Laboratory studies:

Hemoglobin	8.5 g/dL (85 g/L)
Mean corpuscular volume	68 fL
Platelet count	400,000/μL (400 × 10⁹/L)
Reticulocyte count	6% of erythrocytes
Bilirubin, total	2.0 mg/dL (34.2 μmol/L)
Lactate dehydrogenase	300 U/L
Iron studies	
Ferritin	450 ng/mL (450 μg/L)
Iron	60 μg/dL (11 μmol/L)
Total iron-binding capacity	300 μg/dL (54 μmol/L)
Hemoglobin electrophoresis	
Hemoglobin A	94% (slightly low)
Hemoglobin A₂	4% (increased)
Hemoglobin F	2% (increased)
Hemoglobin S	0% (normal)

Numerous target cells are seen on a peripheral blood smear.

Which of the following is the most likely diagnosis?

(A) Anemia of chronic disease

(B) Iron malabsorption

(C) α-Thalassemia

(D) β-Thalassemia

Item 18

A 68-year-old man is evaluated for a 3-year history of dyspnea on exertion. He experiences no headaches or blurred vision. Medical history is notable for a stroke 2 years ago. He is a smoker with an 80-pack-year smoking history. Medications are hydrochlorothiazide, lisinopril, aspirin, and simvastatin.

On physical examination temperature is 36.7 °C (98.0 °F), blood pressure is 145/84 mm Hg, pulse rate is 88/min, and respiration rate is 16/min. Oxygen saturation breathing ambient air is 88%. He has facial plethora. He has no carotid bruits. Cardiac sounds are distant. Pulmonary examination reveals distant breath sounds with scattered wheezing. No hepatosplenomegaly is palpated. No digital clubbing is observed.

Laboratory studies show a hemoglobin level of 18.2 g/dL (182 g/L), leukocyte count of 8000/μL (8 × 10⁹/L) with a normal differential, and platelet count of 225,000/μL (225 × 10⁹/L). Erythropoietin level is 30 mU/mL (30 U/L).

The patient is advised to quit smoking.

Which of the following is the most appropriate next step in management?

(A) Bone marrow biopsy

(B) *JAK2 V617F* testing

(C) Phlebotomy

(D) Supplemental oxygen

Item 19

A 73-year-old woman is evaluated for increasing dyspnea on exertion and left buttock pain of 1 week's duration. She reports pain with standing straight or sitting down. She has no history of trauma. Family history is unremarkable, and she takes no medications.

On physical examination, the patient is pale and displays significant distress by bending over and grasping the back of the chair. Temperature is 36.6 °C (98.1 °F), blood pressure is 140/80 mm Hg, pulse rate is 108/min, and respiration rate is 19/min. A 10-cm hematoma is noted on the left buttock with tracking down the back of the thigh, with smaller ecchymoses scattered over her arms and shins. She has no bleeding of the gums or nose. A stool sample is guaiac negative.

Laboratory studies:

Hematocrit	35%
Leukocyte count	9100/μL (9.1 × 10⁹/L)
Mean corpuscular volume	89 fL
Platelet count	310,000/μL (310 × 10⁹/L)
Activated partial thrombo-plastin time (aPTT)	90 seconds
Prothrombin time	10.3 seconds
aPTT following 1:1 mixing study with normal plasma	45 seconds
Factor VIII activity	3% (normal, 50%-150%)
Factor VIII inhibitor	Markedly elevated

Which of the following is the most appropriate management?

(A) Administer desmopressin

(B) Administer factor VIII

(C) Administer recombinant activated factor VII

(D) Measure lupus anticoagulant

Item 20

A 52-year-old man is evaluated in follow-up. He was admitted to the hospital 2 weeks ago with a new diagnosis of acute myeloid leukemia. He has received induction chemotherapy with daunorubicin and cytarabine. Medical history is remarkable for an urticarial reaction to a platelet transfusion that resolved promptly with diphenhydramine. Other medications are posaconazole, valacyclovir, and cefepime.

On physical examination, temperature is 37.4 °C (99.3 °F), blood pressure is 132/72 mm Hg, pulse rate is 84/min, and respiration rate is 18/min. Oxygen saturation is 94% breathing ambient air. Oropharyngeal examination is unremarkable. He has scattered petechiae over both ankles and an ecchymosis at the insertion site of his central venous catheter.

Laboratory studies show he is neutropenic and has a platelet count of 12,000/μL (12×10^9/L).

Which of the following is the most appropriate management of this patient's thrombocytopenia?

(A) Transfuse leukoreduced, irradiated platelets
(B) Transfuse leukoreduced, irradiated, HLA-matched platelets
(C) Transfuse leukoreduced, irradiated, washed platelets
(D) Recheck platelet count in 24 hours

Item 21

A 77-year-old woman is evaluated for frequently fluctuating INRs (<1.8 to >3.5) while taking warfarin therapy. She has undergone INR testing every 1 to 2 weeks and frequent warfarin dose adjustments. She reports a consistent dietary intake. Medical history is notable only for recurrent deep venous thrombosis. She takes no other medications.

On physical examination, vital signs are normal, as is the remainder of the examination.

Which of the following is the most appropriate next step in management?

(A) Daily low-dose vitamin K supplementation
(B) Genetic testing for cytochrome P-450 2C9 and vitamin K epoxide reductase complex-1 polymorphisms
(C) Genetic testing for factor V Leiden
(D) Warfarin cessation and aspirin initiation

Item 22

A 24-year-old woman is evaluated in the emergency department for dyspnea on exertion and severe fatigue. Medical history is significant for sickle cell anemia, with a hospital admission for acute chest syndrome last year. She reports that her 4-year-old son had a high fever 1 week ago. She takes stable doses of hydroxyurea and a folic acid supplement.

On physical examination, she appears breathless and pale. Temperature is 38.4 °C (101.1 °F), blood pressure is 95/61 mm Hg, pulse rate is 104/min, and respiration rate is 14/min. Scleral icterus is observed. Lungs are clear. Cardiac examination reveals tachycardia with a prominent flow murmur.

Laboratory studies:

Hemoglobin	3.4 g/dL (34 g/L)
Leukocyte count	14,000/μL (14×10^9/L)
Platelet count	222,000/μL (222×10^9/L)
Reticulocyte count	0.1% of erythrocytes

Which of the following is the most likely cause of this patient's findings?

(A) Cytomegalovirus
(B) Epstein-Barr virus
(C) Influenza A virus
(D) Parvovirus B19

Item 23

A 35-year-old woman is evaluated for the recent onset of a rash on her legs. She has no other symptoms. She does not drink alcohol. Medications are an oral contraceptive and a multivitamin.

On physical examination, vital signs are normal. Nonpruritic, nonblanching red macules are noted on the lower extremities. Abdominal examination reveals no splenomegaly.

Laboratory study results show a hematocrit of 38%, leukocyte count of 7000/μL (7×10^9/L), and platelet count of 78,000/μL (78×10^9/L).

The peripheral blood smear is shown.

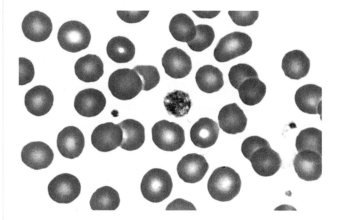

Which of the following is the most appropriate management?

(A) Anti-D immune globulin
(B) Prednisone
(C) Repeat complete blood count in 1 week
(D) Rituximab
(E) Splenectomy

Item 24

A 43-year-old man is evaluated for a 2-day history of painful swelling of the left thigh just below the groin. He reports no preceding trauma, immobility, surgery, hospital stay, or long-distance airline travel. Medical history is notable for well-controlled hypertension. His only medication is losartan.

On physical examination, vital signs are normal. BMI is 28. An approximately 6-cm area of erythema and tenderness with a palpable cord is present overlying the greater saphenous vein on the proximal medial aspect of the left thigh up to the inguinal crease, consistent with superficial thrombophlebitis. Examination of the distal extremities is normal, without swelling or asymmetry. The remainder of the examination is unremarkable.

Which of the following is the most appropriate next step in management?

(A) Low-dose aspirin

(B) Serum D-dimer testing

(C) Venous duplex ultrasonography of the left thigh

(D) Warm compresses and NSAIDs

Item 25

A 79-year-old woman is diagnosed with new-onset anemia during a routine examination. Medical history is significant for an ischemic stroke 8 weeks ago, which resulted in residual right-sided weakness and admission to a rehabilitation facility. At that time, her complete blood count was normal. She has been eating poorly while in the facility. Her medications are aspirin, lisinopril, and simvastatin.

On physical examination, temperature is 37.1 °C (98.8 °F), blood pressure is 120/70 mm Hg, pulse rate is 82/min, and respiration rate is 12/min; BMI is 27. Right-sided motor strength is 3/4 and sensation is normal.

Laboratory studies:

Hemoglobin	10.1 g/dL (101 g/L)
Mean corpuscular volume	102 fL
Folate	2.5 ng/mL (5.7 nmol/L)
Homocysteine	10.2 mg/L (75.4 µmol/L)
Methylmalonic acid	Normal

Which of the following is the most likely diagnosis?

(A) Folate deficiency

(B) Iron deficiency

(C) α-Thalassemia trait

(D) Vitamin B$_{12}$ deficiency

Item 26

A 67-year-old man is evaluated during follow-up consultation after a diagnosis of essential thrombocythemia discovered incidentally on a routine health maintenance examination. His medical history is otherwise unremarkable, and he takes no medications.

On physical examination, he is afebrile, blood pressure is 115/72 mm Hg, pulse rate is 72/min, and respiration rate is 18/min. Cardiac evaluation reveals a regular rate and rhythm with no murmurs.

Results of laboratory studies show a hemoglobin level of 15 g/dL (150 g/L), leukocyte count of 5600/µL (5.6×10^9/L), and platelet count of 770,000/µL (770 × 10^9/L). Follow-up testing confirms a diagnosis of essential thrombocythemia.

Which of the following is the most appropriate treatment?

(A) Anagrelide plus low-dose aspirin

(B) Hydroxyurea plus low-dose aspirin

(C) Ruxolitinib

(D) Warfarin

(E) Observation

Item 27

A 78-year-old woman is evaluated for progressive fatigue and dyspnea with exertion over the past 6 months. She has otherwise felt well with no nausea, vomiting, or changes in stool. Medical history is significant for hypertension and an aortic valve replacement at age 67 years. Medications are metoprolol and warfarin.

On physical examination, the patient appears well. Temperature is 37.0 °C (98.6 °F), blood pressure is 135/55 mm Hg, pulse rate is 65/min, and respiration rate is 14/min. BMI is 28. She has mild scleral icterus. The lungs are clear to auscultation. Examination of the heart reveals a mechanical S$_2$, a grade 3/6 systolic murmur at the right upper sternal border radiating to the carotid arteries, and a soft diastolic murmur heard at the left sternal border. The spleen is not palpable, and no pedal edema is present. Stool guaiac testing is negative.

Laboratory studies:

Haptoglobin	32 mg/dL (320 mg/L)
Hemoglobin	6.5 g/dL (65 g/L)
Leukocyte count	5500/µL (5.5 × 10^9/L)
Mean corpuscular volume	71 fL
Platelet count	290,000/µL (290 × 10^9/L)
Reticulocyte count	2.9% of erythrocytes
Bilirubin, total	2.7 mg/dL (46.2 µmol/L)
Bilirubin, direct	1.0 mg/dL (17.1 µmol/L)
Ferritin	3.6 ng/mL (3.6 µg/L)
Lactate dehydrogenase	1200 U/L

Peripheral blood smear shows 3+ schistocytes and microcytic, hypochromic cells.

Which of the following is the most appropriate diagnostic test to perform next?

(A) ADAMTS-13 assay

(B) D-dimer measurement

(C) Direct antiglobulin (Coombs) test

(D) Echocardiography

Item 28

A 42-year-old man arrives for follow-up consultation. Three months ago he developed a proximal right leg deep venous thrombosis following a skiing-related fracture of the right tibia. Although not recommended by guidelines, a thrombophilia evaluation was performed, which revealed an elevated plasma homocysteine level, and subsequent genetic testing revealed that he is homozygous for the C677T methylene tetrahydrofolate reductase (*MTHFR*) polymorphism. He is otherwise healthy, and his medical history is unremarkable. He has a 12-year-old son. There is no family history of thrombotic disorders. His only medication is warfarin.

Which of the following is the most appropriate next step in management?

(A) Folic acid and vitamin B$_{12}$ administration

(B) Indefinite continuation of warfarin

(C) *MTHFR* polymorphism testing of first-degree relatives

(D) Warfarin discontinuation

Item 29

A 45-year-old man is evaluated following a recent diagnosis of hereditary hemochromatosis. He was screened after a relative was diagnosed with hereditary hemochromatosis. He is asymptomatic and has no clinical or laboratory evidence of liver disease, diabetes mellitus, or cardiomyopathy. Medical history is otherwise negative, and he takes no medications.

On physical examination, vital signs are normal. The examination is unremarkable.

Weekly phlebotomy is planned.

Which of the following dietary constituents should this patient be advised to avoid?

(A) Calcium supplements
(B) Raw or undercooked seafood
(C) Red meat
(D) Vitamin C–containing fruits and vegetables

Item 30

A 26-year-old woman is evaluated during consultation for concerns about a possible hypercoagulable state. Her mother was recently diagnosed with heterozygous factor V Leiden mutation following multiple episodes of venous thromboembolic disease. The patient is concerned with her own risk of thrombosis. Medical history is unremarkable, with no venous thromboembolism or abnormal bleeding. She takes no medications.

The physical examination is unremarkable.

Which of the following is the most appropriate diagnostic test?

(A) Activated protein C resistance assay
(B) Factor V activity level
(C) Factor V Leiden genetic test
(D) No testing

Item 31

A 43-year-old woman is admitted to the hospital for fatigue of 4 weeks' duration, easy bruising and bleeding gums of 1 week's duration, and a 1-day fever of 38.9 °C (102.0 °F).

On physical examination, the patient appears ill. Temperature is 39.4 °C (103.0 °F), blood pressure is 105/62 mm Hg, pulse rate is 115/min, and respiration rate is 22/min. She has gingival bleeding, bleeding around her intravenous insertion site, and multiple ecchymoses and petechiae. Hepatomegaly is also noted.

Laboratory studies:

Activated partial thromboplastin time	65 s
Hemoglobin	7.6 g/dL (76 g/L)
Leukocyte count	32,000/μL (32 × 10⁹/L)
Platelet count	25,000/μL (25 × 10⁹/L)
Prothrombin time	24 s
Fibrinogen	97 mg/dL (0.97 g/L)

A peripheral blood smear shows 80% immature blasts with prominent Auer rods phenotypically consistent with promyelocytes.

Which of the following is the most appropriate initial management?

(A) All-*trans* retinoic acid
(B) Chemotherapy
(C) t(9;22) testing
(D) t(15;17) testing

Item 32

A 25-year-old woman is evaluated for worsening shortness of breath that began 2 to 3 days ago. A week before the onset of these symptoms, she developed a flulike syndrome of fever, myalgia, arthralgia, and transient facial rash. Medical history is significant for anemia. Her father also has anemia. She takes no medications.

On physical examination, the patient appears pale. Temperature is 36.9 °C (98.5 °F), blood pressure is 100/60 mm Hg, pulse rate is 100/min, and respiration rate is 24/min. BMI is 24. Scleral icterus is noted. On palpation, her spleen is enlarged. Cardiopulmonary examination reveals tachycardia.

Laboratory studies:

Hematocrit	18%
Leukocyte count	8300/μL (8.3 × 10⁹/L)
Platelet count	200,000/μL (200 × 10⁹/L)
Lactate dehydrogenase	500 U/L
Direct antiglobulin (Coombs) test	Negative

A peripheral blood smear is shown.

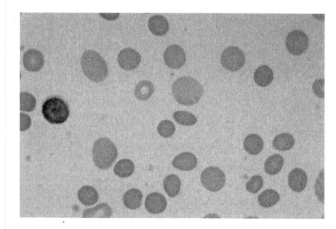

Which of the following is the most appropriate diagnostic test?

(A) Diagnostic trial of prednisone
(B) Flow cytometry
(C) Glucose-6-phosphate dehydrogenase activity
(D) Osmotic fragility test

Item 33

A 45-year-old man is evaluated in follow-up for iron deficiency anemia discovered during routine evaluation 1 week ago. His complete blood count was normal when he was last evaluated 1 year ago. He feels well, his medical history is unremarkable, and he takes no medications.

The physical examination performed 1 week ago was normal.

A fecal occult blood test is negative.

Iron replacement is initiated.

Which of the following is the most appropriate management?

(A) Colonoscopy and upper endoscopy
(B) Repeat iron studies in 1 month
(C) Tissue transglutaminase IgA antibody assay
(D) Wireless capsule endoscopy

Item 34

A 24-year-old woman undergoes routine evaluation. She is pregnant at 12 weeks' gestation. Medical history is notable for homozygous sickle cell anemia (Hb SS). She has had multiple uncomplicated painful crises treated at home with hydration, nonopioid analgesia, and incentive spirometry. She requires hospital management for these episodes approximately twice per year. She has declined the use of hydroxyurea. Her only other medication is folic acid.

On physical examination, vital signs are normal. Mild scleral icterus is noted. A grade 2/6 early systolic flow murmur is heard at the cardiac base. The examination is otherwise normal.

Laboratory results show a hemoglobin level of 7.5 g/dL (75 g/L).

Which of the following is the most appropriate management?

(A) Erythrocyte transfusion to maintain hemoglobin level at 10 g/dL (100 g/L)
(B) Erythropoiesis-stimulating agent
(C) Exchange transfusion
(D) No transfusion at this time

Item 35

A 73-year-old woman is evaluated in the emergency department following a fall in her home. She tripped and fell over a rug. She did not lose consciousness but is experiencing left hip pain. Medical history is remarkable for atrial fibrillation. Her only medication is warfarin.

On physical examination, the patient is afebrile, blood pressure is 137/88 mm Hg, pulse rate is 105/min and irregular, and respiration rate is 14/min. The lungs are clear to auscultation, and the cardiac examination is significant only for an irregular rate. She has mild tenderness to palpation over the left hip. No hematoma or other bleeding is evident. The remainder of the examination is unremarkable.

Laboratory studies show a normal hemoglobin level and an INR of 10.2.

Radiographs of the left hip are negative for fracture.

In addition to withholding warfarin, which of the following is the most appropriate management of this patient's anticoagulation?

(A) 4-Factor prothrombin complex concentrate
(B) Fresh frozen plasma
(C) Oral vitamin K
(D) No additional therapy

Item 36

A 52-year-old man is evaluated for low back pain of 3 months' duration that is nonradiating, progressive, and worse with ambulation. He reports no preceding injury. Medical history is notable for smoldering multiple myeloma diagnosed 1 year ago; he has been stable since that time. His only medication is as-needed acetaminophen.

On physical examination, temperature is 36.8 °C (98.2 °F), blood pressure is 132/82 mm Hg, pulse rate is 70/min, and respiration rate is 14/min. No focal neurologic findings are noted. He has pain to palpation of the lower lumbar spine. The remainder of the examination is unremarkable.

Laboratory studies show a hemoglobin level of 13 g/dL (130 g/L), serum creatinine level of 1.0 mg/dL (88.4 µmol/L), and serum calcium level of 9.8 mg/dL (2.5 mmol/L).

Plain radiographs of the lumbosacral spine demonstrate degenerative disk changes in the lumbar spine but no lytic lesions or fractures.

Which of the following is the most appropriate management?

(A) Chemotherapy
(B) MRI of the lumbar spine
(C) Symptomatic treatment and routine follow-up
(D) Zoledronic acid

Item 37

A 19-year-old woman is evaluated for progressive weakness and dyspnea during exercise. Medical history is notable for heavy menses since menarche that last approximately 8 days. She had abnormal bleeding with wisdom tooth extraction 5 years ago. Her mother and sister have heavy menses. Her only medication is a multivitamin.

On physical examination, she appears pale. Temperature is 36.8 °C (98.2 °F), blood pressure is 110/65 mm Hg, pulse rate is 100/min, and respiration rate is 18/min. Pale conjunctivae are noted. A grade 2/6 systolic murmur is heard at the cardiac base. The lung fields are clear. The remainder of the examination is normal.

Laboratory studies:

Hematocrit	25%
Leukocyte count	5700/µL (5.7 × 10⁹/L)
Mean corpuscular volume	71 fL
Platelet count	490,000/µL (490 × 10⁹/L)
Activated partial thromboplastin time	25 s
Prothrombin time	10 s

Which of the following is the most likely diagnosis?

(A) Factor VII deficiency
(B) Factor XI deficiency
(C) Factor XII deficiency
(D) Hemophilia A
(E) von Willebrand disease

Item 38

A 73-year-old woman undergoes follow-up warfarin monitoring. She takes warfarin for atrial fibrillation and her INRs have previously been stable. Five days ago, she was prescribed a 3-day course of trimethoprim-sulfamethoxazole for an uncomplicated urinary tract infection. Three weeks ago, her INR was 2.9; this morning, her INR is 8.2. She has no history of major bleeding.

On physical examination, vital signs are normal. No bruising or bleeding is evident. The cardiac examination reveals an irregular rhythm but is otherwise unremarkable.

Laboratory studies show a hemoglobin level of 13.6 g/dL (136 g/L) and platelet count of 178,000/μL (178 × 10⁹/L).

Which of the following is the most appropriate management?

(A) Fresh frozen plasma infusion
(B) Oral vitamin K and repeat INR in 24 hours
(C) Prothrombin complex concentrate administration
(D) Warfarin interruption

Item 39

A 58-year-old man is evaluated in the hospital for thrombocytopenia. He recently underwent multiple orthopedic procedures for repair of traumatic injuries experienced 3 days ago. He received 12 units of packed red blood cells throughout trauma resuscitation and surgical procedures. Except for postoperative pain, the patient reports no focal symptoms. Medical history is otherwise unremarkable. Medications are as-needed acetaminophen and oxycodone for pain relief and subcutaneous unfractionated heparin for venous thromboembolism prophylaxis.

On physical examination, temperature is 37.2 °C (99.0 °F), blood pressure is 135/85 mm Hg, pulse rate is 89/min, and respiration rate is 18/min. Multiple healing surgical incisions are clean and dry, without evidence of infection. No lower extremity edema is present. The remainder of the examination is unremarkable.

Laboratory studies show a hemoglobin level of 11.5 g/dL (115 g/L), leukocyte count of 9800/μL (9.8 × 10⁹/L), and platelet count of 115,000/μL (115 × 10⁹/L) (previously 160,000/μL [160 × 10⁹/L]).

Which of the following is the most appropriate next step in management?

(A) 4T pretest probability scoring
(B) Heparin-induced platelet aggregation assay
(C) Platelet factor 4 enzyme-linked immunosorbent assay
(D) Serotonin release assay

Item 40

A 65-year-old man was admitted to the hospital 10 days ago with community-acquired pneumonia requiring intubation, mechanical ventilation, and fluids and vasopressors for persistent hypotension. He has since been extubated and his blood pressure has stabilized;

he no longer requires vasopressor therapy. Oxygen saturation is 90% with 3 L/min oxygen via nasal cannula. He has a resolving cough and improving fatigue. Medical history is otherwise unremarkable. Medications in the hospital are levofloxacin, heparin, and omeprazole.

Laboratory studies:

Hemoglobin	7.4 g/dL (74 g/L) (10.6 g/dL [106 g/L] on admission)
Reticulocyte count	2.0% of erythrocytes; absolute: 58,000/μL (58 × 10⁹/L)
Creatinine	2.8 mg/dL (248 μmol/L) (4.5 mg/dL [398 μmol/L] on admission)
Iron studies	
Ferritin	410 ng/mL (410 μg/L)
Iron, serum	30 μg/dL (5.4 μmol/L)
Total iron-binding capacity	144 μg/dL (26 μmol/L)

Electrocardiography reveals no ST- or T-wave changes.

Which of the following is the most appropriate management of this patient's anemia?

(A) Erythrocyte transfusion
(B) Erythropoiesis-stimulating agent
(C) Intravenous iron
(D) Continue current management

Item 41

A 45-year-old man presents to the emergency department with a 1-week history of fever, chills, hypotension, cough, progressive dyspnea, and lethargy. Medical history is remarkable for hepatitis C virus infection with cirrhosis. Medications are omeprazole and propranolol.

On physical examination, the patient is in moderate respiratory distress. Temperature is 39.2 °C (102.6 °F), blood pressure is 74/42 mm Hg, pulse rate is 144/min, and respiration rate is 26/min. Oxygen saturation is 76% breathing ambient air. He has no jugular venous distention. Chest examination reveals decreased breath sounds over the lower left lung field. Mild abdominal distention is present without a fluid wave. The spleen tip is palpable below the left costal margin.

Laboratory studies:

Activated partial thromboplastin time	42.4 s
Hemoglobin	11.8 g/dL (118 g/L)
Leukocyte count	10,500/μL (10.5 × 10⁹/L)
Platelet count	63,000/μL (63 × 10⁹/L)
Prothrombin time	16.6 s
INR	1.4
Fibrinogen	154 mg/dL (1.5 g/L)

A chest radiograph shows opacity of the left lower lobe and a moderate left-sided pleural effusion.

The patient is admitted to the ICU. Placement of an internal jugular central venous catheter is planned for medication administration.

CONT.

Which of the following is the most appropriate next step in management before catheter placement?

(A) Cryoprecipitate transfusion

(B) Fresh frozen plasma transfusion

(C) Platelet transfusion

(D) No transfusion

Item 42

A 35-year-old woman is evaluated following a recent diagnosis of iron deficiency anemia secondary to menorrhagia. She began an oral contraceptive to control bleeding and oral iron sulfate 6 weeks ago. She has no other medical conditions and takes no additional medications.

On physical examination, vital signs are normal. The conjunctivae are pink. No petechiae or purpura is evident. The remainder of the examination is normal.

Laboratory studies show a hematocrit level of 39%, leukocyte count of 5800/µL (5.8 × 10⁹/L), and platelet count of 35,000/µL (35 × 10⁹/L).

The peripheral blood smear is shown.

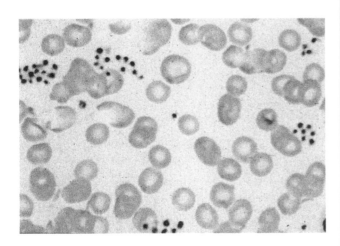

Which of the following is the most appropriate management?

(A) Antinuclear antibody and HIV testing

(B) Plasma exchange

(C) Prednisone

(D) Repeat complete blood count with a citrated tube

Item 43

A 45-year-old woman is evaluated before surgery; she is scheduled to undergo elective hysterectomy for fibroid tumors. Her medical history is significant for type 1 von Willebrand disease (vWD), long-standing iron deficiency anemia, and heavy menstrual bleeding. Family history is notable for vWD in the patient's father, sister, and two sons. Her only medication is iron sulfate.

On physical examination, vital signs are normal. The patient has palpable lower abdominal masses along the midline consistent with fibroids.

Which of the following is the most appropriate perioperative treatment?

(A) Cryoprecipitate

(B) Fresh frozen plasma

(C) Recombinant factor VIII

(D) Tranexamic acid

(E) von Willebrand factor–containing factor VIII concentrates

Item 44

A 55-year-old man is evaluated for fatigue and gradually increasing dyspnea of 1 month's duration. He has otherwise felt well and has no other symptoms, although he reports an occasional bluish tint to his fingers while at work. He is employed as a frozen food handler in a grocery store. Medical history is unremarkable, and he takes no medications.

On physical examination, the patient appears pale. Temperature is 37.0 °C (98.6 °F), blood pressure is 130/65 mm Hg, pulse rate is 98/min, and respiration rate is 18/min. BMI is 26. Mild scleral icterus is noted. A grade 2/6 systolic murmur is heard at the left costal margin without radiation. The lungs are clear to auscultation. No lymphadenopathy is noted, but the spleen tip is palpable below the left costal margin.

Laboratory studies:

Hematocrit	23%
Leukocyte count	13,200/µL (13.2 × 10⁹/L) with normal differential
Platelet count	355,000/µL (355 × 10⁹/L)
Reticulocyte count	14% of erythrocytes
Lactate dehydrogenase	978 U/L

Peripheral blood smear is shown.

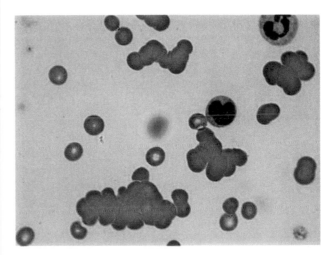

Which of the following is the most appropriate diagnostic test to perform next?

(A) Direct antiglobulin (Coombs) test

(B) Flow cytometry for CD55 or CD59

(C) Hemoglobin electrophoresis

(D) Indirect antiglobulin (Coombs) test

Item 45

A 50-year-old man is evaluated for anemia following a diagnosis of osteomyelitis of the right foot. Complete blood counts before the osteomyelitis diagnosis have been normal. Medical history is notable for type 2 diabetes mellitus. His only medication is metformin.

On physical examination, vital signs are normal; BMI is 30. No cardiopulmonary findings attributable to the anemia are noted. The right foot has a small, deep open wound through which bone can be detected with a metal probe.

Laboratory studies:

Erythrocyte sedimentation rate	60 mm/h
Hemoglobin	8.5 g/dL (85 g/L)
Leukocyte count	15,000/µL (15 × 10⁹/L)
Mean corpuscular volume	80 fL
Reticulocyte count	0.5% of erythrocytes
Iron studies	
Ferritin	500 ng/mL (500 µg/L)
Iron	50 µg/dL (9 µmol/L)
Total iron-binding capacity	225 µg/dL (40 µmol/L)
Transferrin saturation	30%

Appropriate antibiotics are initiated.

Which of the following is the most appropriate management of this patient's anemia?

(A) Bone marrow aspiration
(B) Erythropoiesis-stimulating agent therapy
(C) Oral iron supplementation
(D) Continue current management

Item 46

A 24-year-old man is evaluated for a 2-month history of frequent upper respiratory tract infections, easy bruising, and worsening endurance. Medical and family histories are unremarkable. He takes no medications.

On physical examination, the patient appears fatigued, but not acutely ill. Temperature is 36.7 °C (98.0 °F), blood pressure is 105/62 mm Hg, pulse rate is 108/min, and respiration rate is 14/min. Pallor and several 3- to 4-cm ecchymoses on the lower extremities are noted. He has no hepatosplenomegaly.

Laboratory studies:

Haptoglobin	40 mg/dL (400 mg/L)
Hemoglobin	7.2 g/dL (72 g/L)
Leukocyte count	1000/µL (1 × 10⁹/L) with 5% neutrophils
Platelet count	7000/µL (7 × 10⁹/L)
Lactate dehydrogenase	150 U/L

Bone marrow aspirate demonstrates less than 5% blasts and no dysplastic changes. Results of a bone marrow biopsy are shown (see top of next column).

Which of the following is the most likely diagnosis?

(A) Acute lymphoblastic leukemia
(B) Acute myeloid leukemia
(C) Aplastic anemia
(D) Myelodysplastic syndrome
(E) Paroxysmal nocturnal hemoglobinuria

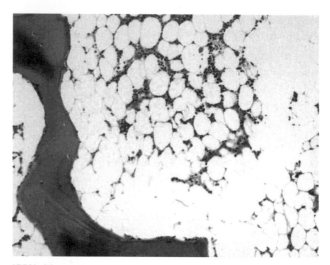

ITEM 46

Item 47

A 56-year-old woman is evaluated for an elevated serum protein level discovered during a routine examination for a life insurance policy. She is asymptomatic. Medical and family histories are unremarkable, and she takes no medications.

On physical examination, vital signs are normal, and the remainder of the examination is unremarkable.

Laboratory studies:

Hemoglobin	13.4 g/dL (134 g/L)
Leukocyte count	6400/µL (6.4 × 10⁹/L)
Platelet count	224,000/µL (224 × 10⁹/L)
Calcium	9.6 mg/dL (2.4 mmol/L)
Creatinine	0.7 mg/dL (61.9 µmol/L)
IgA	2080 mg/dL (20.8 g/L)

Serum protein electrophoresis and immunofixation reveal a monoclonal IgA κ band measuring 1.8 g/dL. A 24-hour urine protein electrophoresis reveals 80 mg of total protein and trace monoclonal free κ light chains that are too low to quantify.

A bone marrow aspirate and biopsy reveals clonal plasma cells representing 8% of the overall marrow cellularity. A skeletal survey demonstrates no lytic lesions, osteopenia, or fractures.

Which of the following is the most appropriate diagnostic test to perform next?

(A) MRI of the cervical, thoracic, and lumbar spine
(B) Serum β₂-microglobulin measurement
(C) Serum free light chain testing
(D) Serum lactate dehydrogenase measurement

Item 48

A 63-year-old man is evaluated for severe mid-upper back pain following a minor fall 1 day ago. He also notes progressive fatigue of 6 months' duration and a 6.8-kg (15 lb) weight loss. Medical history is notable for an 80-pack-year smoking history, although he is currently a nonsmoker.

On physical examination, temperature is 37.3 °C (99.1 °F), blood pressure is 112/74 mm Hg, pulse rate is 98/min, and respiration rate is 18/min. BMI is 22. The cardiopulmonary examination is unremarkable. He has no lymphadenopathy or hepatosplenomegaly. Point tenderness to palpation is noted over the mid thoracic spine. No skin changes or peripheral edema are observed.

Laboratory studies:

Hemoglobin	11 g/dL (110 g/L)
Leukocyte count	4800/µL (4.8 × 10⁹/L) with a normal differential
Platelet count	155,000/µL (155 × 10⁹/L)
Albumin	2.8 g/dL (28 g/L)
Calcium	11.8 mg/dL (3.0 mmol/L)
Creatinine	3.1 mg/dL (274 µmol/L)
Total protein	6.3 g/dL (63 g/L)
Urinalysis	Trace protein, no blood, 0 erythrocytes/hpf, no casts
Urine protein-creatinine ratio	2300 mg/g

A chest radiograph shows no infiltrates and a normal cardiac silhouette. Radiographs of the thoracic spine reveal osteopenia with a compression fracture of T6.

Which of the following is the most appropriate diagnostic test to perform next?

(A) 1,25-Dihydroxyvitamin D (calcitriol) measurement

(B) Intact parathyroid hormone measurement

(C) Parathyroid hormone–related protein measurement

(D) Serum protein electrophoresis and free light chain test

Item 49

A 48-year-old man is evaluated in the emergency department for fever and cough of 7 days' duration. Medical history is notable for an aortic valve replacement. His only regular medication is warfarin, although he reports taking acetaminophen every 2 to 3 hours to relieve his fever and chest pain as a result of coughing.

On physical examination, the patient appears ill and slightly jaundiced. Temperature is 38.9 °C (102.0 °F), blood pressure is 90/45 mm Hg, pulse rate is 120/min, and respiration rate is 24/min. Oxygen saturation is 91% breathing ambient air. Coarse breath sounds with rhonchi in the right lung base are heard on auscultation. Cardiac examination reveals regular tachycardia and a mechanical S₂ but no other findings. Right upper quadrant tenderness and multiple ecchymoses are noted.

Laboratory studies:

D-dimer	5800 µg/mL (5800 mg/L)
Leukocyte count	22,000/µL (22 × 10⁹/L)
Platelet count	95,000/µL (95 × 10⁹/L)
Prothrombin time	58 s
Fibrinogen	110 mg/dL (1.1 g/L)
INR	8.8 (6 weeks ago, 2.5)
Factor V	20% (normal, 50%-150%)
Factor VII	5% (normal, 50%-150%)
Factor VIII	200% (normal, 50%-150%)

Chest radiograph shows a right lower lobe infiltrate.

Which of the following is the most likely cause of the patient's coagulation abnormality?

(A) Disseminated intravascular coagulation

(B) Liver failure

(C) Vitamin K deficiency

(D) Warfarin overdose

Item 50

A 34-year-old man is evaluated for a 3-month history of fatigue, early satiety, and a 10-kg (22 lb) weight loss. Medical history is notable for hypertension, which is well controlled with hydrochlorothiazide.

On physical examination, temperature is 36.7 °C (98.0 °F), blood pressure is 135/81 mm Hg, pulse rate is 114/min, and respiration rate is 13/min. Cardiac and pulmonary examinations are normal, and no lymphadenopathy is noted. The spleen is palpable 10 cm below the costal margin.

Laboratory studies show a hemoglobin level of 8.4 g/dL (84 g/L), leukocyte count of 314,000/µL (314 × 10⁹/L), and platelet count of 622,000/µL (622 × 10⁹/L).

A peripheral blood smear is shown.

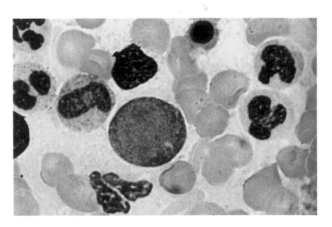

Which of the following is the most likely genetic mutation to explain this patient's findings?

(A) *BCR-ABL*

(B) *IGH/CD1*

(C) *JAK2 V617F*

(D) *PML-RAR*

Item 51

A 30-year-old man with acute lymphoblastic leukemia is evaluated for fever, chills, rigors, and dyspnea, which started toward the end of a platelet transfusion given for chemotherapy-induced thrombocytopenia.

On physical examination, the patient is lethargic, flushed, and clammy. Temperature is 39.4 °C (102.9 °F), blood pressure is 90/42 mm Hg, pulse rate is 150/min, and respiration rate is 24/min (before transfusion, temperature was 37.2 °C [99.0 °F], blood pressure was 140/76 mm Hg, and pulse rate was 90/min). Oxygen saturation is 94% breathing ambient air. Rigors are noted, and skin is warm

CONT.

to the touch without skin changes. Head, neck, and pulmonary examinations are unremarkable. Cardiac examination reveals tachycardia but no murmurs.

In addition to stopping the transfusion and administering intravenous fluids, which of the following is the most appropriate treatment?

- (A) Diphenhydramine, acetaminophen, and meperidine
- (B) Epinephrine
- (C) Vancomycin and cefepime
- (D) No additional treatment

Item 52

A 61-year-old man is evaluated in the emergency department for diffuse, mild, left calf pain without swelling of 10 days' duration, which has worsened in the past 2 days. The patient reports no provoking injury or incident. He feels well otherwise. Medical and family histories are unremarkable. He takes no medications.

On physical examination, temperature is 37.2 °C (99.0 °F), blood pressure is 132/82 mm Hg, pulse rate is 75/min, and respiration rate is 16/min. BMI is 32. He is in no acute distress, but he scores his leg pain as 3/10 in intensity. Mild to moderately deep palpation of the calf muscles provokes diffuse discomfort. The left leg is not discolored, and no edema is present, but it feels slightly fuller than the right and is 1 cm in circumference larger than the right at the midcalf level.

Which of the following is the most appropriate management?

- (A) Anticoagulant therapy for 3 months
- (B) Blood D-dimer test
- (C) Duplex ultrasonography of the leg
- (D) Magnetic resonance venography of the leg

Item 53

A 23-year-old man is admitted to the hospital for severe right upper quadrant pain of 2 days' duration. Medical history is significant for homozygous sickle cell anemia (Hb SS). His only medication is folic acid.

On physical examination, temperature is 37.8 °C (100.0 °F), blood pressure is 115/70 mm Hg, pulse rate is 100/min, and respiration rate is 24/min. Oxygen saturation is 98% breathing ambient air. Palpation confirms a tender right upper quadrant. The remainder of the examination is normal.

Laboratory studies reveal a hemoglobin level of 7.5 g/dL (75 g/L) and a platelet count of 415,000/μL (415 × 10⁹/L).

Abdominal ultrasonography confirms a diagnosis of cholecystitis, and a laparoscopic cholecystectomy is planned before hospital discharge.

In addition to antibiotics, which of the following is the most appropriate preoperative management?

- (A) Erythrocyte exchange transfusion to a target hemoglobin S of less than 30%
- (B) Erythrocyte transfusion to a hemoglobin level of 10 g/dL (100 g/L)
- (C) Erythrocyte transfusion to a hemoglobin level of 12 g/dL (120 g/L)
- (D) Erythrocyte transfusion for symptomatic anemia

Item 54

A 65-year-old woman is evaluated in the emergency department for a 1-day history of pain and swelling in her left leg. Medical history is significant for coronary artery bypass graft surgery 8 days ago with vein harvesting from the right leg. She also has hypertension and hyperlipidemia. Medications are atorvastatin, atenolol, clopidogrel, and aspirin.

On physical examination, temperature is 37.0 °C (98.6 °F), blood pressure is 115/68 mm Hg, pulse rate is 65/min, and respiration rate is 18/min. Oxygen saturation breathing ambient air is 96%. Her sternotomy incision is healing well. The cardiopulmonary examination is normal. The left leg is swollen to the mid-thigh.

Laboratory studies reveal a hematocrit of 33%, leukocyte count of 12,000/μL (12 × 10⁹/L), and platelet count of 55,000/μL (55 × 10⁹/L).

Duplex ultrasonography of the left leg shows acute thrombus in the common femoral vein.

Which of the following is the most appropriate next step in management?

- (A) Await platelet factor 4 immunoassay before initiating anticoagulation
- (B) Await serotonin release assay before initiating anticoagulation
- (C) Initiate argatroban
- (D) Initiate heparin
- (E) Initiate warfarin

Item 55

A 32-year-old woman is evaluated for anticoagulation management after an uncomplicated vaginal delivery of a healthy newborn. She was diagnosed with a bilateral pulmonary embolism at 25 weeks' gestation and was treated with therapeutic low-molecular-weight heparin (LMWH). The LMWH was discontinued at the onset of labor and was restarted 6 hours after delivery. Medical history is otherwise unremarkable, and her only medication is full-dose LMWH.

Anticoagulation for 3 months is planned. The patient wishes to breastfeed her newborn.

Which of the following is the most appropriate anticoagulation option for this patient?

- (A) Apixaban
- (B) Dabigatran
- (C) Fondaparinux
- (D) Rivaroxaban
- (E) Warfarin

Item 56

A 72-year-old woman is evaluated in follow-up for a recent diagnosis of multiple myeloma. She presented with an

8-month history of progressive fatigue and dyspnea with exertion, but has had no other symptoms. Medical history is unremarkable, and she takes no medications.

On physical examination, temperature is 37.6 °C (99.7 °F), blood pressure is 142/86 mm Hg, pulse rate is 90/min, and respiration rate is 14/min. No focal neurologic deficits are observed. Cardiopulmonary examination is normal, and the remainder of the physical examination is unremarkable.

Initial laboratory studies showed a hemoglobin level of 9.2 g/dL (92 g/L), serum calcium level of 10.2 mg/dL (2.6 mmol/L), and serum creatinine level of 1.3 mg/dL (115 μmol/L).

A monoclonal IgG κ band of 4.2 g/dL was seen on serum protein electrophoresis and immunofixation, and myeloma was confirmed with a bone marrow aspirate and biopsy showing clonal plasma cells representing 70% of the overall cellularity.

A skeletal survey demonstrates diffuse osteopenia and a T12 compression fracture with 50% height loss. No lytic lesions are seen.

In addition to starting chemotherapy, which of the following is the most appropriate treatment?

(A) Balloon kyphoplasty to the T12 vertebra
(B) Radiation therapy to the thoracic spine
(C) Zoledronic acid
(D) No additional treatment

Item 57

A 22-year-old woman is evaluated for a 2-month history of increasing fatigue and dyspnea, which is most noticeable with exercise. She otherwise feels well. She notes no gastrointestinal symptoms, although she believes that her urine sometimes appears darker than usual. She eats a normal diet, menstruation is of usual duration and flow, and she is physically active as a distance runner. Medical and family histories are otherwise unremarkable; her only medication is ibuprofen as needed.

On physical examination, temperature is 37.0 °C (98.6 °F), blood pressure is 100/55 mm Hg, pulse rate is 65/min, and respiration rate is 16/min. She has no muscle tenderness or weakness. The remainder of the physical examination is normal. A stool sample is guaiac negative.

Laboratory studies:

Haptoglobin	Undetectable
Hematocrit	25%
Leukocyte count	5500/μL (5.5 × 10⁹/L)
Mean corpuscular volume	72 fL
Platelet count	430,000/μL (430 × 10⁹/L)
Reticulocyte count	1.2% of erythrocytes
Creatine kinase	165 U/L
Ferritin	3 ng/mL (3 μg/L)
Lactate dehydrogenase	1400 U/L
Urinalysis	Dipstick positive for 4+ blood; 0-1 leukocytes/hpf, and 0 erythrocytes/hpf

Peripheral blood smear shows hypochromic microcytic erythrocytes without schistocytes or spherocytes.

Which of the following is the most likely cause of this patient's anemia?

(A) Exercise-induced hematuria
(B) Exercise-induced hemolysis
(C) Inflammatory myopathy
(D) Rhabdomyolysis

Item 58

A 27-year-old woman is evaluated during a follow-up visit. She was evaluated 3 months previously for symptoms of fatigue of 9 months' duration and a craving for ice. She experiences heavy, irregular menstrual cycles, but has no history of other bleeding. Medications are oral contraceptive pills and daily iron, which were initiated 3 months ago.

On physical examination, vital signs are normal; BMI is 31. No splenomegaly is noted.

Laboratory studies:

	3 Months Ago	2 Months Ago	Current
Ferritin	6 ng/mL (6 μg/L)	16 ng/mL (16 μg/L)	45 ng/mL (45 μg/L)
Hemoglobin	8.7 g/dL (87 g/L)	10.1 g/dL (101 g/L)	13 g/dL (130 g/L)
Mean corpuscular volume	71 fL	77 fL	88 fL
Platelet count	800,000/μL (800 × 10⁹/L)	790,000/μL (790 × 10⁹/L)	775,000/μL (775 × 10⁹/L)

Which of the following is the most appropriate diagnostic test to perform next?

(A) *BCR-ABL* genetic analysis
(B) *JAK2 V617F* analysis
(C) Prothrombin time and activated partial thromboplastin time
(D) von Willebrand factor antigen

Item 59

An 18-year-old woman is evaluated in follow-up after routine evaluation 3 months ago revealed iron deficiency thought to be related to menorrhagia. She is African and emigrated from the Ivory Coast 6 months ago. Medical history is remarkable for a 2-year history of chronic dyspepsia treated occasionally with a liquid antacid. Her other medications are an oral contraceptive pill and oral ferrous sulfate three times daily.

On physical examination, vital signs are normal. She appears healthy.

Laboratory studies:

	3 Months Ago	Current
Hematocrit	30%	33%
Mean corpuscular volume	70 fL	70 fL
Platelet count	525,000/μL (525 × 10⁹/L)	500,000/μL (500 × 10⁹/L)

Reticulocyte count	–	0.4% of erythrocytes
Red cell distribu-tion width	17.5% (normal, 14.6%-16.5%)	17%
Iron studies		
Ferritin	10 ng/mL (10 µg/L)	10 ng/mL (10 µg/L)
Iron	15 µg/dL (2.7 µmol/L)	15 µg/dL (2.7 µmol/L)
Total iron-binding capacity	425 µg/dL (76 µmol/L)	400 µg/dL (71.6 µmol/L)
Transferrin saturation	12%	13%

Which of the following is the most appropriate management?

(A) Add ascorbic acid
(B) Perform *Helicobacter pylori* stool antigen assay
(C) Perform IgG antigliadin assay
(D) Switch to ferrous gluconate

Item 60

A 63-year-old man is scheduled for recommended repeat colonoscopy in follow-up of adenomatous polyps detected on screening 3 years ago. Medical history is significant for an unprovoked pulmonary embolism 5 years ago. He was initially treated with warfarin but switched to rivaroxaban 1 year ago because of fluctuating INR values with warfarin. He is otherwise healthy and has had no bleeding.

Laboratory studies show a normal complete blood count and a serum creatinine level of 0.8 mg/dL (70.7 µmol/L).

Which of the following is the most appropriate management of this patient's anticoagulation for undergoing colonoscopy?

(A) Continue rivaroxaban without interruption
(B) Stop rivaroxaban 1 day before colonoscopy without bridging
(C) Stop rivaroxaban 1 day before colonoscopy and bridge with low-molecular-weight heparin
(D) Stop rivaroxaban 5 days before colonoscopy without bridging
(E) Stop rivaroxaban 5 days before colonoscopy and bridge with low-molecular-weight heparin

Item 61

An 18-year-old woman is evaluated following the discovery of anemia on a precollege physical examination. She is asymptomatic. She has regular menstrual cycles every 28 days, which last 5 to 6 days with heavy bleeding on the first 2 days. Medical history is otherwise unremarkable; however, her mother has anemia that is refractory to oral iron therapy. Her only medication is oral iron, which she began taking independently after her anemia diagnosis.

The physical examination is unremarkable.

Laboratory studies:

Erythrocyte count	$6.0 \times 10^6/\mu L$ ($6.0 \times 10^{12}/L$)
Hematocrit	33%
Hemoglobin	11 g/dL (110 g/L)
Leukocyte count	6000/µL ($6 \times 10^9/L$)
Mean corpuscular volume	70 fL
Platelet count	150,000/µL ($150 \times 10^9/L$)
Reticulocyte count	2.3% of erythrocytes
Red cell distribution width	15 (normal range, 14.6-16.5)
Iron studies	
Ferritin	100 ng/mL (100 µg/L)
Iron	60 µg/dL (11 µmol/L)
Total iron-binding capacity	250 µg/dL (45 µmol/L)

A peripheral blood smear is shown.

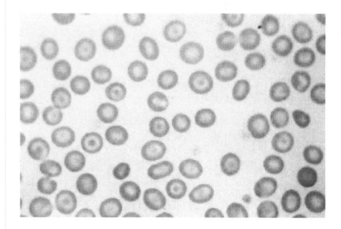

Which of the following is the most appropriate management?

(A) Discontinuation of oral iron supplementation
(B) Fecal occult blood test
(C) Oral contraceptive pill
(D) Parenteral iron supplementation

Item 62

A 19-year-old woman is seen for counseling regarding contraceptives. Medical history is unremarkable; she is nulliparous and has never taken prescription contraceptives. Her father had a pulmonary embolism at age 47 years, which was associated with arthroscopic knee surgery, and her 23-year-old sister experienced a deep venous thrombosis 3 weeks after delivering her first child. The patient does not smoke and takes no medications.

On physical examination, she appears well. Vital signs are normal; BMI is 31. The remainder of the examination is unremarkable.

She states that she does not want to use a copper intra-uterine device (IUD).

Which of the following contraceptive methods would be most appropriate for this patient?

(A) Estrogen-progestin vaginal ring
(B) Low-dose combination estrogen-progestin pill
(C) Progestin-releasing IUD
(D) Transdermal estrogen-progestin patch

Item 63

A 63-year-old man is evaluated in the emergency department for significant shortness of breath and pleuritic anterior chest pain of 48 hours' duration. Three days ago, he completed a 12-hour flight from Asia to the United States. Medical history is otherwise unremarkable and he takes no medications.

On physical examination, he is in mild respiratory distress. He is afebrile, blood pressure is 135/87 mm Hg, pulse rate is 108/min, and respiration rate is 18/min. Oxygen saturation breathing ambient air is 94%. The remainder of the physical examination is unremarkable.

Electrocardiography shows nonspecific ST- and T-wave changes. Echocardiography shows normal right ventricular function. CT angiography of the chest demonstrates multiple pulmonary artery filling defects in the distal branches of the right pulmonary artery consistent with pulmonary embolism.

Which of the following is the most appropriate next step in management?

(A) Catheter-directed thrombolysis
(B) Inpatient anticoagulation
(C) Outpatient anticoagulation
(D) Systemic thrombolysis

Item 64

A 67-year-old man is evaluated for progressive lower extremity swelling and dyspnea with exertion of 12 months' duration and orthopnea of 2 months' duration. He is black. Medical history is otherwise unremarkable, and he takes no medications.

On physical examination, temperature is 36.8 °C (98.2 °F), blood pressure is 118/64 mm Hg, pulse rate is 84/min, and respiration rate is 18/min. He has jugular venous distention, a summation gallop, and dullness to percussion and decreased breath sounds at the lung bases. Bilateral lower extremity pitting edema extends to the mid-calf level. The remainder of the physical examination is normal.

On laboratory testing, complete blood count is normal. Comprehensive metabolic profile reveals only an elevated total serum protein level. Serum protein electrophoresis and immunofixation reveal a monoclonal IgG κ band measuring 0.9 g/dL. A 24-hour urine protein electrophoresis and immunofixation reveal no monoclonal protein and no albuminuria.

Chest radiograph shows cardiomegaly and bilateral pleural effusions. Transthoracic echocardiography reveals severe symmetric left ventricular and septal thickening with a small ventricular cavity and reduced systolic function. Bone marrow aspirate and biopsy shows clonal plasma cells representing 8% of the total cellularity. Although a bone marrow biopsy is negative, a Congo red stain of a fat pad aspirate is positive for amyloid deposits.

Which of the following is the most appropriate management?

(A) Amyloid typing
(B) Autologous hematopoietic stem cell transplantation
(C) Chemotherapy
(D) Transmyocardial biopsy

Item 65

A 24-year-old woman with hemoglobin SS sickle cell disease is evaluated in the emergency department for extremity and chest pain of 24 hours' duration. She is 24 weeks pregnant. She reports the pain is similar to her usual vasoocclusive pain located in her legs and low back but is not sufficiently relieved by morphine taken at home. She experiences pain episodes approximately two to three times per year, which she often manages at home. Medical history is otherwise unremarkable. Her only other medication is a folic acid supplement.

On physical examination, the patient appears uncomfortable and pale, with slight scleral icterus. She is afebrile, blood pressure is 120/70 mm Hg, pulse rate is 110/min, and respiration rate is 24/min and unlabored. Oxygen saturation is 94% breathing ambient air. Cardiac examination reveals regular heart sounds with a grade 2/6 systolic murmur. The lungs are clear to auscultation.

Laboratory studies:

Hemoglobin	5.9 g/dL (59 g/L) (prepregnancy baseline: 7-8 g/dL [70-80 g/L]; during pregnancy: 6-7 g/dL [60-70 g/L])
Alanine aminotransferase	35 U/L
Aspartate aminotransferase	32 U/L
Creatinine	0.7 mg/dL (35.4 µmol/L)

Fetal examination reveals no fetal distress.

Which of the following is the most appropriate treatment?

(A) Erythrocyte transfusion
(B) Exchange transfusion
(C) Hydroxyurea
(D) Intravenous fluids and narcotic analgesics

Item 66

A 65-year-old man is evaluated in the emergency department for a 3-day history of abdominal pain. The pain began acutely and is constant. Medical history is remarkable only for a 4-month history of generalized progressive pruritus without a skin rash. He does not drink alcohol or smoke cigarettes and has no risk factors for chronic hepatitis. He takes no medications.

On physical examination, vital signs are normal. He has a plethoric complexion. Cardiopulmonary examination is normal. Tender hepatomegaly and splenomegaly are present.

Laboratory evaluation discloses erythrocytosis, leukocytosis, thrombocytosis, and markedly elevated serum aminotransferase levels.

Abdominal ultrasonography reveals hepatomegaly, splenomegaly, ascites, and a lack of blood flow in two of the hepatic veins, compatible with Budd-Chiari syndrome.

Which of the following is the most appropriate diagnostic test to perform next?

(A) Bone marrow biopsy

(B) Factor V Leiden genetic test

(C) Flow cytometry for CD55 and CD59

(D) *JAK2 V617F* mutation analysis

Item 67

A 58-year-old woman is diagnosed with acute deep venous thrombosis (DVT) of the proximal left leg. Low-molecular-weight heparin (LMWH) and warfarin are initiated. Medical history is otherwise nonsignificant, and she takes no other medications.

When should LMWH be discontinued?

(A) In 3 days if the INR is therapeutic

(B) In 3 days if the INR is therapeutic for 24 hours

(C) In 5 days if the INR is therapeutic

(D) In 5 days if the INR is therapeutic for 24 hours

Item 68

A 30-year-old woman is evaluated for progressive difficulty walking and numbness in both feet of 1 to 2 months' duration. She is otherwise healthy. She has followed a vegan diet for the past several years. Her only medication is an oral contraceptive pill.

On physical examination, temperature is 37.0 °C (98.6 °F), blood pressure is 120/66 mm Hg, pulse rate is 76/min, and respiration rate is 12/min; BMI is 25. She has decreased sensation and vibratory sense in both legs below the knees. No other neurologic deficits are observed.

Laboratory studies:

Hemoglobin	10.4 g/dL (104 g/L)
Leukocyte count	2800/µL (2.8 × 10⁹/L)
Mean corpuscular volume	105 fL
Vitamin B$_{12}$	210 pg/mL (155 pmol/L)

A peripheral blood smear is shown.

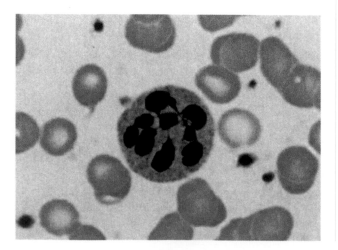

Which of the following is the most appropriate diagnostic test to perform next?

(A) Bone marrow biopsy

(B) Folate level measurement

(C) Homocysteine level measurement

(D) Methylmalonic acid level measurement

Item 69

A 72-year-old man is evaluated for a 6-month history of progressive fatigue, dyspnea with exertion, intermittent drenching night sweats, and a 6.8-kg (15 lb) weight loss. Medical history is unremarkable, and he takes no medications.

On physical examination, the patient appears fatigued. Temperature is 37.0 °C (98.6 °F), blood pressure is 148/86 mm Hg, pulse rate is 88/min, and respiration rate is 16/min. BMI is 24. Neurologic and funduscopic examinations are normal. Lungs are clear to auscultation. Rubbery, 1.5- to 2.5-cm lymph nodes are palpable in the bilateral anterior cervical lymph node chains, right axilla, and bilateral inguinal regions. The spleen is palpable 2 cm below the mid left costal margin.

Laboratory studies:

Hemoglobin	9.4 g/dL (94 g/L)
Leukocyte count	5400/µL (5.4 × 10⁹/L)
Platelet count	184,000/µL (184 × 10⁹/L)
Reticulocyte count	1.5% of erythrocytes
Blood urea nitrogen	20 mg/dL (7.1 mmol/L)
Creatinine	1.1 mg/dL (97.2 µmol/L)
Immunoglobulins	
IgG	540 mg/dL (5.4 g/L)
IgA	80 mg/dL (0.8 g/L)
IgM	3882 mg/dL (38.8 g/L)
Lactate dehydrogenase	120 U/L
Protein, total	9.3 g/dL (93 g/L)

A blood smear is unremarkable with the exception of a reduced number of erythrocytes. A direct antiglobulin (Coombs) test is negative. Serum protein electrophoresis and immunofixation reveal a monoclonal IgM κ band measuring 3.2 g/dL.

A bone marrow aspirate and biopsy reveals clonal plasma cells, plasmacytoid lymphocytes, and mature B cells, representing 50% of the overall marrow cellularity without erythroid hyperplasia. CT of the neck, chest, abdomen, and pelvis demonstrates splenomegaly and cervical, axillary, mesenteric, and inguinal lymphadenopathy with lymph nodes measuring up to 3 cm. The lung fields are clear.

Which of the following is the most appropriate management?

(A) Cold agglutinin titer

(B) Plasma exchange

(C) Rituximab plus chemotherapy

(D) Serum viscosity testing

Item 70

A 25-year-old man is evaluated in the emergency department for a 1-day history of brown urine, fatigue, and shortness of breath. He was diagnosed with a urinary tract infection 4 days ago, for which he was prescribed trimethoprim-sulfamethoxazole. Medical history is otherwise unremarkable. He is black.

On physical examination, temperature is 37.2 °C (99.0 °F), blood pressure is 110/75 mm Hg, pulse rate is 90/min, and respiration rate is 24/min. BMI is 23. Scleral icterus is apparent. Abdominal examination is normal with no indication of hepatosplenomegaly.

Laboratory studies:

Hematocrit	21%
Platelet count	215,000/µL (215 × 10⁹/L)
Reticulocytes	10% of erythrocytes
Bilirubin, total	5.0 mg/dL (85.5 µmol/L)
Lactate dehydrogenase	350 U/L

A peripheral blood smear is shown.

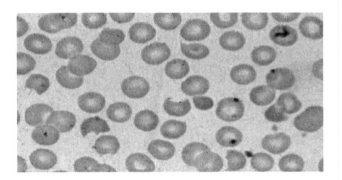

Trimethoprim-sulfamethoxazole is discontinued.

Which of the following is the most appropriate diagnostic test to perform next?

(A) ADAMTS-13 activity assay
(B) Direct antiglobulin (Coombs) test
(C) Glucose-6-phosphate dehydrogenase activity
(D) Osmotic fragility test

Item 71

A 35-year-old woman is evaluated in the emergency department for a 3-day history of worsening dyspnea on exertion. She reports no chest pain. Medical history is notable for systemic lupus erythematosus, which is well controlled with hydroxychloroquine. She takes no other medications.

On physical examination, the patient appears pale and fatigued. Temperature is 37.0 °C (98.6 °F), blood pressure is 110/72 mm Hg, pulse rate is 100/min, and respiration rate is 18/min. Oxygen saturation is 97% breathing ambient air. Neurologic examination is normal. Scleral icterus is noted. She has no lymphadenopathy. A grade 2/6 crescendo-decrescendo systolic murmur is auscultated at the upper right sternal border, and the lung fields are clear bilaterally. Abdominal examination reveals no hepatosplenomegaly or tenderness. Rectal examination shows no masses, and a stool sample is guaiac negative.

Laboratory studies:

Hemoglobin	6.2 g/dL (62 g/L)
Leukocyte count	15,000/µL (15 × 10⁹/L)
Mean corpuscular volume	101 fL
Platelet count	280,000/µL (280 × 10⁹/L)
Reticulocyte count	18% of erythrocytes
Bilirubin, total	2.3 mg/dL (39.3 µmol/L)
Creatinine	Normal
Lactate dehydrogenase	980 U/L
Direct antiglobulin (Coombs) test	Positive for C3 and IgG

Peripheral blood smear shows spherocytes and polychromatophilic erythrocytes but is otherwise normal.

Which of the following is the most appropriate management?

(A) Erythrocyte transfusion
(B) Prednisone
(C) Rituximab
(D) Splenectomy
(E) Vitamin B₁₂

Item 72

A 54-year-old man is evaluated during follow-up consultation regarding laboratory studies completed for a life insurance policy. He reports no symptoms.

On physical examination, temperature is 37.2 °C (99.0 °F), blood pressure is 131/76 mm Hg, pulse rate is 88/min, and respiration rate is 15/min. No splenomegaly is noted.

Laboratory studies:

Hemoglobin	8.9 g/dL (89 g/L)
Leukocyte count	3000/µL (3.0 × 10⁹/L) with 30% neutrophils, 10% monocytes, and 60% lymphocytes
Mean corpuscular volume	105 fL
Platelet count	75,000/µL (75 × 10⁹/L)
Folate	Normal
Vitamin B₁₂	Normal

A bone marrow biopsy shows trilineage dysplasia with 1% blasts. Results of cytogenetic testing show loss of the Y chromosome (−Y).

These findings are compatible with low-risk disease by the International Prognostic Scoring System – Revised criteria.

Which of the following is the most appropriate management?

(A) 5-Azacytidine
(B) Allogeneic hematopoietic stem cell transplantation
(C) Erythropoietin
(D) Observation

Item 73

A 73-year-old man develops acute respiratory distress near the completion of a transfusion of 1 unit of erythrocytes following a total hip arthroplasty. Medical history is significant for hypertension, type 2 diabetes mellitus complicated by

CONT. nephropathy, and hyperlipidemia. Medications are amlodipine, insulin, atorvastatin, and subcutaneous unfractionated heparin.

On physical examination, temperature is 36.8 °C (98.2 °F), blood pressure is 184/72 mm Hg, pulse rate is 114/min, and respiration rate is 24/min. Oxygen saturation is 86% breathing ambient air. Jugular venous pressure is 8 cm H₂O. Crackles are heard halfway up both lung fields. Cardiac examination reveals tachycardia but no murmurs. Trace bilateral pedal edema is noted.

Laboratory studies:

Hemoglobin	7.7 g/dL (77 g/L) (6.8 g/dL [68 g/L] before transfusion)
Bilirubin, total	1.2 mg/dL (20.5 µmol/L)
Creatinine	2.8 mg/dL (248 µmol/L) (2.7 mg/dL [239 µmol/L] before transfusion)
Lactate dehydrogenase	90 U/L
Urinalysis	Negative for protein or blood

Electrocardiography demonstrates sinus tachycardia but shows no evidence of ST-segment or T-wave abnormalities. A chest radiograph reveals bibasilar airspace opacities.

Which of the following is the most likely diagnosis?

(A) Acute hemolytic transfusion reaction
(B) Transfusion-associated circulatory overload
(C) Transfusion-related acute lung injury
(D) Transfusion-transmitted sepsis

Item 74

A 47-year-old woman is evaluated for fatigue and easy bruising of 6 weeks' duration. Medical and family histories are unremarkable, and she takes no medications.

On physical examination, temperature is 36.7 °C (98.0 °F), blood pressure is 131/76 mm Hg, pulse rate is 95/min, and respiration rate is 15/min. Pallor and scattered lower extremity bruising are noted.

Laboratory studies:

Hemoglobin	7.6 g/dL (76 g/L)
Leukocyte count	2000/µL (2 × 10⁹/L) with 30% neutrophils, 20% monocytes, and 50% lymphocytes
Mean corpuscular volume	103 fL
Platelet count	35,000/µL (35 × 10⁹/L)
Folate	Normal
Vitamin B₁₂	Normal

A bone marrow aspirate and biopsy show trilineage dysplasia with 7% blasts. Cytogenetic testing results indicate a complex karyotype.

These findings define high-risk disease by the International Prognostic Scoring System – Revised criteria.

Which of the following is the most appropriate management?

(A) 5-Azacytidine
(B) Allogeneic hematopoietic stem cell transplantation
(C) Erythropoietin
(D) Observation

Item 75

A 65-year-old man is evaluated for shortness of breath with light activity. Medical history is significant for type 2 diabetes mellitus with associated chronic kidney disease; progressive anemia has also been noted. He has no evidence of gastrointestinal bleeding. His only medication is glipizide.

On physical examination, temperature is 37.1 °C (98.7 °F), blood pressure is 140/80 mm Hg, pulse rate is 86/min, and respiration rate is 20/min; BMI is 30.

Laboratory studies:

Hemoglobin	8 g/dL (80 g/L)
Mean corpuscular volume	90 fL
Reticulocyte count	1% of erythrocytes
Creatinine	2.3 mg/dL (203 µmol/L)
Folate	Normal
Ferritin	550 ng/mL (550 µg/L)
Transferrin saturation	40%
Vitamin B₁₂	Normal
Glomerular filtration rate	25 mL/min/1.73 m²

Which of the following is the most appropriate management?

(A) Erythrocyte transfusion
(B) Erythropoiesis-stimulating agent therapy
(C) Erythropoietin level measurement
(D) Iron replacement

Item 76

A 23-year-old woman is evaluated in the emergency department for profound shortness of breath, which developed earlier in the day. She reports no chest pain but feels very weak. Medical history is significant for homozygous sickle cell anemia (Hb SS). She was evaluated in the emergency department 1 week ago for symptomatic anemia; she received a transfusion of 2 units of packed red blood cells, her hemoglobin level increased to 8.5 g/dL (85 g/L), and she was sent home. Her only medication is folic acid.

On physical examination, she appears pale and weak. Temperature is 37.1 °C (98.8 °F), blood pressure is 100/60 mm Hg, pulse rate is 110/min, and respiration rate is 32/min. Oxygen saturation is 96% breathing ambient air. Scleral icterus is noted. Cardiac examination reveals a grade 3/6 early systolic murmur at the base of the heart. Lungs are clear. Abdominal palpation reveals no hepatosplenomegaly.

Laboratory studies:

Hemoglobin	3.5 g/dL (35 g/L)
Platelet count	415,000/µL (415 × 10⁹/L)
Reticulocyte count	8% of erythrocytes
Bilirubin, total	7.7 mg/dL (132 µmol/L)
Lactate dehydrogenase	650 U/L

Which of the following is the most likely diagnosis?

(A) Aplastic crisis
(B) Delayed hyperhemolytic transfusion reaction
(C) Hepatic sequestration crisis
(D) Splenic sequestration crisis

Item 77

A 46-year-old woman is evaluated for a 3-week history of increasing fatigue and new lymphadenopathy. Medical history is remarkable for a 3-year history of rheumatoid arthritis. Medications are methotrexate and ibuprofen as needed.

On physical examination, temperature is 37.5 °C (99.5 °F), blood pressure is 128/78 mm Hg, pulse rate is 92/min, and respiration rate is 18/min. Bilateral axillary lymph nodes are palpable. The spleen is palpable 1 cm below the left costal margin. Other than changes of rheumatoid arthritis apparent in the hands and feet, the remainder of the physical examination is normal.

Laboratory studies show a hemoglobin level of 12.5 g/dL (125 g/L); a leukocyte count of 2000/µL (2×10^9/L) with 70% lymphocytes, 10% monocytes, and 20% neutrophils; and a platelet count of 155,000/µL (155×10^9/L).

A peripheral blood smear is shown.

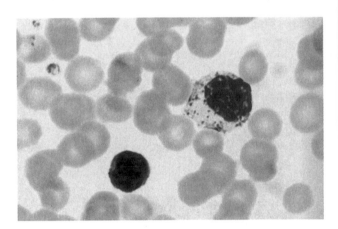

Which of the following is the most likely diagnosis?

(A) Aplastic anemia
(B) Autoimmune neutropenia
(C) Felty syndrome
(D) Paroxysmal nocturnal hemoglobinuria

Oncology Questions

Item 78

A 28-year-old woman is evaluated in the emergency department for a 1-week history of progressive headache associated with nausea and vomiting. Medical history is significant for HIV infection. She is nonadherent to her antiretroviral therapy regimen and takes no other medications.

On physical examination, she is awake and oriented. The patient is afebrile, blood pressure is 130/80 mm Hg, pulse rate is 100/min, and respiration rate is 16/min. No enlarged lymph nodes are palpated. The liver and spleen are not enlarged. The remainder of her physical examination is unremarkable, and her neurologic examination shows papilledema but no other focal findings.

Results of a complete blood count and serum chemistry panel, including toxoplasmosis titer measured at the time of HIV diagnosis, are normal.

CT scan of the head is shown (see top of next column).

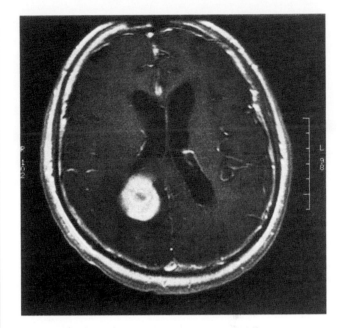

Which of the following is the most appropriate next step in management?

(A) Combination chemotherapy
(B) High-dose intravenous glucocorticoids
(C) Intracranial pressure monitoring
(D) Stereotactic radiation therapy

Item 79

A 68-year-old woman is evaluated in the emergency department for a 1-week history of polyuria, polydipsia, and progressive confusion. She has a 2-year history of multiple myeloma that was treated 1 year ago with chemotherapy. Her medical history is otherwise noncontributory, and she takes no medications.

On physical examination, the patient is afebrile, blood pressure is 100/60 mm Hg, pulse rate is 100/min, and respiration rate is 14/min. The patient's skin and mucous membranes are dry. She appears confused, and her reflexes are hyporeactive. The remainder of her examination is unremarkable.

Laboratory studies:

Blood urea nitrogen	60 mg/dL (21.4 mmol/L)
Calcium	14.5 mg/dL (3.6 mmol/L)
Creatinine	3.5 mg/dL (309.4 µmol/L) (baseline 1.2 mg/dL [106.1 µmol/L])

Intravenous high-volume normal saline and high-dose glucocorticoids are started.

Which of the following is the most appropriate next step in treatment?

(A) Cinacalcet
(B) Hemodialysis
(C) Intravenous bisphosphonate
(D) Multiagent chemotherapy

Item 80

A 58-year-old man undergoes follow-up evaluation for cancer of the ascending colon diagnosed 3 weeks ago. Colonoscopy at that time revealed a fungating mass in the ascending colon. Biopsy revealed adenocarcinoma, and additional studies showed no evidence of metastatic disease. Right hemicolectomy was performed. The pathology report showed a 4-cm primary adenocarcinoma with clear margins at resection, full-thickness penetration through the colonic wall into pericolonic fat, and 4/21 lymph nodes involved (stage III). Medical history is otherwise unremarkable, and the patient takes no medications.

On physical examination, vital signs are normal. Examination of the abdomen shows well-healed surgical scars but is otherwise normal.

Which of the following is the most appropriate management at this time?

(A) Leucovorin, 5-fluorouracil, and oxaliplatin (FOLFOX)
(B) Radiation therapy
(C) Radiation therapy and capecitabine followed by capecitabine plus oxaliplatin (CAPOX)
(D) Observation

Item 81

A 70-year-old man is hospitalized for new-onset abdominal pain and nausea. He has had little to eat or drink for the past 24 hours. The patient had a cerebrovascular accident 1 year ago and since then has resided in a nursing home. He has long-standing congestive cardiomyopathy, hypertension, type 1 diabetes mellitus with peripheral neuropathy, and chronic kidney disease. He is mostly bedbound but is able to sit in a chair with assistance for several hours each day. Medications are amlodipine, enalapril, furosemide, insulin, and metoprolol.

On physical examination, the patient appears chronically ill. Temperature is 37.7 °C (99.9 °F), blood pressure is 150/85 mm Hg, pulse rate is 80/min, and respiration rate is 12/min. BMI is 21. The sclerae are icteric, and mucous membranes are dry. There are crackles at the bilateral lung bases. Heart examination is significant for an S_3 heart sound. The abdomen is moderately distended with diffuse mild tenderness but without rebound or guarding. The liver edge is palpable. There is bilateral pitting edema of the extremities.

The patient's Eastern Cooperative Oncology Group/World Health Organization performance status level is assessed to be 4 (completely disabled, totally confined to a bed or chair, and unable to do any self-care).

The serum albumin level is 2.8 g/dL (28 g/L), the serum total bilirubin level is 2.3 mg/dL (39.3 µmol/L), and the serum creatinine level is 2.6 mg/dL (229.8 µmol/L).

A CT scan of the abdomen without contrast shows hepatomegaly with multiple metastatic lesions, enlarged retroperitoneal lymph nodes, abdominal carcinomatosis, moderate ascites, and a nonobstructing mass lesion in the cecum. A diagnostic paracentesis is performed, and 2 liters of bloody ascitic fluid are removed; cytology samples are positive for adenocarcinoma.

Gentle intravenous hydration is begun, and the patient is given parenteral morphine, which provides adequate relief of pain.

Which of the following is the most appropriate management?

(A) Leucovorin, 5-fluorouracil, and oxaliplatin (FOLFOX)
(B) Single-agent, low-dose 5-fluorouracil
(C) Surgical resection of the cecal mass
(D) Supportive, comfort-oriented care

Item 82

A 55-year-old man is evaluated for a 3-month history of cough and unexplained weight loss and a 2-week history of shortness of breath. He has never smoked cigarettes.

On physical examination, vital signs are normal. Breath sounds are decreased, and there is dullness to percussion over the right lung field. Examination findings are otherwise unremarkable.

Chest radiograph shows a right pleural effusion and right hilar mass. CT scan of the chest reveals a large right pleural effusion, a right upper lobe mass with associated consolidation, hilar and mediastinal lymphadenopathy, and an irregular right adrenal mass. A CT-guided transthoracic biopsy of the right upper lobe mass shows adenocarcinoma.

Which of the following is the most appropriate management?

(A) EGFR mutation testing
(B) K-*ras* mutation testing
(C) PET scanning
(D) Surgical resection

Item 83

A 68-year-old woman is evaluated for a 1-month history of a painful lump underneath the tongue. She has a 45-pack-year smoking history and continues to smoke.

On physical examination, vital signs are normal. An ulcerated lesion measuring approximately 1 cm is seen on the anterior floor of the mouth.

The lesion is resected. Pathology specimens identify poorly differentiated squamous cell carcinoma with negative margins.

The patient is encouraged to stop smoking. Following discussion of the benefits and risks, she is enrolled in a lung cancer screening program utilizing low-dose CT scanning.

Which of the following surveillance tests should also be recommended for this patient?

(A) CT scans
(B) PET/CT scan
(C) Oral examinations and direct laryngoscopy
(D) No additional follow-up

Item 84

A 55-year-old woman is evaluated in the emergency department for a 3-day history of diarrhea. She reports seven to eight stools daily without vomiting. She also notes abdominal cramping without vomiting and has been able to maintain adequate fluid intake. Medical history is significant for metastatic malignant melanoma, for which she recently completed the third of four planned doses of ipilimumab therapy. She has no history of inflammatory bowel disease, recent antibiotic use, recent travel, or consumption of uncooked foods. The remainder of the medical history is noncontributory, and she takes no other medications.

On physical examination, temperature is 37.5 °C (99.5 °F), blood pressure is 125/85 mm Hg, pulse rate is 90/min without orthostatic changes, and respiration rate is 14/min. The abdomen is soft and nontender with increased bowel sounds. The remainder of the physical examination is normal.

Laboratory studies:

Hemoglobin	12.2 g/dL (122 g/L)
Leukocyte count	9300/µL (9.3 × 10⁹/L) with normal differential
Alanine aminotransferase	120 U/L
Aspartate aminotransferase	160 U/L
Creatinine	1.2 mg/dL (106.1 µmol/L)
Fecal occult blood test	Negative

A chest radiograph is normal and abdominal films show nondilated bowel loops with no free air.

In addition to discontinuing the ipilimumab and providing supportive care, which of the following is the most appropriate next step in treatment?

(A) Broad-spectrum intravenous antibiotics

(B) Granulocyte-macrophage colony-stimulating factor

(C) High-dose intravenous glucocorticoids

(D) Observation

Item 85

A 33-year-old woman was diagnosed with *BRCA1* mutation 2 months ago. Her paternal aunt was diagnosed with breast cancer at age 45 years and was found to have a deleterious *BRCA1* mutation. She has no family history of ovarian cancer. She has one child and would like to have another child in the next year. She seeks advice on when to have prophylactic bilateral salpingo-oophorectomies (BSO). She is in good health and has no active medical problems.

Physical examination shows no worrisome breast masses. Pelvic examination is normal. The remainder of the physical examination is normal.

Laboratory studies are normal. Results of a mammogram 1 month ago, a transvaginal ultrasound 2 weeks ago, and a breast MRI 1 week ago are normal.

Which of the following is the most appropriate management?

(A) Recommend immediate BSO

(B) Recommend prophylactic BSO by age 35 years

(C) Defer prophylactic BSO until age 40 years

(D) Semi-annual pelvic ultrasound until age 50 years

Item 86

A 68-year-old man is evaluated for a 4-month history of fatigue, weight loss, and night sweats. He is a farmer and has been unable to work since his symptoms developed. Medical history is significant for hypertension, type 2 diabetes mellitus, and an anterior ST-elevation myocardial infarction. Medications are ramipril, glipizide, metoprolol, and low-dose aspirin.

On physical examination, the patient is afebrile, blood pressure is 140/88 mm Hg, pulse rate is 60/min, and respiration rate is 16/min. BMI is 30. Enlarged axillary lymph nodes are palpated.

Laboratory studies:

Hemoglobin	10.5 g/dL (105 g/L)
Lactate dehydrogenase	Elevated
HIV	Negative
Epstein-Barr virus	Negative
Hepatitis B virus	Negative
Hepatitis C virus	Negative

CT scans show axillary, mediastinal, and pelvic lymphadenopathy. Echocardiogram shows a left ventricular ejection fraction of 30%.

Lymph node and bone marrow biopsies reveal diffuse large B-cell lymphoma.

Which of the following factors most strongly correlates with overall survival in this patient after treatment?

(A) Revised International Prognostic Index score

(B) Presence of anemia

(C) Presence of B symptoms

(D) Presence of type 2 diabetes mellitus

Item 87

A 42-year-old woman is evaluated for postcoital bleeding and intermittent pelvic pain. She otherwise feels well. The patient is premenopausal and has two children.

On physical examination, vital signs are normal. General examination is normal. An ulcerating 2-cm cervical mass is visible on speculum examination. Bimanual pelvic examination shows a bulky mass in the cervix that is fixed to the left pelvic side wall and is not mobile.

Results of complete blood count and serum chemistry panel are normal.

CT scan of the abdomen and pelvis shows a 4.5-cm mass involving the lower uterus and extending to the left pelvic side wall. Left hydronephrosis and hydroureter are present. No disease is detected outside the pelvis. Biopsy of the cervical mass shows poorly differentiated invasive squamous cell carcinoma. Chest CT is normal.

Which of the following is the most appropriate treatment?

(A) Radiation therapy

(B) Radiation therapy with concurrent chemotherapy

(C) Radical hysterectomy

(D) Radical hysterectomy followed by chemotherapy

(E) Simple hysterectomy with ovarian preservation

Item 88

A 70-year-old man is evaluated for a 3-month history of fatigue, weight loss, fever, and night sweats. He has a long-standing history of Crohn disease treated with infliximab.

On physical examination, temperature is 38.0 °C (100.4 °F), blood pressure is 110/60 mm Hg, pulse rate is 105/min, and respiration rate is 16/min. Fixed cervical, axillary, and inguinal lymphadenopathy is present on palpation. There is no splenomegaly. The remainder of the examination is unremarkable.

Chest radiograph is normal. CT scans show extensive cervical, axillary, abdominal, and pelvic lymphadenopathy; there is no mediastinal lymphadenopathy.

Which of the following is the most likely diagnosis?

(A) Non-Hodgkin lymphoma
(B) Sarcoidosis
(C) Testicular cancer
(D) Tuberculosis

Item 89

A 78-year-old man is hospitalized for a 1-week history of progressive and severe back pain and weakness in both legs. He describes a sense of "heaviness" in his legs and has had increasing difficulty climbing stairs and getting out of a chair. Medical history is significant for asymptomatic multiple myeloma that has been followed with periodic examinations and laboratory studies; his last assessment was 3 months ago and was stable.

On physical examination, vital signs are normal. He has point tenderness over the T10 and T11 vertebral bodies, decreased lower extremity muscle strength (3$^+$/5), increased reflexes isolated to both lower extremities, and bilateral extensor plantar responses. The remainder of the physical examination is unremarkable.

Laboratory studies are significant for a serum hemoglobin level of 6.5 g/dL (65 g/L) and a serum calcium level of 13 mg/dL (3.2 mmol/L).

MRI of the thoracic and lumbar spine shows a vertebral body mass with extension into the epidural space at T12 and compression of the spinal cord.

Which of the following is the most appropriate initial step in treatment?

(A) Biopsy of the epidural mass
(B) Decompressive surgery
(C) Intravenous glucocorticoids
(D) Multiagent chemotherapy
(E) Radiation therapy

Item 90

A 55-year-old woman is evaluated for a mass in her left breast. She otherwise feels well. She is postmenopausal. Medical and family histories are otherwise negative and she takes no medications.

On physical examination, vital signs are normal. A firm, mobile mass measuring 2.5 × 2.0 cm is palpated in the upper outer quadrant of the left breast, adjacent to the areola. There is no right breast mass. The remainder of the examination is unremarkable.

Mammogram of the left breast shows a 2.9-cm spiculated mass at the site of the palpable lesion. Ultrasound examination shows a 3.5-cm mass. Ultrasound-guided biopsy specimens reveal grade 3 invasive ductal carcinoma that is estrogen receptor negative, progesterone receptor negative, and *HER2* positive. No lymphovascular invasion is noted.

A preoperative echocardiogram is normal; the left ventricular ejection fraction is 65%.

The patient desires breast-conserving surgery, but the surgeon believes that the mass is too large to resect with a lumpectomy because of her small breast size, the moderately large size of the cancer, and its central location.

Which of the following is the most appropriate management?

(A) Mastectomy with postoperative chemotherapy
(B) Neoadjuvant anastrozole
(C) Neoadjuvant trastuzumab-based chemotherapy
(D) Staging CT and bone scans

Item 91

An 80-year-old woman is hospitalized after a mechanical fall. She has a history of stage I estrogen receptor–positive and progesterone receptor–positive left breast cancer diagnosed 13 years ago; *HER2* testing was not done at that time. She was treated with breast-conserving surgery, primary breast radiation, and adjuvant tamoxifen for 5 years. She is not having any current bone pain or headaches.

On physical examination, vital signs are normal. A large palpable lesion is present over the left frontal skull. There is no lymphadenopathy. Examination of the left breast shows a healed incision with no masses. There are no right breast masses. The remainder of the examination is unremarkable.

Serum alkaline phosphatase level is elevated at 264 U/L (normal 36-92 U/L) and serum CA 15-3 level is 100.2 U/mL (normal <30 U/mL). Remaining laboratory studies, including serum calcium level, are normal.

CT scan of the head done in the emergency room shows a 3-cm lytic lesion in the left frontal skull. MRI of the brain confirms the presence of a large frontal skull lesion but shows no brain metastases. Bone and CT scans show lesions in the spine, skull, sternum, and bilateral ilium bones consistent with metastases. No visceral disease is present.

Biopsy of a lytic lesion in the right ilium shows metastatic adenocarcinoma consistent with primary breast cancer (estrogen receptor positive, progesterone receptor positive, and *HER2* negative).

Which of the following is the most appropriate treatment?

(A) Anastrozole
(B) Chemotherapy
(C) Radiation to areas of bone involvement
(D) Radium-223 isotope

Item 92

A 57-year-old woman undergoes follow-up evaluation. The patient underwent bilateral breast reduction surgery 3 months ago. The initial pathology report noted bilateral atypical ductal hyperplasia. Examination of additional pathology specimens showed no evidence of carcinoma. A mammogram obtained 2 months prior to the breast reduction surgery was normal.

The patient has been taking continuous conjugated estrogen and medroxyprogesterone hormone replacement therapy (HRT) since menopause at age 50 years. HRT has been tapered since the diagnosis of atypical ductal hyperplasia, and plans are to discontinue therapy in 1 month. There is no family history of breast or ovarian cancer.

On physical examination, vital signs are normal. Well-healed mastopexy incisions with mild induration are present. There are no breast masses. The remainder of the examination is unremarkable.

Which of the following is the most appropriate breast cancer prevention strategy?

(A) Begin antiestrogen chemoprevention therapy
(B) Begin vitamin D supplementation
(C) Bilateral prophylactic mastectomy
(D) Continue hormone replacement therapy

Item 93

A 70-year-old man undergoes follow-up evaluation for a recent diagnosis of colorectal cancer. He underwent left hemicolectomy and a bulky 8-cm tumor of the sigmoid colon was removed. Pathology reports revealed a poorly differentiated adenocarcinoma penetrating into pericolonic fat, with 1/22 resected lymph nodes involved with cancer (T3N1; stage III). The patient recovered well from surgery and completed 6 months of adjuvant chemotherapy.

Findings on physical examination today, including vital signs, are unremarkable.

The patient is scheduled to have physical examination and carcinoembryonic antigen monitoring every 3 to 6 months. Colonoscopy could not be performed preoperatively because of obstruction and is therefore scheduled to be done 6 months after surgery and repeated at 3- to 5-year intervals.

Which of the following surveillance imaging studies should also be done?

(A) Chest/abdomen CT scans annually for 3 to 5 years
(B) Chest/abdomen CT scans annually for 10 years
(C) PET/CT scans annually for 5 years
(D) No additional imaging studies

Item 94

A 35-year-old man undergoes follow-up evaluation. The patient is asymptomatic. Testicular cancer was diagnosed recently and was treated with radical inguinal orchiectomy and adjuvant bleomycin/etoposide/cisplatin chemotherapy. Treatment was completed 3 months ago. Medical history is otherwise noncontributory, and the patient takes no medications.

On physical examination, vital signs are normal. The remainder of the examination is unremarkable.

Which of the following treatment-related conditions is this patient most likely to develop?

(A) Gastric ulcer
(B) Metabolic syndrome
(C) Obstructive uropathy
(D) Soft-tissue sarcoma

Item 95

A 48-year-old woman is evaluated for a 6-week history of fatigue and an enlarged right cervical lymph node. She has no significant medical history and takes no medications.

On physical examination, vital signs are normal. A 4-cm firm, enlarged right cervical lymph node is palpated. There is no other lymphadenopathy and no splenomegaly. The remainder of the examination is unremarkable.

Laboratory studies, including complete blood count, erythrocyte sedimentation rate, serum lactate dehydrogenase level, and serum β_2-microglobulin level, are normal.

Lymph node biopsy reveals effacement of the normal architecture by sheets of atypical lymphoid cells. Flow cytometry results are positive for B antigens CD19, CD20, CD22, and CD79a, consistent with diffuse large B-cell lymphoma. CT scans of the chest, abdomen, and pelvis show an isolated enlarged right cervical lymph node but are otherwise normal.

Which of the following is the most appropriate treatment?

(A) Allogeneic hematopoietic stem cell transplantation
(B) Autologous hematopoietic stem cell transplantation
(C) Involved-field radiation therapy
(D) Rituximab plus cyclophosphamide, doxorubicin, vincristine, and prednisone (R-CHOP)

Item 96

A 62-year-old man is evaluated for a 1-month history of nausea, anorexia, right upper quadrant abdominal pain, and a 4.5-kg (10-lb) weight loss. A superficial spreading melanoma of the left thigh, 2.2 mm deep, with one positive sentinel lymph node was diagnosed 1 year ago. The patient declined adjuvant interferon alfa therapy.

On physical examination, vital signs are normal. There is a well-healed 4-cm incision on the upper left anterior thigh and a healed incision in the left inguinal area. Abdominal examination reveals mild right upper quadrant tenderness to palpation, and the liver is palpable 4 cm below the costochondral margin with a nodular, firm edge. The remainder of the examination is normal.

Laboratory studies are significant for alanine aminotransferase of 211 U/L, aspartate aminotransferase of 156 U/L, and serum bilirubin of 1.6 mg/dL (27.4 µmol/L).

CT scan of the abdomen and pelvis shows an enlarged liver with five hypodense lesions in both lobes measuring up to 2.5 cm that are consistent with metastases. There are no ascites, abdominal lymphadenopathy, or splenomegaly.

Ultrasound-guided liver biopsy specimens show metastatic melanoma. CT scan of the chest is normal.

Which of the following is the most appropriate next step in management?

(A) *BRAF* V600 mutation analysis
(B) Dacarbazine-based chemotherapy
(C) High-dose interferon alfa
(D) Immunotherapy with ipilimumab

Item 97

A 61-year-old woman undergoes routine follow-up evaluation. Stage II colon cancer was diagnosed 3 years ago and was treated with surgical resection. The patient now feels well. She works full time and exercises regularly. Medical history is otherwise unremarkable, and she takes no medications.

Findings on physical examination, including vital signs, are normal.

Routine surveillance CT scans of the chest and abdomen show three new hypodense lesions in the right lobe of the liver, ranging in size from 1 to 3 cm. No other abnormalities are seen.

Which of the following is the most appropriate management?

(A) CT-guided needle biopsy of a liver lesion
(B) Hepatic artery embolization
(C) Palliative systemic chemotherapy
(D) Radiation therapy to the liver
(E) Right hepatectomy

Item 98

A 62-year-old man is evaluated for a 4- to 6-week history of passing bright red blood stool. He has no other symptoms. Medical history is unremarkable, and he takes no medications.

On physical examination, vital signs are normal. Abdominal examination is normal; the liver and spleen are not enlarged. Digital rectal examination reveals brown stool that is positive for occult blood.

Colonoscopy reveals a nonobstructing polypoid mass in the sigmoid colon. The remainder of the colon, from the ileocecal valve to the anus, is normal. Biopsy of the mass shows adenocarcinoma.

Which of the following diagnostic studies should be performed next?

(A) Bone scan
(B) CT colonography
(C) CT of the chest, abdomen, and pelvis
(D) PET/CT

H Item 99

A 27-year-old man is evaluated in the emergency department for a 1-week history of bruising and gingival bleeding with flossing. He has no significant medical history and takes no medications.

On physical examination, temperature is 37.5 °C (99.5 °F), blood pressure is 110/80 mm Hg, pulse rate is 80/min, and respiration rate is 14/min. Scattered ecchymoses and cutaneous petechiae are present. There is no lymphadenopathy or splenomegaly.

Laboratory studies:

Leukocyte count	150,000/µL (150 × 10⁹/L)
Platelet count	20,000/µL (20 × 10⁹/L)
Creatinine	4 mg/dL (353.6 µmol/L)
Fibrinogen	Normal
Phosphorus	8 mg/dL (2.58 mmol/L)
Urate	12 mg/dL (0.71 mmol/L)

Peripheral blood smear shows 70% circulating myeloblasts.

Which of the following is the most appropriate treatment?

(A) Fresh frozen plasma
(B) High-volume normal saline hydration and rasburicase
(C) Multiagent chemotherapy
(D) Platelet transfusion

Item 100

A 32-year-old woman undergoes postoperative follow-up evaluation. The patient was diagnosed with a 1.9-cm, stage II, estrogen receptor–positive, progesterone receptor–positive, *HER2*-positive grade 3 invasive ductal carcinoma of the left breast, with 2/6 positive lymph nodes. She underwent breast excision 2 weeks ago. Medical history is otherwise noncontributory. She and her husband have one child and wish to have additional children.

On physical examination, vital signs are normal. There is a healing left breast incision. There is no lymphadenopathy. The remainder of the examination is unremarkable.

Laboratory studies are normal.

Which of the following is the most appropriate next step in the management of this patient?

(A) Begin adjuvant chemotherapy without trastuzumab
(B) Delay chemotherapy until after further childbearing
(C) Recommend embryo cryopreservation before chemotherapy
(D) Advise against further pregnancies

Item 101

A 64-year-old man is evaluated for a 2-month history of increasing abdominal discomfort, right upper quadrant abdominal pain, and decreased appetite. He has lost 2.5 kg (5.5 lb) during this time. Medical history is unremarkable, and he takes no medications.

On physical examination, vital signs are normal. BMI is 29. A 3-cm left supraclavicular lymph node is palpated. The abdomen is moderately distended, soft, and nontender. The liver is enlarged on palpation. Testicular examination is unremarkable. A digital rectal examination shows a normal rectum and moderately enlarged prostate without nodularity. A stool sample is negative for occult blood.

Laboratory studies are significant for a serum alkaline phosphatase level of 340 U/L, serum total bilirubin level of 1.3 mg/dL (22.2 µmol/L), and serum creatinine level of 0.7 mg/dL (61.9 µmol/L).

CT scans of the chest, abdomen, and pelvis show extensive metastases scattered throughout the liver, with enlarged periportal and retroperitoneal lymph nodes measuring up to 4 cm in diameter and no bony metastases. CT-guided needle biopsy of the liver shows moderately differentiated adenocarcinoma. Upper endoscopy and colonoscopy are normal.

Treatment for which of the following malignancies would be most appropriate?

(A) Gastrointestinal
(B) Germ cell (testicular)
(C) Lung
(D) Neuroendocrine
(E) Prostate

Item 102

A 60-year-old woman is evaluated for a 5-year history of asymptomatic, intermittently enlarged lymph nodes. She has no other significant medical history and takes no medications.

On physical examination, the patient is afebrile, blood pressure is 140/85 mm Hg, pulse rate is 76/min, and respiration rate is 12/min. Enlarged cervical, axillary, and epitrochlear lymph nodes are palpated. There is no splenomegaly. The remainder of the examination is unremarkable.

Complete blood count and peripheral blood smear are normal. Chest radiograph is normal. CT scans show no evidence of mediastinal, abdominal, or pelvic lymphadenopathy.

A lymph node biopsy reveals a CD20-positive grade II follicular lymphoma, and a bone marrow biopsy shows infiltration with small CD20-positive lymphocytes representing 20% of the cellular elements. Fluorescence in situ hybridization analysis shows the presence of the *BCL2* oncogene.

Which of the following is the most appropriate treatment?

(A) Lenalidomide
(B) Rituximab plus cyclophosphamide, doxorubicin, vincristine, and prednisone (R-CHOP)
(C) Rituximab
(D) Rituximab plus involved-field radiation therapy
(E) Observation

Item 103

A 44-year-old woman is evaluated for a 2-month history of a painless right neck mass. Medical history is unremarkable, and she takes no medications. She is a lifelong nonsmoker.

On physical examination, vital signs are normal. A 5-cm right anterior neck mass is palpated. The remainder of the examination is unremarkable.

An initial CT scan of the neck shows a 4.5-cm, partially necrotic, right-sided lymph node. Asymmetric thickening

of the right base of the tongue is also seen. Subsequent laryngoscopy shows an ulcerated mass involving the right base of the tongue. Biopsy of the tongue mass identifies poorly differentiated invasive squamous cell carcinoma. PET/CT scans show no evidence of distant metastases.

Which of the following studies should be performed next?

(A) Bone scan
(B) Human papillomavirus immunohistochemistry testing
(C) MRI of the brain
(D) Right cervical lymph node biopsy

Item 104

A 72-year-old man is evaluated in the emergency department for a 3-week history of headache and facial swelling and a 2-week history of shortness of breath.

On physical examination, the patient is afebrile, blood pressure is normal, pulse rate is 104/min, and respiration rate is 22/min. Oxygen saturation is 90% on ambient air. Diffuse facial erythema is present, and neck veins are dilated bilaterally.

CT scan of the chest shows a 7-cm medial left lung mass and bulky mediastinal lymphadenopathy. Superior vena cava compression with associated collateral vessels is also identified. MRI of the brain is negative.

Which of the following is the most appropriate management?

(A) Biopsy of the lung mass
(B) Immediate radiation therapy
(C) Placement of a superior vena cava stent
(D) Venography

Item 105

A 65-year-old woman is evaluated for aching pain in the bilateral hips, knees, and ankles.

Two years ago she was diagnosed with estrogen and progesterone receptor–positive, *HER2*-negative, stage IIIA cancer of the left breast, with 4 positive lymph nodes. She received adjuvant chemotherapy, breast radiation, and anastrozole. After eight months of anastrozole, she experienced severe arthralgia in her knees, hips, and ankles, worse in the morning and after sitting. Anastrozole was stopped for 3 weeks, and her symptoms markedly improved. Letrozole was then started. Now 4 months after beginning letrozole, her joint pains have recurred and are again debilitating. NSAIDs do not provide relief.

On physical examination, vital signs are normal. Well-healed bilateral mastectomy incisions are present without nodularity. There is no lymphadenopathy. The remainder of the physical examination is unremarkable.

In addition to discontinuing the letrozole, which of the following is the most appropriate management?

(A) Obtain PET scan
(B) Prednisone
(C) Restart anastrozole
(D) Start tamoxifen

Item 106

A 76-year-old woman is evaluated for a 3-month history of abdominal pain and weight loss. She has also had a nonproductive cough for several weeks. Medical history is unremarkable, and she takes no medications.

On physical examination, vital signs are normal. BMI is 22. A firm 3-cm left supraclavicular lymph node is palpated. Abdominal examination reveals a liver edge that is palpable 3 cm below the right costal margin. On digital rectal examination, a stool sample is positive for trace occult blood.

Contrast-enhanced CT scans of the chest and abdomen show multiple lung and liver metastases and a mass in the transverse colon. Biopsy of the mass obtained during colonoscopy reveals adenocarcinoma.

Which of the following diagnostic studies should be performed next?

(A) K-*ras* and N-*ras* genotyping of the tumor
(B) Measurement of serum dihydropyrimidine dehydrogenase (DPD) level
(C) Measurement of serum *UGT1A1* level
(D) Multigene array analysis of the tumor for prognostic markers

Item 107

A 68-year-old man requests evaluation for prostate cancer. He is asymptomatic. Following a discussion of the risks and benefits of prostate cancer screening, the patient decides to be screened.

Physical examination findings are normal. Digital rectal examination is normal.

Serum prostate-specific antigen level is 5.8 ng/mL (5.8 µg/L).

Transrectal ultrasound–guided prostate biopsy is done and shows adenocarcinoma in 2/12 cores, confined to the right lobe (Gleason score: 3 + 3 = 6).

Which of the following diagnostic imaging studies should be done next?

(A) Bone scan
(B) CT of the chest, abdomen, and pelvis
(C) Immunoscintigraphy
(D) PET/CT
(E) No imaging studies are needed

Item 108

A 38-year-old man is evaluated for a pigmented lesion on his upper left back. The lesion has been increasing in size over the past 2 months. He is otherwise asymptomatic. Medical history is unremarkable.

On physical examination, vital signs are normal. A 1.8-cm, irregular, dark, pigmented, slightly raised papule with irregular borders is present on his upper back. There are no adjacent lesions and no associated lymphadenopathy. The remainder of the examination is unremarkable.

Skin biopsy shows malignant melanoma, superficial spreading type, and measuring 1.4 mm in thickness, with invasion into the reticular dermis but not into the subcuta-

neous tissue. Dermal mitotic figures are not identified, and there is no lymphovascular invasion. Tumor extends to the lateral and deep margins of the excision. There is evidence of a vertical growth phase.

In addition to complete excision with a 2-cm margin, which of the following is the most appropriate treatment?

(A) Adjuvant chemotherapy
(B) Adjuvant interferon alfa
(C) Sentinel lymph node biopsy
(D) No further therapy

Item 109

A 69-year-old man undergoes follow-up evaluation. He was diagnosed with stage II colon cancer 3 years ago, and surgical resection was performed. The patient has been followed since then without additional treatment. He has no other medical problems and takes no medications.

Physical examination findings, including vital signs, are normal.

Follow-up contrast-enhanced CT scans of the chest and abdomen show two new hypodense lesions (6 cm and 4 cm) confined to the right lobe of the liver, with the larger lesion located close to hilum but without evidence of vascular invasion. No other metastases or additional abnormalities are identified.

The patient is evaluated by an experienced liver surgeon who believes that the larger lesion is unresectable due to its close proximity to the middle hepatic vein.

Laboratory studies, including measures of liver and kidney function, are normal.

Which of the following is the most appropriate approach to providing chemotherapy in this patient?

(A) Adjuvant chemotherapy
(B) Conversion chemotherapy
(C) Neoadjuvant chemotherapy
(D) Palliative chemotherapy
(E) No chemotherapy

Item 110

A 49-year-old woman is evaluated for a 3-month history of abdominal discomfort and fatigue. She has recently noted increasing abdominal girth despite a decreased appetite. Medical history is unremarkable, and she takes no medications.

On physical examination, vital signs are normal. BMI is 29. Cardiopulmonary examination is normal. The abdomen is moderately distended, soft, and nontender with shifting dullness consistent with ascites.

CT scans of the chest, abdomen, and pelvis are consistent with abdominal carcinomatosis with omental masses and ascites. No adnexal masses are seen.

Which of the following is the most appropriate management?

(A) Cytoreductive surgery followed by systemic chemotherapy
(B) Intraperitoneal chemotherapy

(C) Omental mass biopsy followed by pelvic radiation therapy and chemotherapy

(D) Ovarian biopsy followed by systemic chemotherapy

(E) Supportive comfort-oriented care

Item 111

A 70-year-old man undergoes follow-up evaluation to determine treatment options following a third occurrence of bladder cancer. High-grade transitional cell carcinoma of the bladder was initially diagnosed 7 months ago following cystoscopy to evaluate painless hematuria. Transurethral resection of the bladder tumor (TURBT) was performed followed by administration of intravesical bacillus Calmette-Guérin (BCG). Three months later, surveillance cystoscopy identified recurrent superficial high-grade transitional cell carcinoma in the same location that was again treated with TURBT and BCG. Now, 4 months following the second episode, high-grade transitional cell carcinoma is again diagnosed. This time, the cancer is in the same location with an additional focus near the trigone. No evidence of invasion into the muscle layer of the bladder has ever been identified.

Physical examination findings, including vital signs, are normal.

CT scans of the abdomen and pelvis (done at the time of the second recurrence) identified no evidence of significant bladder wall thickening, regional lymphadenopathy, or evidence of metastatic disease.

Which of the following is the most appropriate treatment at this time?

(A) Chemotherapy

(B) Cystectomy

(C) External-beam radiation therapy

(D) TURBT followed by intravesical BCG

Item 112

A 48-year-old man is evaluated for a 3-month history of dyspepsia, increasing episodes of nausea, and fatigue. He is maintaining adequate caloric intake and is continuing to work and participate in all routine daily activities, albeit with some increased fatigue.

On physical examination, the patient is afebrile, blood pressure is 115/70 mm Hg, pulse rate is 72/min, and respiration rate is 10/min. BMI is 26. A firm liver edge is palpated 5 cm below the right costal margin. The remainder of the examination is unremarkable.

Upper endoscopy reveals a mass arising in the wall of the proximal stomach just below the gastroesophageal junction. Biopsy of the mass reveals adenocarcinoma. CT scans of the chest and abdomen show multiple liver metastases and evidence of peritoneal carcinomatosis.

Before selecting a systemic chemotherapy regimen, which of the following information about the tumor biopsy specimen would be most helpful?

(A) *BRAF* mutational status

(B) Estrogen and progesterone receptor status

(C) *HER2* expression status

(D) K-*ras* mutational status

Item 113

A 34-year-old woman is evaluated for a 4-week history of tenderness in her left lower breast. Her paternal grandmother died of ovarian cancer at age 54 years. There is no family history of breast cancer. She has a 2-cm palpable left lower outer breast mass on exam. The remainder of the examination is unremarkable.

Results of complete blood count and serum chemistry panel are normal. A mammogram shows increased density and calcifications at the site of the palpable mass. Ultrasound examination reveals a 1.9-cm hypoechoic mass. Ultrasound-guided needle biopsy specimens show a high-grade invasive ductal carcinoma, estrogen receptor–negative, progesterone receptor–negative, and negative for *HER2* amplification.

Which of the following is the most appropriate initial management?

(A) Bilateral mastectomy

(B) *BRCA1/2* testing

(C) Left mastectomy

(D) Lumpectomy with sentinel lymph node biopsy

Item 114

A 54-year-old woman undergoes an examination. She feels well and is asymptomatic. The patient asks to be screened for ovarian cancer. She is postmenopausal and has two children. She used oral contraceptives from age 20 to 35 years. There is no family history of breast, ovarian, colon, endometrial, or gastric cancer.

On physical examination, vital signs are normal. Other findings on physical examination, including pelvic and rectal examinations, are normal.

Which of the following is the most appropriate ovarian cancer screening option for this patient?

(A) Serum CA-125 testing

(B) Transvaginal ultrasound

(C) Transvaginal ultrasound and serum CA-125 testing

(D) No screening studies are indicated

Item 115

A 60-year-old woman is evaluated for right-sided flank pain. Medical history is unremarkable.

Findings on physical examination, including vital signs, are normal.

CT scan of the abdomen and pelvis identifies a 6-cm right upper pole kidney mass. The lesion is resected with negative margins. Pathology specimens show clear cell carcinoma with evidence of renal vein involvement.

Which of the following is the most appropriate management after surgery?

(A) Adjuvant sunitinib

(B) Adjuvant temsirolimus

(C) Radiation therapy

(D) Observation

Item 116

A 52-year-old woman is evaluated for a 3-month history of enlarged bilateral axillary lymph nodes. She has also recently developed fever, weight loss, and night sweats. Medical history is unremarkable, and she takes no medications.

On physical examination, temperature is 38.5 °C (101.3 °F), blood pressure is 100/60 mm Hg, pulse rate is 90/min, and respiration rate is 14/min. Firm bilateral axillary lymph nodes are palpated. Splenomegaly is present. The remainder of the examination is unremarkable.

Laboratory studies:

Hemoglobin	9.0 g/dL (90 g/L)
Leukocyte count	18,000/µL (18×10^9/L)
Platelet count	70,000/µL (70×10^9/L)
Lactate dehydrogenase	Elevated
β_2-microglobulin	Elevated

CT scans of the chest, abdomen, and pelvis show bilateral enlarged axillary and intra-abdominal lymph nodes and an enlarged spleen. Axillary lymph node excisional biopsy reveals diffuse infiltration with small monoclonal lymphoid cells with CD20+ and cyclin D1 overexpression. Subsequent colonoscopy is performed, and biopsy indicates mucosal infiltration with lymphoid cells expressing B-cell markers.

Which of the following is the most likely diagnosis?

(A) Diffuse large B-cell lymphoma

(B) Follicular lymphoma

(C) Hodgkin lymphoma

(D) Mantle cell lymphoma

Item 117

A 62-year-old woman undergoes follow-up evaluation. Stage II ovarian cancer was diagnosed 5 months ago. No residual cancer was identified after debulking surgery. Postoperative chemotherapy was given and resulted in complete remission. The patient currently reports feeling well.

Medical history includes stage I endometrial cancer diagnosed at age 42 years for which the patient underwent hysterectomy without bilateral salpingo-oophorectomy. Family history is significant for endometrial cancer in her maternal grandmother and colon cancer in her mother and maternal uncle.

On physical examination, vital signs are normal. A well-healed abdominal midline incision is present. Remaining examination findings are unremarkable.

Results of complete blood count, serum chemistry panel, and serum CA-125 level are normal.

Which of the following studies should be done next?

(A) *BRCA1/2* testing

(B) Serial CT scans of abdomen and pelvis

(C) Serum CA-125 monitoring

(D) Testing for Lynch syndrome

Item 118

A 48-year-old man is evaluated for a 7-year history of spreading plaques associated with dry, itchy skin. He has no other significant medical history and takes no medications.

On physical examination, vital signs are normal. Skin lesions are present on the arms, back, and legs. Representative skin findings on the back are shown.

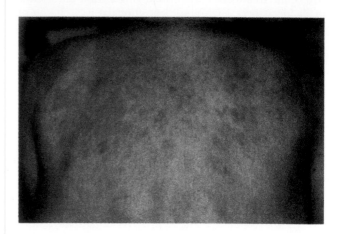

There is no lymphadenopathy or hepatosplenomegaly. The remainder of the examination is unremarkable. Results of complete blood count and serum chemistry panel are normal.

Chest radiograph is normal. Skin biopsy reveals infiltration with CD4-positive T cells with cerebriform-appearing nuclei consistent with mycosis fungoides.

Which of the following is the most appropriate management?

(A) Cyclophosphamide, doxorubicin, vincristine, and prednisone (CHOP) chemotherapy

(B) Psoralen plus ultraviolet A (PUVA) therapy

(C) Topical glucocorticoids

(D) Rituximab

Item 119

A 69-year-old woman is evaluated for a 3-month history of intermittent rectal bleeding and increasing fatigue. Medical history is unremarkable, and she takes no medications. Her father died of metastatic colon cancer at age 78 years.

On physical examination, vital signs are normal. The abdomen is soft and nontender. Bowel sounds are normal, and the liver and spleen are not enlarged. Digital rectal examination discloses blood-streaked stool.

Colonoscopy reveals a nonobstructing 4-cm mass in the mid rectum, approximately 8 cm from the anal verge. Biopsy findings show adenocarcinoma. Pelvic MRI shows tumor penetration into, but not through, the rectal wall (TNM stage T2); no abnormal lymph nodes are seen (TNM stage N0). Contrast-enhanced CT scans of the chest and abdomen are normal.

Which of the following is the most appropriate treatment at this time?

(A) Chemotherapy
(B) Radiation plus chemotherapy
(C) Radiation plus chemotherapy followed by surgical resection
(D) Surgical resection

Item 120

A 58-year-old woman is undergoes a routine cervical cancer screening examination. She is asymptomatic. The patient is postmenopausal and has two children. Medical history is unremarkable. Her mother was diagnosed with breast cancer at age 72 years.

On physical examination, vital signs are normal. An ovarian mass, measuring approximately 8 cm, is palpated on pelvic examination. Remaining examination findings are unremarkable.

Laboratory studies show a normal complete blood count, chemistry panel, and serum CA-125 level.

Transvaginal ultrasound shows a 12.8-cm complex mass in the cul de sac extending to both adnexa. No ascites are present. CT scan of the pelvis shows a 13.4-cm complex left pelvic mass and a 5.8-cm right pelvic mass but no liver lesions, ascites, peritoneal masses, or pleural effusions. Chest radiograph and chest CT scans are normal.

Which of the following is the most appropriate management?

(A) CT-guided biopsy of the mass
(B) Exploratory surgery
(C) MRI of the abdomen and pelvis
(D) *BRCA1/2* testing

Item 121

A 54-year-old man is evaluated for a 3-month history of worsening dyspepsia, gastric bloating, and abdominal discomfort. His dyspepsia has so far been treated with ranitidine. The patient is allergic to penicillin.

On physical examination, the patient is afebrile, blood pressure is 112/70 mm Hg, pulse rate is 83/min, and respiration rate is 14/min. BMI is 25. No palpable lymphadenopathy is present. Abdominal examination reveals mild epigastric tenderness. The remainder of the examination is unremarkable.

The hemoglobin level is 11.5 g/dL (115 g/L). Complete blood count and differential are otherwise normal. Results of fecal occult blood testing are positive.

Upper endoscopy shows several small gastric ulcers. Histopathologic studies reveal evidence of *Helicobacter pylori* infection and small clonal mucosa-associated B cells expressing the CD20 antigen consistent with mucosa-associated lymphoid tissue lymphoma. A CT scan of the abdomen shows no evidence of lymphadenopathy.

Ranitidine is discontinued.

Which of the following is the most appropriate management?

(A) Begin omeprazole, metronidazole, and clarithromycin
(B) Begin rituximab
(C) Obtain bone marrow biopsy
(D) Obtain PET/CT scan

Item 122

A 61-year-old man is evaluated in follow-up after surgical resection of a tongue base tumor.

A neck CT showed asymmetric thickening of the left tongue base and a 2-cm lymph node on the left. Biopsy identified moderately differentiated invasive squamous cell carcinoma. Preoperative PET/CT showed no distant metastatic disease. At surgery, the mass was resected with one positive margin; left modified radical neck dissection identified 3/31 positive lymph nodes, with one lymph node with extracapsular extension.

On physical examination, vital signs are normal. The tongue base resection is well healed and the oral cavity is otherwise normal. The neck incisions are clean and dry, and no lymphadenopathy is detected.

Which of the following is the most appropriate postsurgical management?

(A) Cetuximab alone
(B) Chemotherapy alone
(C) Chemotherapy and radiation therapy
(D) Radiation therapy followed by chemotherapy
(E) Observation

Item 123

A 24-year-old man is evaluated after he felt a mass in his right testicle. The patient is asymptomatic and is otherwise healthy.

On physical examination, vital signs are normal. A 2- to 3-cm solid mass is palpated in the right testicle. The remainder of the examination is unremarkable.

Serum α-fetoprotein level is normal, serum lactate dehydrogenase (LDH) level is 450 U/L, and serum β-human chorionic gonadotropin level is less than 5 U/L.

Testicular ultrasound confirms the presence of a hypoechoic solid right testicular mass.

Right radical inguinal orchiectomy is performed, and pathological examination reveals seminoma. Subsequent CT scan of the abdomen and pelvis shows no lymphadenopathy or evidence of metastatic disease. The tumor is stage I based on surgical and radiographic findings and tumor marker studies. LDH is normal following orchiectomy.

Which of the following is the most appropriate management for this patient?

(A) Active surveillance
(B) Hematopoietic stem cell transplantation
(C) Platinum-based chemotherapy
(D) Retroperitoneal lymph node dissection

Item 124

A 59-year-old woman undergoes follow-up evaluation for management of limited-stage small cell lung cancer diagnosed during care for an episode of pneumonia.

The patient was treated with a course of chemotherapy and radiation therapy. CT scan of the chest following treatment showed near-complete resolution of the lung mass and lymphadenopathy.

On physical examination, vital signs are normal. Auscultation of the chest is unremarkable, and the remainder of her examination is normal.

Which of the following is the most appropriate next step in the management of this patient?

(A) Maintenance chemotherapy
(B) PET/CT scan
(C) Prophylactic cranial irradiation
(D) Surgical removal of the residual lung mass

Item 125

A 68-year-old man undergoes follow-up evaluation. The patient has stage IIIB nodular sclerosing Hodgkin lymphoma that was initially diagnosed 3 years ago. Complete remission was achieved following administration of six cycles of doxorubicin, bleomycin, vinblastine, and dacarbazine (ABVD) chemotherapy. Two months ago, stage IIIB Hodgkin lymphoma was again diagnosed. Salvage chemotherapy was initiated with dexamethasone, ifosfamide, cisplatin, and etoposide (DICE). The patient has now completed two cycles of DICE chemotherapy.

On physical examination, the patient is afebrile, blood pressure is 142/80 mm Hg, pulse rate is 80/min, and respiration rate is 12/min. There is no palpable lymphadenopathy. The remainder of the examination is unremarkable. Results of a complete blood count and serum chemistry panel are normal.

PET/CT imaging shows no residual disease.

Which of the following is the most appropriate treatment at this time?

(A) Allogeneic hematopoietic stem cell transplantation
(B) Autologous hematopoietic stem cell transplantation
(C) Continued salvage DICE chemotherapy
(D) Involved-field radiation therapy

Item 126

A 44-year-old woman undergoes follow-up evaluation. Stage I cancer of the left breast was diagnosed 3 years ago (1.4-cm, grade 2 invasive ductal carcinoma, estrogen receptor positive, progesterone receptor positive, *HER2* negative, 0/2 positive sentinel lymph nodes, and a low score on 21-gene recurrence score testing). *BRCA1/2* testing results were negative. She underwent breast-conserving surgery and radiation therapy and then started tamoxifen. The patient is concerned about her risk of recurrence. Menses are irregular. She has occasional hot flushes and night sweats on tamoxifen but otherwise feels well. There is no family history of breast or ovarian cancer.

On physical examination, vital signs are normal. BMI has remained stable at 22.4. Well-healed left breast and left axilla incisions are present. There are no breast masses or lymphadenopathy. The remainder of the examination is unremarkable.

Results of a bilateral mammogram obtained 1 month ago were normal.

Which of the following is the most appropriate next step in the management of this patient?

(A) Bilateral breast MRI
(B) Complete blood count, liver chemistry studies, and CEA and CA 15-3 measurement
(C) CT of the chest, abdomen, and pelvis and bone scan
(D) No diagnostic studies at this time

Item 127

A 72-year-old man undergoes follow-up examination for prostate cancer. The patient was diagnosed with prostate cancer 2 years ago and was treated with external-beam radiation therapy. Six months ago, androgen deprivation therapy was added in response to a rising prostate-specific antigen level in the absence of local disease progression.

More recently, the patient developed worsening back and chest pain. A bone scan showed multifocal osseous metastases in the thoracic spine, lumbar spine, and ribs. CT scans of the chest, abdomen, and pelvis did not show enlarged lymph nodes or visceral metastases. His symptoms remain poorly controlled on opioid medications. Medications are extended-release morphine, oxycodone-acetaminophen, leuprolide, and flutamide.

On physical examination, blood pressure is 140/82 mm Hg, pulse rate is 97/min, and respiratory rate is 20/min. Physical examination reveals multiple tender areas involving the thoracic and lumbar spine. The remainder of the physical examination, including neurological examination, is normal.

In addition to a bisphosphonate, which of the following is the most appropriate treatment?

(A) Bilateral orchiectomy
(B) Estrogen therapy
(C) External-beam radiation to the lumbar spine
(D) Radium-223

Item 128

A 51-year-old woman undergoes a follow-up evaluation. The patient recently required surgery for stage I cancer of the right breast confirmed as a grade 3 invasive ductal carcinoma that was estrogen receptor negative, progesterone receptor negative, and *HER2* negative. Sentinel lymph nodes were negative. The patient currently states that she feels well. Medical history is otherwise unremarkable, and she is perimenopausal.

On physical examination, vital signs are normal. Healed incisions of the right breast and right axilla are present. There are no masses in either breast and no lymphadenopathy. The remainder of the examination is unremarkable.

Which of the following is the most appropriate next step in management?

(A) Anastrozole

(B) Anthracycline-based chemotherapy

(C) Autologous hematopoietic stem cell transplantation

(D) Bevacizumab

Item 129

A 38-year-old woman undergoes routine follow-up evaluation. The patient was treated with mantle irradiation for stage IIA Hodgkin lymphoma at age 19 years. She has done well and has no evidence of recurrence. Personal and family medical histories are noncontributory.

On physical examination, vital signs are normal. A healed incision from a previous lymph node biopsy is present in the right supraclavicular area. There is no lymphadenopathy, and breast examination is normal. The remainder of the examination is unremarkable.

No recent imaging studies have been obtained.

Which of the following is the recommended cancer screening program for this patient?

(A) Begin annual mammograms now

(B) Begin annual mammogram and breast MRIs now

(C) Begin annual mammograms at age 40 years

(D) Begin monthly breast self-examination now

Item 130

A 55-year-old woman undergoes follow-up evaluation for a recent diagnosis of lung cancer. Initial evaluation included a plain chest radiograph that showed a right middle lobe mass confirmed as a 3-cm spiculated mass on chest CT. PET/CT identified hypermetabolic uptake in the mass but was otherwise normal.

On surgical resection, the tumor was identified as an intermediate-grade adenocarcinoma with clear margins and was negative for molecular genetic abnormalities. One hilar lymph node was positive, and 10/10 mediastinal lymph nodes were negative for tumor.

She has never smoked. Medical history is otherwise negative, and she takes no medications.

On physical examination, vital signs are normal. Her right thoracic surgical incisions are clean and dry. The lung fields are clear. The remainder of her examination is unremarkable.

Which of the following is the most appropriate next step in this patient's management?

(A) Chemotherapy

(B) Erlotinib

(C) Radiation therapy

(D) Observation

Item 131

A 58-year-old woman is evaluated for a 6-month history of progressive lymphadenopathy. She is otherwise asymptomatic. Medical history is unremarkable, and she takes no medications.

On physical examination, vital signs are normal. Cervical and axillary lymphadenopathy is palpated. Abdominal examination reveals splenomegaly; the liver is not enlarged. The remainder of the examination is unremarkable.

Laboratory studies indicate a leukocyte count of 12,000/μL (12.0 × 10⁹/L), with 65% lymphocytes.

CT scans show diffuse cervical, axillary, abdominal, and pelvic lymphadenopathy and splenomegaly.

Which of the following diagnostic studies should be performed next?

(A) Bone marrow biopsy

(B) Excisional biopsy of an enlarged lymph node

(C) Fine-needle lymph node biopsy

(D) Lumbar puncture

(E) PET/CT scan

Item 132

A 79-year-old man is evaluated for a recent diagnosis of prostate cancer following detection of a left-sided prostate nodule during evaluation for worsening prostatic hyperplasia symptoms. Biopsy of the prostate nodule showed adenocarcinoma with a Gleason score of 3 + 4 = 7; additional core samples were negative for cancer. Medical history is also significant for myocardial infarction and heart failure. The patient has been hospitalized three times in the past 12 months because of exacerbations of heart failure. Medications are carvedilol, lisinopril, metoprolol, aspirin, furosemide, tamsulosin, and finasteride.

On physical examination, vital signs are normal. Mild bibasilar crackles are auscultated and there is trace lower extremity edema. The remainder of the physical examination is unremarkable.

Serum prostate-specific antigen level prior to biopsy was 4.9 ng/mL (4.9 μg/L).

Which of the following is the most appropriate management?

(A) Active surveillance

(B) Cryotherapy

(C) External-beam radiation therapy

(D) Radical prostatectomy

(E) Observation

Item 133

A 77-year-old woman is evaluated for new-onset fatigue and anemia. She otherwise feels well. Medical history is unremarkable, and she takes no medications.

Physical examination findings, including vital signs, are normal. BMI is 22.

Colonoscopy identifies a 7-cm mass in the transverse colon. Biopsy of the mass shows poorly differentiated adenocarcinoma. Contrast-enhanced CT scans of the chest, abdomen, and pelvis show the mass, but no other abnormalities are identified.

Which of the following is likely to be the most important factor in determining this patient's prognosis?

(A) Degree of differentiation of the tumor
(B) Patient's performance status
(C) Size of the tumor
(D) Stage of the tumor

Item 134

A 48-year-old woman is evaluated for a 6-month history of rectal pain and bright red blood per rectum upon defecation. She has a long-standing history of genital warts. Medical history is otherwise unremarkable, and she takes no medications.

On physical examination, vital signs are normal. Abdominal examination reveals no masses. Bowel sounds are normal, and the liver and spleen are not enlarged. Digital rectal examination reveals a hard, tender mass in the anal canal measuring approximately 2.5 cm in diameter. There is no inguinal lymphadenopathy.

Laboratory studies are unremarkable.

Contrast-enhanced CT scan of the pelvis confirms the anal mass and shows no associated lymphadenopathy or other abnormalities. Contrast-enhanced CT scans of the chest and abdomen are normal. Biopsy of the anal mass shows invasive squamous cell carcinoma.

Which of the following is the most appropriate treatment?

(A) Radiation therapy
(B) Radiation therapy with concurrent chemotherapy
(C) Radiation therapy with concurrent chemotherapy followed by surgical resection
(D) Surgical resection

Item 135

A 62-year-old man undergoes follow-up evaluation. The patient received an examination 2 weeks ago following a minor bicycle accident during which a firm, nontender, palpable liver edge 2 cm below the right costal margin was found incidentally. Examination findings were otherwise unremarkable.

A contrast-enhanced CT scan of the abdomen showed a slightly enlarged liver with numerous (>10) hypodense lesions ranging in size from 0.5 to 1.5 cm. Needle biopsy of a liver lesion showed a low-grade, well-differentiated neuroendocrine tumor with fewer than 2 mitoses per 50/hpf. An indium-111 pentetreotide scan (radiolabeled octreotide scan) confirmed the presence of multiple small-volume liver lesions, as well as an approximately 1-cm area of increased avidity in the mesentery consistent with a small bowel carcinoid primary tumor.

Medical history is otherwise unremarkable. He has not had diarrhea, constipation, flushing of the skin, or wheezing. He takes no medications.

On physical examination, vital signs are normal. The remainder of the examination is unremarkable except for the palpable liver edge.

Laboratory studies:

Alkaline phosphatase	115 U/L
Alanine aminotransferase	Normal
Aspartate aminotransferase	Normal
Total bilirubin	Normal
Serotonin	Normal

Which of the following is the most appropriate management?

(A) Hepatic artery embolization
(B) Octreotide therapy
(C) Radiofrequency ablation of the liver lesions
(D) Repeat abdominal imaging in 3 to 4 months
(E) Systemic chemotherapy

Item 136

A 55-year-old man is evaluated for a 1-year history of postprandial indigestion. Associated symptoms are nausea, oily stools, and a 4.5-kg (10.0-lb) weight loss over the past 6 months. His medical history is significant for a recent diagnosis of prediabetes. His current medications are ibuprofen, acetaminophen, and omeprazole.

On physical examination, vital signs are normal; BMI is 25. Scleral icterus is present. Abdominal examination reveals epigastric abdominal pain without guarding or rebound. The remainder of the examination is normal.

Upper endoscopy is normal. Contrast-enhanced CT scan shows a solid 2.5-cm hypoattenuating lesion suspicious for pancreatic adenocarcinoma confined to the head of the pancreas. Dilation of the upstream pancreatic duct and common bile duct is noted. There is no regional lymphadenopathy. The liver parenchyma appears normal.

Which of the following is the most appropriate management?

(A) Endoscopic ultrasound-guided fine needle aspiration
(B) Measurement of CA 19-9
(C) Percutaneous needle biopsy
(D) Surgical resection of the pancreatic mass

Item 137

A 63-year-old woman is evaluated for a 2-month history of pain in her right chest and right ribs as well as right upper abdominal discomfort. Medical history is significant for stage II cancer of the right breast diagnosed 4 years ago and identified as an estrogen receptor–positive, progesterone receptor–negative, HER2-negative invasive ductal carcinoma with negative sentinel lymph nodes. She was treated with breast-conserving therapy, primary breast radiation therapy, and adjuvant chemotherapy and has been receiving adjuvant anastrozole since completing radiation.

On physical examination, vital signs are normal. There is tenderness over the anterior lower right ribs, but no mass or bone defects are present. There are no breast masses or lymphadenopathy. Abdominal examination shows no epigastric mass or tenderness. The liver and spleen are not palpable.

Chest and rib radiographs are normal. CT scans of the abdomen and pelvis show two liver lesions and lytic bone lesions in the spine and pelvis consistent with metastases.

Which of the following is the most appropriate management?

(A) Anthracycline-based chemotherapy

(B) Biopsy of a liver lesion

(C) Exemestane combined with everolimus

(D) PET/CT scan

Item 138

A 70-year-old woman is hospitalized for worsening generalized weakness, anorexia for several days associated with weight loss, and back pain responsive to NSAID administration. The patient recently completed chemotherapy for poorly differentiated adenocarcinoma of the right lung and metastasis-related pathologic compression of the L3 vertebral body without cord compression. Her Eastern Cooperative Oncology Group/World Health Organization performance status is 3 (confined to bed or chair more than 50% of waking hours).

At the time of diagnosis, the patient was treated with four cycles of carboplatin/paclitaxel chemotherapy. CT scans after completing chemotherapy showed an increase in the right lung mass, a new right pleural effusion, increased size of hilar and mediastinal lymph nodes, and new lesions in the liver, consistent with metastases.

On physical examination, the patient is afebrile, blood pressure is 95/57 mm Hg, pulse rate is 90/min, and respiration rate is 20/min. Oxygen saturation is 94% on ambient air. Decreased breath sounds are auscultated over the right lower lung field. There is tenderness over the lumbosacral area. Neurological examination is normal.

Which of the following is the most appropriate next step in management?

(A) Comprehensive palliative care assessment

(B) Initiation of a different chemotherapy regimen

(C) Initiation of artificial nutrition support

(D) Placement of a thoracostomy tube

(E) Radiation therapy to the L3 vertebral body

Item 139

A 78-year-old man is evaluated for headaches, blurred vision, facial flushing, and mild right midback discomfort. The patient is a lifelong nonsmoker.

On physical examination, blood pressure is 150/95 mm Hg; other vital signs are normal. Oxygen saturation is 99% on ambient air. Facial plethora is present. There is no hepatosplenomegaly. The remainder of the examination is unremarkable.

Laboratory studies:

Erythropoietin	150 mU/mL (150 U/L)
Hematocrit	55.2%
Hemoglobin	18.2 g/dL (182 g/L)
Leukocyte count	8200/µL (8.2×10^9/L)
Platelet count	312,000/µL (312×10^9/L)

Urinalysis reveals microscopic hematuria.

Which of the following diagnostic studies should be performed next?

(A) Bone marrow biopsy

(B) CT of the abdomen and pelvis

(C) *JAK2* mutation testing

(D) Peripheral blood flow cytometry

Item 140

A 42-year-old man is evaluated for a 3-month history of dyspepsia and increasing episodes of nausea. Medical history is unremarkable, and he takes no medications.

On physical examination, vital signs are normal. Examination of the abdomen is normal.

Upper endoscopy discloses a large (6-cm) mass in the wall of the proximal duodenum. Biopsy reveals a gastrointestinal stromal tumor staining positive for KIT protein (CD117). Contrast-enhanced CT scans of the chest and abdomen show no other abnormalities.

The patient undergoes complete resection of the mass with clear margins. The final pathology report confirms the original diagnosis and notes a high mitotic rate of 5 to 10 mitoses per 50/hpf. The tumor is classified as being at higher risk for recurrence on the basis of its mitotic rate, large size, and location in the small intestine.

Which of the following is the most appropriate adjuvant treatment?

(A) Epirubicin, cisplatin, and 5-fluorouracil

(B) Imatinib

(C) Radiation therapy

(D) Observation

Item 141

A 37-year-old woman is evaluated in the emergency department for fever and rigors of 4 hours' duration. Medical history is significant for acute lymphoblastic leukemia for which she completed multiagent chemotherapy 10 days ago. Her medical history is otherwise noncontributory, and she takes no other medications.

On physical examination, temperature is 38.8 °C (101.8 °F), blood pressure is 110/60 mm Hg, pulse rate is 100/min, and respiration rate is 16/min. On pulmonary

CONT.

examination, the lungs are clear. The remainder of the physical examination is unremarkable.

Laboratory studies indicate a leukocyte count of $0.3/\mu L$ ($0.0003 \times 10^9/L$) with 0 neutrophils. The remaining laboratory studies are normal.

A chest radiograph is normal. Blood and urine cultures are obtained.

Which of the following is the most appropriate next step in management?

(A) Administer granulocyte-macrophage colony-stimulating factor

(B) Await culture results before starting antimicrobial therapy

(C) Begin piperacillin-tazobactam

(D) Begin vancomycin

Item 142

A 61-year-old man undergoes follow-up evaluation for prostate cancer diagnosed 6 months ago that was treated with radical prostatectomy. CT scans of the chest, abdomen, and pelvis at the time of diagnosis were normal. Bone scan at that time showed no evidence of metastatic disease. The serum prostate-specific antigen (PSA) level at the time of surgery was 12 ng/mL ($12 \mu g/L$), decreasing to 0.6 ng/mL ($0.6 \mu g/L$) 6 weeks after surgery.

Physical examination findings are unremarkable.

Serum PSA measurement obtained at the time of this visit is 10 ng/mL ($10 \mu g/L$). Repeat imaging studies were obtained, and no evidence of metastatic disease was identified.

Which of the following is the most appropriate management?

(A) Androgen deprivation therapy

(B) Chemotherapy

(C) Continued monitoring of the serum PSA level

(D) Salvage radiotherapy

Item 143

A 72-year-old man is evaluated for a 4-month history of pain in the left side of his throat. He also has pain when swallowing and a 2-month history of dysphagia. The patient has a 15-pack-year smoking history but stopped smoking 5 years ago. Medical history is otherwise unremarkable, and he takes no medications.

On physical examination, vital signs are normal. There is no palpable cervical adenopathy and there are no abnormalities on inspection or palpation of the oral pharynx and tongue.

Laryngoscopy identifies a mass centered in the left tongue base. Biopsy of the mass identifies moderately differentiated invasive squamous cell carcinoma. PET/CT scans show hypermetabolic uptake in the tongue base mass without any evidence of cervical lymph node involvement or distant metastasis. On PET/CT the tongue base mass measures 2.1 cm.

Which of the following is the most appropriate treatment approach for this patient?

(A) Concurrent cisplatin-based chemotherapy followed by radiation

(B) Radiation followed by adjuvant chemotherapy

(C) Radiation therapy plus cetuximab

(D) Radiation therapy or surgery alone

Item 144

A 55-year-old man undergoes follow-up evaluation for pancreatic cancer. He underwent a pancreaticoduodenectomy (Whipple procedure), with the pathology report showing stage II pancreatic cancer. Because of postoperative complications and a slow recuperation period, he did not receive postoperative therapy. Nine months postoperatively, the patient was able to resume all activities, including full-time work and regular exercise. Three months later, however, he developed right upper quadrant pain. A CT scan showed postsurgical changes in the pancreatic bed and multiple liver metastases. The patient remains medically fit, has good oral intake, and maintains all activities. Medical history is otherwise unremarkable, and he takes no medications.

On physical examination, vital signs are normal. BMI is 27. The abdomen is soft and nontender with normal bowel sounds. The liver is enlarged. The remainder of the examination is unremarkable.

Laboratory studies:

Hemoglobin	12.8 g/dL (128 g/L)
Leukocyte count	7200/μL (7.2×10^9/L)
Platelet count	302,000/μL (302×10^9/L)
Albumin	Normal
Total bilirubin	Normal
Creatinine	Normal

Which of the following is the most appropriate management?

(A) Multiagent systemic chemotherapy

(B) Single-agent systemic chemotherapy

(C) Radiation therapy to the liver

(D) Transarterial chemoembolization of liver lesions

Item 145

A 32-year-old man is evaluated in the emergency department for fever, neck pain, and a rapidly enlarging right cervical lymph node. The patient first noticed the lymph node 3 weeks ago. He has no significant medical history and takes no medications.

On physical examination, temperature is 38.5 °C (101.3 °F), blood pressure is 120/70 mm Hg, pulse rate is 110/min, and respiration rate is 17/min. A 16-cm firm, enlarged right cervical lymph node is palpated. There is no other lymphadenopathy and no splenomegaly. The remainder of the examination is unremarkable.

Laboratory studies:

Complete blood count	Normal
Creatinine	1.2 mg/dL (106.1 μmol/L)
Lactate dehydrogenase	830 U/L
Phosphorus	5.4 mg/dL (1.74 mmol/L)
Potassium	5.0 mEq/L (5.0 mmol/L)
Urate	8.0 mg/dL (0.47 mmol/L)

CONT.

CT scans of the chest, abdomen, and pelvis reveal a 20-cm enlarged right cervical lymph node that is displacing the trachea to the left. Biopsy of the node shows CD20-positive Burkitt lymphoma. Treatment with hydration, furosemide, and allopurinol are initiated.

Which of the following is the most appropriate additional treatment?

(A) Involved-field radiation therapy

(B) Clarithromycin, amoxicillin, plus omeprazole

(C) Rituximab plus hyperfractionated cyclophosphamide, vincristine, doxorubicin, and dexamethasone (R-hyper-CVAD)

(D) Surgical debulking followed by radiation therapy

Item 146

A 45-year-old man undergoes follow-up evaluation for chronic lymphocytic leukemia. He was diagnosed 1 year ago after presenting with profound fatigue, decreased performance status, diffuse lymphadenopathy, and splenomegaly. He has been treated with rituximab, fludarabine, cyclophosphamide, and prednisone since the time of diagnosis without significant improvement in his symptoms or blood counts. He continues to complain of marked fatigue but minimal symptoms associated with lymphadenopathy or splenic enlargement. He reports no abnormal bleeding. Current medications are alemtuzumab and gamma globulin. Family history is significant for a mother with transfusion-dependent myelodysplastic syndrome and a sister and brother who are well.

On physical examination, vital signs are normal. Enlarged cervical, axillary, and inguinal lymph nodes are palpated. Splenomegaly extending 15 cm below the costal margin at the anterior axillary line is present. The remainder of the examination is unremarkable.

Laboratory studies show a hemoglobin level of 9.5 g/dL (95 g/L), a leukocyte count of 30,000/µL (30 × 10⁹/L) with 70% small mature lymphocytes, and a platelet count of 40,000/µL (40 × 10⁹/L).

Flow cytometry studies show small mature B cells co-expressing CD5 and CD23. Fluorescence in situ hybridization indicates a chromosome 17p deletion.

Chest radiograph is normal. CT scans show extensive cervical, axillary, abdominal, and pelvic lymphadenopathy and splenomegaly.

Which of the following is the most appropriate next step in treatment?

(A) Hematopoietic stem cell transplantation

(B) Leukapheresis

(C) Lymph node radiation

(D) Splenectomy

Item 147

A 76-year-old man is evaluated for a 1-month history of increasing fatigue, abdominal pain, decreased appetite,

and a 4.5-kg (10-lb) weight loss. He does not have cough, dyspnea, or chest pain. Medical history is unremarkable, and he takes no medications. The patient is a lifelong nonsmoker.

On physical examination, the patient is afebrile, blood pressure is 130/80 mm Hg, pulse rate is 84/min, and respiration rate is 12/min. Abdominal examination reveals hepatomegaly. The remainder of the examination is unremarkable.

The serum alkaline phosphatase level is 225 U/L, the serum total bilirubin level is 2.0 mg/dL (34.2 µmol/L), and the serum creatinine level is 0.9 mg/dL (79.6 µmol/L).

Contrast-enhanced CT scans of the abdomen and pelvis show multiple liver metastases with 50% liver replacement and several metastases in the ribs and pelvic bones. CT-guided needle biopsy of the liver reveals high-grade poorly differentiated neuroendocrine cancer. A subsequent chest CT scan shows no evidence of tumor.

Which of the following is the most appropriate treatment?

(A) Hepatic artery embolization

(B) Octreotide

(C) Platinum-based systemic chemotherapy

(D) Radiation therapy for bone metastases

(E) Radiofrequency ablation of liver metastases

Item 148

A 43-year-old woman undergoes follow-up evaluation following a recent diagnosis of estrogen receptor-positive, progesterone receptor–positive, HER2-negative, grade 2 invasive ductal carcinoma of the left breast. The patient was treated with surgery, adjuvant chemotherapy, and radiation therapy. This is her first postradiation visit. She currently takes no medications. She is premenopausal.

On physical examination, vital signs are normal. Well-healed incisions of the left breast and left axilla are present. There is no lymphadenopathy and no right breast masses. The remainder of the examination is unremarkable.

Results of a complete blood count and serum chemistry panel are normal.

Which of the following is the most appropriate therapy?

(A) Exemestane alone

(B) Tamoxifen alone

(C) Maintenance chemotherapy with oral capecitabine

(D) No additional adjuvant therapy

Item 149

A 65-year-old man is seen in follow-up for a recent diagnosis of non–small cell lung cancer. He presented 2 weeks ago with a 3-month history of worsening shortness of breath, fatigue, and reduced appetite with a 35-pound weight loss. Medical history is notable for COPD with baseline shortness of breath with exertion, but no supplemental oxygen requirement. Medications are tiotropium and as-needed albuterol metered dose inhalers.

Physical examination at the time of diagnosis revealed decreased breath sounds in the left lung field. Chest radiograph showed near complete obliteration of the left lung field. CT scan of the chest confirmed the presence of a large left-sided pleural effusion and showed evidence of multiple hepatic and osseous metastatic lesions. He underwent left-sided large volume thoracentesis, and cytology confirmed squamous cell carcinoma.

He currently notes that despite fluid drainage, his breathing has not improved significantly and he is now using home oxygen. He remains weak, spending significant time in bed and requiring assistance in performing many of his daily self-care activities.

Chest auscultation reveals a clear improvement in left-sided breath sounds, and a chest radiograph shows a small amount of residual pleural fluid on the left.

Which of the following is the most appropriate management?

(A) Palliative care assessment

(B) Platinum-based chemotherapy

(C) Pleurodesis

(D) Radiation to bone metastases

Answers and Critiques

Hematology Answers

Item 1   Answer: C

Educational Objective: Diagnose thrombotic thrombocytopenic purpura.

The most appropriate diagnostic test to perform at this time is a peripheral blood smear. This patient likely has thrombotic thrombocytopenic purpura (TTP). TTP should be suspected in patients who have microangiopathic hemolytic anemia, characterized by schistocytes on the peripheral blood smear and increased serum lactate dehydrogenase levels, and thrombocytopenia. A peripheral blood smear is essential to determine whether the anemia is caused by a microangiopathic hemolytic process as indicated by the presence of schistocytes. Patients may also have fever; kidney manifestations such as hematuria, elevated creatinine level, and proteinuria; and fluctuating neurologic manifestations, but the absence of these symptoms does not exclude the diagnosis.

Assays for ADAMTS-13 activity and inhibitor titer are available but are best used for prognosis rather than to guide therapy, because TTP requires immediate treatment that cannot be delayed until laboratory test results are available. Low activity levels and a positive inhibitor titer confer a higher risk for relapse.

An osmotic fragility test is used to evaluate for hereditary spherocytosis, which can produce hemolysis in the setting of an acute infection. However, hereditary spherocytosis does not cause thrombocytopenia, kidney injury, or mental status changes.

TTP can overlap with hemolytic uremic syndrome (HUS), which usually occurs in children. HUS may be precipitated by an infectious diarrheal illness, especially *Escherichia coli* O157:H7 or *Shigella* species. These bacteria elaborate a toxin that resembles antigens on renal endothelial cells and bind and cause renal cell death. It is not clinically helpful to attempt to distinguish between TTP and HUS, because many patients with HUS respond to plasma exchange, the treatment for TTP.

KEY POINT

- Thrombotic thrombocytopenic purpura is a clinical diagnosis that requires the presence of thrombocytopenia and microangiopathic hemolytic anemia, which is confirmed by schistocytes on the peripheral blood smear.

Bibliography

Crawley JT, Scully MA. Thrombotic thrombocytopenic purpura: basic pathophysiology and therapeutic strategies. Hematology Am Soc Hematol Educ Program. 2013;2013:292-9. [PMID: 24319194]

Item 2   Answer: A

Educational Objective: Treat a patient for major bleeding who is taking warfarin.

The patient should be given 4-factor prothrombin complex concentrate (4f-PCC) in addition to intravenous vitamin K and fluids. He is experiencing major bleeding complicated by warfarin therapy and requires immediate anticoagulation reversal. 4f-PCC is a plasma-derived product that contains all four vitamin K–dependent coagulation factors (factors II, VII, IX, and X). Unlike fresh frozen plasma (FFP), 4f-PCC is stored at room temperature, does not require ABO typing, and can be infused quickly because of its small volume, thus reducing the time to delivery of therapy. Compared with FFP, 4f-PCC has been shown to more rapidly achieve hemostasis in patients with visible or musculoskeletal bleeding with less risk of fluid overload and no difference in thromboembolic events. This agent has therefore been approved by the FDA for urgent reversal of coagulation factor deficiencies related to vitamin K antagonist therapy for adult patients with acute major bleeding, as well as for adult patients in need of urgent surgery or an invasive procedure.

Activated factor VII (factor VIIa) has been evaluated in case series for the treatment of vitamin K antagonist–related bleeding. Although factor VIIa can correct the INR quickly in most instances, it is unclear if this is associated with achievement of optimal hemostasis considering factors II, IX, and X are not replaced with this agent. A low dose of factor VIIa may be used in conjunction with 3-factor PCCs (which contain very little factor VII) for treatment of major vitamin K antagonist–associated bleeding in situations when 4f-PCCs are not available and the patient has a contraindication to the use of FFP (for example, uncompensated heart failure).

Cryoprecipitate is rich in fibrinogen and is used to treat inherited or acquired fibrinogen deficiency or dysfibrinogenemia. It has no role in the management of vitamin K antagonist–related bleeding.

FFP can be used when 4f-PCC is not readily available. However, 4f-PCC is also less likely than FFP to induce transfusion-associated circulatory overload, an important consideration in patients with heart failure or transfusion-related acute lung injury. Furthermore, 4f-PCC goes through viral inactivation, which reduces the incidence of transfusion-transmitted infectious diseases.

KEY POINT

- Major bleeding associated with vitamin K antagonists should be treated by reversing anticoagulation with 4-factor prothrombin complex concentrate in addition to intravenous vitamin K.

Bibliography

Sarode R, Milling TJ Jr, Refaai MA, et al. Efficacy and safety of a 4-factor prothrombin complex concentrate in patients on vitamin K antagonists presenting with major bleeding: a randomized, plasma-controlled, phase IIIb study. Circulation. 2013 Sep 10;128(11):1234-43. [PMID: 23935011]

Item 3   Answer: D

Educational Objective: Diagnose chronic thromboembolic pulmonary hypertension in a patient with a previous pulmonary embolism.

A radionuclide ventilation-perfusion (V/Q) lung scan is the preferred and recommended initial study to evaluate for possible chronic thromboembolic pulmonary hypertension (CTEPH), which is likely in this patient. CTEPH is defined as a mean pulmonary artery pressure of greater than 25 mm Hg, with normal pulmonary capillary wedge pressure, left atrial pressure, and left ventricular end-diastolic pressure. It typically occurs within 2 years following a pulmonary embolism (PE), affecting 3.8% of patients, although only about 50% of these have a history of clinically detected PE. Patients with CTEPH often present with persistent shortness of breath or progressively worsening dyspnea, especially on exertion. For a patient in whom pulmonary hypertension is suspected, a V/Q scan can help determine if the patient's pulmonary hypertension is due to obstruction of medium-sized or larger pulmonary arteries (as is characteristic of CTEPH), because V/Q mismatches would be seen. In nonthromboembolic pulmonary hypertension, a V/Q scan would be normal. If the V/Q scan suggests CTEPH, confirmatory right heart catheterization with pulmonary artery pressure measurements and pulmonary arteriography is indicated.

Pulmonary CT angiography (CTA) is not sensitive for diagnosing chronic PE and often appears normal despite chronic perfusion defects, primarily because CTEPH involves chronic changes in the pulmonary vasculature owing to organization of thrombus and recanalization and is not associated with distinct intraluminal filling defects. V/Q scanning is more sensitive for detecting these changes, with a reported sensitivity of CTEPH detection of more than 96% compared with 51% with CTA.

Serum D-dimer testing is not a sensitive marker to detect CTEPH. The pulmonary changes associated with CTEPH involve organization of clots and are not clearly associated with active thrombosis. Therefore, D-dimer levels are unable to provide diagnostic information.

Similarly, venous Doppler ultrasonography would be helpful in evaluating for active thrombosis in the legs but would not provide helpful diagnostic information for evaluation of pulmonary hypertension.

KEY POINT

- Ventilation-perfusion lung scanning is appropriate for determining chronic thromboembolic pulmonary hypertension in patients with a history of pulmonary embolism and persistent or progressive dyspnea.

Bibliography

Kim NH, Delcroix M, Jenkins DP, et al. Chronic thromboembolic pulmonary hypertension. J Am Coll Cardiol. 2013 Dec 24;62(25 Suppl):D92-9. [PMID: 24355646]

Item 4   Answer: D

Educational Objective: Diagnose paroxysmal nocturnal hemoglobinuria.

The most likely diagnosis is paroxysmal nocturnal hemoglobinuria (PNH). PNH is an acquired clonal stem cell disorder that should be considered in patients presenting with hemolytic anemia, pancytopenia, or unprovoked atypical thrombosis. Mutations in the *PIG-A* gene lead to the reduction or absence of glycosylphosphatidylinositol, an important erythrocyte-anchoring protein. Hemolysis is caused by the absence of decay-accelerating factor (CD55) and the membrane inhibitor of reactive lysis (CD59), which are glycosylphosphatidylinositol-dependent complement regulatory proteins. Diagnosis of PNH is based on flow cytometry results, which can detect CD55 and CD59 deficiency on the surface of peripheral erythrocytes or leukocytes.

The patient does not have aplastic anemia (AA). Although AA often has small PNH clones present, thrombosis and hemolysis are not features of this disease. In patients with AA, however, annual screening for the presence of PNH clones by flow cytometry is recommended.

The myelodysplastic syndromes (MDS) are clonal hematopoietic stem cell disorders characterized by ineffective hematopoiesis. Although MDS may present with a hypocellular bone marrow approximately 10% of the time, thrombosis and hemolysis are not typical symptoms. MDS usually presents with anemia or pancytopenia and a hypercellular marrow with dysplastic changes in cell precursors.

Myeloproliferative neoplasms (MPNs) can present with splanchnic thrombosis and should be considered in the differential diagnosis of unusual blood clots. However, the peripheral blood counts do not suggest MPN (no cell lines are elevated), and hemolysis is not a prominent clinical feature. Additionally, the marrow in MPNs is typically hypercellular or fibrotic.

KEY POINT

- Findings diagnostic of paroxysmal nocturnal hemoglobinuria include hemolytic anemia, hypocellular bone marrow, and lack of CD55 and CD59.

Bibliography

Parker CJ. Paroxysmal nocturnal hemoglobinuria. Curr Opin Hematol. 2012 May;19(3):141-8. [PMID: 22395662]

Item 5   Answer: C

Educational Objective: Diagnose Budd-Chiari syndrome associated with *JAK2 V617F* activating mutation.

Testing for the *JAK2 V617F* activating mutation is the most appropriate next step. This patient presents with acute portal hypertension caused by thrombosis of the hepatic veins, or Budd-Chiari syndrome (BCS), which is one of the few noncirrhotic causes of portal hypertension. Clinically, this syndrome can present acutely as fulminant hepatic failure or subacutely with tender hepatomegaly and rapid-onset ascites, as in this patient. Upon discovery of the *JAK2* activating mutation in 2005, it became apparent that up to half of patients with idiopathic BCS had an acquired mutation in *JAK2*, without overt suggestion of a myeloproliferative neoplasm. Therefore, testing for *JAK2* is part of the diagnostic testing protocol that includes consideration of paroxysmal nocturnal hemoglobinuria in the differential diagnosis of splanchnic vein thrombosis.

Antiphospholipid antibodies have been associated with BCS, but they are notoriously nonspecific, and much of the literature concerning antiphospholipid antibodies was written before more specific acquired causes were discerned. Diagnosis of antiphospholipid antibody syndrome requires persistent elevation of antibodies in association with a clinically consistent clot. Because deep venous thrombosis (DVT) and pulmonary embolism (PE), arterial thrombosis, and placental clots are more commonly associated with antiphospholipid antibody syndrome than splanchnic vein thrombosis, testing for this disorder is not indicated until other more likely diagnoses are excluded.

Factor V Leiden most characteristically presents as DVT, with or without PE. Less commonly, patients may experience cerebral, mesenteric, and portal vein thrombosis.

Patients with the prothrombin gene mutation (G20210A) are at increased risk for DVT and, less commonly, cerebral vein thrombosis. In patients with splanchnic vein thrombosis, testing for the more common *JAK2* mutation is the most appropriate initial step.

KEY POINT

- A *JAK2* activating mutation occurs in approximately half of patients with idiopathic Budd-Chiari syndrome.

Bibliography

Yonal I, Pinarbasi B, Hindilerden F, et al. The clinical significance of JAK2V617F mutation for Philadelphia-negative chronic myeloproliferative neoplasms in patients with splanchnic vein thrombosis. J Thromb Thrombolysis. 2012 Oct;34(3):388-96. [PMID: 22569900]

Item 6   Answer: B

Educational Objective: Diagnose hemophilia A.

The patient should undergo factor VIII testing. He has had abnormal bleeding following a surgical procedure and dental extractions. The activated partial thromboplastin time (aPTT) is prolonged but corrects fully in a 1:1 mixing study. This could occur with clotting factor deficiencies VIII, IX, and XI; however, this patient's bleeding disorder appears to be familial. Because his maternal grandfather may have had a bleeding disorder resulting in intracerebral bleeding at a young age, and his brother had abnormal bleeding, the likely inheritance pattern is X-linked recessive; only hemophilia A and B are

inherited in this fashion. Hemophilia A results from factor VIII deficiency and hemophilia B from factor IX deficiency; both produce a prolongation of the aPTT that fully corrects in a mixing study. Persons with severe hemophilia have less than 1% factor VIII or IX activity; they will have severe recurrent hemarthroses as well as retroperitoneal and intramuscular bleeding. Central nervous system hemorrhage is especially hazardous and is a leading cause of death. Mild hemophilia may present in adulthood and is characterized by posttraumatic or surgical bleeding.

The bleeding time test is performed by blotting away excess blood, which tests primary hemostasis rather than fibrin formation. The bleeding time is prolonged in patients with platelet dysfunction, von Willebrand disease (vWD), thrombocytopenia, and anemia. The bleeding time will be abnormal in this patient because of his anemia and will not assist in establishing the diagnosis.

Patients with factor XI deficiency will have a prolonged aPTT, as in this patient, but the inheritance pattern is autosomal recessive, not X-linked. Additionally, bleeding is not spontaneous, tends to be milder in degree, and typically affects mucocutaneous surfaces. It is highly unlikely to cause an intracerebral hemorrhage in a younger person, such as this patient's grandfather.

The antiphospholipid syndrome is defined by the presence of antiphospholipid antibodies and typical clinical manifestations. This disorder may occur as an independent syndrome (primary antiphospholipid syndrome) or secondary to underlying systemic lupus erythematosus. Antiphospholipid antibodies include anticardiolipin, anti-β_2-glycoprotein I, and the lupus anticoagulant. The lupus anticoagulant does prolong the aPTT, but the aPTT will not correct in a 1:1 mixing study. Lupus anticoagulant is also more likely to lead to abnormal thrombosis rather than bleeding.

KEY POINT

- Hemophilia A results from factor VIII deficiency and hemophilia B from factor IX deficiency; both produce a prolongation of the activated partial thromboplastin time that fully corrects in a mixing study.

Bibliography

Carcao MD. The diagnosis and management of congenital hemophilia. Semin Thromb Hemost. 2012 Oct;38(7):727-34. [PMID: 23011791]

Item 7   Answer: C

Educational Objective: Diagnose hypereosinophilic syndrome.

The most likely diagnosis is hypereosinophilic syndrome (HES). This patient presents with cardiac complications of HES, an elevated eosinophil count (>1500/µL [1.5 × 10^9/L]) without a secondary cause, and evidence of organ involvement. The causes of eosinophilia are described in the CHINA mnemonic (connective tissue diseases, helminthic infection, idiopathic [HES], neoplasia, allergy). The most common organs affected by HES include the skin, lungs, gastrointestinal tract, and heart. HES may or may not be associated with mutations in the tyrosine kinase receptor gene, but such involvement is important to identify, because treatment with imatinib is effective in such cases.

Acute eosinophilic leukemia is characterized by increases in immature eosinophils in blood and bone marrow and infiltration of tissues with immature eosinophils. Like HES, cardiac dysfunction can develop, but findings of an acute leukemic syndrome are pronounced and include anemia, thrombocytopenia, and infection.

Chronic myeloid leukemia (CML) is a clonal hematopoietic stem cell disorder characterized by myeloid proliferation. In chronic-phase CML, the leukocyte count is high, the hemoglobin level is low or normal, and the platelet count is normal or high. CML may be associated with an absolute eosinophilia, but tissue or organ dysfunction is not common. Detection of the (9;22) translocation by routine cytogenetics or fluorescence in situ hybridization or of the *BCR-ABL* fusion transcript by reverse transcriptase-polymerase chain reaction is diagnostic.

Systemic mastocytosis with eosinophilia is characterized by urticaria pigmentosa, a unique identifying clinical finding. Urticaria pigmentosa findings include pruritic yellow to red or brown macules, papules, plaques, and nodules. The most common noncutaneous findings are gastrointestinal and include symptoms such as abdominal pain, diarrhea, nausea, and vomiting.

KEY POINT

- An elevated eosinophil count (>1500/µL [1.5×10^9/L]) without a secondary cause and evidence of organ involvement are diagnostic of hypereosinophilic syndrome.

Bibliography
Tefferi A, Gotlib J, Pardanani A. Hypereosinophilic syndrome and clonal eosinophilia: point-of-care diagnostic algorithm and treatment update. Mayo Clin Proc. 2010 Feb;85(2):158-64. [PMID: 20053713]

Item 8   Answer: A
Educational Objective: Manage thrombocytopenia in pregnancy.

The most appropriate management for this patient's thrombocytopenia is immediate delivery of the fetus, because she has HELLP (Hemolysis, Elevated Liver enzymes, and Low Platelets) syndrome. Although she has a history of immune thrombocytopenic purpura (ITP), and her platelet counts have been low throughout the pregnancy, her markedly decreased platelet count is worrisome and could indicate development of another condition. Worsening anemia, right upper quadrant pain, hypertension, proteinuria, and elevated liver enzymes are more consistent with a microangiopathy of pregnancy (HELLP syndrome, preeclampsia, thrombotic thrombocytopenic purpura [TTP]) rather than worsening ITP. Her clinical picture is more consistent with preeclampsia (new-onset hypertension at >20 weeks' gestation) with proteinuria or the

HELLP syndrome. The relationship between preeclampsia and HELLP syndrome is unclear; HELLP syndrome occurs in 10% to 20% of women with preeclampsia but occasionally in some patients without hypertension or proteinuria. The primary treatment for both conditions, particularly in advanced pregnancy, is urgent delivery. Platelet counts tend to recover quickly after delivery; persistent thrombocytopenia several days after delivery should raise concern for another diagnosis, such as thrombotic thrombocytopenic purpura–hemolytic uremic syndrome (TTP-HUS).

Administering intravenous immune globulin is not indicated as a treatment for thrombocytopenia associated with preeclampsia and HELLP syndrome.

Plasma exchange can be undertaken if TTP is present earlier in the pregnancy before delivery is a viable option, but would not be a preferred treatment strategy in a patient in whom delivery is appropriate. Plasma exchange would be indicated if thrombocytopenia persisted after delivery and TTP-HUS were diagnosed.

Glucocorticoids such as prednisone are not indicated for microangiopathy of pregnancy. Additionally, if used as a treatment for ITP, prednisone typically takes 48 to 72 hours for effectiveness. Therefore, treatment with prednisone would not be appropriate in this patient.

KEY POINT

- Immediate delivery of the fetus is the best management approach for pregnant women experiencing thrombotic microangiopathy of pregnancy.

Bibliography
Bockenstedt PL. Thrombocytopenia in pregnancy. Hematol Oncol Clin North Am. 2011 Apr;25(2):293-310. [PMID: 21444031]

Item 9   Answer: A
Educational Objective: Determine duration of anticoagulation in a patient with venous thromboembolism.

This patient should continue anticoagulation therapy indefinitely. Because his venous thromboembolism (VTE) was unprovoked, he is at relatively high risk for recurrence if he stops anticoagulation. Based on his history, stable INR values, absence of comorbidities, and age, his bleeding risk is low. He also does not have a strong preference to discontinue anticoagulation. The decision to treat him for an extended period of time is consistent with the American College of Chest Physicians guidelines, which suggest extended anticoagulant therapy in patients with unprovoked proximal leg deep venous thrombosis (DVT) or pulmonary embolism who have low or moderate bleeding risk. Re-evaluation of this indication based on periodic risk/benefit assessments, new clinical study data, and new anticoagulation drug availability is appropriate.

Short-term anticoagulant therapy (3 months) is suggested for patients with VTE associated with a major transient risk factor, such as major surgery, trauma, or immobility; patients with unprovoked distal leg DVT; and patients with unprovoked proximal leg DVT who are at high risk for bleeding. Therefore, 3 months of therapy, or extending treatment to 6 months, would not be optimal treatment for this patient with an unprovoked proximal DVT.

Because identification of an inherited thrombophilia often does not change treatment decisions in a patient with VTE (does not reliably predict risk of recurrence or influence duration of recommended anticoagulation), evidence-based guidelines recommend against routine thrombophilia testing. In this patient with an unprovoked proximal DVT, the recommendation for long-term anticoagulation would not be altered by the results of such testing, thus, it would not be helpful. Testing may be indicated, however, in patients with VTE at intermediate risk for recurrence by traditional predictors in whom finding a strong thrombophilic risk might alter therapeutic decisions.

KEY POINT

- Long-term anticoagulation therapy is recommended for patients with unprovoked proximal leg deep venous thrombosis or pulmonary embolism who have low or moderate bleeding risk.

Bibliography

Kearon C, Akl EA, Comerota AJ, et al; American College of Chest Physicians. Antithrombotic therapy for VTE disease: antithrombotic therapy and prevention of thrombosis, 9th ed: American College of Chest Physicians evidence-based clinical practice guidelines [erratum in Chest. 2012 Dec;142(6):1698-704]. Chest. 2012 Feb;141(2 Suppl):e419S-94S. [PMID: 22315268]

Item 10   Answer: C

Educational Objective: Treat anemia in a patient with Hodgkin lymphoma.

The patient should receive leukoreduced, irradiated erythrocytes. She has pancytopenia with symptomatic anemia likely because of her chemotherapy. Her bone marrow erythrocyte production cannot be efficiently increased because of her cancer treatment, so an erythrocyte transfusion is clinically indicated. However, immunocompromised patients (those with severe, inherited T-cell immunodeficiency syndromes or Hodgkin lymphoma or recipients of allogeneic or autologous hematopoietic stem cell transplantation, purine analog–based chemotherapy [fludarabine, cladribine, deoxycoformycin], alemtuzumab, or rabbit antithymocyte globulin therapy) are at increased risk of developing transfusion-associated graft-versus-host disease (ta-GVHD). ta-GVHD occurs when the recipient's immune system is unable to eradicate contaminating donor lymphocytes in the transfused erythrocyte or platelet product; the transfused lymphocytes mount an immune response toward the recipient that may result in a maculopapular skin rash, gastrointestinal symptoms, cough and dyspnea, and pancytopenia due to marrow aplasia. Irradiation of the cellular product inactivates contaminating lymphocytes and prevents this complication. ta-GVHD may also occur when partial HLA matching occurs, in which the recipient is heterozygous for an HLA haplotype for which the donor is homozygous. In such a situation, the recipient's immune

system will not recognize the donor lymphocytes as foreign and will fail to mount an immune response. As such, all HLA-matched products require irradiation (that is, HLA-matched platelets for patients with platelet transfusion refractoriness owing to alloimmunization), regardless of the competency of the recipient's immune system.

The patient would benefit from leukoreduced erythrocytes, thus minimizing the risk of febrile nonhemolytic transfusion reactions, as well as HLA alloimmunization and subsequent platelet transfusion refractoriness. Although leukoreduction alone likely reduces the risk of ta-GVHD, it does not eliminate the risk of this complication.

This patient has a positive cytomegalovirus (CMV) IgG antibody and thus has already been exposed to this infectious agent. Therefore, a CMV-negative product is not required. Furthermore, the current generation of prestorage leukocyte filters has significantly decreased the risk of CMV transmission as a result of erythrocyte and platelet transfusion. As such, not all transfusion centers use CMV-negative products for recipients who are CMV seronegative.

Washed erythrocytes are considered for patients with a history of severe allergic reactions to transfusions, which this patient does not have.

KEY POINT

- Leukoreduced and irradiated erythrocytes should be used when transfusing select patients who are immunocompromised to reduce the risk of transfusion-associated graft-versus-host disease and febrile nonhemolytic transfusion reaction.

Bibliography

Treleaven J, Gennery A, Marsh J, et al. Guidelines on the use of irradiated blood components prepared by the British Committee for Standards in Haematology blood transfusion task force. Br J Haematol. 2011 Jan;152(1): 35-51. [PMID: 21083660]

Item 11   Answer: B

Educational Objective: Manage Philadelphia chromosome–positive acute lymphoblastic leukemia in an older patient.

This patient has acute lymphoblastic leukemia (ALL), and the most appropriate treatment is dasatinib with dexamethasone. Diagnosis requires the presence of 25% or more lymphoblasts on bone marrow examination. Cytochemical stains and flow cytometry can help distinguish ALL from acute myeloid leukemia (AML) and B-cell from T-cell ALL. The prognosis for an older patient with ALL has traditionally been poor, with Philadelphia chromosome [t(9;22)] positivity indicating worse outcomes. Twenty-five percent of all adults with ALL and up to 50% of those older than 70 years are positive for t(9;22). With the advent of tyrosine kinase inhibitor (TKI) therapy, medications like imatinib and dasatinib have become the backbone of therapy for Philadelphia chromosome–positive ALL and can be used alone or with chemotherapy. The most significant advance in the treatment of older patients with

CONT.

Philadelphia chromosome–positive disease is TKI therapy. The results of dasatinib and dexamethasone therapy are better than those for traditional chemotherapy, with less toxicity. For older patients who have Philadelphia chromosome–negative ALL, no clear standard cytotoxic chemotherapy regimen exists. However, TKI therapy can provide disease control for greater than 1 year with much less toxicity.

Based on encouraging progress in intensive pediatric regimens, asparaginase has been incorporated into care for adolescents and young adults with ALL. However, use in older adult patients does not improve outcomes and multiplies toxicity.

Anthracyclines (such as daunorubicin), vincristine, and dexamethasone are part of traditional chemotherapy for pediatric and adult patients with ALL; however, results in older patients are disappointing. Therefore, none of these medications would be the best treatment option for this older patient. Combination regimens such as hyperfractionated cyclophosphamide, vincristine, doxorubicin, and dexamethasone (Hyper-CVAD) can cure adults with ALL, but are too toxic for use in elderly populations. The paradox of ALL in older adults is that although less aggressive regimens are less toxic, they compromise the ability to control the leukemia.

KEY POINT

- Tyrosine kinase inhibitor therapy, such as dasatinib, provides a significant advance in the treatment of older patients with Philadelphia chromosome-positive acute lymphoblastic leukemia.

Bibliography

Foà R, Vitale A, Vignetti M, et al; GIMEMA Acute Leukemia Working Party. Dasatinib as first-line treatment for adult patients with Philadelphia chromosome-positive acute lymphoblastic leukemia. Blood. 2011 Dec 15; 118(25):6521-8. [PMID: 21931113]

Item 12   Answer: D

Educational Objective: Determine indications for thrombophilia testing in a patient with a first thromboembolic event.

No thrombophilia testing is indicated in this patient. No evidence indicates that identification of a thrombophilia in this patient would influence the duration or intensity of anticoagulant therapy. Consequently, the American Society of Hematology recommends against thrombophilia testing in patients who develop a venous thromboembolism (VTE) in the setting of a major transient risk factor (surgery, trauma, or prolonged immobility). The appropriate duration of anticoagulation for this patient with VTE due to recent trauma and major surgery is 3 months, regardless of identification of a thrombophilia. It is unclear which patients benefit from thrombophilia testing. It may be appropriate to consider evaluation for a strong thrombophilia in a patient with VTE who is at intermediate risk for recurrent VTE by traditional recurrence risk factors. These are patients with a thromboembolism associated with

minor VTE risk factors, such as women with hormone- or pregnancy-associated VTE or men or women with VTE associated with minor immobility or minor surgery. Finding a strong thrombophilia in these patients may be one of the indications for long-term anticoagulation.

Antiphospholipid antibodies (APLAs) impart a greater risk of arterial and venous thromboembolism. Although the prothrombin time (PT) and activated partial thromboplastin time (aPTT) may be elevated in patients with APLAs, they are not adequately sensitive or specific to indicate the presence or absence of this cause of thrombophilia. If antiphospholipid syndrome is suspected, APLA tests (lupus anticoagulant, anticardiolipin antibodies, and anti-β_2-glycoprotein I antibodies) should be ordered, independent of whether the PT and aPTT are normal or prolonged. Testing for any of these conditions is not indicated in this patient.

If thrombophilia testing is indicated, evaluation should be based on the circumstances, location, and extent of the thrombosis, possibly with input from a coagulation subspecialist. Factor V Leiden and the prothrombin G20210A mutation are the most common inherited thrombophilias and are associated with a mildly increased risk for VTE.

KEY POINT

- Thrombophilia testing is not indicated in patients who develop a venous thromboembolism in the setting of a major transient risk factor (major surgery or trauma or prolonged immobility), because results would not influence duration or intensity of anticoagulation therapy.

Bibliography

Hicks LK, Bering H, Carson KR, et al. The ASH Choosing Wisely® campaign: five hematologic tests and treatments to question. Blood. 2013 Dec 5;122(24):3879-83. [PMID: 24307720]

Item 13   Answer: D

Educational Objective: Manage an acute, uncomplicated vaso-occlusive pain episode with opioids.

The most appropriate pain regimen for this patient is scheduled morphine. Pain is the most common complication of sickle cell disease (SCD) and may be the initial presenting symptom in patients who subsequently develop more severe complications, such as acute chest syndrome (ACS) or multiorgan failure. Patients commonly have musculoskeletal symptoms, but vaso-occlusion can occur in any organ system. No reliable physical or laboratory findings serve as useful surrogate markers for excluding vaso-occlusion; therefore, managing a painful episode in SCD is based on symptoms. Management of an uncomplicated painful episode includes hydration, nonopioid and opioid analgesia, and incentive spirometry to avoid ACS. Morphine and hydromorphone are the opioid analgesics of choice. During hospitalization, opioid analgesia is most effectively delivered by regularly scheduled opioid administration or by patient-controlled analgesia pumps that include a basal rate and a demand option.

CONT.

Meperidine is generally avoided because of its short half-life and lowered seizure threshold.

NSAIDs such as ketoprofen may be useful in the outpatient management of a painful vaso-occlusive crisis in patients with stable kidney function, but are probably inadequate as single agents for patients with severe pain requiring hospitalization. In addition, randomized studies have demonstrated no benefit of adding an NSAID to an opioid for the treatment of acute vaso-occlusive crisis in hospitalized patients.

KEY POINT

- During hospitalization, opioid analgesia is most effectively delivered by regularly scheduled opioid administration or by patient-controlled analgesia pumps.

Bibliography

Yale SH, Nagib N, Guthrie T. Approach to the vaso-occlusive crisis in adults with sickle cell disease [erratum in Am Fam Physician. 2001 Jul 15;64(2):220]. Am Fam Physician. 2000 Mar 1;61(5):1349-56, 1363-4. [PMID: 10735342]

Item 14   Answer: C

Educational Objective: Diagnose suspected pulmonary embolism in a pregnant woman.

This patient, who is pregnant and has a clinical suspicion for pulmonary embolism (PE), should undergo lower extremity venous duplex ultrasonography. Because anticoagulant therapy for PE and deep venous thrombosis (DVT) is similar, diagnosing a DVT noninvasively through ultrasonography would allow immediate initiation of therapy and avoid fetal exposure to radiation and contrast, which are involved in other studies for diagnosing PE. However, a normal lower extremity study for DVT does not exclude the presence of a PE in a patient with a reasonable pretest probability based on clinical features, such as this woman. If her ultrasound is normal, a ventilation-perfusion (V/Q) lung scan is the next preferred modality. If a V/Q scan is unavailable, CT pulmonary angiography is the next diagnostic choice.

Unfortunately, no validated clinical prediction rules exist for assessing pretest probability of PE in pregnant women. Additionally, D-dimer levels are normally elevated during pregnancy. Therefore, D-dimer testing has minimal clinical utility in evaluating for the presence of PE or DVT.

KEY POINT

- The preferred initial diagnostic test to perform in a pregnant patient with possible pulmonary embolism is lower extremity venous duplex ultrasonography to assess for the presence of deep venous thrombosis, which, if present, would obviate the need for radiation and contrast exposure associated with other diagnostic studies.

Bibliography

James AH. Prevention and treatment of venous thromboembolism in pregnancy. Clin Obstet Gynecol. 2012 Sep;55(3):774-87. [PMID: 22828110]

Item 15   Answer: B

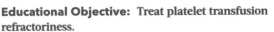

Educational Objective: Treat platelet transfusion refractoriness.

This patient should receive HLA-matched platelets. She meets criteria for platelet transfusion refractoriness, defined as an increase in the platelet count less than 10,000/µL (10×10^9/L) measured 10 to 60 minutes after transfusion on at least two separate occasions. Nonimmune causes include sepsis, fever, disseminated intravascular coagulation, splenomegaly, and medications that decrease platelet half-life. This patient has no features suggesting a nonimmune cause. She is most likely alloimmunized from her previous pregnancies. Such patients are ideally treated with HLA-matched platelets. A systematic review demonstrated improved 1-hour posttransfusion platelet counts with HLA typing. However, the effects on 24-hour platelet counts were more varied, and the impact of this practice on bleeding and mortality is unclear. If HLA-matched platelets are not available, other strategies can be used, including transfusion of HLA-compatible platelets, in which the transfused platelets are missing the antigen to which the patient's alloantibodies are directed, or platelet crossmatching, in which the patient's serum is incubated with donor platelets.

ABO-matched platelets lead to a slightly higher platelet increment in patients who are not alloimmunized but are not likely to have a significant impact on someone who is truly alloimmunized.

Washed platelets are typically reserved for patients who have had severe allergic reactions to platelet transfusion (such as patients who are IgA deficient).

Studies have shown that prophylactic platelet transfusion for a platelet count less than 10,000/µL (10×10^9/L) is superior to platelet transfusions administered at the onset of clinical bleeding, thus decreasing the incidence of clinically significant bleeding. As such, observation without platelet transfusion is inappropriate.

KEY POINT

- Patients experiencing platelet transfusion refractoriness because of alloimmunization should receive HLA-matched platelets.

Bibliography

Pavenski K, Rebulla P, Duquesnoy R, et al; International Collaboration for Guidelines Development, Implementation and Evaluation for Transfusion Therapies (ICTMG) Collaborators. Efficacy of HLA-matched platelet transfusions for patients with hypoproliferative thrombocytopenia: a systematic review. Transfusion. 2013 Oct;53(10):2230-42. [PMID: 23550773]

Item 16   Answer: B

Educational Objective: Manage a patient with acute venous thromboembolism who experienced a major bleeding episode.

Inferior vena cava (IVC) filter placement is indicated; this patient cannot safely undergo anticoagulation because of his

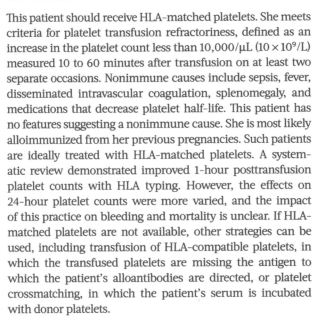

recent major gastrointestinal bleed. He is at increased risk for bleeding owing to the presence of a coagulopathy, likely secondary to his liver disease, and thrombocytopenia, likely due to hypersplenism from an enlarged spleen resulting from portal hypertension. Despite having prolonged coagulation parameters, patients with liver disease are not "autoanticoagulated" and may experience venous thromboembolism (VTE), because procoagulant and anticoagulant protein production is deficient in unpredictable ratios, making it nearly impossible to predict if the patient is most at risk for bleeding or thrombosis. Because of this, anticoagulation in patients with liver disease should be undertaken with caution because of the risk for bleeding. This patient's bleeding risk is very high because of the recent episode of bleeding varices. When IVC filters are necessary, retrievable filters are strongly recommended rather than permanent filters. Whether IVC filters are beneficial for patients with pulmonary embolism (PE) despite appropriate therapeutic anticoagulation is unclear; a possible indication is massive PE with poor cardiopulmonary reserve. No evidence supports the use of IVC filters in the primary prophylaxis of VTE. If the bleeding risk resolves, a conventional course of anticoagulant therapy is recommended with consideration of filter removal.

Considering this patient's risk for bleeding, no anticoagulant (such as heparin, argatroban, rivaroxaban) can safely be given. Additionally, rivaroxaban and argatroban are partially cleared by the liver and are contraindicated in severe liver disease.

KEY POINT

- In patients who cannot safely undergo anticoagulation therapy for venous thromboembolism, such as those with recent bleeding, an inferior vena cava filter should be used until the bleeding risk resolves.

Bibliography
Kearon C, Akl EA, Comerota AJ, et al; American College of Chest Physicians. Antithrombotic therapy for VTE diseaseAntithrombotic Therapy for VTE: antithrombotic therapy and prevention of thrombosis, 9th ed: American College of Chest Physicians evidence-based clinical practice guidelines. Chest. 2012 Feb;141(2 Suppl):e419S-94S. [PMID: 22315268]

Item 17   Answer: D
Educational Objective: Diagnose β-thalassemia.

This patient's most likely diagnosis is β-thalassemia intermedia. She has erythrocyte parameters typical for thalassemia (hemolytic anemia, microcytosis, target cells), a common genetic disorder caused by a mutation in one or more α-globin or β-globin genes leading to a quantitative deficiency in the synthesis of that globin chain. The imbalance in globin-chain synthesis leads to impaired production of hemoglobin and ineffective erythropoiesis, with intramedullary hemolysis and often chronic anemia. α-Thalassemia and β-thalassemia are usually differentiated by hemoglobin electrophoresis, with β-thalassemia associated with a slightly increased hemoglobin A_2 and some residual hemoglobin F. Because of this patient's increased hemoglobin A_2 level, she most likely has β-thalassemia. Because of the low-level hemolysis associated

with either type of thalassemia, patients with thalassemia (and other chronic hemolytic anemias) can commonly have low folate levels even if dietary intake is inadequate, leading to worsening of chronic anemia.

Although most patients with β-thalassemia intermedia are anemic at baseline, most are physiologically adjusted to a hemoglobin level between 7 and 10 g/dL (70-100 g/L). This is not an anemia associated with chronic inflammation.

The patient's iron studies do not indicate iron deficiency; in fact, her ferritin level is elevated, which is often seen in thalassemia. Therefore, she is unlikely to be experiencing iron malabsorption.

KEY POINT

- Hemolytic anemia, microcytosis, and target cells are typical of β-thalassemia, which is associated with slightly increased hemoglobin A_2 and some residual hemoglobin F.

Bibliography
Peters M, Heijboer H, Smiers F, et al. Diagnosis and management of thalassaemia. BMJ. 2012 Jan 25;344:e228. [PMID: 22277544]

Item 18   Answer: D
Educational Objective: Evaluate erythrocytosis.

The patient should receive supplemental oxygen. He probably has secondary erythrocytosis due to hypoxic lung disease and may benefit from oxygen therapy based on his documented hypoxemia (arterial Po_2 ≤55 mm Hg [7.3 kPa] or arterial oxygen saturation ≤88%). The erythropoietin level is elevated owing to hypoxemia, causing an erythrocyte mass. No splenomegaly is present on physical examination, and the lung examination suggests COPD.

Because of the patient's elevated erythropoietin level and hypoxemia, a bone marrow biopsy is not required to exclude polycythemia vera (PV). No leukocytosis, basophilia, or thrombocytosis is seen on laboratory studies, all of which are common in PV.

The *JAK2 V617F* activating mutation defines PV, and 95% of PV harbors this mutation, with the other 5% presenting with variations of the mutation. No *JAK2*-negative PV exists. However, *JAK2* testing is expensive and is not required when a clear cause of secondary erythrocytosis is apparent.

The appropriate management of secondary erythrocytosis is control of the underlying cause. In most circumstances, therapeutic phlebotomy is not recommended for secondary erythrocytosis, because the increased erythrocyte mass is compensating for an unmet tissue oxygenation need.

KEY POINT

- Secondary erythrocytosis can be caused by hypoxemia, so patients may benefit from oxygen supplementation.

Bibliography
Kremyanskaya M, Mascarenhas J, Hoffman R. Why does my patient have erythrocytosis? Hematol Oncol Clin North Am. 2012 Apr;26(2):267-83. [PMID: 22463827]

Item 19   Answer: C

Educational Objective: Manage acquired hemophilia.

The patient should be given recombinant activated factor VII (VIIa). She is an older adult with no bleeding history and no family history of bleeding disorders who now has intramuscular and cutaneous bleeding, which suggests an acquired bleeding disorder. Acquired hemophilia (acquired factor VIII deficiency) causes bleeding with an isolated prolongation of the activated partial thromboplastin time (aPTT). It is associated with the postpartum state, malignancy, or autoimmune conditions, but 50% of cases are idiopathic. Patients have no history of bleeding, but bleeding at presentation can be severe. Unlike congenital hemophilia, bleeding in acquired hemophilia tends to be mucocutaneous and intramuscular. Factor VIII levels are reduced, and mixing study results show unsuccessful correction consistent with an inhibitor. Test results for the lupus anticoagulant are negative.

Patients with low titers of inhibitor (measured in Bethesda units) may be treated with factor VIII concentrates. Patients with high inhibitor titers (>5 Bethesda units) require treatment with recombinant factor VIIa or prothrombin complex concentrates designed to activate factor X and secure hemostasis independent of factor VIII and the intrinsic pathway. Patients may require immunosuppression for inhibitor eradication.

Mild bleeding associated with low inhibitor titers may be treated with desmopressin. However, this patient's hematocrit is low, she has tachycardia possibly related to volume depletion, and her inhibitor level is elevated, making desmopressin a less suitable treatment than recombinant factor VIIa.

Lupus anticoagulants can interfere with the coagulation cascade, causing a prolongation of the aPTT or prothrombin time not corrected by a mixing study. Although they prolong in vitro coagulation tests, they are associated with an increased risk for venous and arterial thromboembolism, not a bleeding tendency. This patient's cutaneous and intramuscular bleeding is inconsistent with the presence of a lupus anticoagulant.

KEY POINT

- Recombinant activated factor VII is used to treat the bleeding episodes of acquired hemophilia associated with high titers of inhibitor.

Bibliography

Franchini M, Mannucci PM. Acquired haemophilia A: a 2013 update. Thromb Haemost. 2013 Dec;110(6):1114-20. [PMID: 2400830]

Item 20   Answer: D

Educational Objective: Manage thrombocytopenia in a patient with acute myeloid leukemia.

The platelet count should be rechecked in 24 hours. Although this patient is significantly thrombocytopenic, phase III clinical trial data do not support the use of prophylactic platelet transfusions for patients with acute myeloid leukemia (AML) whose platelet count is 10,000/µL (10×10^9/L) or higher. Randomized studies have been published comparing a platelet transfusion threshold of 10,000/µL (10×10^9/L) to 20,000/µL (20×10^9/L) in stable patients with AML undergoing induction or consolidation chemotherapy; all have demonstrated equivalent outcomes with respect to clinically significant bleeding, need for erythrocyte transfusions, and mortality during induction chemotherapy. Therefore, these data support and guidelines recommend a threshold of 10,000/µL (10×10^9/L) for prophylactic platelet transfusion in hospitalized patients with thrombocytopenia due to decreased bone marrow production. Patients with acute promyelocytic leukemia (APL), fever, clinically significant bleeding, or a need for invasive procedures were not evaluated in these studies and are typically transfused at a threshold of 20,000/µL (20×10^9/L).

Transfusion of leukoreduced, irradiated platelets would be appropriate if the patient's platelet count decreases to less than 10,000/µL (10×10^9/L). HLA-matched platelets would only be used if the patient had a history of platelet transfusion refractoriness attributed to platelet alloantibodies. Washing of platelets leads to loss of platelet numbers and function and is reserved for patients with a history of a severe allergic reaction to a transfused blood product (such as anaphylaxis in a patient with IgA deficiency).

KEY POINT

- Clinically stable patients with chemotherapy-induced thrombocytopenia who are not bleeding do not benefit from platelet transfusion when the platelet count is 10,000/µL (10×10^9/L) or greater.

Bibliography

Estcourt L, Stanworth S, Doree C, et al. Prophylactic platelet transfusion for prevention of bleeding in patients with haematological disorders after chemotherapy and stem cell transplantation. Cochrane Database Syst Rev. 2012 May 16;5:CD004269. [PMID: 22592695]

Item 21   Answer: A

Educational Objective: Manage warfarin therapy with vitamin K supplementation.

The patient should begin daily low-dose vitamin K supplementation. In 2007, a double-blind randomized trial compared the effects of low-dose vitamin K (100-150 µg/d) and placebo on INR stability in 70 patients receiving chronic warfarin therapy. Vitamin K supplementation resulted in 19 of 35 patients achieving the predefined criteria for stable control of anticoagulation compared with only 7 of 35 patients receiving placebo. It was hypothesized that low-dose vitamin K reduced the day-to-day variation in dietary vitamin K intake in patients with unexplained INR fluctuations.

Polymorphisms in the genes transcribing enzymes involved in the metabolism of vitamin K antagonists, such as cytochrome P-450 2C9 and vitamin K epoxide reductase complex-1, contribute to the variability in dose requirements among patients but do not explain day-to-day or week-to-week INR fluctuations in individual patients. Therefore, genetic testing would not be helpful in this situation.

A factor V Leiden mutation would not explain INR fluctuations. The only thrombophilia that might cause INR fluctuations over time is the presence of a lupus anticoagulant; however, such frequent fluctuations as this patient is experiencing would not be expected with any thrombophilia. Thus, a thrombophilia evaluation would not be indicated.

Aspirin alone will not provide the same protective benefit as warfarin for this patient with recurrent deep venous thrombosis.

KEY POINT

- In some patients with fluctuating INRs while taking warfarin, daily supplementation with low-dose vitamin K (100-150 µg/d) can stabilize the INR.

Bibliography

Sconce E, Avery P, Wynne H, Kamali F. Vitamin K supplementation can improve stability of anticoagulation for patients with unexplained variability in response to warfarin. Blood. 2007 Mar 15;109(6):2419-23. [PMID: 17110451]

Item 22   Answer: D

Educational Objective: Diagnose the cause of an aplastic crisis.

The patient has parvovirus B19 infection. She has chronic hemolytic anemia due to sickle cell anemia and presents with severe anemia and a completely inadequate reticulocyte response 1 week after being exposed to a child with a febrile illness, which was likely caused by parvovirus B19. Hydroxyurea could lead to worsening anemia in a patient with sickle cell anemia but would not cause the acute signs or symptoms found in this patient. A subsequent bone marrow examination would demonstrate pure red cell aplasia (PRCA). Parvovirus has a tropism for erythrocyte precursors and is a known cause of aplastic crisis in patients with underlying sickle cell disease (SCD). Immune competent patients and those without chronic hemolysis have a milder hematologic response to parvovirus infection and are more likely to recover spontaneously.

Cytomegalovirus could cause constitutional symptoms and could trigger a painful crisis, but it is not associated with direct destruction of erythrocyte precursors. Cytomegalovirus may cause retinitis, gastroenteritis, or hepatitis in an immunocompromised patient, none of which are seen in this patient. Adults with SCD are functionally asplenic.

Epstein-Barr virus is unlikely owing to its lack of association with PRCA. However, viral illnesses are the frequent underlying causes that precipitate vaso-occlusive crises or acute chest syndrome in patients with SCD.

Influenza A virus is an unlikely diagnosis because the patient has no typical symptoms. Although influenza A could cause severe viral pneumonia and could lead to acute chest syndrome, its association with PRCA is not strong.

KEY POINT

- Parvovirus B19 infection can cause acquired pure red cell aplasia in an otherwise functionally asplenic patient with sickle cell disease.

Bibliography

Young NS, Brown KE. Parvovirus B19. N Engl J Med. 2004 Feb;350(6):586-97. [PMID: 14762186]

Item 23   Answer: C

Educational Objective: Manage asymptomatic immune thrombocytopenic purpura.

The patient most likely has immune thrombocytopenic purpura (ITP) and should have another complete blood count performed in 1 week. Although ITP is a diagnosis of exclusion, supportive clinical findings include an otherwise normal blood count and the absence of additional organ dysfunction. Platelets on the peripheral blood smear are large because they typically have been recently released from the marrow, and the enhanced hemostatic function of these young platelets may account for less severe bleeding symptoms than those associated with other diseases with a similar platelet count. Not all patients with ITP require therapy, and monitoring for signs of bleeding or further declines in platelet counts may be appropriate. Asymptomatic patients without evidence of bleeding and platelet counts greater than 30,000 to 40,000/µL (30-40 ×10⁹/L) have less than a 15% chance of developing more severe thrombocytopenia requiring treatment. In such patients, the most appropriate course of action is to provide counseling on potential bleeding symptoms and repeat the complete blood count at a designated interval, generally 1 to 2 weeks, until the course of the illness is determined.

In adults with ITP, therapy may be required for patients with platelet counts lower than 30,000 to 40,000/µL (30-40 × 10⁹/L) or with bleeding. Initial therapy consists of glucocorticoids. Patients who do not respond to glucocorticoid therapy should be treated with an additional agent such as intravenous immune globulin or anti-D immune globulin or rituximab.

Splenectomy leads to a sustained remission in 75% of patients. Because of this patient's lack of symptoms and platelet count greater than 30,000/µL (30 ×10⁹/L), therapy is unnecessary at this time, and the patient may be safely observed.

KEY POINT

- Patients with immune thrombocytopenic purpura without evidence of bleeding and platelet counts greater than 30,000 to 40,000/µL (30-40 ×10⁹/L) have less than a 15% chance of developing more severe thrombocytopenia requiring treatment and can be managed with careful observation.

Bibliography

Neunert C, Lim W, Crowther M, Cohen A, Solberg L Jr, Crowther MA; American Society of Hematology. The American Society of Hematology 2011 evidence-based practice guideline for immune thrombocytopenia. Blood. 2011 Apr 21;117(16):4190-207. [PMID: 21325604]

Item 24   Answer: C

Educational Objective: Manage unprovoked proximal leg superficial thrombophlebitis.

This patient should undergo venous duplex ultrasonography of the left thigh to evaluate for deep venous thrombosis (DVT) associated with his superficial venous thrombophlebitis (SVT). DVT or pulmonary embolism (PE) develops in up to 3.3% of patients with isolated SVT. The risk increases in patients with SVT of the great or small saphenous vein, with extremity swelling more pronounced than would be expected from the SVT alone, and with progressive symptoms. In these situations, such as with this patient, duplex ultrasonography is indicated to assess for the possibility of an associated DVT.

The effectiveness of low-dose aspirin to treat or prevent propagation of clots in SVT has not been established. Additionally, the use of other anticoagulants for treatment of SVT is controversial. Some evidence indicates that patients with extensive SVT may benefit from a short course of anticoagulant therapy. However, because of a lack of additional data, the specific patients for whom treatment is indicated, the optimal duration of anticoagulation, and the appropriate drug dose and choice are unknown.

D-dimer testing has no utility for differentiating superficial from deep venous thrombosis because levels may be elevated in both conditions. It would, therefore, not be useful in this patient.

Nonextensive SVT, defined as less than 5 cm in length and not near the deep venous system, may be treated with only symptomatic therapy consisting of analgesics, anti-inflammatory medications, and warm or cold compresses for symptom relief, because the risk of progression into the deep venous system and of PE is low.

KEY POINT

- Duplex ultrasonography is indicated to assess for the possibility of an associated deep venous thrombosis (DVT) in patients with isolated superficial venous thrombophlebitis (SVT), because DVT or pulmonary embolism risk increases in patients with SVT of the great or small saphenous vein, with extremity swelling more pronounced than would be expected from the SVT alone, and with progressive symptoms.

Bibliography

Quéré I, Leizorovicz A, Galanaud JP, et al; Prospective Observational Superficial Thrombophlebitis (POST) Study Investigators. Superficial venous thrombosis and compression ultrasound imaging. J Vasc Surg. 2012 Oct;56(4):1032-8. [PMID: 22832262]

Item 25   Answer: A

Educational Objective: Diagnose folate deficiency.

This patient has folate deficiency. Folate deficiency caused by decreased folate consumption occurs infrequently, because normal diets are replete with folate. However, patients with folate-deficient diets, especially those with generalized malnutrition or poor nutrition, can become folate deficient in weeks to months because of relatively limited stores of folate in the body. Other less common causes of folate deficiency include conditions such as hemolytic anemia (for example, sickle cell disease), desquamating skin disorders (for example, psoriasis), and other conditions associated with increased cellular turnover. Measuring serum folate levels is typically unreliable in diagnosing folate deficiency, because folate levels increase rapidly after a single folate-containing meal. Plasma homocysteine levels increase in folate deficiency, whereas homocysteine and methylmalonic acid levels are increased in cobalamin deficiency. An elevated homocysteine level has a sensitivity of greater than 90% in the diagnosis of folate deficiency, making homocysteine measurement a reasonable test when the disorder is suspected but the serum folate level is normal.

In addition to peripheral blood smear findings of microcytosis and anisopoikilocytosis (abnormalities in erythrocyte size and shape), patients with iron deficiency have reduced serum iron and ferritin levels, increased total iron-binding capacity, and reduced transferrin saturation (iron/total iron-binding capacity). The patient's macrocytosis and high homocysteine level make iron deficiency an unlikely cause of her anemia.

α-Thalassemia trait (or α-thalassemia minor) is associated with mild anemia, microcytosis, hypochromia, target cells on the peripheral blood smear, and, in adults, normal hemoglobin electrophoresis results. The (-α/-α) variant is found in 2% to 3% of all black persons and is often mistaken for iron deficiency. The patient's new-onset macrocytic anemia is not consistent with an inherited hemoglobinopathy associated with microcytosis.

Vitamin B_{12} deficiency usually develops over several months, not weeks. Furthermore, homocysteine and methylmalonic acid levels are elevated in vitamin B_{12} deficiency, but this patient's methylmalonic acid level is normal.

KEY POINT

- An elevated homocysteine level is 90% sensitive for folate deficiency, making this measurement the most sensitive diagnostic marker in suspected folate deficiency when the serum folate level is normal.

Bibliography

Kaferle J, Strzoda CE. Evaluation of macrocytosis. Am Fam Physician. 2009 Feb 1;79(3):203-8. [PMID: 19202968]

Item 26   Answer: B

Educational Objective: Treat essential thrombocythemia based on risk stratification.

Hydroxyurea plus low-dose aspirin is the most appropriate treatment for patients with essential thrombocythemia (ET) in whom treatment is indicated. Treatment of ET requires reduction of the platelet count; however, when and whom to treat remain controversial. Although the exact platelet count does not determine the risk for thrombosis, lowering the platelet count in patients at risk for thrombosis will decrease this risk and, possibly, the risk for secondary myelofibrosis. Patients do not require treatment if they are younger than 60 years, have a platelet count less than 1 million/μL (1000 × 10^9/L), and have no history of thrombosis. Hydroxyurea plus low-dose aspirin is the best treatment option for ET when treatment is required in patients older than 60 years, those with a platelet count greater than 1 million/μL (1000 × 10^9/L), or those with a history of thrombosis or an increased risk for thrombosis because of cardiovascular risk factors such as hypertension and diabetes mellitus. Hydroxyurea plus low-dose aspirin reduces the risk for arterial thrombosis and bleeding (regardless of the platelet count achieved) in patients with ET.

Anagrelide is another platelet-lowering agent used to manage ET, but in a randomized trial comparing anagrelide with hydroxyurea, anagrelide was found to have a less favorable side effect profile. Likewise, hydroxyurea, but not anagrelide, decreases thrombotic risk independent of platelet-count lowering.

Ruxolitinib is an inhibitor of constitutively active *JAK2 V617F*. Although 50% of patients with ET demonstrate this mutation, ruxolitinib has a therapeutic role only in alleviating the splenomegaly and systemic symptoms of primary myelofibrosis.

Warfarin has not been studied for primary prophylaxis of ET; therefore, it would not be an appropriate treatment choice for this patient.

The patient's age is an important factor in initiating therapy, making observation an inappropriate choice.

KEY POINT

- Hydroxyurea plus low-dose aspirin is the best treatment option for essential thrombocythemia when treatment is required in patients older than 60 years, those with a platelet count greater than 1 million/μL (1000 × 10^9/L), or those with a history of thrombosis.

Bibliography

Passamonti F, Thiele J, Girodon F, et al. A prognostic model to predict survival in 867 World Health Organization-defined essential thrombocythemia at diagnosis: a study by the International Working Group on Myelofibrosis Research and Treatment. Blood. 2012 Aug 9;120(6):1197-201. [PMID: 22740446]

Item 27   Answer: D

Educational Objective: Diagnose macroangiopathic hemolytic anemia caused by a mechanical heart valve.

This patient should be further evaluated with echocardiography; she likely has hemolysis due to her mechanical aortic valve. She has evidence of hemolytic anemia based on her low serum haptoglobin and high lactate dehydrogenase levels. The peripheral blood smear shows schistocytes, which are often found in clinical conditions in which erythrocytes are

damaged in small blood vessels (microangiopathic hemolytic anemia), but schistocytes may also occur from trauma in larger blood vessels (macroangiopathic hemolytic anemia). The patient has a mechanical heart valve with a significant murmur, suggesting possible valve dysfunction, and, in the absence of other likely causes of a microangiopathic hemolytic anemia, this is likely the cause of her hemolysis. Therefore, echocardiography to identify a regurgitant jet or paravalvular leak, suggested by the murmur present in this patient, would be the most appropriate next diagnostic study. In patients with suspected valve-associated hemolysis, transesophageal echocardiography is the preferred study because of its ability to effectively visualize the aortic valve structures for this potential complication. Patients with chronic intravascular hemolysis may ultimately develop iron deficiency anemia as the heme iron released from the hemolysis passes through the kidneys and is lost in the urine.

Thrombotic thrombocytopenic purpura (TTP) is a cause of microangiopathic hemolytic anemia and should be considered in this patient. However, her normal platelet count and the slowly progressive onset of her symptoms make this diagnosis unlikely. In patients with TTP, an ADAMTS-13 assay may be helpful in estimating prognosis, but would not be an appropriate study in this patient.

Disseminated intravascular coagulation (DIC) is an acquired form of microangiopathic hemolytic anemia. Acute DIC is associated with evidence of accelerated fibrinolysis, including increased fibrin degradation products and D-dimer. However, this patient has no other clinical findings consistent with DIC (such as bleeding or thrombocytopenia), making this an unlikely diagnosis and a D-dimer measurement unnecessary.

The direct antiglobulin (Coombs) test is used to determine an autoimmune cause of hemolytic anemia. However, neither warm nor cold autoimmune hemolytic anemia causes schistocytes as seen in this patient's blood smear, making this diagnosis unlikely. Therefore, this test would be of low diagnostic yield.

KEY POINT

- Patients with suspected macroangiopathic hemolytic anemia caused by a mechanical heart valve should be diagnosed using transesophageal echocardiography.

Bibliography

Shapira Y, Vaturi M, Sagie A. Hemolysis associated with prosthetic heart valves: a review. Cardiol Rev. 2009 May-Jun;17(3):121-4. [PMID: 19384085]

Item 28   Answer: D

Educational Objective: Manage anticoagulation in a patient with an elevated plasma homocysteine level and methylene tetrahydrofolate reductase polymorphism.

This patient's warfarin should be discontinued. Patients who have experienced a single venous thromboembolism (VTE) due to a major transient risk factor only require short-term anticoagulation for 3 months. This patient experienced a deep venous thrombosis following a traumatic tibia fracture. Generally, the clinical setting of a thrombotic event (unprovoked versus provoked) provides greater prognostic information regarding recurrence risk than the results of thrombophilia testing. Therefore, in most instances, thrombophilia testing results will not influence treatment duration and testing is not indicated. If thrombophilia testing is considered, it should be targeted to persons in whom finding a strong thrombophilia may influence length of anticoagulant treatment or have an impact on other family members if they also tested positive for the higher risk thrombophilia. However, consensus is limited on what defines higher risk thrombophilias.

Elevated plasma homocysteine levels are associated with an increased risk for a first venous or arterial thromboembolic event. Homocysteine levels can be lowered with folic acid, vitamin B_6, and vitamin B_{12}. However, this does not change the risk of a first thromboembolic event, which this patient has already experienced, nor of recurrent VTE.

Homozygosity for the methylene tetrahydrofolate reductase (*MTHFR*) C677T polymorphism can be associated with elevated homocysteine levels but alone is not a risk factor for VTE. Thus, no clinical indication exists for testing for the *MTHFR* polymorphism in patients or first-degree relatives.

KEY POINT

- Thrombophilia test results typically do not influence treatment duration, so testing is not indicated, especially for patients with only a single venous thromboembolism resulting from a major transient risk factor.

Bibliography

Gatt A, Makris M. Hyperhomocysteinemia and venous thrombosis. Semin Hematol. 2007 Apr;44(2):70-6. [PMID: 17433898]

Item 29   Answer: B

Educational Objective: Diagnose infectious complications of iron overload syndromes.

This patient should be advised to avoid eating raw or undercooked seafood. Patients with iron overload syndromes, including those with hereditary hemochromatosis, are at risk for a number of infections with organisms whose virulence is increased in the presence of excess iron. Although the exact mechanisms of increased susceptibility to specific infections are not known, pathogens require mobilization of tissue iron from the host, which is increased in iron overload syndromes. Additionally, excess iron appears to impair host defenses against certain infections, such as decreasing the chemotactic response and compromising the ability of phagocytic cells. The result is increased virulence among specific infectious organisms in patients with iron overload, including *Vibrio* species *(vulnificus, cholerae)*, *Escherichia coli*, *Yersinia enterocolitica*, *Listeria monocytogenes*, cytomegalovirus, hepatitis B and C viruses, and HIV. Fungi include *Aspergillus fumigatus* and mucor. *V. vulnificus* infection is associated with ingestion of raw seafood, especially oysters,

and the risk of sepsis and death is significantly increased in persons with hemochromatosis; therefore, these foods should be specifically avoided by these patients.

Oral calcium supplements may bind iron in the gut and inhibit iron absorption and are acceptable to take if needed for another indication. However, this inhibitory effect is small relative to the removal of iron by phlebotomy. Therefore, supplementation for treatment of hemochromatosis in those undergoing phlebotomy is not usually required.

Although red meat contains iron, and excessive meat intake should be avoided, consumption of moderate amounts of meat by those being treated with phlebotomy is reasonable for nutritional purposes. The amount of iron removed by phlebotomy far exceeds the iron content of a moderate intake of meat.

Vitamin C (ascorbic acid) may interact with tissue iron and lead to generation of oxidative radicals with the potential for tissue damage. However, the amount of vitamin C contained in fruits and vegetables is relatively low, and their consumption as part of a normal diet should not be discouraged.

KEY POINT

- *Vibrio vulnificus* infection is associated with ingestion of raw seafood, especially oysters, and the risk of sepsis and death is increased in persons with hereditary hemochromatosis.

Bibliography

Khan FA, Fisher MA, Khakoo RA. Association of hemochromatosis with infectious diseases: expanding spectrum. Int J Infect Dis. 2007 Nov;11(6): 482-7. [PMID: 17600748]

Item 30   Answer: D

Educational Objective: Manage testing of family members for factor V Leiden mutation.

This patient should not undergo further testing for a factor V Leiden (FVL) mutation. FVL is the most common inherited thrombophilia, resulting from a point mutation in the factor V gene that causes it to be resistant to inactivation by activated protein C (APC). FVL prevalence in the United States is 3% to 8% in whites and 1.2% in blacks, but it rarely occurs in African and Asian populations. Homozygous FVL carries an 18-fold increased risk of first-time venous thromboembolism (VTE), whereas FVL heterozygosity only carries a 2.7-fold increased risk. Although this patient's mother has a known inherited thrombophilia with recurrent episodes of VTE, no evidence indicates testing for inherited thrombophilia is beneficial in an asymptomatic child, particularly with heterozygous FVL, which is not considered a strong thrombophilia.

In patients in whom testing for FVL is indicated, the presence of FVL can be detected by an APC resistance assay that assesses the ability of protein C to inactivate factor Va. This is a very sensitive study that effectively excludes FVL if normal and is the preferred initial screening test, mainly because it is typically less expensive than the FVL genetic test. An abnormal result suggests heterozygous or homozygous FVL, depending on the degree of abnormality, but should be followed by confirmatory genetic polymerase chain reaction testing of the FVL gene that assesses for the point mutation in genetic material from leukocytes from the peripheral blood.

Factor V deficiency is an extremely rare inherited disorder that causes abnormal bleeding as a result of failure of thrombin generation because of inadequate amounts of factor V. This patient has no evidence of a bleeding disorder, so testing factor levels is not indicated.

KEY POINT

- Routine testing for factor V Leiden (FVL) mutation in offspring of a patient with FVL is not indicated.

Bibliography

Middeldorp S. Is thrombophilia testing useful? Hematology Am Soc Hematol Educ Program. 2011;2011:150-5. [PMID: 22160027]

Item 31   Answer: A

Educational Objective: Treat acute promyelocytic leukemia.

All-*trans* retinoic acid (ATRA) should be administered as soon as possible, followed by chemotherapy, for this patient with acute promyelocytic leukemia (APL). APL is a clinically and biologically distinct variant of acute myelocytic leukemia characterized by the presence of a (15;17) gene translocation, which gives rise to the promyelocytic leukemia–retinoic acid receptor-α fusion transcript and arrest of leukemic cells at the promyelocyte stage. Adding ATRA to standard induction and consolidation chemotherapy releases the block in promyelocyte maturation and produces cure in up to 80% of patients. If APL is suspected, ATRA should be initiated without waiting for confirmation. This patient's symptoms and laboratory studies strongly suggest APL, with prominent Auer rods on the peripheral blood smear and bleeding out of proportion to thrombocytopenia. She also has biochemical evidence of disseminated intravascular coagulation, which is a defining clinical clue to APL. In addition to appropriate blood product transfusion support, early ATRA administration is required to help patients survive induction chemotherapy. The greatest mortality risk from APL accrues in the first 2 weeks, with delay in ATRA administration being one of several root causes.

Testing for the t(9;22) would not be helpful in this patient, because it would identify the Philadelphia chromosome, which only has relevance in chronic myeloid leukemia or acute lymphoblastic leukemia.

Testing for the t(15;17) would confirm a diagnosis of APL and can be accomplished in less than 24 hours using fluorescence in situ hybridization. However, enough clinical clues are already provided to strongly suspect the diagnosis, and ATRA should be initiated at the point of clinical suspicion to improve early survival.

KEY POINT

- Immediate administration of all-*trans* retinoic acid is important in preventing early mortality in suspected acute promyelocytic leukemia.

Bibliography

Altman JK, Rademaker A, Cull E, et al. Administration of ATRA to newly diagnosed patients with acute promyelocytic leukemia is delayed contributing to early hemorrhagic death. Leuk Res. 2013 Sep;37(9):1004-9. [PMID: 23768930]

Item 32   Answer: D

Educational Objective: Diagnose hereditary spherocytosis.

This patient should undergo an osmotic fragility test. She most likely has hereditary spherocytosis. Inheritance is usually autosomal dominant with variable penetrance but may occasionally be sporadic. Alternations in membrane structure destabilize the erythrocyte, leading to a spherocytic shape, reduced deformability, trapping, and subsequent destruction in the spleen. Hereditary spherocytosis should be suspected in patients with a personal or family history of anemia, jaundice, splenomegaly, or gallstones. Some patients, such as this patient, may come to medical attention because of an aplastic crisis precipitated by an acute parvovirus B19 infection. Spherocytes are present on the peripheral blood smear, and the direct antiglobulin (Coombs) test (DAT) is negative. The osmotic fragility test with 24-hour incubation is a key step in diagnosis, demonstrating increased erythrocyte fragility in hypotonic saline compared with control erythrocytes.

Patients with warm autoimmune hemolytic anemia (WAIHA) may present with rapid or insidious symptoms of anemia or jaundice; mild splenomegaly is often present. Spherocytes are seen on the peripheral blood smear. The DAT is used to diagnose WAIHA. In less than 10% of patients, the DAT may be normal, in which case more sensitive diagnostic testing through a reference laboratory or blood center is required. First-line therapy for WAIHA is glucocorticoids; however, a trial period of prednisone is not indicated in this patient with a negative DAT and a family history of anemia.

Paroxysmal nocturnal hemoglobinuria (PNH) is an acquired clonal progenitor cell disorder characterized by hemolytic anemia, pancytopenia, or unprovoked thrombosis. Diagnosis is based on flow cytometry results, which can detect CD55 and CD59 deficiency on the surface of peripheral erythrocytes or leukocytes. In the absence of pancytopenia and a history of thrombosis, flow cytometry is not indicated in this patient

Glucose-6-phosphate dehydrogenase (G6PD) deficiency is caused by various mutations on the X chromosome and occurs more commonly in men, often in blacks. During an acute hemolytic episode, bite cells may be seen on the peripheral blood smear, and a brilliant cresyl blue stain may reveal Heinz bodies (denatured oxidized hemoglobin). These findings are not present in the patient's peripheral blood smear, so measuring the G6PD activity is not indicated.

- The osmotic fragility test with 24-hour incubation is a key step in diagnosing hereditary spherocytosis.

Bibliography

Bolton-Maggs PH, Langer JC, Iolascon A, Tittensor P, King MJ; General Haematology Task Force of the British Committee for Standards in Haematology. Guidelines for the diagnosis and management of hereditary spherocytosis-2011 update. Br J Haematol. 2012 Jan;156(1):37-49. [PMID: 22055020]

Item 33   Answer: A

Educational Objective: Evaluate the cause of iron deficiency anemia with colonoscopy and upper endoscopy.

This patient should undergo evaluation by colonoscopy and upper endoscopy. Iron deficiency can result from blood loss or malabsorption. In men and nonmenstruating women, gastrointestinal blood loss is always the presumed cause of iron deficiency unless proven otherwise and may develop secondary to an undiagnosed colonic neoplasm. Colon cancer is the most commonly detected cancer causing iron deficiency anemia.

Remeasuring iron stores in 1 month will not be helpful and is not an appropriate choice without assessing the cause of the iron deficiency. In patients who receive adequate treatment for iron deficiency anemia, reticulocytosis can be expected within 7 to 10 days, and the hemoglobin level can be expected to increase in 1 to 2 days. Iron stores are not expected to normalize for 6 months.

Iron malabsorption can result from celiac disease, inflammatory bowel disease, or surgical resection (affecting the duodenum, as in gastric bypass). Some malabsorption syndromes, such as celiac disease, are not accompanied by diarrhea, steatorrhea, or weight loss. In developed nations, gastrointestinal bleeding is the most common cause of iron deficiency; iron malabsorption is much less common. Considering this patient's complete blood count was normal 1 year ago, celiac disease is an unlikely cause of iron deficiency, and screening for celiac disease with tissue transglutaminase IgA antibody is not appropriate at this time.

Wireless capsule endoscopy is an effective technology that provides visualization of the small bowel. Unlike angiography or technetium scans, wireless capsule endoscopy is effective even in the absence of active bleeding. It detects the source of occult bleeding in 50% to 75% of patients. In those with iron deficiency anemia, in whom bleeding can be episodic, capsule endoscopy is another way to investigate potential sources of blood loss after other investigations have been unrevealing. Wireless capsule endoscopy should not precede colonoscopy and upper endoscopy as the first diagnostic tests for adult patients with iron deficiency anemia and presumed gastrointestinal blood loss.

- In men and nonmenstruating women, gastrointestinal blood loss is the presumed cause of iron deficiency unless proven otherwise; because it may develop secondary to an undiagnosed colonic neoplasm, colonoscopy and upper endoscopy are recommended.

Bibliography

Kim SJ, Ha SY, Choi BM, et al. The prevalence and clinical characteristics of cancer among anemia patients treated at an outpatient clinic. Blood Res. 2013 Mar;48(1):46-50. [PMID: 23589795]

Item 34   Answer: D

Educational Objective: Manage transfusion in an asymptomatic pregnant patient with sickle cell anemia.

The patient should not receive an erythrocyte transfusion at this time. Erythrocyte transfusion in sickle cell disease (SCD) is appropriate only for specific indications, including stroke, symptomatic anemia, acute chest syndrome (ACS), surgical interventions, secondary prevention of stroke or ACS, and, possibly, prevention of priapism, pulmonary hypertension, and nonhealing ulcers. Transfusion is not indicated for uncomplicated pregnancy, routine painful episodes, minor surgery not requiring anesthesia, or asymptomatic anemia. Erythrocyte exchange transfusion is indicated for acute ischemic stroke, ACS with significant hypoxia, and multiorgan failure/hepatopathy as well as in persons in whom simple transfusion would increase the hemoglobin level to greater than 10 g/dL (100 g/L). Chronic transfusion can lead to iron overload, alloimmunization, and an increased risk for a delayed hemolytic transfusion reaction. Erythrocytes used in transfusion should be leukoreduced, hemoglobin S negative, and phenotypically matched for the E, C, and K antigens as well as for any known alloantibodies. Hemoglobin targets should remain less than 10 g/dL (100 g/L) to avoid hyperviscosity.

In a randomized trial, transfusion reduced the risk of pain crisis in pregnant women with SCD but showed no clear improvement in maternal mortality, perinatal mortality, or severe maternal morbidity (pulmonary embolism, chronic heart failure, ACS). Transfusion should be provided based on symptoms of anemia and not hemoglobin levels.

Erythropoiesis-stimulating agents (ESAs) are used to treat anemia in conditions in which bone marrow stimulation of erythrocyte production is inadequate, such as chronic kidney disease. However, in SCD, erythropoietin levels are typically high to augment bone marrow erythrocyte production in response to chronic hemolysis. Therefore, ESAs are not indicated for treatment of the anemia associated with SCD.

- In patients with sickle cell disease, including pregnant patients, transfusion is not indicated for uncomplicated pregnancy, routine painful episodes, minor surgery not requiring anesthesia, or asymptomatic anemia.

Bibliography

Okusanya BO, Oladapo OT. Prophylactic versus selective blood transfusion for sickle cell disease in pregnancy. Cochrane Database Syst Rev. 2013 Dec 3;12:CD010378. [PMID: 24297507]

Item 35   Answer: C

Educational Objective: Manage a supratherapeutic INR in a patient receiving vitamin K antagonist therapy.

This patient should be treated with oral vitamin K for a supratherapeutic INR without evidence of active bleeding. Elevation of the INR beyond the desired therapeutic range is common in patients taking vitamin K antagonists. Recommended management depends on the level of INR elevation and whether active bleeding or bleeding risk factors are present. In patients without bleeding, management involves withholding warfarin and possibly administering oral vitamin K, depending on the level of INR elevation. For a supratherapeutic INR less than 5.0, withholding warfarin and restarting at a lower dose are usually adequate. For an INR of 5.0 to 9.0, a similar management strategy is appropriate, although administration of 1 to 2.5 mg of oral vitamin K is reasonable in patients at risk for bleeding. In patients with an INR greater than 9.0, such as this patient, administration of 2.5 to 5 mg of oral vitamin K is indicated to more rapidly reduce the INR to the desired range.

In patients with serious bleeding, active reversal of anticoagulation is indicated regardless of the INR level. Use of intravenous vitamin K and 4-factor prothrombin complex concentrate (PCC) (or 3-factor PCC and fresh frozen plasma [FFP] or recombinant activated factor VII) is preferred. FFP alone is an option if factor concentrates are unavailable. These treatments are not indicated in this patient who does not have evidence of active bleeding.

Because the risk of bleeding increases with the level of INR elevation, not providing additional treatment for this patient with a significantly supratherapeutic INR would be inappropriate.

KEY POINT

- In patients taking a vitamin K antagonist who have an INR greater than 9 and no evidence of bleeding, oral vitamin K and withholding warfarin are indicated to rapidly reduce the INR.

Bibliography

Ageno W, Gallus AS, Wittkowsky A, Crowther M, Hylek EM, Palareti G; American College of Chest Physicians. Oral anticoagulant therapy: antithrombotic therapy and prevention of thrombosis, 9th ed: American College of Chest Physicians evidence-based clinical practice guidelines. Chest. 2012 Feb;141(2 Suppl):e44S-88S. [PMID: 22315269]

Item 36   Answer: B

Educational Objective: Manage low back pain in a patient with smoldering multiple myeloma.

This patient should undergo MRI of the lumbar spine. He has a diagnosis of smoldering (asymptomatic) multiple myeloma, which is defined as an M protein level of 3 g/dL or more or clonal plasma cells representing 10% or more of the total marrow cellularity on bone marrow biopsy but the absence of disease-specific signs or symptoms. Most patients with smoldering myeloma eventually develop symptomatic disease, with a median time to progression of 4.8 years. Therefore, surveillance in these patients is necessary. The CRAB (hyperCalcemia, Renal failure, Anemia, Bone disease) criteria for a diagnosis of multiple myeloma requiring therapy are commonly used to determine the need to start chemotherapy. Although this patient does not have hypercalcemia, kidney disease (renal failure), or anemia, he is experiencing unexplained lower back pain with nonspecific findings on plain radiographic imaging. Therefore, additional imaging is warranted to better determine the cause of the pain. Although plain radiography remains an important component of the initial evaluation of patients with multiple myeloma, more than 30% of trabecular bone must be lost before lytic lesions are evident by plain radiographs. MRI is a more sensitive imaging modality for detecting lytic bone lesions of myeloma, and would be the preferred next imaging study in this patient. Additional imaging techniques that may be used in multiple myeloma include CT or PET/CT.

The role of chemotherapy in patients with smoldering myeloma is unclear. Although lenalidomide and dexamethasone have been shown to delay disease progression, the optimal patient population for these agents has not been identified, and early initiation of chemotherapy for smoldering myeloma is not routinely utilized.

Although most patients with acute low-back pain may be treated conservatively without imaging, symptomatic treatment of this patient's low back pain with routine follow-up would not be appropriate because of his diagnosis of multiple myeloma and the possibility that his back pain is secondary to disease progression.

Bisphosphonates are a key component of therapy for patients with multiple myeloma requiring therapy. Zoledronic acid has been shown to reduce the risk of skeletal-related events and improve progression-free survival. However, the patient has yet to be diagnosed with symptomatic myeloma. No role exists for the routine use of bisphosphonates for patients with smoldering myeloma.

KEY POINT

- An MRI or CT is more sensitive at detecting lytic bone lesions than plain radiographs in patients with multiple myeloma and should be considered when bone pain is present and plain radiographs are unrevealing.

Bibliography

Dimopoulos M, Terpos E, Comenzo RL, et al. International myeloma working group consensus statement and guidelines regarding the current role of imaging techniques in the diagnosis and monitoring of multiple myeloma. Leukemia. 2009;23(9):1545-1556. [PMID: 19421229]

Item 37　　Answer:　E

Educational Objective: Diagnose von Willebrand disease.

The patient most likely has von Willebrand disease (vWD). vWD is an autosomal codominant disorder. Von Willebrand factor (vWF) protects factor VIII from degradation, and factor VIII levels can be low enough in vWD to cause slight prolongation of the activated partial thromboplastin time (aPTT), although typically the prothrombin time (PT) and aPTT are normal. Hemorrhagic manifestations of vWD are characterized by mucocutaneous bleeding, not hemarthroses as in hemophilia. Many women with vWD have significant menorrhagia, endometriosis, and postpartum hemorrhage. Mild vWD may not be detected by the Platelet Function Analyzer-100 (PFA-100®) assay, necessitating measurement of vWF antigen and activity levels for diagnosis. Additionally, levels of vWF fluctuate in response to estrogens, stress, exercise, inflammation, and bleeding, and repeated assays may be required to make the diagnosis.

Factor VII deficiency may be inherited or acquired as a result of vitamin K deficiency or warfarin therapy. Patients with factor VII deficiency will have an abnormal prolongation of the PT but a normal aPTT, which is incompatible with this patient's findings.

Factor XI deficiency is an autosomal recessive bleeding disorder and may be associated with a prolonged aPTT and significant bleeding with surgery or trauma. Severe factor XI deficiency is much more frequent in persons of European Jewish descent. Severe factor XI deficiency will prolong the aPTT and is not associated with spontaneous bleeding or with the classic bleeding manifestations of hemophilia, such as hemarthrosis or soft-tissue bleeding, making this diagnosis unlikely.

Factor XII deficiency also produces a normal PT and markedly prolonged aPTT but is not associated with bleeding manifestations and, therefore, is not a likely diagnosis for this patient.

Factor VIII deficiency is responsible for hemophilia A, an X-linked recessive disorder. Severe hemophilia A is characterized by recurrent hemarthroses resulting in chronic, crippling degenerative joint disease unless treated prophylactically with factor replacement. Mild hemophilia may present in adulthood, characterized by posttraumatic or surgical bleeding and a prolonged aPTT. This patient's clinical presentation of mucocutaneous bleeding, normal aPTT, and apparent inheritance pattern of bleeding are not compatible with hemophilia.

KEY POINT

- Symptoms of von Willebrand disease typically include easy bruising, postsurgical bleeding, and heavy menstrual bleeding in women in conjunction with normal prothrombin and normal to minimally prolonged activated partial thromboplastin times.

Bibliography

Lillicrap D. von Willebrand disease: advances in pathogenetic understanding, diagnosis, and therapy. Hematology Am Soc Hematol Educ Program. 2013;2013:254-60. [PMID: 24319188]

Item 38　　Answer:　D

Educational Objective: Manage an elevated INR in a patient taking warfarin.

Because the patient is not bleeding and is not at high risk for bleeding, interruption of warfarin therapy is appropriate. Concomitant antibiotic and warfarin use can result in INR elevation. A population-based study revealed that the over-anticoagulation risk was most strongly increased by amoxicillin, clarithromycin, norfloxacin, and trimethoprim-sulfamethoxazole. Changes in the INR were often noted in the first 3 days of antibiotic use. This patient's elevated INR is most likely related to her concomitant use of warfarin and trimethoprim-sulfamethoxazole. The appropriate treatment for patients taking warfarin whose INR is supratherapeutic depends on the absolute INR value, the absence or presence of bleeding risk factors or active bleeding, and the seriousness of bleeding, if present. Increased age, actively bleeding lesions, coagulation disorders, and use of antiplatelet drugs increase the bleeding risk while taking warfarin. If the INR is less than 5.0 and no bleeding is apparent, the next dose of warfarin is withheld and the subsequent maintenance dose is reduced. If the INR is 9.0 or less and the risk of bleeding is low, the next one or two doses of warfarin are withheld and the INR is repeated in 48 hours; in these patients who have no evidence of bleeding, the American College of Chest Physicians (ACCP) recommends against the routine use of vitamin K. If the INR is greater than 9.0, warfarin is withheld and 2.5 to 5 mg of oral vitamin K is administered.

Patients with an elevated INR and serious bleeding (or those requiring rapid anticoagulation reversal) are treated by withholding warfarin and administering 10 mg of vitamin K intravenously. For patients with critical need of anticoagulation reversal (for example, intracerebral bleeding), the ACCP recommends administration of 4-factor prothrombin complex concentrate rather than fresh frozen plasma.

KEY POINT

- In patients without evidence of bleeding whose INR is 9.0 or less while taking warfarin, the next one or two dose(s) should be withheld, but the American College of Chest Physicians recommends against the routine use of vitamin K.

Bibliography

Holbrook A, Schulman S, Witt DM, et al. Evidence-based management of anticoagulant therapy: antithrombotic therapy and prevention of thrombosis, 9th ed: American College of Chest Physicians evidence-based clinical practice guidelines. Chest. 2012 Feb;141(2 Suppl):e152S-84S. [PMID: 22315259]

Answers and Critiques

Item 39   Answer: A

Educational Objective: Evaluate a patient for heparin-induced thrombocytopenia.

Performing 4T pretest probability scoring for the possibility of heparin-induced thrombocytopenia (HIT) is the most appropriate next step in management. This patient's platelet count decreased following a recent exposure to heparin, raising concern for the possibility of HIT. The 4T score is used to estimate the pretest probability of HIT based on clinical factors, including degree of thrombocytopenia, timing of the decrease in platelet count, presence of any potential sequelae of HIT (such as thrombosis), and whether another potential cause for thrombocytopenia exists. Possible point values range from 0 to 8; scores of 0 to 3 indicate low probability, 4 or 5 indicate intermediate probability, and 6 to 8 represent high pretest probability. The 4T score has been validated in a study of more than 3000 patients with a negative predictive value of 99.8% in those with low probability scores. Although specific decisions must be made for individual patients based on their clinical status, many physicians reserve further evaluation for patients with intermediate or high pretest probability scores, with close clinical observation in those with low probability scores. This patient has a 4T score of 1 based on a possible alternative explanation for his thrombocytopenia (blood transfusion), indicating a low pretest probability of HIT; therefore, observation without additional testing for HIT would be reasonable.

Confirmatory testing for antiplatelet antibodies may be done by direct antibody testing or by functional assays that test the ability of serum from patients with HIT to activate test platelets. Direct antibody testing is typically performed by enzyme-linked immunosorbent assay (ELISA) that detects antibodies directed toward heparin-platelet factor 4 complexes. The two commonly used functional assays are the serotonin release assay (SRA) and the heparin-induced platelet aggregation (HIPA) assay. SRA is considered the gold standard study for HIT with a sensitivity and specificity of more than 95%; HIPA is also very specific but has a lower sensitivity than SRA. However, no clear indication exists for confirmatory testing for HIT considering this patient's low pretest probability.

KEY POINT

- Assessing the pretest probability of heparin-induced thrombocytopenia by using a risk scoring system, such as the 4T score, is helpful in guiding therapy in patients at low risk for it.

Bibliography
Lee GM, Arepally GM. Diagnosis and management of heparin-induced thrombocytopenia. Hematol Oncol Clin North Am. 2013 Jun;27(3):541-63. [PMID: 23714311]

 Item 40   Answer: D

Educational Objective: Manage anemia in a critically ill hospitalized patient.

Continuing current management is appropriate. The patient is asymptomatic and displays no end-organ

compromise as a result of reduced oxygen-carrying capacity. A randomized phase III study was performed in euvolemic patients whose hemoglobin level decreased to less than 9 g/dL (90 g/L) within 72 hours of admission to an ICU. Patients were assigned to a liberal transfusion strategy targeting a hemoglobin level of 10 to 12 g/dL (100-120 g/L), in which they were transfused when their hemoglobin level decreased to less than 10 g/dL (100 g/L), or a restrictive approach, in which they were transfused for a hemoglobin level less than 7 g/dL (70 g/L) (target 7-9 g/dL [70-90 g/L]). Mortality rates were at least as good for those assigned to the restrictive transfusion approach. However, a subset analysis revealed that patients with ischemic heart disease had a trend toward higher mortality with a restrictive transfusion practice that was not statistically significant, suggesting that patients with ischemic heart disease should be evaluated on a case-by-case basis until further phase III data dictate otherwise.

Although the patient has an elevated creatinine level, this is likely the result of sepsis and appears to be improving with volume repletion and correction of hypotension. As such, there is no role for an erythropoiesis-stimulating agent (ESA). Furthermore, ESAs have not been studied for this indication.

The patient has iron indices typical of an inflammatory anemia (low serum iron, low total iron-binding capacity, normal transferrin saturation, elevated ferritin), likely due to sepsis and not iron deficiency anemia (low serum iron, high-normal to high total iron-binding capacity, low transferrin saturation, low ferritin). Therefore, intravenous iron is not indicated.

KEY POINT

- In hospitalized patients without symptoms or end-organ damage, a restrictive treatment strategy for hemoglobin levels less than 7 g/dL (70 g/L) and targeting 7 to 9 g/dL (70-90 g/L) is appropriate.

Bibliography
Hébert PC, Wells G, Blajchman MA, et al. A multicenter, randomized, controlled clinical trial of transfusion requirements in critical care. Transfusion Requirements in Critical Care Investigators, Canadian Critical Care Trials Group [erratum in N Engl J Med. 1999 Apr 1;340(13):1056]. N Engl J Med. 1999 Feb 11;340(6):409-17. [PMID: 9971864]

Item 41   Answer: D

Educational Objective: Manage mild coagulopathy in a patient undergoing central venous catheter placement.

No transfusion is needed before central venous catheter insertion. This patient has modest coagulopathy and thrombocytopenia resulting from hepatitis C–related liver disease. Previous retrospective studies have shown that central venous catheter insertion is safe in patients with a prolonged prothrombin time and INR, including those with liver disease. In a prospective audit of 580 internal jugular and subclavian vein cannulations in patients with chronic liver

CONT.

disease and an INR of 1.5 or greater, only one major vascular complication was noted.

Although his fibrinogen level is slightly low, cryoprecipitate is typically reserved for patients with clinically significant bleeding and a fibrinogen level less than 100 mg/dL (1.0 g/L). Cryprecipitate in the prophylaxis of bleeding for patients with low fibrinogen levels undergoing procedures has not been evaluated.

Numerous studies have shown that fresh frozen plasma (FFP) is overutilized in nonbleeding patients with mild coagulopathies, which is a significant problem given the risks associated with FFP use, including transfusion-related acute lung injury, transfusion-transmitted infection, transfusion-associated circulatory overload, allergic reactions, and hemolysis. The role of FFP in the prevention of bleeding complications for nonbleeding patients undergoing procedures is unclear. However, it is known that FFP is ineffective at correcting a minimally elevated INR (<1.85).

Most procedures and surgeries can be safely performed with a platelet count of at least 50,000/µL (50 × 10^9/L), although a platelet count of at least 100,000/µL (100 × 10^9/L) is recommended for neurosurgical intervention. Thus, a platelet transfusion is not indicated for this patient.

KEY POINT

- Patients with mild coagulopathy requiring central venous catheter insertion do not need to receive fresh frozen plasma or other transfusions before the procedure.

Bibliography

Yang L, Stanworth S, Hopewell S, Doree C, Murphy M. Is fresh-frozen plasma clinically effective? An update of a systematic review of randomized controlled trials. Transfusion. 2012 Aug;52(8):1673-86. [PMID: 22257164]

Item 42   Answer: D

Educational Objective: Manage pseudothrombocytopenia.

The patient's blood should be redrawn using a citrated tube. She has pseudothrombocytopenia as shown on the peripheral blood smear, a condition that leads to the formation of platelet clumps in vitro. This in vitro occurrence is caused by the presence of ethylenediaminetetra-acetic acid (EDTA) agglutinins, which naturally occur in approximately 0.1% of the population and lead to platelet clumping. The automated platelet counter does not recognize the clumps as masses of platelets, and the platelet count is, therefore, spuriously low. Drawing a complete blood sample into a citrate- or heparin-anticoagulated tube may resolve the clumping.

Prednisone and methylprednisolone are first-line agents for treating adults with immune (or idiopathic) thrombocytopenic purpura (ITP) who require therapy. ITP is an acquired autoimmune condition in which autoantibodies are directed against platelet surface proteins, leading to platelet destruction that may be only partially counteracted

by increased bone marrow platelet production. Variants of ITP may be drug induced or part of a broader illness of abnormal immune regulation, as with systemic lupus erythematosus, HIV infection, or lymphoproliferative malignancies. Therapy may be required for patients with platelet counts lower than 30,000 to 40,000/µL (30-40 × 10^9/L) or with bleeding. Because this patient most likely does not have ITP, diagnostic testing for systemic lupus erythematosus with antinuclear antibody or HIV testing is not indicated.

Plasma exchange would not benefit this patient. Thrombotic thrombocytopenic purpura (TTP) is a process characterized by abnormal activation of platelets and endothelial cells, deposition of fibrin in the microvasculature, and peripheral destruction of erythrocytes and platelets. Most patients with the typical sporadic form of TTP have developed autoantibodies directed against the protease that cleaves the high-molecular-weight multimers of von Willebrand factor. Initial treatment consists of plasma exchange. Because this patient has platelet clumping on the peripheral blood smear and no evidence of schistocytes characteristic of TTP-associated microangiopathic hemolysis, the diagnosis of TTP is unlikely and plasma exchange is unnecessary.

KEY POINT

- Platelet clumping signifies pseudothrombocytopenia, which will resolve if blood is redrawn using a citrated or heparinized tube.

Bibliography

Lippi G, Plebani M. EDTA-dependent pseudothrombocytopenia: further insights and recommendations for prevention of a clinically threatening artifact. Clin Chem Lab Med. 2012 Aug;50(8):1281-5. [PMID: 22868791]

Item 43   Answer: E

Educational Objective: Manage von Willebrand disease perioperatively.

The most appropriate perioperative treatment for this patient is von Willebrand factor (vWF)–containing factor VIII concentrates. She has type 1 von Willebrand disease (vWD) and is scheduled for abdominal surgery. The best products to give are the vWF-containing factor VIII concentrates. These so-called "intermediate purity," plasma-derived products have undergone viral inactivation (of viruses such as HIV and hepatitis B and C), and their use has not led to transmission of any serious illness. Desmopressin, which leads to release of vWF and factor VIII from endothelial cells and thus provides hemostasis, can be used for less invasive procedures. However, unless a trial of desmopressin shows a robust, sustained response, it should not be used for a major surgery.

Cryoprecipitate contains a concentrated source of factor VIII, vWF, factor XIII, fibronectin, and fibrinogen and is the treatment of choice in bleeding patients with hypofibrinogenemia from liver disease, thrombolytic therapy, or disseminated intravascular coagulation (DIC). Cryoprecipitate is not virally inactivated and is therefore not a first-line agent for this patient with vWD.

Fresh frozen plasma (FFP) contains all the blood clotting factors and is indicated for warfarin reversal in actively bleeding patients (alone or concomitantly with a 3-factor prothrombin complex concentrate), treatment of thrombotic thrombocytopenic purpura, dilutional coagulopathy during massive transfusion, and in bleeding patients with several factor deficiencies such as in DIC or liver disease. However, the concentration of vWF in FFP is too low to correct the patient's vWF levels without producing volume overload. Other risks include viral transmission, transfusion-related acute lung injury, and febrile, allergic, and anaphylactic reactions.

Recombinant factor VIII is used to treat patients with hemophilia A. Recombinant factor VIII is devoid of any vWF and would not improve hemostasis in this patient with vWD.

Fibrinolytic agents such as ε-aminocaproic acid and tranexamic acid can be used in patients with mild vWD to prevent dissolution of the hemostatic plug, particularly those associated with mucocutaneous bleeding. Prolonged use of these agents is associated with the potential for thrombosis, especially in patients with an underlying thrombophilia. Used as a single agent, tranexamic acid is unlikely to provide sufficient hemostasis for a patient undergoing abdominal surgery.

KEY POINT

- Patients with von Willebrand disease scheduled to undergo major surgery should be treated with factor VIII concentrates containing von Willebrand factor.

Bibliography

Lillicrap D. von Willebrand disease: advances in pathogenetic understanding, diagnosis, and therapy. Hematology Am Soc Hematol Educ Program. 2013;2013:254-60. [PMID: 24319188]

Item 44   Answer: A

Educational Objective: Diagnose cold agglutinin disease.

A direct antiglobulin (Coombs) test is the most appropriate next diagnostic step for this patient with cold agglutinin disease. Autoimmune hemolytic anemias are characterized by the presence of antibodies directed toward antigens on the surface of erythrocytes; they are further classified by the type of immunoglobulin involved and the resulting tendency of hemolysis to occur in warm or cold environments. Direct IgG optimally binds erythrocytes at temperatures of 37.0 °C (98.6 °F), causing warm autoimmune hemolytic anemia. The immune response to the bound IgG causes erythrocytes to become spherocytic, resulting in hemolysis. Direct IgM binds more effectively at temperatures colder than 32.0 °C (89.6 °F), typically in the fingers, toes, and nose, causing cold agglutinin disease. IgM-coated erythrocytes agglutinate in the microvasculature, leading to cyanosis and ischemia in the cold extremities. The IgM antibodies fix complement and then detach from erythrocytes when they return to the warmer body core. This patient likely has cold agglutinin disease because he has

an acquired hemolytic anemia associated with cold exposure and supported by his peripheral blood smear, showing agglutinated erythrocytes that disappear when warmed. Cold agglutinin disease may occur as a primary disorder or may be associated with a lymphoproliferative disorder or certain infections, such as *Mycoplasma pneumoniae* or Epstein-Barr virus. The primary treatment for cold agglutinin disease is avoidance of cold exposure.

Flow cytometry to detect the absence of specific cell surface antigens (CD55 and CD59) is useful in diagnosing paroxysmal nocturnal hemoglobinuria, which is another potential cause of hemolytic anemia. However, testing for this disorder is indicated only in patients without evidence of an autoimmune cause of hemolysis. Therefore, such testing would be inappropriate for this patient.

Multiple congenital hemoglobinopathies are associated with hemolysis, although this patient's clinical picture is consistent with an acquired hemolytic anemia. Therefore, hemoglobin electrophoresis would not likely be helpful in establishing the cause of his hemolysis.

The indirect antiglobulin test detects antierythrocyte antibodies in the serum and is used primarily before blood transfusion and in prenatal testing of pregnant women. It would not provide significant diagnostic information in this patient.

KEY POINT

- Cold agglutinin disease, identified by characteristic erythrocyte clumping that disappears when a peripheral blood sample is warmed, can be confirmed by direct antiglobulin (Coombs) testing.

Bibliography

Swiecicki PL, Hegerova LT, Gertz MA. Cold agglutinin disease. Blood. 2013 Aug 15;122(7):1114-21. [PMID: 23757733]

Item 45   Answer: D

Educational Objective: Manage inflammatory anemia.

The only management the patient requires at this time is observation. He has inflammatory anemia (previously anemia of chronic disease), which does not usually require treatment. Chronic infections such as tuberculosis or osteomyelitis, malignancies, and collagen vascular diseases are associated with anemia. In response to inflammatory states, erythropoietin production is inhibited and the erythroid precursor response to erythropoietin is blunted. Inflammation leads to increased levels of inflammatory cytokines, including tumor necrosis factor-α, interleukin (IL)-6, IL-1, and interferon, which lead to altered erythropoietin responsiveness. In particular, IL-6 causes hepatic synthesis of the small peptide hepcidin, which is pivotal in regulating iron absorption. Hepcidin causes decreased iron absorption from the gastrointestinal tract and decreased iron release by macrophages by inducing internalization and proteolysis of the transporter protein ferroportin. No laboratory test is commercially available for measuring hepcidin levels.

A peripheral blood smear may be normal in patients with inflammatory anemia, or, over time, may show microcytic hypochromic erythrocytes such as in iron deficiency. Typically, inflammatory anemia is characterized by a hemoglobin level greater than 8 g/dL (80 g/L). Because of erythrocyte underproduction, the reticulocyte count is typically low for the degree of anemia. The serum iron level is initially normal but decreases over time, the total iron-binding capacity is low, and the ferritin level is typically elevated.

Although bone marrow evaluation is seldom necessary, ample stainable iron would be present. However, it is not indicated for diagnosis in classic cases of inflammatory anemia.

Erythropoiesis-stimulating agents may improve inflammatory anemia but are associated with thrombosis and other effects that impede safe use.

Iron replacement is unlikely to alleviate the patient's symptoms, because he is not iron deficient. Iron deficiency would present with a low ferritin level of less than 100 ng/mL (100 µg/L) even in the setting of chronic inflammation. Additionally, total iron-binding capacity in iron deficiency tends to be elevated and not decreased. However, the transferrin saturation is normal in inflammatory anemia.

KEY POINT

- Inflammatory anemia typically requires no treatment other than for the underlying condition.

Bibliography

Weiss G, Goodnough LT. Anemia of chronic disease. N Engl J Med. 2005 Mar 10;352(10):1011-23. [PMID: 15758012]

Item 46   Answer: C

Educational Objective: Diagnose aplastic anemia.

The patient has aplastic anemia (AA). He presents with an insidious clinical course and has severe pancytopenia. The absolute neutrophil count is only 50/µL (0.05 × 10⁹/L). Despite severe neutropenia, AA may present with clinically unimpressive infections. This contrasts with the acute leukemias. The bone marrow biopsy demonstrating less than 10% cellularity confirms the diagnosis of aplasia. AA may occur secondary to infections or toxins. However, it usually presents without preceding insult. Such patients respond to immunosuppressive therapy, and allogeneic hematopoietic stem cell (HSC) transplantation can be curative in young otherwise healthy patients.

Acute lymphoblastic leukemia (ALL) is a reasonable consideration in this patient, because ALL is more common in adolescents and young adults. It can present with pancytopenia rather than hyperleukocytosis. However, the bone marrow biopsy excludes ALL, because leukemic blasts more typically cause marrow hypercellularity; very few blood-making cells are present on this patient's biopsy. For the same reason, acute myeloid leukemia can be excluded.

The myelodysplastic syndromes (MDS) are clonal HSC disorders characterized by ineffective hematopoiesis and a variable rate of transformation to acute myeloid leukemia. MDS can present with pancytopenia, although it occurs less commonly in younger patients. However, the bone marrow in MDS is classically hypercellular. Although hypocellular MDS exists, crossover with AA is considerable, and the decrease in marrow cellularity is not this striking.

Paroxysmal nocturnal hemoglobinuria (PNH) is an acquired HSC disorder that should be considered in patients presenting with hemolytic anemia, pancytopenia, or unprovoked atypical thrombosis. The bone marrow is usually hypocellular with PNH, but other features such as hemolysis and thrombosis are present, distinguishing it from AA. Likewise, the degree of hypocellularity is not as severe as that of AA.

KEY POINT

- Aplastic anemia is characterized by severe hypocellularity of the bone marrow and pancytopenia.

Bibliography

Devitt KA, Lunde JH, Lewis MR. New onset pancytopenia in adults: a review of underlying pathologies and the associated clinical and laboratory findings. Leuk Lymphoma. 2014 May;55(5):1099-105. [PMID: 23829306]

Item 47   Answer: C

Educational Objective: Diagnose monoclonal gammopathy of undetermined significance.

Serum free light chain (FLC) testing should be performed. This patient meets criteria for a diagnosis of monoclonal gammopathy of undetermined significance (MGUS), because clonal plasma cells represent less than 10% of the total marrow cellularity, and she does not meet CRAB (hyperCalcemia, Renal failure, Anemia, Bone disease) criteria for a diagnosis of multiple myeloma requiring therapy. MGUS is common, affecting 3.2% of persons 50 years or older and 5.3% of persons 70 years or older. The risk of progression to a clinically symptomatic disease is approximately 1% per year. Risk factors for progression include a non-IgG M protein, an M protein level of at least 1.5 g/dL, and an abnormal serum FLC ratio. A few FLCs (not bound to immunoglobulin) circulate normally and can be measured in serum. The FLC ratio measures the κ and λ FLCs, expressed as the κ/λ FLC ratio. Persons without a plasma cell dyscrasia have normal ratios; abnormal ratios suggest a disproportionate production of a monoclonal κ or λ chain. An abnormal FLC ratio is prognostically helpful, because it suggests a more virulent plasma cell clone that may be at higher risk of transforming into overt multiple myeloma. This patient has two risk factors identified thus far (M protein level ≥1.5 g/dL and an IgA M protein). Serum free κ and λ light chain level measurement and κ/λ FLC ratio determination are essential parts of the evaluation of MGUS; they help delineate the risk of progression to clinically symptomatic disease and dictate the frequency of follow-up. Patients with zero, one, two, or three risk factors have a risk of progression to clinically symptomatic disease over 20 years of 5%, 21%, 37%, and 58%, respectively.

MRI imaging of the spine and whole spine MRI have not been shown to further risk stratify patients with MGUS. However, in patients with smoldering (asymptomatic) multiple myeloma, more than one focal bone lesion on MRI is associated with a greater risk of progression to multiple myeloma requiring therapy.

The β_2-microglobulin and lactate dehydrogenase levels are useful tools for determining the prognosis of multiple myeloma requiring therapy but are not routinely performed in MGUS.

KEY POINT

- Risk factors for progression of monoclonal gammopathy of undetermined significance to multiple myeloma include a non-IgG M protein, an M protein level of at least 1.5 g/dL, and an abnormal serum free light chain ratio.

Bibliography

Kyle RA, Durie BG, Rajkumar SV, et al; International Myeloma Working Group. Monoclonal gammopathy of undetermined significance (MGUS) and smoldering (asymptomatic) multiple myeloma: IMWG consensus perspective risk factors for progression and guidelines for monitoring and management. Leukemia. 2010 Jun;24(6):1121-7. [PMID:20410922]

Item 48　　Answer:　D

Educational Objective: Diagnose multiple myeloma requiring therapy.

Serum protein electrophoresis and serum free light chain (FLC) testing should be performed in this patient with likely multiple myeloma; together, these have a diagnostic sensitivity approaching 100% for multiple myeloma requiring therapy. This patient has several findings suspicious for this disease as the cause of his hypercalcemia, including osteopenia with a thoracic compression fracture, anemia, and kidney dysfunction. However, kidney dysfunction can occur as a direct result of hypercalcemia, regardless of its underlying cause. An important clue in this patient is the discordance between the degree of proteinuria assessed by the urinalysis compared with the urine protein-creatinine ratio. A routine dipstick urinalysis will detect albuminuria but is relatively insensitive at detecting other urine proteins. However, a urine protein-creatinine ratio measures all proteins in the urine, including immunoglobulins, if present. This discrepancy should raise suspicion for monoclonal FLCs in the urine (Bence-Jones proteinuria) and potential cast nephropathy. Similarly, a sulfosalicylic acid test will detect all urine proteins, including light chains, and can be performed for suspected myeloma cast nephropathy. In FLC myeloma, the serum protein electrophoresis may only reveal hypogammaglobulinemia and no monoclonal band or a low-level monoclonal band because of its insensitivity at detecting monoclonal FLCs. However, the serum FLC test, an antibody-based assay that can detect low levels of FLCs, will demonstrate an elevated level of the affected monoclonal FLC and an abnormal serum κ/λ FLC ratio.

Increased 1,25-dihydroxyvitamin D (calcitriol) levels may result from ingestion of calcitriol or increased 25-hydroxyvitamin D (calcidiol) activation to calcitriol as a result of underlying granulomatous disease (for example, sarcoidosis) or lymphoma, thus leading to hypercalcemia. This patient has no history of calcitriol ingestion and no physical examination or radiographic features of granulomatous disease or lymphoma. Increased calcitriol levels do not explain his anemia, osteopenia and thoracic compression fracture, or kidney dysfunction with nonalbumin proteinuria.

Primary hyperparathyroidism can present with hypercalcemia, bone mineral density loss with increased compression fracture risk, and, when hypercalcemia is severe enough or long-standing, kidney dysfunction. However, primary hyperparathyroidism is uncommonly associated with anemia and does not explain the proteinuria, so measuring the intact parathyroid hormone level is not indicated.

Hypercalcemia associated with myeloma results from osteoclast activation, not secretion of parathyroid hormone-related protein (PTHrP). PTHrP is produced more commonly in solid tumors, such as squamous cell (head and neck, lung); renal cell; and bladder, breast, and ovarian carcinomas. Although the patient has an extensive smoking history, no findings on physical examination or chest radiograph suggest the presence of a solid tumor. Additionally, PTHrP-mediated hypercalcemia from an occult solid tumor would not explain this patient's proteinuria.

KEY POINT

- Combination serum protein electrophoresis and free light chain testing has a sensitivity approaching 100% for diagnosing multiple myeloma requiring therapy.

Bibliography

Katzmann JA, Kyle RA, Benson J, et al. Screening panels for detection of monoclonal gammopathies. Clin Chem. 2009;55(8):1517-1522. [PMID: 19520758]

Item 49　　Answer:　B　　

Educational Objective: Diagnose coagulopathy of liver disease.

The patient most likely has liver failure resulting from excessive acetaminophen use as the cause of his coagulopathy. He takes chronic warfarin therapy but presents with a significant coagulopathy of unclear cause. Specific factor level measurement is useful when it is clinically helpful to understand the basis of a coagulation disorder to guide therapy. A panel of factors, including factor V, factor VII, and factor VIII, may be checked when it is important to distinguish between liver failure, disseminated intravascular coagulation, or vitamin K deficiency/warfarin overdose. In liver failure, all clotting factor activity levels are low except for factor VIII, which is synthesized in all endothelial cells rather than only hepatic endothelial cells. Additionally, good hepatic function is required for factor VIII clearance, thus factor VIII levels increase in liver disease. Patients with severe liver failure (and on occasion those with acute liver failure) will have prolonged prothrombin and activated partial thromboplastin times because of decreased levels of coagulation factors. This is called the coagulopathy of liver disease. The elevated D-dimer level is also consistent with liver disease, because D-dimers are cleared by the liver; a high D-dimer level does not automatically indicate disseminated intravascular coagulation (DIC).

DIC begins with abnormal thrombin generation, rapid consumption of clotting factors and platelets, and accelerated fibrinolysis. Although hemorrhage may result from low levels of clotting factors and platelets, histopathologic examination of affected tissues shows a fibrin clot in the microvasculature. A thrombotic microangiopathy may ensue, and schistocytes develop in 30% of patients. An elevated factor VIII level, as seen in this patient, rules out DIC.

Factor V levels can be used to distinguish between liver disease and vitamin K deficiency, because factor V is synthesized in the liver but is not a vitamin K–dependent factor. Thus, someone with vitamin K deficiency will have normal levels of factor V, whereas a patient with liver failure will have low factor V levels. This patient's low factor V level rules out warfarin overdose as well as vitamin K deficiency, because normal levels would be expected in vitamin K deficiency.

KEY POINT

- Coagulopathy of liver disease is characterized by prolonged prothrombin and activated partial thromboplastin times and increased factor VIII level.

Bibliography
Tripodi A, Primignani M, Chantarangkul V, et al. An imbalance of pro- vs anti-coagulation factors in plasma from patients with cirrhosis. Gastroenterology. 2009 Dec;137(6):2105-11. [PMID: 19706293]

Item 50   Answer: A

Educational Objective: Diagnose chronic myeloid leukemia.

This patient is most likely to have a *BCR-ABL* genetic mutation predisposing him to chronic myeloid leukemia (CML). He has the classic presentation for CML with the insidious onset of fatigue; early satiety and progressive weight loss associated with splenomegaly; and a peripheral blood smear demonstrating myelocytes, metamyelocytes, and basophils. The peripheral blood smear of CML is commonly described as mimicking a bone marrow aspirate. Basophilia is a general clue to the presence of a myeloproliferative neoplasm (MPN).

IGH/CD1 is the mutation associated with mantle cell lymphoma (MCL). MCL can present with hyperleukocytosis and massive splenomegaly, but myeloid precursors and basophilia would not be seen on peripheral blood smear.

The *JAK2* gene mutation is associated with polycythemia vera, essential thrombocytosis (ET), and primary myelofibrosis but not CML. Because CML is a more likely diagnosis, especially because of the prominence and degree of leukocytosis, *BCR-ABL* mutation should be excluded first in this patient.

PML-RAR protein mutation is associated with acute promyelocytic leukemia (APL). APL does not demonstrate basophilia or transitional myeloid precursors on the peripheral blood smear. Additionally, it is clinically associated with disseminated intravascular coagulation and thrombocytopenia rather than thrombocytosis, and splenomegaly is uncommon in APL.

KEY POINT

- Patients with suspected chronic myeloid leukemia should be tested for an underlying *BCR-ABL* mutation.

Bibliography
Tefferi A, Vardiman JW. Classification and diagnosis of myeloproliferative neoplasms: the 2008 World Health Organization criteria and point-of-care diagnostic algorithms. Leukemia. 2008 Jan;22(1):14-22. [PMID: 17882280]

Item 51   Answer: C

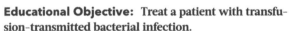

Educational Objective: Treat a patient with transfusion-transmitted bacterial infection.

In addition to stopping the transfusion and resuscitating the patient, broad-spectrum antibiotics such as vancomycin and cefepime should be started, and blood cultures should be drawn to determine the infecting organism. The patient is most likely experiencing sepsis as a result of transfusion-transmitted bacterial infection. Clinical criteria for a possible septic transfusion reaction include any of the following within 5 hours of completion of a transfusion: temperature greater than 39.0 °C (102.2 °F) or temperature two degrees higher than pretransfusion, rigors, pulse rate greater than 120/min or more than 40/min higher than pretransfusion, or a decrease or increase in blood pressure of greater than 30 mm Hg. Transfusion-transmitted bacterial infection remains an important cause of transfusion-related morbidity and mortality with rates of all septic reactions and fatal septic reactions reaching 1:74,807 and 1:498,711 per distributed platelet component. The majority of infections are due to staphylococcal species, although gram-negative organisms are also implicated. The blood product bag should be sealed and sent to the microbiology laboratory for culture.

Acetaminophen, diphenhydramine, and meperidine may be used as symptomatic treatment of a febrile nonhemolytic transfusion reaction. However, febrile nonhemolytic transfusion reactions are not typically associated with hypotension.

Epinephrine should only be used to treat anaphylaxis, which is less likely than sepsis in this patient. Anaphylaxis is associated with hypotension and respiratory distress, but this patient has no dermatologic (pruritus, urticaria, angioedema), pulmonary (wheezing, cough), or gastrointestinal (nausea, vomiting, abdominal cramping, diarrhea) manifestations suggesting anaphylaxis. Additionally, anaphylaxis is not associated with fever.

Considering the high morbidity and mortality associated with a septic transfusion reaction, stopping the transfusion and volume resuscitation alone are insufficient. This patient needs broad spectrum antibiotics to treat his transfusion-associated infection.

KEY POINT

- Transfusion should be stopped immediately and intravenous fluids and antibiotics should be given to patients experiencing transfusion-transmitted bacterial infection.

Bibliography

Eder AF, Kennedy JM, Dy BA, et al; American Red Cross Regional Blood Centers. Bacterial screening of apheresis platelets and the residual risk of septic transfusion reactions: the American Red Cross experience (2004-2006). Transfusion. 2007 Jul;47(7):1134-42. [PMID: 17581147]

Item 52   Answer: B

Educational Objective: Choose the appropriate diagnostic test for a patient with a low pretest probability of deep venous thrombosis.

A blood D-dimer test should be performed. American College of Chest Physicians guidelines suggest that a clinical pretest probability assessment of deep venous thrombosis (DVT) should be the first part of the diagnostic process for a first lower extremity DVT, rather than performing an imaging study in all patients. The pretest probability that this patient has a DVT is low. Applying the Wells criteria for DVT, this patient's score is 0, making DVT an unlikely diagnosis. The criteria include a medical history indicating increased risk for venous thromboembolism (VTE) (such as previously documented DVT; paralysis, paresis, recent cast immobilization of legs; recent bedridden state for ≥3 days; major surgery) and leg symptoms highly suggestive of DVT (calf swelling ≥3 cm; swelling of the entire leg; unilateral pitting edema; localized tenderness along the deep venous system). Because this patient has none of these factors and no alternative explanation for his leg symptoms, obtaining a D-dimer test is an appropriate next step. If the test is negative, no further testing is needed, because a VTE has been ruled out. However, if the D-dimer is positive, an imaging study is then indicated. The imaging test of choice is duplex ultrasonography of the leg. When using the D-dimer test for pretest probability assessments, a moderately or highly sensitive assay should be used. Physicians must be aware of the sensitivity of the test used in local laboratories. Lower sensitivity assays have not been validated as useful for predicting pretest probability.

Long-term anticoagulants should not be prescribed without a confirmed diagnosis of VTE. However, in a patient with high or intermediate clinical suspicion of DVT, beginning anticoagulation while awaiting diagnostic test results is appropriate. In a patient with low clinical suspicion of acute DVT, such as this patient, withholding anticoagulant therapy while awaiting the test result is suggested.

If a D-dimer test is not available or is positive, performing duplex ultrasonography would be the appropriate next step.

Magnetic resonance venography is a noninvasive diagnostic method that is as accurate as contrast venography for DVT diagnosis. However, it is not the study of choice for DVT diagnosis because of the complexities of performing the test and its high cost relative to duplex ultrasonography. Additionally, initial imaging is not indicated in this patient with a low risk of DVT before further assessment with D-dimer testing.

KEY POINT

- A blood D-dimer test using a moderately or highly sensitive assay should be the first step in the diagnosis of deep venous thrombosis in a patient with low pretest probability.

Bibliography

Bates SM, Jaeschke R, Stevens SM, et al; American College of Chest Physicians. Diagnosis of DVT: antithrombotic therapy and prevention of thrombosis, 9th edition: American College of Chest Physicians evidence-based clinical practice guidelines. Chest. 2012 Feb;141(2 Suppl):e351S-418S. [PMID: 22315267]

Item 53   Answer: B

Educational Objective: Manage transfusion in a patient with sickle cell disease who requires cholecystectomy.

This patient should receive an erythrocyte transfusion to a target hemoglobin level of 10 g/dL (100 g/L). He has homozygous sickle cell anemia (Hb SS) and must undergo laparoscopic cholecystectomy, a surgical procedure of low to moderate risk. Patients requiring surgery should undergo transfusion before their procedure to avoid complications. Transfusion to a hemoglobin level of 10 g/dL (100 g/L) has been shown to be equivalent to exchange transfusion for low- to medium-risk surgeries. The recent TAPS study showed that, for this surgical risk group, significantly more clinically important complications occurred in the group that did not receive preoperative transfusion (39%) than the group that did receive transfusion (15%). Significantly more serious events were also recorded in the nontransfusion group (30%) than in the transfusion group (3%), most of which were acute chest syndrome (ACS). Erythrocyte transfusions must be given with care in patients with sickle cell disease, because these transfusions are associated with iron overload. In some patients, "hyperhemolysis" occurs because of alloimmune responses to erythrocyte antigens, which leads to a delayed transfusion reaction characterized by hyperbilirubinemia and anemia. Additionally, erythrocyte transfusions that result

CONT.

in hemoglobin levels greater than 10 g/dL (100 g/L) can increase blood viscosity and potentially cause thrombotic complications.

Several multicenter studies have documented the clinical efficacy of transfusion to 10 g/dL (100 g/dL) compared with the more aggressive strategy of exchange transfusion targeting a hemoglobin S level of 30%. Transfusion and exchange transfusion are associated with similar serious surgery-related complications and ACS, but transfusion is associated with fewer transfusion-related complications and exposure to less blood.

KEY POINT

- Patients with sickle cell disease undergoing low- to moderate-risk surgery should receive erythrocyte transfusion, which has been shown to be equivalent to exchange transfusion, targeting a hemoglobin level of 10 g/dL (100 g/L) before the procedure to avoid complications.

Bibliography

Howard J, Malfroy M, Llewelyn C, et al. The Transfusion Alternatives Preoperatively in Sickle Cell Disease (TAPS) study: a randomised, controlled, multicentre clinical trial. Lancet. 2013 Mar 16;381(9870):930-8. [PMID: 23352054]

 Item 54   Answer: C

Educational Objective: Manage heparin-induced thrombocytopenia.

This patient most likely has heparin-induced thrombocytopenia (HIT) with thrombosis after being exposed to heparin during coronary artery bypass graft surgery, so the most appropriate next step is to initiate argatroban, a direct thrombin inhibitor used for anticoagulation in HIT. Patients who receive heparin during cardiothoracic surgery or after orthopedic surgery are more likely to develop HIT than are patients who receive heparin for dialysis or deep venous thrombosis prophylaxis. HIT develops 5 to 10 days after exposure to heparin, with a decrease in platelet counts of 50% or more and, in a subset of patients, paradoxical arterial or venous thrombotic events despite the presence of thrombocytopenia. The "4T score" has been devised to help clinicians decide the pretest probability for diagnosing HIT based on clinical factors, including degree of thrombocytopenia, timing of the decrease in platelet count, presence of potential sequelae of HIT (such as thrombosis), and whether another potential cause for thrombocytopenia exists. Possible point values range from 0 to 8; scores of 0 to 3 indicate low probability, 4 or 5 indicate intermediate probability, and 6 to 8 represent high probability. The patient's 4T score is 8 (2 points each for timing of platelet count decrease, presence of thrombosis, timing of thrombocytopenia, and no other cause of the thrombocytopenia), indicating a high pretest probability of HIT. In patients with a high pretest probability, immediate cessation of any heparin-containing products is indicated, with initiation of a nonheparin anticoagulant;

the only anticoagulant approved for the treatment of HIT is argatroban.

Confirmatory testing for presumed HIT is performed by HIT antibody testing. Immunoassays detect the presence of a HIT antibody (such as those directed toward platelet factor 4) in a patient's serum. Functional assays measure the ability of a HIT antibody from a patient's serum to activate test platelets (such as by measuring the release of serotonin). Because of the high risk of thrombosis associated with HIT and the possible delay associated with obtaining these studies, anticoagulation with a heparin alternative should be started before performing confirmatory testing.

Heparin cessation and treatment with a nonheparin anticoagulant are mandatory when a high pretest probability of HIT exists, because 30% to 50% of patients experience thromboses with heparin withdrawal alone. This patient already has evidence of thrombosis and must start treatment immediately to prevent extension and embolization.

Warfarin initiation alone is inadequate, because it may take 3 to 5 days to achieve a therapeutic anticoagulation effect. Additionally, starting warfarin before the platelet count has normalized in patients with HIT or starting warfarin without a bridging anticoagulant has been associated with development of warfarin skin necrosis and clot progression.

KEY POINT

- Heparin cessation and immediate treatment with a nonheparin alternative anticoagulant (lepirudin, argatroban, danaparoid) are mandatory when a high pretest probability of heparin-induced thrombocytopenia is present.

Bibliography

Lee GM, Arepally GM. Heparin-induced thrombocytopenia. Hematology Am Soc Hematol Educ Program. 2013;2013:668-74. [PMID: 24319250]

Item 55   Answer: E

Educational Objective: Treat a patient with venous thromboembolism who wishes to breastfeed.

Warfarin would be the most appropriate anticoagulation option for this patient. Warfarin is avoided during pregnancy because it crosses the placenta, causes fetal anticoagulation throughout the pregnancy, and is a teratogen. Because heparins do not cross the placenta and do not cause fetal anticoagulation, patients receiving chronic warfarin therapy are typically transitioned to either unfractionated or low-molecular-weight heparin (LMWH) during pregnancy. However, warfarin is not present in breast milk in any substantial amount and does not induce an anticoagulant effect in the breastfed infant. It is, therefore, a good option for anticoagulation in this patient. Similarly, heparins are minimally excreted in breast milk, and any drug ingested by an infant is unlikely to have any clinically relevant effect because of the very low bioavailability of oral heparins. Thus, LMWH and warfarin are both appropriate anticoagulant options for women who want to breastfeed.

It is unknown whether apixaban, dabigatran, or rivaroxaban are excreted in human milk. Therefore, known safe alternatives to these new oral anticoagulants should be used in women intending to breastfeed.

Fondaparinux has been demonstrated to be excreted in the milk of lactating rats. It is unknown whether it is excreted in human milk. Therefore, an alternative anticoagulant rather than fondaparinux is recommended for women who breastfeed.

KEY POINT

- Warfarin and low-molecular-weight heparin are considered safe for use by women requiring anticoagulant therapy who wish to breastfeed.

Bibliography

Bates SM, Greer IA, Middeldorp S, et al. VTE, thrombophilia, antithrombotic therapy, and pregnancy: antithrombotic therapy and prevention of thrombosis, 9th ed: American College of Chest Physicians evidence-based clinical practice guidelines. Chest. 2012 Feb;141(2 Suppl):e691S-736S. [PMID: 22315276]

Item 56   Answer: C

Educational Objective: Treat multiple myeloma–related bone disease.

In addition to chemotherapy, this patient should be treated with a bisphosphonate such as zoledronic acid. She has multiple myeloma requiring therapy with anemia and myeloma-related bone disease manifested by osteopenia with a T12 compression fracture. Studies have shown that bisphosphonates inhibit osteoclast-mediated osteolysis, reduce the risk of skeletal-related events (pathologic fracture, need for radiation therapy or surgery to bone, spinal cord compression), decrease bone-related pain, and improve median overall survival. The risk of skeletal-related events was reduced in patients with or without evidence of lytic bone disease on plain radiographs. Bisphosphonates therefore represent a critical aspect of care for patients with myeloma requiring therapy, and guidelines call for the use of zoledronic acid or pamidronate in all patients with newly diagnosed multiple myeloma.

Although vertebroplasty has not been shown to be beneficial in the management of osteoporotic vertebral body compression fractures, a small randomized study comparing balloon kyphoplasty with nonsurgical management of painful vertebral body compression fractures in patients with multiple myeloma and solid tumors demonstrated improved short-term physical functioning, pain control, and quality of life for those undergoing kyphoplasty. However, data on long-term outcomes with kyphoplasty are lacking in patients with cancer, and no role has been established for the procedure in the absence of pain.

Radiation therapy is typically reserved for pain related to lytic bone disease, particularly in patients with increasingly chemotherapy-resistant disease, and would not be appropriate in this patient.

Because of the documented efficacy of bisphosphonate therapy in patients with multiple myeloma requiring therapy, it would be inappropriate not to provide further treatment for this patient.

KEY POINT

- The bisphosphonates pamidronate and zoledronic acid should be used for all patients with newly diagnosed multiple myeloma requiring therapy.

Bibliography

Terpos E, Morgan G, Dimopoulos MA, et al. International myeloma working group recommendations for the treatment of multiple myeloma-related bone disease. J Clin Oncol. 2013;31(18):2347-57. [PMID: 23690408]

Item 57   Answer: B

Educational Objective: Diagnose exercise-induced hemolysis.

This patient likely has exercise-induced hemolysis, also known as march hemoglobinuria or runner's hemolysis. This is caused by erythrocyte damage through repetitive mechanical trauma such as running or marching, resulting in intravascular hemolysis. Hemolysis leads to increased levels of free hemoglobin in the plasma, which is filtered by the kidneys, resulting in hemoglobinuria. Urinalysis findings show evidence of blood in the urine by dipstick but no erythrocytes, as seen in this patient. With prolonged intravascular hemolysis, patients may become secondarily iron deficient through iron loss in the urine. Patients with this entity may show iron deficiency anemia with evidence of urine iron loss, indicated by the presence of hemosiderin in sloughed tubular cells by Prussian blue staining. Exercise-induced hemolysis is considered a benign condition and is treated by removal or reduction of the traumatic cause of erythrocyte injury.

Strenuous exercise is a well-described cause of either gross or microscopic hematuria. Although the mechanism for hematuria associated with exercise has not been fully elucidated, it is considered a benign condition and should resolve with termination of exercise. This patient has evidence of myoglobinuria but not of hematuria given the lack of erythrocytes in her urine, making this a less likely diagnosis.

An inflammatory myopathy, such as polymyositis, may cause muscle damage and the finding of positive blood on the urine dipstick without significant hematuria. However, inflammatory myopathies are usually associated with muscle weakness and tenderness and an elevated creatine kinase level, which are absent in this patient.

Rhabdomyolysis is caused by injury and necrosis of muscle with release of intracellular muscle contents into the circulation; myoglobin may be detected in the urine as hemoglobin in the absence of erythrocytes. However, rhabdomyolysis is usually associated with muscle pain and significant elevations in circulating muscle enzyme levels, including creatine kinase. This patient has no muscle tenderness and her creatine kinase level is normal, making this diagnosis unlikely.

KEY POINT

- Exercise-induced hemolysis (march hemoglobinuria or runner's hemolysis) is caused by erythrocyte damage through repetitive mechanical trauma such as running or marching, resulting in intravascular hemolysis with loss of iron in the urine

Bibliography

Dang CV. Runner's anemia. JAMA. 2001 Aug 8;286(6):714-6. [PMID: 11495622]

Item 58   Answer: B

Educational Objective: Diagnose essential thrombocythemia.

Mutational analysis for *JAK2 V617F* should be conducted. The patient presented with iron deficiency anemia and thrombocytosis. Thrombocytosis is often associated with iron deficiency anemia, particularly if bleeding is the cause of the anemia. However, when the patient's anemia was corrected with oral iron and oral contraceptive pills for better regulation of menstruation, thrombocytosis persisted, suggesting a disorder in platelet regulation. Iron deficiency is the most common cause of reactive thrombocytosis, which corrects within weeks of correcting the iron deficiency. Infection, inflammation, and malignancy are other causes. With iron deficiency ruled out as a cause and no other causes clinically apparent, essential thrombocythemia (ET) becomes more probable. Her lack of splenomegaly is fairly typical. The *JAK2* activating mutation is present in 50% of patients with ET, so a negative result would not exclude the diagnosis, but a positive result supports the diagnosis of a myeloproliferative neoplasm (polycythemia vera, ET, or primary myelofibrosis).

BCR-ABL testing, then bone marrow aspiration and biopsy, would be performed if the platelet count remained persistently elevated after correction of serum iron levels with a negative *JAK2* mutation status, because myeloproliferative neoplasms other than ET can less commonly elevate the platelet count. In ET, general hypercellularity and megakaryocyte hyperplasia would be seen on the bone marrow examination.

Testing the prothrombin and activated partial thromboplastin times would not be the most appropriate choice, because it focuses the diagnosis on a bleeding diathesis rather than thrombocytosis. Similarly, von Willebrand factor antigen testing does not address the patient's persistently elevated platelet count.

KEY POINT

- A patient with iron deficiency and isolated thrombocytosis that persists after correction of iron deficiency should undergo *JAK2 V617F* mutational analysis as part of the evaluation for essential thrombocythemia.

Bibliography

Tefferi A. Polycythemia vera and essential thrombocythemia: 2013 update on diagnosis, risk-stratification, and management. Am J Hematol. 2013 Jun;88(6):507-16. [PMID: 23695894]

Item 59   Answer: B

Educational Objective: Manage refractory iron deficiency.

The most appropriate management is to perform a stool antigen assay for *Helicobacter pylori* infection. This patient has iron deficiency anemia. Iron deficiency is a common problem because of the precarious balance between iron intake and use. Women of reproductive age may lose enough iron through normal menstrual blood loss to become iron deficient in the absence of uterine or gastrointestinal disease. Iron malabsorption is a relatively uncommon cause of iron deficiency but should be considered when no other cause of iron deficiency is apparent and particularly when the deficiency is refractory to adequate iron replacement therapy. It is usually caused by generalized malabsorption conditions such as celiac disease, achlorhydria secondary to atrophic gastritis or proton pump inhibitor therapy, or, occasionally, *H. pylori* infection. This patient's history of chronic dyspepsia and refractoriness to oral iron therapy suggest the possibility of *H. pylori* infection. *H. pylori* infection is endemic in many developing countries. Patients treated for underlying *H. pylori* infection may have improved iron absorption, making oral iron replacement an effective treatment.

Although ascorbic acid can facilitate iron absorption, no convincing data suggest the addition of this agent is worth the increase in cost or gastrointestinal toxicity.

Celiac disease is an immunologic response to dietary gliadins in patients genetically at risk as deemed by the presence of *HLA-DQ2* or *HLA-DQ8*. The typical features of celiac disease are diarrhea, bloating, and weight loss; it is diagnosed mainly in whites of northern European ancestry and would be an unusual cause of refractory iron deficiency anemia in a woman of African descent with dyspepsia. Antigliadin assays have poor sensitivity and specificity and a high false-positive rate, so they are not recommended for diagnosing celiac disease.

Iron deficiency is most easily treated with oral iron salts. Oral ferrous sulfate is the least expensive preparation. Each 325-mg tablet of ferrous sulfate contains 66 mg of iron, 1% to 2% of which is absorbed. Although other oral iron salts such as ferrous gluconate or ferrous fumarate are available, none of these have proved superior to ferrous sulfate in tolerability or efficacy.

KEY POINT

- Iron malabsorption is usually caused by generalized malabsorption conditions such as celiac disease, achlorhydria, or *Helicobacter pylori* infection.

Bibliography

Righetti AA, Koua AY, Adiossan LG, et al. Etiology of anemia among infants, school-aged children, and young non-pregnant women in different settings of South-Central Cote d'Ivoire. Am J Trop Med Hyg. 2012 Sep;87(3):425-34. [PMID: 22848097]

Item 60   Answer: B

Educational Objective: Manage a patient undergoing colonoscopy and taking a new oral anticoagulant.

The patient should stop rivaroxaban, a new oral anticoagulant (NOAC), the day before his scheduled colonoscopy. Because polypectomy or biopsy of lesions may become necessary during this patient's colonoscopy, interruption of anticoagulation is suggested in patients who are not at high risk for thromboembolic events, which includes this patient, because his thrombotic event occurred more than 3 months ago. Compared with warfarin, it is not yet known at what residual drug level procedures and surgeries can be safely performed without undue bleeding risk in patients taking an NOAC. In the absence of clinical data about when to stop these drugs before surgery, the half-life of the anticoagulant is the most frequently used parameter to decide when to stop the drug. Reported half-lives are 14 to 17 hours for dabigatran, 7 to 11 hours for rivaroxaban, 8 to 14 hours for apixaban, and 5 to 11 hours for edoxaban. For surgical procedures with standard risk for bleeding, the NOAC should be discontinued 2 to 3 half-lives beforehand, and in procedures with high bleeding risk, 4 to 5 half-lives beforehand. Close attention to kidney function is needed, because kidney impairment leads to prolonged half-lives of the NOACs. In this patient with normal kidney function, stopping rivaroxaban 24 to 36 hours before the procedure would be appropriate.

Bridging with low-molecular-weight heparin (LMWH) is not indicated, because LMWHs have half-lives of 4 to 7 hours, not much shorter than the NOACs. Additionally, this patient is not at high risk for thromboembolism and would not need preprocedural bridging even if he were taking warfarin.

KEY POINT

- The new oral anticoagulants should be stopped 24 to 36 hours before surgeries with standard risk for bleeding and 2 to 4 days before surgeries with a high risk for bleeding in patients with normal kidney function.

Bibliography

ASGE Standards of Practice Committee, Anderson MA, Ben-Menachem T, Gan SI, et al. Management of antithrombotic agents for endoscopic procedures. Gastrointest Endosc. 2009 Dec;70(6):1060-70. [PMID: 19889407]

Item 61   Answer: A

Educational Objective: Manage α-thalassemia.

This patient should discontinue her oral iron supplementation, because she does not have iron deficiency. She likely has α-thalassemia trait presenting with a mild microcytic anemia. Microcytic hypochromic erythrocytes and target forms may be seen on the peripheral blood smear in α- and β-thalassemia, which can only be differentiated by hemoglobin electrophoresis, in which α-thalassemia shows a normal pattern and β-thalassemia typically has a slightly increased hemoglobin A_2 band. α-Thalassemia trait (or α-thalassemia minor, double gene deletion -α/-α or --/αα) is associated with mild anemia, microcytosis, hypochromia, target cells on the peripheral blood smear, and, in adults, normal hemoglobin electrophoresis results. The (-α/-α) variant is often mistaken for iron deficiency. Microcytic anemia associated with a normal or slightly increased erythrocyte count is characteristic of thalassemia but not of iron deficiency. The red cell distribution width (RDW) is also useful in distinguishing between thalassemia and iron deficiency, because the RDW is often elevated in iron deficiency but normal in thalassemia. No treatment or monitoring is necessary for α-thalassemia trait.

The mild anemia of α-thalassemia is often confused with iron deficiency anemia, especially in a patient who could have a plausible cause for iron deficiency from menstrual blood loss. However, this patient's iron values are not consistent with iron deficiency, and the normal RDW argues against iron deficiency and the need for iron replacement therapy. This also rules out the need for evaluation for gastrointestinal blood loss with fecal occult blood testing.

Starting an oral contraceptive pill could potentially lessen the patient's menstrual bleeding, but because she is not iron deficient, oral contraceptives would not correct her mild anemia.

KEY POINT

- α-Thalassemia trait (or α-thalassemia minor), which is associated with mild anemia, microcytosis, hypochromia, target cells on the peripheral blood smear, and, in adults, normal hemoglobin electrophoresis results, requires no treatment.

Bibliography

Harteveld CL, Higgs DR. Alpha-thalassaemia. Orphanet J Rare Dis. 2010 May 28;5:13. [PMID: 20507641]

Item 62   Answer: C

Educational Objective: Determine the appropriate contraceptive choice for a woman at increased risk for venous thromboembolism.

A progestin-releasing intrauterine device (IUD) would be most appropriate for this patient. Other choices include the progestin-only pill, depot injection, or implanted rod. She is at increased risk for venous thromboembolism (VTE) because of her family history of VTE in two first-degree relatives and her obesity. Progestin-releasing IUDs do not appear to increase VTE risk, so they are a good contraceptive choice for women who are at increased risk for VTE. It is uncertain if oral progestin-only contraceptives (min-ipill) lead to an increased risk of VTE; however, the risk appears to be more clearly increased if additional VTE risk factors are present (obesity, immobility, surgery). Injectable progestins do appear to increase the risk of VTE.

Oral contraceptive pills (OCPs) include combination estrogen-progestin products and progestin-only pills. Combinations with lower estrogen doses are as effective with fewer side effects. Combined products are also available as a patch and a vaginal ring. Contraindications to combination products include history or increased risk of thrombosis, liver disease, breast cancer, migraine with aura, and uncontrolled hypertension. Women older than 35 years who smoke more than 15 cigarettes per day should not be prescribed estrogen-containing preparations because of an increased risk of stroke. Because this patient is at increased risk for thrombosis, she should not use any method of contraception containing estrogen.

KEY POINT

- Progestin-releasing intrauterine devices are the most appropriate contraceptive option for women at increased risk for venous thromboembolism (VTE) because they are not associated with increasing the VTE risk further, whereas progestin-only pills, implants, and injections may slightly increase the risk for thrombosis.

Bibliography

Mantha S, Karp R, Raghavan V, Terrin N, Bauer KA, Zwicker JI. Assessing the risk of venous thromboembolic events in women taking progestin-only contraception: a meta-analysis. BMJ. 2012 Aug 7;345:e4944. [PMID: 22872710]

Item 63   Answer: C

Educational Objective: Manage pulmonary embolism with outpatient anticoagulation.

This patient can receive anticoagulant therapy in the outpatient setting. When treating acute pulmonary embolism (PE), it is essential to initiate anticoagulation immediately and achieve therapeutic levels of anticoagulation within 24 hours; failure to do so correlates with an increased risk of clinical progression and recurrence. Anticoagulation can be achieved with unfractionated heparin (either intravenous or subcutaneous), subcutaneous low-molecular-weight heparin (LMWH), or the pentasaccharide fondaparinux. Outpatient management is safe for up to 50% of patients with PE, including some with mild right heart strain on cardiac echocardiography. However, hospital admission is appropriate for patients who are too ill to be managed at home (those needing supplemental oxygen or requiring intravenous pain medications) and those with comorbid conditions that may contribute to rapid clinical deterioration (for example, high bleeding risk).

A 2012 guideline from the American College of Chest Physicians (ACCP) recommends thrombolytic therapy for patients with PE and a systolic blood pressure less than 90 mm Hg and without contraindications (for example, high bleeding risk). Thrombolytic therapy does not appear to have therapeutic benefit in unselected patients with acute PE and is associated with an increased risk for major hemorrhage. No clear evidence indicates thrombolytic therapy should be used in patients with evidence of pulmonary hypertension or right ventricular dysfunction detected by echocardiography, positive cardiac enzymes, or both. This patient has no indications for thrombolytic therapy. If thrombolytic therapy were appropriate, the ACCP's guidelines recommend systemic administration rather than catheter-directed thrombolysis.

KEY POINT

- Outpatient anticoagulation management is possible for patients with pulmonary embolism, unless they require supplemental oxygen, intravenous pain medications, or management of comorbid conditions that may contribute to rapid clinical deterioration or if home circumstances make outpatient therapy unfeasible.

Bibliography

Kearon C, Akl EA, Comerota AJ, et al. Antithrombotic therapy for VTE disease: antithrombotic therapy and prevention of thrombosis, 9th ed: American College of Chest Physicians evidence-based clinical practice guidelines. Chest. 2012 Feb;141(2 Suppl):e419S-94S. [PMID: 22315268]

Item 64   Answer: A

Educational Objective: Diagnose amyloidosis.

This patient should undergo amyloid typing to classify his amyloidosis (for example, immunoglobulin light chain [AL], hereditary, or secondary [AA] amyloidosis). Amyloid typing can be accomplished by protein sequencing of the amyloid material from an involved biopsy specimen or by immunofluorescence or immunohistochemistry. He has an IgG κ monoclonal gammopathy, evidence of cardiac infiltration shown by diffuse myocardial thickening, and amyloid deposition seen on a fat pad aspirate; these findings suggest amyloid cardiomyopathy. The presence of an IgG κ monoclonal gammopathy suggests the possibility of AL amyloidosis. However, hereditary amyloidosis with incidental monoclonal gammopathy of undetermined significance (MGUS) must also be considered. The most common variant of hereditary cardiac amyloidosis is characterized by a Val-122Ile mutation in transthyretin. It is present in 3.5% of black persons and is associated with late onset cardiac involvement, typically after the age of 50 years, without evidence of other end-organ damage related to amyloidosis. Mass spectroscopy, which has 98% sensitivity and specificity, can be used to sequence and identify the composition of the amyloid deposits. Amyloid typing to establish the correct type of amyloidosis syndrome is absolutely critical, particularly in light of the high prevalence of MGUS, to avoid exposing a patient to inappropriate and potentially difficult therapy.

Chemotherapy and autologous hematopoietic stem cell transplantation (HSCT) are appropriate therapies for a patient with an established diagnosis of AL amyloidosis but not hereditary amyloidosis. A diagnosis of AL amyloidosis requires initiation of chemotherapy or pursuit of autologous HSCT, whereas a diagnosis of Val122Ile transthyretin-mutated amyloidosis is treated supportively. Patients with earlier onset hereditary amyloidosis characterized by more extensive or severe organ involvement would be considered for liver transplantation.

Although a transmyocardial biopsy would show evidence of amyloid deposition in the heart, this invasive procedure is unnecessary in patients with a typical clinical presentation, consistent noninvasive cardiac imaging findings, and documented amyloid deposition on biopsy from a noncardiac site, as seen in this patient.

KEY POINT

- Patients with amyloidosis should undergo amyloid typing of amyloid deposits to further classify the type of amyloidosis present.

Bibliography

Vrana JA, Gamez JD, Madden BJ, Theis JD, Bergen HR 3rd, Dogan A. Classification of amyloidosis by laser microdissection and mass spectrometry-based proteomic analysis in clinical biopsy specimens. Blood. 2009 Dec 3;114(24):4957-9. [PMID: 19797517]

Item 65   Answer: D

Educational Objective: Treat vaso-occlusive pain in a pregnant patient with sickle cell disease.

This patient should receive intravenous fluids and narcotic analgesics. She is experiencing a vaso-occlusive pain episode that does not differ greatly from those she typically experiences. Because no reliable physical findings or laboratory markers can objectively establish the vaso-occlusion, the diagnosis of vaso-occlusive pain is based on subjective reports by the patient. She has no signs of acute chest syndrome (ACS) (no fever or hypoxia [oxygen saturation >90% breathing room air]) or other end-organ damage (her creatinine and aminotransferase levels are normal). No randomized studies have been conducted on the effectiveness or harms of standard therapy for vaso-occlusive crisis during pregnancy. Expert opinion recommends this patient should receive the same treatment as nonpregnant patients with sickle cell disease, which includes rest, relaxation, warmth, NSAIDs (which are considered safe before 30 weeks' gestation), oral and intravenous hydration, and narcotic analgesia. Narcotics are safe to use during pregnancy, and she will benefit from hydration, which will theoretically correct any dehydration contributing to the vaso-occlusive episode.

Because neither the patient nor the fetus is displaying symptoms of anemia (significant shortness of breath, dizziness, and chest pain in the mother or fetal distress), transfusion is not indicated. The patient's hemoglobin level is slightly lower now than her prepregnancy baseline; however, neither transfusion nor exchange transfusion is indicated in asymptomatic patients without signs of end-organ damage. Neither has been shown to decrease maternal morbidity or mortality during pregnancy, but both would predispose the patient to iron overload and erythrocyte antibody production. Transfusion would be appropriate to treat symptomatic anemia or signs of end-organ involvement (stroke symptoms, kidney failure, ACS, hepatic involvement).

Hydroxyurea therapy results in decreased mortality in hemoglobin SS sickle cell anemia and is indicated in patients with recurrent painful episodes, ACS, and symptomatic anemia. However, because of its potential teratogenicity, hydroxyurea should not be administered during pregnancy. Proper contraception before hydroxyurea initiation should be discussed with the nonpregnant patient.

KEY POINT

- Expert opinion recommends that pregnant patients should receive the same treatment for acute vaso-occlusive crisis as nonpregnant patients with sickle cell disease.

Bibliography

Martí-Carvajal AJ, Peña-Martí GE, Comunián-Carrasco G, Martí-Peña AJ. Interventions for treating painful sickle cell crisis during pregnancy. Cochrane Database Syst Rev. 2009 Jan 21;(1):CD006786. [PMID: 19160301]

Item 66   Answer: D

Educational Objective: Diagnose polycythemia vera as a cause of Budd-Chiari syndrome.

The appropriate next step would be to test for the *JAK2 V617F* mutation. This patient likely has polycythemia vera (PV), a myeloproliferative neoplasm (MPN). Symptoms include generalized pruritus that often worsens after bathing, erythromelalgia (a burning sensation in the palms and soles), and hypermetabolic symptoms such as fever, weight loss, and sweating. On physical examination, patients may have plethora and hepatosplenomegaly. Twenty percent of patients experience arterial or venous thrombosis as their initial symptom. PV and the other MPNs predispose to the development of the Budd-Chiari syndrome (BCS), which is characterized by hepatic venous outflow tract obstruction (including the suprahepatic inferior vena cava) and other intra-abdominal thromboses, such as thrombosis of the portal, superior mesenteric, or splenic vein. Abdominal pain, ascites, liver and spleen enlargement, and portal hypertension occur with symptomatic BCS. Ninety-five percent of patients with PV have the *JAK2* mutation, so it is an appropriate confirmatory test for suspected PV. Anticoagulant therapy is recommended for all patients with BCS regardless of whether an underlying prothrombotic disorder is discovered. Phlebotomy to normalize the hematocrit (goal <45% in men, <42% in women) is indicated, and adding the myelosuppressive agent hydroxyurea to phlebotomy decreases thrombotic events in patients with PV.

Bone marrow aspirate and biopsy findings are nonspecific in PV; they may show an increased number of megakaryocytes in a moderately to markedly hypercellular marrow and an increase in reticulin. Because they are not diagnostic and the procedure is invasive, bone marrow biopsy is typically unnecessary and is not an appropriate early diagnostic test.

Although factor V Leiden is a risk factor for venous thromboembolism, it would not explain the patient's erythrocytosis, leukocytosis, or thrombocytosis. Therefore, it is not a helpful test to perform in this patient.

Paroxysmal nocturnal hemoglobinuria (PNH) is an acquired clonal stem cell disorder that should be considered in patients with hemolytic anemia, pancytopenia, or unprovoked atypical thrombosis. Thrombotic complications of PNH may occur in atypical locations, such as the hepatic veins (BCS) or mesenteric or cerebral circulation, and develop more frequently in patients with large PNH clones. PNH is diagnosed by flow cytometry, which can detect CD55 and CD59 deficiency on the surface of peripheral erythrocytes or leukocytes. Erythrocytosis, leukocytosis, thrombocythemia, and generalized pruritus are not typical for PNH.

KEY POINT

- Arterial or venous thrombosis is the initial symptom in 20% of patients with polycythemia vera (PV) and should prompt testing for the *JAK2 V617F* mutation, which is found in nearly 100% of patients with PV.

Bibliography
Tefferi A. Polycythemia vera and essential thrombocythemia: 2013 update on diagnosis, risk-stratification, and management. Am J Hematol. 2013 Jun;88(6):507-16. [PMID: 23695894]

Item 67   Answer: D
Educational Objective: **Treat a patient with venous thromboembolism with an initial combination of a parenteral anticoagulant and warfarin.**

Heparin should be given for no less than 5 days and only discontinued at that time if the INR is therapeutic for 24 hours. Warfarin may be initiated on the first or second day of heparin therapy. Because factor II and X levels require at least 5 days to decline sufficiently, parenteral anticoagulation should overlap with warfarin for at least 5 days and until an INR of 2 or more is achieved.

The initial warfarin dose may be based on a patient's predicted maintenance dose using available calculators, and a patient's nutritional status, comorbid diseases, and age must be considered. Excessively high initial doses should be avoided because they can lead to supratherapeutic INR values and premature discontinuation of parenteral therapy. Patients should be followed closely with frequent INR studies at the initiation of therapy to achieve values consistently within the desired range. After patients achieve consistently stable INR levels with an established dose, INR monitoring may eventually be extended to every 12 weeks for the duration of treatment, but testing frequency should be determined individually. The duration of warfarin therapy is determined by the type of thrombotic event and the presence or absence of situational triggers (provoked versus unprovoked), thrombophilic states, active cancer, and a history of thrombotic events.

KEY POINT

- Parenteral anticoagulant administration must overlap with warfarin for at least 5 days and until the INR is greater than 2 for 24 hours.

Bibliography
Ageno W, Gallus AS, Wittkowsky A, et al. Oral anticoagulant therapy: antithrombotic therapy and prevention of thrombosis, 9th ed: American College of Chest Physicians evidence-based clinical practice guidelines. Chest. 2012 Feb;141(2 Suppl):e44S-88S. [PMID: 22315269]

Item 68   Answer: D
Educational Objective: **Diagnose cobalamin (vitamin B$_{12}$) deficiency.**

The most appropriate diagnostic test is to measure the methylmalonic acid level. This patient likely has cobalamin (vitamin B$_{12}$) deficiency, which she is at risk for based on following a vegan diet for several years. Compared with folate deficiency, which develops within weeks, cobalamin deficiency develops over months to years. She also has neurologic findings typical of and concerning for cobalamin deficiency. If left untreated, neurologic function could continue to decrease. A macrocytic anemia is characteristic of cobalamin deficiency, and the peripheral blood smear shows a typical hypersegmented neutrophil, a result of ineffective myelopoiesis. In many patients with suspected cobalamin deficiency, vitamin B$_{12}$ levels will be in the normal range, and further testing is indicated to obtain better sensitivity. Methylmalonic acid is elevated in 98% of people with cobalamin deficiency; therefore, this would be a sensitive and specific test to determine deficiency.

Cobalamin deficiency can occasionally present with pancytopenia, which could prompt a bone marrow examination; however, a bone marrow biopsy is not needed to diagnose suspected cobalamin deficiency. The patient's neutropenia will likely resolve as the cobalamin deficiency is corrected.

This patient is unlikely to have isolated folate deficiency considering her neurologic symptoms, which are commonly seen with cobalamin, but not folate, deficiency. Testing the methylmalonic acid level concomitantly rules out folate deficiency and diagnoses cobalamin deficiency, because methylmalonic acid levels will be normal in cases of folate deficiency.

Homocysteine levels are elevated in cobalamin deficiency, but they can also be elevated in folate deficiency, so checking the homocysteine level is not the best test to perform. Evaluating the methylmalonic acid level will more accurately provide a diagnosis.

KEY POINT

- The methylmalonic acid level is elevated in 98% of patients with cobalamin deficiency, making it a sensitive and specific laboratory test to use in determining deficiency.

Bibliography

Stabler SP. Clinical practice. Vitamin B12 deficiency. N Engl J Med. 2013 Jan 10;368(2):149-60.[PMID: 23301732]

Item 69   Answer: C

Educational Objective: Manage Waldenström macroglobulinemia.

This patient should begin combination rituximab plus chemotherapy. He has symptomatic Waldenström macroglobulinemia, demonstrated by a neoplastic infiltrate consisting of clonal lymphocytes, plasmacytoid lymphocytes, plasma cells, and immunoblasts comprising 10% or more of the bone marrow cellularity with disease-related manifestations, including night sweats, weight loss, anemia, lymphadenopathy, and splenomegaly. Management of this low-grade, mature B-cell, non-Hodgkin lymphoma consists of the anti-CD20 monoclonal antibody, rituximab, as single agent therapy or combined with chemotherapy. Considering this patient's degree of symptoms and tumor burden, along with his otherwise good health, combined rituximab and chemotherapy would be highly appropriate. The chemotherapy regimen may consist of an alkylating agent base (such as cyclophosphamide) or purine analog base (such as fludarabine).

Management of anemia should be directed at treating the underlying cause, in this case the Waldenström macroglobulinemia. Plasma exchange is essential for patients presenting with symptomatic hyperviscosity and is occasionally used as adjunctive therapy for cold agglutinin disease, an autoimmune hemolytic anemia that can be associated with Waldenström macroglobulinemia. However, it would not be appropriate in this patient, who does not have symptoms of hyperviscosity. Although the patient is anemic and has an elevated lactate dehydrogenase level, the reticulocyte count is low considering the degree of anemia, no erythrocyte clumps appear on the peripheral blood smear, and the direct antiglobulin (Coombs) test is negative, making a diagnosis of cold agglutinin disease highly unlikely. Furthermore, the patient does not have any clinical manifestations of this disorder (such as acrocyanosis), so a cold agglutinin titer would not be appropriate.

The patient has no symptoms of hyperviscosity (blurry vision, headache, hearing loss, tinnitus, vertigo, dizziness, altered mental status) or findings on physical examination to suggest hyperviscosity (dilated, tortuous retinal veins on funduscopic examination). In the absence of signs and symptoms of hyperviscosity and an M protein of less than 4 g/dL, serum viscosity testing is of no significant value.

KEY POINT

- Initial therapy for Waldenström macroglobulinemia may consist of rituximab as monotherapy or combined with chemotherapy, which may include an alkylating agent or a purine analog.

Bibliography

Gertz MA. Waldenström macroglobulinemia: 2013 update on diagnosis, risk stratification, and management. Am J Hematol. 2013 Aug;88(8):70-11. [PMID: 23784973]

Item 70   Answer: C

Educational Objective: Diagnose glucose-6-phosphate dehydrogenase deficiency.

This patient's glucose-6-phosphate dehydrogenase (G6PD) activity should be measured in 2 months. G6PD deficiency is an X-linked disease and occurs more commonly in men, often in blacks. This variant typically leads to episodic hemolysis in response to oxidant stressors (for example, infections or drugs such as dapsone, trimethoprim-sulfamethoxazole, and nitrofurantoin). Elevated levels of G6PD are found in normal young reticulocytes, and levels may appear falsely normal during an acute hemolytic episode, causing a missed diagnosis. Consequently, G6PD levels should be checked a few months after the occurrence of an acute event. During an acute hemolytic episode, bite cells may be seen on the peripheral blood smear, as are apparent in this patient's peripheral blood smear.

Thrombotic thrombocytopenic purpura (TTP) should be suspected in patients who have anemia, schistocytes on the peripheral blood smear, increased serum lactate dehydrogenase level, and thrombocytopenia. TTP can be triggered by drugs, especially quinine, ticlopidine, mitomycin C, cyclosporine, or gemcitabine. The mechanism of disease is thought to be antibodies directed against the protease ADAMTS-13 that is responsible for cleaving the high-molecular-weight multimers of von Willebrand factor. Assays for ADAMTS-13 activity are available but are not needed for a TTP diagnosis and are not indicated in patients who lack the essential diagnostic criteria for TTP.

Hereditary spherocytosis should be suspected in patients with a personal or family history of anemia, jaundice, splenomegaly, or gallstones. Spherocytes are present on the peripheral blood smear, and the direct antiglobulin (Coombs) test is negative. The osmotic fragility test with 24-hour incubation is a key diagnostic step, demonstrating increased erythrocyte fragility in hypotonic saline compared with control erythrocytes. This patient's ethnic background, absence of splenomegaly, and presence of bite cells on the peripheral blood smear do not support a diagnosis of hereditary spherocytosis.

KEY POINT

- Glucose-6-phosphate dehydrogenase deficiency typically leads to episodic hemolysis in response to oxidant stressors (infections or drugs such as dapsone, trimethoprim-sulfamethoxazole, and nitrofurantoin).

Bibliography

Cappellini MD, Fiorelli G. Glucose-6-phosphate dehydrogenase deficiency. Lancet. 2008 Jan 5;371(9606):64-74. [PMID: 18177777]

Item 71   Answer: B

Educational Objective: Treat a patient with warm autoimmune hemolytic anemia.

The patient should be given prednisone. She has warm autoimmune hemolytic anemia (WAIHA), indicated by the high reticulocyte count, elevated bilirubin and lactate dehydrogenase (LDH) levels, the positive direct antiglobulin (Coombs) test, and spherocytes seen on peripheral blood smear. In WAIHA, IgG antibodies are directed against erythrocyte surface membrane molecules, which leads to phagocytosis by macrophages that cause erythrocytes to become progressively more spherocytic. These abnormal erythrocytes are then destroyed in the spleen. WAIHA can manifest as a primary disorder or as a complication of another disorder, including autoimmune conditions (systemic lupus erythematosus) or lymphoproliferative disorders (chronic lymphocytic leukemia). Treatment is immunosuppression to halt the immune-mediated erythrocyte destruction and allow the patient's own bone marrow to regenerate the erythrocytes, if possible. The best initial treatment for this condition is a glucocorticoid such as prednisone.

Transfusion in patients with WAIHA is a topic of debate. Although this patient has severe anemia, she has no organ dysfunction, is not hypoxic, and has no signs or symptoms of heart failure or angina. Additionally, her bone marrow is able to respond to her hemolysis, and her hemoglobin level would be expected to recover with treatment of her hemolytic condition. Additionally, erythrocyte transfusions are complicated in patients with WAIHA, because the antibodies causing hemolysis may crossreact with transfused erythrocytes, making crossmatch-compatible blood difficult to find. Therefore, transfusion in patients with WAIHA should be approached carefully, and if necessary, should be performed with type-specific, crossmatch-incompatible blood. Consultation with a hematologist and transfusion medicine specialist is recommended.

Rituximab and splenectomy are typically reserved to treat patients in whom first-line therapy for WAIHA has failed; they are not used in the acute setting. An inadequate response to glucocorticoids may indicate the need for splenectomy or alternative immunosuppression.

Although the mean corpuscular volume is elevated, this patient's clinical picture is inconsistent with vitamin B_{12} deficiency, which typically includes a low reticulocyte count (although the LDH and total bilirubin levels can be quite elevated because of intramedullary hemolysis). Additionally, no hypersegmented neutrophils are seen, and she has no abnormal neurologic findings.

KEY POINT

- Treatment of warm autoimmune hemolytic anemia is based on initial immunosuppression with glucocorticoids to halt immune-mediated erythrocyte destruction and allow bone marrow to regenerate the erythrocytes.

Bibliography

Crowther M, Chan YL, Garbett IK, Lim W, Vickers MA, Crowther MA. Evidence-based focused review of the treatment of idiopathic warm immune hemolytic anemia in adults. Blood. 2011 Oct 13;118(15):4036-40. [PMID: 21778343]

Item 72   Answer: D

Educational Objective: Manage low-risk myelodysplastic syndrome with observation.

Observation is appropriate for this patient with low-risk myelodysplastic syndrome (MDS), incidentally discovered by a complete blood count showing asymptomatic pancytopenia. The mild macrocytosis is typical. The bone marrow biopsy is appropriate to confirm a suspected diagnosis of myelodysplasia in the setting of the normal vitamin B_{12} and folate levels and to provide important prognostic information. This patient has low-risk disease by the revised International Prognostic Scoring System criteria despite two involved cell lines. The low-risk cytogenetics and low marrow blasts (<2%) indicate very low-risk MDS. Median survival is 8.8 years in a generally older adult population and the median time to 25% acute myeloid leukemia (AML) progression is more than 14 years. No therapy will improve prognosis in this situation.

5-Azacytidine is appropriate therapy for higher risk MDS for the purpose of improving blood counts, delaying AML progression, and extending survival. It would be indicated to lessen transfusion dependence or to improve prognosis for high-risk disease, but is inappropriate in this patient, whose disease is low risk.

Allogeneic hematopoietic stem cell transplantation is not justified, because this patient's disease is very low risk. In contrast, a patient with very high-risk disease has an expected median survival of less than 1 year, justifying the treatment-related morbidity associated with transplantation.

Erythropoietin is inappropriate because this patient is asymptomatic. Recombinant erythropoietin can be effective in approximately 25% of patients with MDS. However, the goal hemoglobin level is 10 g/dL (100 g/L), and targets to higher values have been associated with arterial and venous thrombosis.

KEY POINT

- Myelodysplastic syndrome should be managed based on risk stratification, with patients with low-risk disease requiring no treatment.

Bibliography

Lyons RM. Myelodysplastic syndromes: therapy and outlook. Am J Med. 2012 Jul;125(7 Suppl):S18-23. [PMID: 22735747]

Item 73   Answer: B

Educational Objective: Diagnose transfusion-associated circulatory overload.

The most likely diagnosis is transfusion-associated circulatory overload (TACO). TACO is an underdiagnosed condition that

CONT.

occurs in 0.3% to 8% of patients undergoing transfusion in the hospital and is associated with increased inpatient mortality and a longer length of hospital stay. TACO is defined as the new onset or exacerbation of at least three of the following findings within 6 hours of completing a transfusion: acute respiratory distress, elevated B-type natriuretic peptide (BNP) level, elevated central venous pressure (CVP), evidence of left heart failure, evidence of positive fluid balance, and radiographic evidence of pulmonary edema. Risk factors include age older than 60 years, chronic kidney disease, chronic heart failure, number of blood products transfused, and the volume transfused per hour. Preventive measures include a slower rate of infusion for those at risk (1 mL/kg/hour) and diuretic therapy to maintain euvolemia.

An acute hemolytic transfusion reaction (AHTR) is unlikely. The patient's hemoglobin level increased appropriately after the transfusion (1 g/dL/U [10 g/L/U]), and the lactate dehydrogenase and total bilirubin levels are not elevated. No protein was seen on urinalysis, kidney function is unchanged, and the patient is not hypotensive. Additionally, pulmonary opacities as seen on the radiograph would not be expected with AHTR.

Distinguishing TACO from transfusion-related acute lung injury (TRALI) can be challenging. Fever and hypotension occur in only one third of patients with TRALI. However, TRALI is not associated with signs of volume overload (increased jugular venous pressure, lower extremity edema, elevated CVP). BNP and N-terminal proBNP levels have not been studied in TRALI but are elevated with TACO.

Transfusion-associated sepsis is highly unlikely in the absence of fever and hypotension.

KEY POINT

- Patients experiencing acute respiratory distress, elevated B-type natriuretic peptide level, elevated central venous pressure, evidence of left heart failure, evidence of positive fluid balance, or radiographic evidence of pulmonary edema within 6 hours of transfusion should be diagnosed with transfusion-associated circulatory overload.

Bibliography
Murphy EL, Kwaan N, Looney MR, et al; TRALI Study Group. Risk factors and outcomes in transfusion-associated circulatory overload. Am J Med. 2013 Apr;126(4):357, e29-38. [PMID: 23357450]

Item 74   Answer: B

Educational Objective: Treat high-risk myelodysplastic syndrome with hematopoietic stem cell transplantation.

This patient should undergo allogeneic hematopoietic stem cell transplantation (HSCT). She has myelodysplastic syndrome (MDS), diagnosed by complete blood count results from an investigation of symptomatic pancytopenia. The monocytosis and mild macrocytosis are typical. Bone marrow examination is required to confirm the diagnosis and to provide prognostic information that can inform therapeutic

recommendations. The International Prognostic Scoring System – Revised criteria weigh cytogenetics most heavily when determining risk. A complex karyotype places this patient in a high-risk group. Involvement of three cell lines and more than 5% marrow blasts specifies the highest risk group. In very high-risk disease, median survival is expected to be less than 1 year. Such a prognosis in a younger patient justifies the recommendation for allogeneic HSCT at diagnosis. Although transplantation is associated with significant risks, it is also the only curative therapy for MDS.

5-Azacytidine is appropriate for higher risk MDS but does not have curative potential. In a younger, fit patient, HSCT is a better choice. For older patients (generally older than 60 years) or those with significant comorbidities, 5-azacytidine would be an appropriate option.

Erythropoietic agents, such as epoetin and darbepoetin alfa, may improve hemoglobin levels in patients with symptomatic anemia and lower risk MDS but are not appropriate as single therapy for high-risk disease. This patient is at high risk of transforming from MDS to acute myeloid leukemia (AML); HSCT will mitigate that risk, but treatment with erythropoietin will not.

Because of this patient's high-risk MDS, observation would be inappropriate. The natural history of high-risk MDS is progression to AML. Because secondary AML is much harder to cure, primary therapy before transformation improves prognosis.

KEY POINT

- Younger, fit patients with high-risk myelodysplastic syndrome should receive allogeneic hematopoietic stem cell transplantation, which is the only curative therapy option.

Bibliography
Vaughn JE, Scott BL, Deeg HJ. Transplantation for myelodysplastic syndrome 2013. Curr Opin Hematol. 2013 Nov;20(6):494-500. [PMID: 24104409]

Item 75   Answer: B

Educational Objective: Treat anemia of chronic kidney disease.

This patient should receive erythropoiesis-stimulating agent (ESA) therapy. He has anemia of chronic kidney disease (CKD), which affects 90% of patients with a glomerular filtration rate less than 25 to 30 mL/min/1.73 m². Erythropoietin is made by interstitial peritubular fibroblasts of the kidney, so patients with reduced kidney function may have low erythropoietin levels; however, erythropoietin resistance also occurs. When patients with reduced kidney function develop anemia, evaluation for other causes is appropriate; in particular, relative iron deficiency is common. If iron stores are adequate and other causes have also been eliminated (such as cobalamin and folate deficiency, gastrointestinal bleeding), the anemia can be attributed to CKD. The routine measurement of erythropoietin levels plays no role in CKD, because this expensive test does not aid in the diagnosis or guide treatment decisions. ESAs should be considered for patients with symptomatic anemia attributable to erythropoietin deficiency when the hemoglobin level is less than 10 g/dL (100 g/L). Patients with CKD must be carefully counseled about the risks of ESAs, which include increased risk of thrombotic and cardiovascular events as well as increased blood pressure. Additionally, clinicians should explain that target hemoglobin values are lower than those used in the past, and that patients must be monitored regularly to titrate the dose to a target hemoglobin level of 10 to 11 g/dL (100-110 g/L).

Transfusions are avoided in patients with CKD unless a compelling reason exists, such as tissue ischemia. Transfusions sensitize patients to HLAs, which complicate kidney transplantation options.

Even though many patients benefit from iron replacement, this man has adequate iron stores, so replacement therapy is not indicated.

KEY POINT

- Erythropoiesis-stimulating agents should be considered for patients with chronic kidney disease and symptomatic anemia attributable to erythropoietin deficiency when the hemoglobin level is less than 10 g/dL (100 g/L).

Bibliography

Kidney Disease: Improving Global Outcomes (KDIGO) Anemia Work Group. KDIGO clinical practice guideline for anemia in chronic kidney disease. Kidney Inter Suppl. 2012;2:279-335. www.kdigo.org/clinical_practice_guidelines/pdf/KDIGO-Anemia%20GL.pdf

Item 76   Answer: B

Educational Objective: Diagnose delayed hyperhemolytic transfusion reaction.

This patient has delayed hyperhemolytic transfusion reaction (DHTR). Chronic transfusion in patients with sickle cell disease (SCD) can lead to iron overload, alloimmunization, and an increased risk for DHTR. DHTR is caused by an amnestic response of a preformed erythrocyte alloantibody after re-exposure to an erythrocyte antigen outside the ABO system. Additionally, an autoimmune component could be worsening the hemolysis. Following transfusion, a 1% to 1.6% chance exists of developing these antibodies. DHTR may then occur after re-exposure with subsequent transfusion. Clinical findings, which typically develop approximately 2 to 19 days after erythrocyte transfusion, include anemia, reticulocytosis, jaundice, a significant decrease in hemoglobin level, and increases in hemolytic markers such as lactate dehydrogenase and bilirubin levels, although many patients will be asymptomatic. Patients with SCD may present with a worsening pain crisis. Hemolysis is typically extravascular, and life-threatening complications are rare. Treatment is supportive. Subsequent transfusions should be minimized but not withheld when indicated, such as in situations of severely symptomatic anemia and multiorgan failure.

Transient aplastic crisis can occur when patients with chronic hemolytic anemia and shortened erythrocyte survival are infected with parvovirus B19, which leads to suppression of erythrocyte production identified by anemia and lack of reticulocytosis. Parvovirus B19 infection is a viral syndrome characterized by malaise, fever, and arthralgia; 25% of patients are asymptomatic.

A rare complication of SCD is hepatic sequestration crisis, characterized by large numbers of erythrocytes becoming trapped in the liver. Patients may develop acute anemia, reticulocytosis, hypovolemia, and distributive shock. Prominent symptoms include right upper quadrant pain, hepatomegaly, and anemia. The patient has none of these manifestations.

Splenic sequestration crisis occurs when splenic pooling of erythrocytes causes an acute anemia with reticulocytosis and a rapidly enlarging spleen. Patients may develop hypotension and shock. This condition is found primarily in children who have functional spleens that have not been subjected to multiple infarctions and subsequent development of fibrotic atrophy. This adult patient does not have splenomegaly. Splenic sequestration crisis is not the most likely diagnosis for anemia following a transfusion.

KEY POINT

- Delayed hyperhemolytic transfusion reaction can occur several days after transfusion and is diagnosed by a significant decrease in the hemoglobin level with reticulocytosis and concomitant increases in the bilirubin and lactate dehydrogenase levels.

Bibliography

Scheunemann LP, Ataga KI. Delayed hemolytic transfusion reaction in sickle cell disease. Am J Med Sci. 2010 Mar;339(3):266-9. [PMID: 20051821]

Item 77   Answer: C

Educational Objective: Diagnose Felty syndrome.

This patient has Felty syndrome, which is the clinical triad of rheumatoid arthritis (RA), splenomegaly, and neutropenia. Splenomegaly and lymphadenopathy may occur secondary to connective tissue disorders such as RA. The unusual cell seen on the peripheral blood smear is a large granular lymphocyte (LGL). LGLs may be seen in up to 40% of patients with Felty syndrome; they may also be associated with other collagen vascular diseases and autoimmune neutropenia. LGL leukemia may also occur in patients with rheumatoid arthritis. Because patients with Felty syndrome and LGL leukemia tend to share HLA-DR4 positivity, they are thought to be part of the same disease spectrum in which immune system dysfunction leads to expansion of this type of cell. The mechanism of neutropenia in Felty syndrome is considered partially autoimmune (likely related to the process leading to development of LGLs) and partially owing to sequestration associated with splenomegaly. Felty syndrome is the most appropriate diagnosis for this patient because the clinical triad is present. This is a useful syndrome to recognize clinically, because it may lead to an RA diagnosis when articular involvement is less prominent.

Aplastic anemia refers to conditions in which the bone marrow fails to produce blood cells, resulting in a hypocellular bone marrow and pancytopenia. It can be acquired or congenital and may be classified as moderate, severe, or very severe. This patient only has leukopenia, which is not consistent with aplastic anemia.

Autoimmune neutropenia is an acquired abnormality that may be associated with underlying disorders of immune regulation such as systemic lupus erythematosus or may exist in a more isolated form. The degree of neutropenia is generally not severe enough to be linked with frequent infections, and spontaneous remission may occur in patients with the primary form. Antineutrophil antibodies may be detected, although tests for them, which differ from the antineutrophil cytoplasmic antibody tests used to evaluate vasculitis, may not be widely available and have variable sensitivity and specificity. In patients in whom antineutrophil antibodies are not detected, the diagnosis is established by excluding other causes.

Paroxysmal nocturnal hemoglobinuria (PNH) is an acquired clonal progenitor cell disorder that should be considered in patients presenting with hemolytic anemia, pancytopenia, or unprovoked atypical thrombosis. PNH does not present with isolated leukopenia.

KEY POINT

- Felty syndrome is characterized by rheumatoid arthritis, splenomegaly, and neutropenia.

Bibliography

Liu X, Loughran TP Jr. The spectrum of large granular lymphocyte leukemia and Felty's syndrome. Curr Opin Hematol. 2011 Jul;18(4):254-9. [PMID: 21546829]

Oncology Answers

Item 78   Answer: B

Educational Objective: Manage a patient with suspected central nervous system lymphoma.

In this patient who most likely has a primary central nervous system (CNS) lymphoma with evidence of mass effect, high-dose glucocorticoids should be administered immediately. Because the brain is enclosed in a fixed space, mass effect within the brain causes progressively increased intracranial pressure (ICP) that, if untreated, can lead to diffuse brain injury, permanent disability, and death. Headache is typically the first presenting symptom and is followed by nausea and vomiting; as ICP increases, more advanced findings include altered mental status, focal neurologic deficits (such as papilledema), and loss of consciousness. Because progression can be rapid, emergent CT or MRI imaging of the brain followed by immediate treatment are essential to avoid the late adverse consequences of increased ICP that lead to permanent neurologic dysfunction and death. Glucocorticoids remain the initial therapy of choice because of their rapid anti-inflammatory effect that decreases the edema associated with malignant mass lesions.

Intravenous administration of dexamethasone is standard for later stages of increased ICP (impaired mentation, uncontrolled seizures) with a recommended dose of 8 to 10 mg every 6 hours. Higher-dose dexamethasone (100 mg/d) does not improve the response rate and is associated with more adverse effects.

Metastatic tumors originating from lung cancer and cutaneous melanoma are the most common malignancy-related causes of increased ICP. These tumors, particularly melanoma, are also associated with intracerebral hemorrhage. Other less common causes of increased ICP related to malignancy include lymphoma, primary brain tumors, and germ cell tumors. Because treatment of ICP varies markedly depending on the cause, a tissue diagnosis of the mass lesion is important in guiding subsequent therapy. A primary CNS lymphoma is the most likely diagnosis in this young patient with a brain mass and HIV infection that is not optimally treated. Because lymphomas are extremely glucocorticoid sensitive, early administration may make obtaining a tissue sample difficult by distorting histologic findings; it is therefore preferable to obtain a biopsy in a stable patient with possible or likely CNS lymphoma prior to glucocorticoid therapy if there are minimal sequelae of increased ICP. However, in all patients with more advanced complications of increased ICP such as this patient, immediate glucocorticoid treatment is indicated.

Combination chemotherapy is appropriate only after initial steps are taken to lower the ICP and a tissue diagnosis is established, which has not yet been done in this patient.

Intracranial pressure monitoring is used to follow the effectiveness of therapies intended to decrease pressure in the cranial space and is most often used in association with severe traumatic brain injury. Although the benefit of pressure monitoring needs to be evaluated in an individual patient, it would not be appropriate to delay administration of glucocorticoids while assessing this patient for monitoring.

Either whole brain or stereotactic radiation therapy may be appropriate for some tumors causing increased ICP, but this therapy would be indicated only after the patient receives acute treatment and a tissue diagnosis is established.

KEY POINT

- Patients who have increased intracranial pressure associated with suspected central nervous system lymphoma require immediate high-dose glucocorticoids to treat the mass effect and a brain biopsy to establish the tissue diagnosis.

Bibliography

Patil CG, Pricola K, Garg SK, Bryant A, Black KL. Whole brain radiation therapy (WBRT) alone versus WBRT and radiosurgery for the treatment of brain metastases. Cochrane Database Syst Rev. 2010 Jun 16;(6):CD006121. Update in: Cochrane Database Syst Rev. 2012;9:CD006121. [PMID: 20556764]

Item 79   Answer: C

Educational Objective: Treat a patient with malignancy-associated hypercalcemia.

The most appropriate next step in treatment for this patient with malignancy-associated hypercalcemia is an intravenous bisphosphonate. Initial therapy for hypercalcemia is high-volume normal saline hydration, and in those with kidney failure, forced diuresis with a loop diuretic such as furosemide. This helps restore intravascular volume and decreases serum calcium levels acutely. For tumors that are glucocorticoid-sensitive, such as multiple myeloma and some types of lymphoma, glucocorticoids are indicated to decrease tumor-associated osteoclast activation. Bisphosphonates are powerful inhibitors of osteoclast-mediated bone resorption with an onset of effect occurring several days after administration and a duration of up to several weeks depending on the specific agent used, which allows longer-term control of calcium levels. Hypercalcemia is usually a manifestation of advanced disease, is associated with poor prognosis, and occurs in up to 10% of patients with cancer. Hypercalcemia is most common among patients with multiple myeloma and breast, renal, and lung cancer. Patients initially present with nausea, vomiting, constipation, and polyuria. Polydipsia, diffuse muscle weakness, and confusion follow.

Cinacalcet is a calcimimetic agent that is used to lower the calcium level in patients with primary and tertiary hyperparathyroidism associated with chronic kidney disease. It is not effective or approved for use in malignancy-associated hypercalcemia.

Dialysis is an effective method for lowering serum calcium levels, although it is generally reserved for patients with severe, symptomatic hypercalcemia who have not responded to acute treatment with hydration and other measures or patients in whom aggressive hydration is contraindicated. Dialysis would not be appropriate in this patient whose response to hydration and other initial therapies has not been assessed.

Treatment with chemotherapy or disease-specific targeted agents would be appropriate for long-term control of hypercalcemia but would not be effective for short-term therapy of hypercalcemia.

KEY POINT

- Immediate hydration with large-volume normal saline infusion, forced diuresis with furosemide, glucocorticoid therapy for glucocorticoid-responsive malignancies such as multiple myeloma, and a bisphosphonate is appropriate treatment of malignancy-related hypercalcemia.

Bibliography
Ziegler R. Hypercalcemic crisis. J Am Soc Nephrol. 2001 Feb;12 Suppl 17:S3-9. [PMID: 11251025]

Item 80   Answer: A

Educational Objective: Treat stage III colon cancer with adjuvant chemotherapy.

Chemotherapy with leucovorin, 5-fluorouracil, and oxaliplatin (FOLFOX) is most appropriate for this patient with stage III colon cancer. Stage III colon cancer is potentially curable, and the likelihood of cure is modestly but statisti-

cally significantly increased by the use of adjuvant chemotherapy. Administration of leucovorin plus 5-fluorouracil (5-FU) was established as an appropriate standard adjuvant treatment for stage III colon cancer in the 1990s. However, in 2004, a large randomized trial comparing adjuvant leucovorin and 5-FU with FOLFOX adjuvant chemotherapy showed that the FOLFOX regimen led to improved disease-free and overall survival. Capecitabine is an oral prodrug that is converted to 5-FU in the body. The combination of capecitabine plus intravenous oxaliplatin (CAPOX) is also an acceptable regimen for adjuvant treatment of patients with stage III colon cancer.

Because local recurrence of colon cancer rarely develops and because it can be difficult to isolate the small bowel from the radiation field, radiation therapy, either alone or in combination with chemotherapy, does not have a role in the routine management of patients with stage III colon cancer. In addition, radiation to the small bowel may cause substantial toxicity. However, because local recurrence is a greater problem in patients with rectal cancer and because it is far easier to isolate the small bowel from the radiation field when treating rectal cancer, the combination of radiation therapy and chemotherapy, preferably preoperatively, is routinely used for treating patients with stage II and III rectal cancer.

Stage III colon cancer is potentially curable with surgery and adjuvant chemotherapy. For patients with good performance status, adjuvant chemotherapy with its associated survival advantage is preferred to observation alone.

KEY POINT

- Chemotherapy with capecitabine and oxaliplatin (CAPOX) or leucovorin, 5-fluorouracil, and oxaliplatin (FOLFOX) is appropriate adjuvant therapy for patients with stage III colon cancer.

Bibliography
Haller DG, Tabernero J, Maroun J, et al. Capecitabine plus oxaliplatin compared with fluorouracil and folinic acid as adjuvant therapy for stage III colon cancer. J Clin Oncol. 2011 Apr 10;29(11):1465-71. [PMID: 21383294]

Item 81   Answer: D

Educational Objective: Manage a patient with metastatic cancer and poor performance status.

Supportive, comfort-oriented care is most appropriate for this patient who has advanced metastatic adenocarcinoma in the setting of multiple severe chronic comorbidities and a debilitated medical condition resulting in a poor performance status. A key aspect of managing patients with cancer is an assessment of their performance status, defined as the specific level of well-being and ability to perform daily activities. Several formal measures of performance status are available, such as the Karnofsky score and the Zubrod score (also called the Eastern Cooperative Oncology Group/World Health Organization system). Scores on these measures correlate with the ability of an individual patient to tolerate potential therapeutic interventions. In patients with very low performance measure scores, a less aggressive and more supportive treatment approach is usually warranted based on likely outcomes of therapy. Virtually all oncology clinical trials showing efficacy of chemotherapy exclude patients with poor performance status because toxicity and harm occur more frequently and clinical benefit occurs less frequently in these patients. In addition, this patient has elevated serum bilirubin and creatinine levels. Because liver and kidney function affect metabolism of many oncology drugs, treatment of patients with chronic liver or kidney disease is challenging and is associated with a higher risk of complications. In some cases, poor performance has developed based on tumor-related symptoms and might be expected to improve with treatment of the cancer. However, this patient's poor performance status appears to be due to his chronic illnesses and is not likely to improve significantly following treatment of his cancer.

Combination chemotherapy is contraindicated in a debilitated patient and would likely cause severe and even life-threatening toxicity.

Single-agent, low-dose chemotherapy is highly unlikely to provide any benefit and is still associated with the risk of toxicity.

The patient is a poor candidate for surgery, has no evidence of colonic obstruction, and would likely have considerable postoperative and healing complications with little, if any, chance of benefit.

KEY POINT

- Supportive, comfort-oriented care is appropriate for a frail patient with metastatic cancer, significant medical comorbidities, and a poor performance status.

Bibliography

Proulx K, Jacelon C. Dying with dignity: the good patient versus the good death. Am J Hosp Palliat Care. 2004 Mar-Apr;21(2):116-20. [PMID: 15055511]

Item 82   Answer: A
Educational Objective: Determine need for molecular testing in a patient with adenocarcinoma of the lung.

This patient with stage IV adenocarcinoma of the lung (based on the presence of a likely right adrenal metastasis) should undergo tumor testing for the presence of an epidermal growth factor receptor (EGFR) mutation. Because studies have documented improved survival in patients with EGFR mutations who are treated with an EGFR tyrosine kinase inhibitor (such as erlotinib, gefitinib, or afatinib), testing to identify this mutation is a key component of the initial evaluation of all patients diagnosed with metastatic nonsquamous non–small cell lung cancer (NSCLC). In patients with likely metastatic disease who might be candidates for therapy, ensuring that an adequate tissue sample is obtained (core needle biopsy at a minimum) is essential to allow for needed molecular testing.

Although K-*ras* testing can help determine the prognosis in patients with NSCLC, it is not currently considered a

routine component of evaluation because existing renin-angiotensin system inhibitors used to treat patients with this mutation have not proven to be effective.

PET scanning has a role in evaluating patients who are believed to have potentially resectable disease. However, obtaining a PET scan in a patient who clearly has metastatic disease based on CT imaging is unnecessary.

Because this patient has both a pleural effusion and a likely adrenal metastasis that would classify his disease as stage IV, he is not considered a surgical candidate.

KEY POINT

- Testing to identify an epidermal growth factor receptor (EGFR) mutation is a key component in the initial evaluation of metastatic nonsquamous non–small cell lung cancer due to improved survival in patients with EGFR mutations who are treated with EGFR tyrosine kinase inhibitors.

Bibliography

Rosell R, Carcereny E, Gervais R, et al; Spanish Lung Cancer Group in collaboration with Groupe Français de Pneumo-Cancérologie and Associazione Italiana Oncologia Toracica. Erlotinib versus standard chemotherapy as first-line treatment for European patients with advanced EGFR mutation-positive non-small-cell lung cancer (EURTAC): a multicentre, open-label, randomised phase 3 trial. Lancet Oncol. 2012 Mar;13(3):239-46. [PMID: 22285168]

Item 83   Answer: C
Educational Objective: Manage posttreatment surveillance following therapy for head and neck cancer.

Periodic oral examinations and direct laryngoscopy are indicated for this patient. Following successful treatment of localized squamous cell carcinoma of the head and neck, patients remain at risk for developing both local cancer recurrence and second primary cancers, especially cancers due to tobacco and alcohol use. Tobacco and alcohol act as chemical carcinogens and induce genetic changes in the squamous mucosa of the head and neck that are not limited to the site involved with the cancer. These genetic changes expose patients to ongoing risk for development of second primary cancers. Therefore, surveillance must be directed at identifying both locally recurrent cancer and second primary cancers elsewhere in the head and neck. This is accomplished by assessment of the primary site (for example, in this patient by direct oral examination) and periodic assessment of the remaining squamous mucosa of the head and neck via direct laryngoscopy. In addition, this patient population is at high risk for non–small cell lung cancer, which represents the most commonly diagnosed second cancer in patients with head and neck cancer. This patient also meets the general criteria for lung cancer screening with low-dose CT as she is between the ages of 55 to 74 years with a smoking history of at least 30 pack-years within 15 years of quitting. Inclusion of low-dose CT surveillance for lung cancer should therefore be discussed with any patient being treated for tobacco-related head and neck cancer.

Within the first 6 months following treatment, imaging of the primary tumor site and neck is performed to establish a baseline for future reference. Imaging techniques, including CT, MRI, PET, and ultrasonography, have been used in posttreatment surveillance for locoregional recurrence. Subsequent imaging is generally based on the presence of signs or symptoms. Biannual CT scans are not indicated, and the additional radiation poses an unnecessary danger to the patient.

Providing no posttreatment surveillance is not recommended, as this patient should be evaluated periodically for development of both locally recurrent cancer and a second primary cancer.

KEY POINT

- Posttreatment surveillance of patients with head and neck cancer should be directed toward identifying development of both locally recurrent cancer and a second primary cancer at a more distant site.

Bibliography

Chuang SC, Scelo G, Tonita JM, et al. Risk of second primary cancer among patients with head and neck cancers: A pooled analysis of 13 cancer registries. Int J Cancer. 2008 Nov 15;123(10):2390-6. [PMID: 18729183]

Item 84   Answer: C

Educational Objective: Manage ipilimumab-induced toxicity.

Initiation of high-dose intravenous glucocorticoids and aggressive supportive care in addition to discontinuing the offending medication is the most appropriate treatment for this patient with ipilimumab toxicity with severe diarrhea and evidence of autoimmune hepatitis. Ipilimumab is a new class of antineoplastic therapy that inhibits the function of T-cell checkpoint receptors (ipilimumab or PD-1 and PD-L1 inhibitors), thereby enhancing the function of the immune system and inducing remissions in patients with various solid tumors, particularly metastatic melanoma. However, T-cell checkpoint inhibitors also can cause many potentially permanent and life-threatening organ toxicities that are autoimmune-mediated based on their enhancement of immune function. These include dermatologic (rash, mucositis), gastrointestinal (diarrhea, colitis), liver (autoimmune hepatitis), and endocrine (hypothalamic/pituitary, thyroid, and adrenal insufficiency). Other organ involvement (eye, kidney, hematologic, pulmonary, and neurologic) has also been reported. Because the toxicity results from triggering an exaggerated immune response, treatment of these toxicities involves removing the causative agent and providing immunosuppression, preferably with high-dose glucocorticoids due to their nonspecific immune-suppressing effects and rapid onset of action. Recognition of the autoimmune effect of the treatment is critical since the autoimmune-triggered toxicity from this class of medications can be fatal if immunosuppressive therapy is delayed.

Because the mechanism of toxicity is not directly related to leukopenia and this patient has a normal leukocyte count with no objective evidence of infection, broad-spectrum antibiotics are not indicated, and delayed recognition of the drug-related syndrome from treatment of possible bacterial infection could be detrimental.

Similarly, because the toxicity of T-cell checkpoint inhibitors is not due to leukopenia, treatment with growth factors, such as granulocyte-macrophage colony-stimulating factor, does not have a role in either the prevention or treatment of complications associated with this class of drugs.

Because rapid immunosuppression may reverse the severe autoimmune reactions triggered by ipilimumab, discontinuation of the medication and supportive care alone is inadequate therapy for this patient.

KEY POINT

- Patients with acute ipilimumab toxicity should receive fluid replacement and immediate glucocorticoid therapy to reverse the damage this agent can cause; delay in treatment can be fatal.

Bibliography

Weber JS, O'Day S, Urba W, et al. Phase I/II study of ipilimumab for patients with metastatic melanoma. J Clin Oncol. 2008 Dec 20;26(36):5950-6. [PMID: 19018089]

Item 85   Answer: B

Educational Objective: Determine appropriate timing of prophylactic bilateral salpingo-oophorectomies for a *BRCA1* carrier.

Prophylactic bilateral salpingo-oophorectomies (BSO) by the age of 35 years is recommended for this patient. Patients with *BRCA1/2* mutations are at increased risk for ovarian cancer. The lifetime risk is 35% to 46% in *BRCA1* mutation carriers and 13% to 23% in *BRCA2* carriers. National guidelines recommend risk-reducing BSO in women who carry deleterious *BRCA1/2* mutations between ages 35 and 40 years, once childbearing is complete. A recent registry data analysis of almost 6000 women with *BRCA1* or *BRCA2* mutations proposed that risk-reducing BSO be done by age 35 years in women with *BRCA1* mutations due to a 4% risk of ovarian cancer between ages 35 and 40 years. Women with *BRCA2* mutations in this registry data did not develop ovarian cancers until after age 40 years and had an ovarian cancer risk under 1% if BSO was deferred to age 50 years.

Also shown was an 80% reduction in the risk of ovarian, tubal, or peritoneal cancer after prophylactic BSO and a 77% reduction in all-cause mortality. Previous studies have demonstrated a 48% reduction in breast cancer in *BRCA1/2* carriers who underwent prophylactic oophorectomy while premenopausal.

Hormone replacement can safely be given to healthy *BRCA1/2* carriers after BSO for relief of menopausal symptoms and preservation of bone health if nonhormonal options are not effective. Limited studies have not demonstrated an increased risk of breast cancer with hormone replacement therapy when stopped prior to the normal age of menopause.

At age 33 years, this patient will have two years to pursue further childbearing and still be able to have BSO by age 35 years. It is not necessary to recommend immediate BSO. In the study mentioned above, there was a 0.5% risk of ovarian cancer between the ages of 30 and 34 years and only one occult ovarian cancer found at prophylactic BSO during these ages.

Semi-annual transvaginal ultrasound and serum CA-125 monitoring is recommended for *BRCA1/2* mutation carriers starting at age 30 years, but the evidence shows very limited effectiveness of such screening. Prophylactic BSO is the only method that has been shown to decrease ovarian cancer mortality in women at high risk for ovarian cancer.

KEY POINT

- Risk-reducing bilateral salpingo-oophorectomies are recommended in women who carry deleterious *BRCA1* or *BRCA2* mutations between ages 35 and 40 years, once childbearing is complete.

Bibliography

Finch AP, Lubinski J, Møller P, et al. Impact of oophorectomy on cancer incidence and mortality in women with a BRCA1 or BRCA2 mutation. J Clin Oncol. 2014 May 20;32(15):1547-53. [PMID: 24567435]

Item 86   Answer: A

Educational Objective: Determine the prognosis of a patient with newly diagnosed lymphoma.

Although all of the options listed above affect the prognosis of this patient with an aggressive B-cell lymphoma, the revised International Prognostic Index score (r-IPI) correlates most strongly with his chance of overall survival after standard therapy.

Non-Hodgkin lymphoma (NHL) consists of over 20 subtypes defined by cell surface antigen expression and other morphologic features, including unique molecular profiles. The first major distinction divides NHL into three categories based on immunophenotyping to a B-cell, T-cell, or natural killer (NK) cell lineage. B-cell lymphomas account for 85% of all cases of NHL, T-cell lymphomas for 13%, and NK-cell lymphomas for 2%. A history of farming is not uncommon among newly diagnosed patients with B-cell lymphomas because components in some fertilizers are thought to be causative. Staging of lymphoma consists of structural disease assessment using physical examination findings, CT imaging, biopsy findings of potential disease sites, and disease activity assessment using PET scanning to quantify the standard uptake value. Age, concomitant infection or immunodeficiency, and expression of driver gene mutations can all influence prognoses. The Ann Arbor Staging System criteria can be used for most forms of lymphoma, however, the r-IPI score is most predictive of outcomes in patients with dif-

fuse large B-cell lymphoma. The r-IPI incorporates multiple clinical factors, including the patient's age, performance status, disease stage, degree of extranodal involvement, and serum lactate dehydrogenase level to generate a score that correlates with progression-free and overall survival after standard therapy. This patient has a high r-IPI score due to stage IV disease (bone marrow involvement), a high serum lactate dehydrogenase level, and poor performance status.

The presence of anemia and B symptoms might be indicative of aggressive disease, but are not incorporated into the r-IPI score, which is the best predictor of clinical outcome.

The presence of diabetes appears to have a minimal effect on the outcome of lymphoma and is therefore not an independent predictive factor.

KEY POINT

- The revised International Prognostic Index (r-IPI) score has the greatest influence on the prognosis in patients with diffuse large B-cell lymphoma.

Bibliography

Sehn LH, Berry B, Chhanabhai M, et al. The revised International Prognostic Index (R-IPI) is a better predictor of outcome than the standard IPI for patients with diffuse large B-cell lymphoma treated with R-CHOP. Blood. 2007 Mar 1;109(5):1857-61. [PMID: 17105812]

Item 87   Answer: B

Educational Objective: Treat advanced cervical cancer with chemoradiation therapy.

Radiation therapy and concurrent cisplatin-based chemotherapy is the most appropriate treatment for this patient who has bulky stage III cervical cancer (extending to the pelvic wall and/or involving the lower third of the vagina). Cervical cancer remains the second most common cancer in women worldwide. Early-stage cervical cancer without spread to the pelvic wall or to the lower third of the vagina can be treated successfully with surgery alone, but more locally advanced cancer requires radiation therapy instead of surgery. In 1999, based on five published randomized clinical trials, the National Cancer Institute issued a clinical alert recommending chemoradiation therapy for locally advanced cervical cancer. These initial studies used cisplatin-based chemotherapy during radiation; results showed a decrease in local and distant recurrence compared with radiation therapy alone.

Chemoradiation has since become the standard of care, and weekly cisplatin administration during radiation is the most frequently used regimen, although non–platinum-based chemotherapy regimens also have been shown to be effective. Radiation therapy alone can be used for patients with stage I (confined to the cervix) or nonbulky stage II cervical cancer (invading beyond the uterus but not to the pelvic wall or lower third of the vagina) as an alternative to hysterectomy but should be combined with chemotherapy for patients with bulky stage II, stage III, and stage IVA cervical cancers (spread to adjacent organs but no distant metastases).

Radical hysterectomy is appropriate for patients with stage I or nonbulky stage IIA cervical cancer, which includes invasion beyond the uterus but not extending to the pelvic wall or to the lower third of the vagina. However, radical hysterectomy is not an option for this patient who has bulky disease extending to the pelvic wall (stage III).

There is no benefit to using adjuvant chemotherapy after hysterectomy or to administering chemotherapy prior to surgery. The survival benefit of chemotherapy is proven only when given with concomitant radiation therapy for patients with intermediate- and high-risk cervical cancer.

Patients with stage I cervical cancer may have ovarian preservation if maintaining fertility is desired. For microscopic disease confined to the cervix (stage IA), simple hysterectomy, cone biopsy, or removal of the cervix alone are options, all of which include ovarian preservation.

KEY POINT

- Patients with locally advanced cervical cancer should be treated with radiation therapy and concomitant chemotherapy, as use of chemoradiation is associated with a decrease in local and distant cancer recurrence compared with radiation therapy alone.

Bibliography

Chemoradiotherapy for Cervical Cancer Meta-Analysis Collaboration. Reducing uncertainties about the effects of chemoradiotherapy for cervical cancer: a systematic review and meta-analysis of individual patient data from18 randomized trials. J Clin Oncol. 2008 Dec 10;26(35):5802-12. [PMID: 19001332]

Item 88   Answer: A

Educational Objective: Diagnose immunosuppression-induced non-Hodgkin lymphoma.

This patient, who presents with fixed, palpable lymphadenopathy in multiple sites and systemic B symptoms (night sweats, fever, and weight loss), most likely has non-Hodgkin lymphoma (NHL) associated with immunosuppression due to the long-term administration of infliximab. Viral infections including Epstein-Barr virus, HIV, human T-cell lymphotrophic virus type-1, and hepatitis B and C viruses are all capable of directly driving transformation of lymphoid tissue to lymphoma or contributing indirectly by causing immunodeficiency, a risk factor for lymphoma development. Specific examples include the development of posttransplant lymphoproliferative disorders presenting as high-grade B-cell NHL caused by ongoing immunosuppression with agents such as cyclosporine or tacrolimus to prevent rejection in solid organ transplantation or graft-versus-host disease in allogeneic hematopoietic stem cell transplantation. Excisional biopsy of an adequate tissue sample that preserves the architecture of the lymph node is required for the diagnosis of lymphoma.

Sarcoidosis can present with or without symptoms that include fatigue, weight loss, joint pain, cough, and shortness of breath. Sarcoidosis is believed to be a consequence of an immune reaction to an unknown antigen, and not immunosuppression.

Testicular cancer can occur late in life but usually does not present with fever and night sweats and would not likely be associated with axillary and cervical lymphadenopathy without mediastinal lymphadenopathy.

Tuberculosis occurs more commonly in patients treated with infliximab. A nonreactive tuberculin skin test cannot be used to exclude tuberculosis because of this patient's immunosuppressed state. However, his extensive extra-abdominal lymphadenopathy without mediastinal lymphadenopathy makes tuberculosis unlikely.

KEY POINT

- Patients receiving long-term immunosuppressive therapy are at greater risk for developing non-Hodgkin lymphoma.

Bibliography

Lenz G, Staudt LM. Aggressive lymphomas. N Engl J Med. 2010 Apr 15;362(15):1417-29. [PMID: 20393178]

Item 89   Answer: C

Educational Objective: Treat a patient with spinal cord compression caused by multiple myeloma.

This patient with spinal cord compression should receive immediate administration of intravenous high-dose glucocorticoids to prevent permanent neurologic deficits. This patient has MRI-confirmed spinal cord compression characterized by mid back pain and physical findings of lower extremity hyperreflexia and weakness. His known multiple myeloma with corresponding anemia and hypercalcemia suggest progression of his disease with a plasma cell tumor as the cause of his spinal cord compression. Glucocorticoid therapy is the initial treatment in most cases of malignant spinal cord compression as they decrease inflammation and reduce the mass effect due to edema associated with many tumors. In this case, glucocorticoid therapy has the added benefit of directly treating the hypercalcemia and plasma cell myeloma. Glucocorticoid treatment is then followed with more definitive therapy, often radiation and possible neurosurgical intervention in some cases.

Biopsy of the epidural mass is not necessary because of the patient's known likely causative disease and could delay initiation of glucocorticoids and radiation therapy and increase the risk of permanent nerve damage.

Although neurosurgical intervention consisting of decompressive surgery might be necessary in some patients with spinal cord compression, it would not be appropriate before administration of immediate glucocorticoids.

Definitive treatment with chemotherapy or an immunomodulator may be appropriate but would not have the required immediate effect of glucocorticoids in preventing progressive neurologic damage.

Radiation therapy alone would not address the swelling associated with spinal cord compression nor the hypercalcemia or underlying systemic plasma cell myeloma. However, radiation therapy is often a useful therapy for treating bulky disease.

KEY POINT

- Patients with cancer who develop symptoms of possible spinal cord compression require immediate administration of intravenous high-dose glucocorticoids to prevent permanent neurologic deficits.

Bibliography

Taylor JW, Schiff D. Metastatic epidural spinal cord compression. Semin Neurol. 2010 Jul;30(3):245-53. [PMID: 20577931]

Item 90   Answer: C

Educational Objective: Treat breast cancer with neoadjuvant chemotherapy in a patient who desires breast-conserving surgery.

This patient should receive neoadjuvant trastuzumab-based chemotherapy. Disease-free survival and overall survival are equivalent in patients treated with neoadjuvant and adjuvant chemotherapy. However, neoadjuvant chemotherapy may allow performance of more breast-conserving procedures by decreasing the size of the tumor. In addition, the response to neoadjuvant chemotherapy is predictive of long-term disease-free and overall survival. Cancers with the highest response rate to neoadjuvant chemotherapy are those that are either HER2 positive or triple-negative tumors (tumors that are negative for estrogen receptor, progesterone receptor, and HER2 amplification). Patients with these types of cancer can be offered neoadjuvant chemotherapy even if decreasing the tumor size in order to perform breast-conserving surgery is not needed. After neoadjuvant chemotherapy, pathologic complete response, defined as the absence of any residual invasive cancer in the breast or lymph nodes, occurs in up to 60% of patients with HER2-positive cancers and up to 40% of those with triple-negative cancers and correlates with an excellent long-term disease-free survival.

The regimens used for neoadjuvant chemotherapy are generally the same as those used for postoperative adjuvant chemotherapy. Patients are closely monitored with breast exams during neoadjuvant chemotherapy to make sure they are responding. Unless a patient has tumor progression or is on a clinical trial assessing the response of a new regimen, all of the chemotherapy is usually completed before surgery. A patient with a HER2-positive cancer would receive trastuzumab during the nonanthracycline part of adjuvant chemotherapy, receiving 1 year of trastuzumab in total. Trastuzumab-containing regimens without anthracyclines are an option, particularly for women with a higher risk of cardiomyopathy because of older age or pre-existing hypertension. Pertuzumab is a newly approved anti-HER2 monoclonal antibody that may be used with trastuzumab and

chemotherapy for neoadjuvant treatment of HER2-amplified breast cancers that measure 2 cm or more and/or are sentinel lymph node positive. The NeoSphere study demonstrated improved pathologic complete response rates (46% vs 29%) when pertuzumab was added to trastuzumab and docetaxel for HER2-amplified breast cancers with these higher risk features.

Immediate mastectomy is not required for this patient, who desires breast conservation and is likely to achieve this goal with neoadjuvant chemotherapy.

Neoadjuvant antiestrogen therapy (for example, with anastrozole) is an option for postmenopausal women with large or locally advanced breast cancers that are hormone receptor positive, particularly patients who are not good candidates for adjuvant chemotherapy because of advanced age or medical comorbidities. However, this therapy is not effective in patients with estrogen receptor–negative cancers.

As this patient does not have any worrisome symptoms or signs suggestive of systemic metastases, she does not need CT or bone scans for staging. Current American Society of Clinical Oncology (ASCO) guidelines recommend against performing PET, CT, or radionuclide bone scans in patients with stages 0 to II breast cancer in the absence of findings that would suggest metastatic disease.

KEY POINT

- Neoadjuvant chemotherapy may be indicated for patients with HER2-amplified or triple-negative breast cancers and for patients with larger cancers who desire breast-conserving surgery.

Bibliography

Kaufmann M, Hortobagyi GN, Goldhirsch A, et al. Recommendations from an international expert panel on the use of neoadjuvant (primary) systemic treatment of operable breast cancer: an update. J Clin Oncol. 2006 Apr 20;24(12):1940-9. Erratum in: J Clin Oncol. 2006 Jul 1;24(19):3221. [PMID: 16622270]

Item 91   Answer: A

Educational Objective: Treat metastatic estrogen receptor–positive breast cancer that involves only bone.

Because this patient's metastases involve only bone, her cancer is estrogen receptor positive, and she has had a long disease-free interval, she has a high likelihood of responding to primary antiestrogen therapy with anastrozole. Other aromatase inhibitors such as letrozole or exemestane would be equally effective. Aromatase inhibitors are superior to tamoxifen for first-line treatment of metastatic breast cancer because of improved response rates and disease-free survival. If she becomes resistant to aromatase inhibitor therapy, everolimus is a mammalian target of rapamycin (mTOR) inhibitor that is approved for treatment of metastatic breast cancer in combination with exemestane. If she responds to anastrozole and subsequently develops progressive disease, other antiestrogen agents, including tamoxifen and fulvestrant, could be used sequentially.

Chemotherapy with agents such as paclitaxel is used instead of antiestrogen therapy for treatment of metastatic breast cancer in patients with hormone receptor–negative disease, those with an impending visceral crisis due to extensive metastases, or those who do not respond to anti-estrogen therapy.

Radiation to symptomatic areas of bone metastases is an important palliative treatment. However, patients with asymptomatic or minimally symptomatic bone lesions are not treated with radiation therapy unless bone stability is a concern.

Radium-223 is an alpha particle–emitting isotope that targets bone metastases. It is only used in bone metastases due to castrate-resistant prostate cancer.

KEY POINT

- Patients with estrogen receptor–positive breast cancer who develop metastases limited to bone after a long disease-free interval should be treated initially with an aromatase inhibitor.

Bibliography

Glück S. Extending the clinical benefit of endocrine therapy for women with hormone receptor-positive metastatic breast cancer: differentiating mechanisms of action. Clin Breast Cancer. 2014 Apr;14(2):75-84. [PMID: 24355138]

Item 92   Answer: A

Educational Objective: Prevent breast cancer in a patient with atypical ductal hyperplasia.

This patient with atypical ductal hyperplasia (ADH) should be offered breast cancer chemoprophylaxis, with exemestane being the most effective agent for postmenopausal women. ADH is a breast lesion associated with an increased risk of development of breast cancer. Studies have shown a three- to fivefold increased risk of breast cancer after a diagnosis of ADH, with a cumulative incidence at 30 years of 35%. Patients with ADH are candidates for breast cancer chemoprophylaxis. Among the available chemoprophylactic agents, exemestane is associated with the greatest reduction in breast cancer risk. Exemestane is an aromatase inhibitor that prevents conversion of androgens to estrogens and profoundly suppresses estrogen levels in postmenopausal women. The National Cancer Institute of Canada's Exemestane Prophylaxis Study compared administration of exemestane for 5 years with administration of placebo for the same period in patients with a 5-year risk of breast cancer of at least 1.67%. Patients with ADH were included in this study. At a median follow-up of 3 years, there was a 65% relative reduction in the annual incidence of invasive breast cancer in patients taking exemestane. Toxicities included a low incidence of grade 3 arthralgia and hot flushes. There was no difference in the incidence of skeletal fractures or development of osteoporosis, cardiovascular events, or other cancers in patients taking either exemestane or placebo.

Alternate chemoprophylaxis options include tamoxifen and raloxifene. Tamoxifen decreases the risk of breast cancer by 49% though it has a 0.1% risk per year of endometrial cancer and a 1% risk of vascular events including venous thrombosis and strokes. Raloxifene does not increase the risk of endometrial cancer and has a 25% lower risk of vascular events. It is less effective than tamoxifen, retaining 76% of the benefit of tamoxifen, but is an option in patients who want to decrease toxicities. All three chemoprophylaxis agents (tamoxifen, raloxifene, and exemestane) can be used in postmenopausal women but only tamoxifen is an option in premenopausal or perimenopausal women.

Vitamin D supplementation is being studied for breast cancer prevention, but any benefits are currently unclear. Some studies have shown a mild decrease in breast cancer risk in persons with normal serum vitamin D levels compared with those having low levels, whereas other studies have found no benefit.

Bilateral prophylactic mastectomy is an option for women with a high risk of breast cancer due to inherited syndromes, such as women with *BRCA1/2* mutations, but is not appropriate for women with atypical lesions such as atypical hyperplasia or lobular neoplasia.

Continuing hormone replacement therapy will increase the risk of breast cancer and prevent chemoprophylactic medications such as tamoxifen, raloxifene, and exemestane from decreasing this risk.

KEY POINT

- Patients with newly diagnosed atypical ductal hyperplasia should be offered breast cancer chemoprophylaxis; exemestane is associated with the greatest reduction in breast cancer risk.

Bibliography

Goss PE, Ingle JN, Alés-Martínez JE, et al; NCIC CTG MAP.3 Study Investigators. Exemestane for breast-cancer prevention in postmenopausal women. N Engl J Med. 2011 Jun 23;364(25):2381-91. Erratum in: N Engl J Med. 2011 Oct 6;365(14):1361. [PMID: 21639806]

Item 93   Answer: A

Educational Objective: Manage postoperative surveillance for a patient with stage III colon cancer.

This patient has completed therapy for high-risk stage III colon cancer, and postoperative surveillance should include physical examination and serum carcinoembryonic antigen measurement every 3 to 6 months, as well as CT scans of the chest and abdomen (and pelvis for patients with rectal cancer) annually for 3 to 5 years. Colonoscopy, if done pre-operatively, should be performed 1 year after resection and then repeated at 3- to 5-year intervals. Because this patient was unable to undergo colonoscopy preoperatively, this procedure should be performed initially 6 months after surgery. Postoperative surveillance is done to identify patients with relapse of colorectal cancer that is potentially curable by surgery. The risks of radiation exposure and false-positive findings leading to additional tests and possibly invasive procedures must be balanced against the benefits of surveillance studies.

Routine CT scans annually for 10 years is not indicated because most colorectal cancers recur within the first 3 years after surgery, and scanning beyond 3 to 5 years is therefore not warranted.

PET scans may be useful adjuncts to evaluate equivocal abnormalities seen on CT scans; however, they are not recommended for routine surveillance following resection of colorectal cancer and should not be used for this purpose.

A 2007 Cochrane review of follow-up strategies for patients treated for nonmetastatic colorectal cancer concluded that there is an overall survival benefit by intensifying the follow-up of patients after curative surgery, but because of the wide variations in follow-up programs included in the analysis, no conclusion could be drawn about the best combination and frequency of procedures and tests to maximize benefits and minimize harms. However, the results of this review imply that some intensity of surveillance is more beneficial than observation alone.

KEY POINT

- Postoperative surveillance for patients with colorectal cancer includes physical examination and serum carcinoembryonic antigen measurement every 3 to 6 months, and CT scans of the chest and abdomen (and pelvis for patients with rectal cancer) annually for 3 to 5 years; colonoscopy, if done preoperatively, should be performed 1 year after resection and then repeated at 3- to 5-year intervals.

Bibliography

Meyerhardt JA, Mangu PB, Flynn PJ, et al; American Society of Clinical Oncology. Follow-up care, surveillance protocol, and secondary prevention measures for survivors of colorectal cancer: American Society of Clinical Oncology clinical practice guideline endorsement. J Clin Oncol. 2013 Dec 10;31(35):4465-70. [PMID: 24220554]

Item 94   Answer: B

Educational Objective: Recognize the risk of treatment-related complications following therapy for testicular cancer.

This patient is most likely to develop metabolic syndrome. Following treatment of testicular germ cell tumors, men remain at risk for both recurrent cancer and many other long-term medical complications. Although some complications occur during or soon after treatment, others develop years after initial therapy, particularly as many patients are relatively young at the time of diagnosis. The risks for an individual patient are associated with the type of treatment given. Both radiation therapy and chemotherapy are associated with specific risks. Among these is an increased risk for development of metabolic syndrome (insulin resistance, hypertension, dyslipidemia, abdominal obesity). The risk is particularly increased in men treated with combination chemotherapy. Data indicate that the risk for cardiovascular diseases (such as ischemic coronary disease, heart failure, peripheral vascular disease) is also increased in this patient population. Additional risks associated with treat-

ment of testicular cancer that would be relevant to this specific patient include kidney disease, peripheral neuropathy, chronic pulmonary toxicity, secondary malignancy, and sexual dysfunction. Most of these would be evident either during or soon after completion of treatment. Secondary malignancy typically develops years following treatment.

The risk of gastric and duodenal ulcer disease is increased slightly in men treated with radiation therapy, which this patient did not have.

Obstructive uropathy is only rarely associated with treatment of testicular cancer, and that association occurs only in men treated with radiation therapy.

The risk of secondary solid tumors is increased in patients treated for testicular cancer, with the most common sites of involvement being the lung, colon, bladder, pancreas, and stomach. Soft tissue sarcomas are not commonly reported in these patients in the absence of radiotherapy, which is known to increase the risk of soft tissue sarcoma, typically diagnosed many years after treatment. As the patient in this case was not treated with radiation, he would not be expected to have an increased risk of soft tissue sarcoma.

KEY POINT

- Treatment-related complications in men who had therapy for testicular cancer include cardiovascular disease (specifically metabolic syndrome), kidney disease, peripheral neuropathy, chronic pulmonary toxicity, secondary malignancy, and sexual dysfunction.

Bibliography

Willemse PM, Burggraaf J, Hamdy NA, et al. Prevalence of the metabolic syndrome and cardiovascular disease risk in chemotherapy-treated testicular germ cell tumour survivors. Br J Cancer. 2013 Jul 9;109(1):295-6. Erratum in: Br J Cancer. 2013 Jul 9;109(1):295-6. [PMID: 23660945]

Item 95   Answer: D

Educational Objective: Treat diffuse large B-cell lymphoma with rituximab plus cyclophosphamide, doxorubicin, vincristine, and prednisone (R-CHOP).

Standard therapy for all patients with diffuse large B-cell lymphoma (DLBCL), regardless of disease stage or prognosis, includes rituximab plus cyclophosphamide, doxorubicin, vincristine, and prednisone (R-CHOP). Acceptable management includes chemotherapy alone or a shorter course of chemotherapy with involved-field radiation in early stage disease. The lymphomas are of B-cell or T-cell phenotype. DLBCL is the most common form of lymphoma and, together with the less common T-cell phenotype, represents 30% of all lymphomas. Most patients with DLBCL present with advanced (stage III and IV) disease and have symptoms including fever, night sweats, and weight loss ("B" symptoms). Disease progression is rapid without therapy. The revised International Prognostic Index (r-IPI) score was developed to assist in determining prognosis before therapy. The r-IPI score is based on the patient's age, serum lactate dehydrogenase level, number of extranodal sites, disease stage, and performance status.

Because this patient has limited disease and a low r-IPI score, standard R-CHOP chemotherapy should result in a durable complete remission. Expected cure rates range from less than 20% for patients with advanced disease and a high r-IPI score to greater than 80% for those with localized disease and a low r-IPI score. Studies are ongoing regarding the effectiveness of more aggressive initial therapy for patients with advanced disease associated with high r-IPI scores, such as using rituximab plus hyperfractionated cyclophosphamide, vincristine, doxorubicin, and dexamethasone (R-hyper-CVAD) and adding novel agents, including immunomodulators such as lenalidomide. However, standard R-CHOP chemotherapy is appropriate for this patient at this time.

Allogeneic hematopoietic stem cell transplantation (HSCT) remains investigational as salvage therapy for patients with DLBCL due to the high risk of morbidity.

Autologous HSCT is reserved as salvage therapy for patients who have chemotherapy-sensitive relapsed disease associated with a greater than 1-year disease-free interval from the start of initial therapy. Early relapse patients have poor outcomes after autologous HSPCT and should be considered for clinical trials.

Involved-field radiation therapy is indicated for patients with bulky disease. This patient has no evidence of bulky disease at this time.

KEY POINT

- Standard therapy for all patients with diffuse large B-cell lymphoma, regardless of disease stage or prognosis, is rituximab plus cyclophosphamide, doxorubicin, vincristine, and prednisone (R-CHOP).

Bibliography

Martelli M, Ferreri AJ, Agostinelli C, Di Rocco A, Pfreundschuh M, Pileri SA. Diffuse large B-cell lymphoma. Crit Rev Oncol Hematol. 2013 Aug;87(2):146-71. [PMID: 23375551]

Item 96   Answer: A

Educational Objective: Manage metastatic melanoma with *BRAF* V600 mutation analysis.

The most appropriate next step in management is *BRAF* V600 mutation analysis. Approximately 50% to 70% of cutaneous melanomas carry mutations in *BRAF*, a gene coding for a protein that leads to tumor activation though the mitogen-activated protein kinase (MAPK) pathway; 80% to 90% of these are the V600E mutation, with the remainder being other mutations at the V600 position. Inhibitors of *BRAF* are associated with response rates of over 50% and improved overall and progression-free survival in metastatic melanoma with a V600 mutation. Therefore, all patients with metastatic melanoma should have their tumor tested for the presence of driver V600 *BRAF* mutation to determine whether treatment with a *BRAF* inhibitor is a therapeutic option. Vemurafenib and dabrafenib are the available *BRAF* inhibitors. These agents have a rapid onset of action and are preferred over immunotherapy for initial treatment in patients with poor risk

characteristics, including visceral metastases to sites other than the lung, an elevated serum lactate dehydrogenase, or a poor performance status. If a V600 mutation is present in this patient with liver metastases and an elevated serum lactate dehydrogenase, treatment with a *BRAF* inhibitor should be offered as a treatment option.

Chemotherapy with dacarbazine, the only chemotherapeutic agent approved for treatment of metastatic melanoma, has a response rate of only 7% to 12% and has not been shown to improve overall survival. It is usually reserved for patients who are not candidates for high-dose interleukin-2 (IL-2), ipilimumab, or *BRAF* inhibitor therapy.

High-dose interferon alfa is used as adjuvant therapy for patients with nonmetastatic melanoma who are at high risk for recurrence but is inferior to other immunotherapy options, including ipilimumab and high-dose IL-2, for patients with metastatic melanoma.

Ipilimumab is a monoclonal antibody that targets cytotoxic T-lymphocyte antigen-4 (CTLA-4), which is a normal immune checkpoint molecule that down-regulates pathways of T-cell activation. CTLA-4 inhibition unleashes an immune response against the tumor. In patients with metastatic melanoma, treatment with ipilimumab improves overall survival. However, the response to ipilimumab can be delayed and there can be transient worsening of disease initially. In patients with poor prognostic features and a *BRAF* V600 mutation, the more rapid response of a *BRAF* inhibitor is preferred. If this patient's melanoma does not have a driver *BRAF* mutation, then treatment with ipilimumab would be offered.

KEY POINT

- All patients with metastatic melanoma should have their tumor tested for the presence of a driver V600 *BRAF* mutation. If this mutation is present in patients with poor prognostic features, treatment with a *BRAF* inhibitor is recommended as initial therapy.

Bibliography

Sosman JA, Kim KB, Schuchter L, et al. Survival in BRAF V600-mutant advanced melanoma treated with vemurafenib. N Engl J Med. 2012 Feb 23;366(8):707-14. [PMID: 22356324]

Item 97   Answer: E

Educational Objective: Treat oligometastatic colorectal cancer by surgical resection.

Right hepatectomy is most appropriate for this patient who underwent primary resection for stage II colon cancer 3 years ago and now has three new liver lesions in a surgically resectable pattern. The role of monitoring patients after initial resection is to detect recurrent, surgically curable tumors, such as oligometastatic liver or lung metastases, and monitor for the development of new primary cancer. Monitoring typically includes a physical examination and measurement of serum carcinoembryonic antigen levels every 3 to 6 months for the first 3 years and every 6 months during years 4 and 5. Surveillance CT scans of the chest and abdomen are recommended annually for at least the first 3 years postoperatively. This patient has oligometastatic disease that is potentially curable by surgical resection and should undergo right hepatectomy.

A needle biopsy is not indicated. The clinical presentation is so strongly indicative of metastatic colorectal cancer that a negative needle biopsy would not exclude the diagnosis of cancer and would therefore not alter management. Surgical resection would be warranted regardless of the biopsy results.

Hepatic artery embolization is a palliative technique used to treat patients with more vascular tumors, such as hepatocellular carcinoma and neuroendocrine tumors. It is not routinely used for treatment of metastatic colorectal cancer and would not be an appropriate consideration when a potentially curative alternative such as surgery is available.

Given that this patient's liver metastases are potentially curable, palliative chemotherapy is not indicated.

Radiation therapy is not routinely used to treat liver metastases and would also not be an appropriate consideration for a patient who is a candidate for potentially curative surgery.

KEY POINT

- The development of oligometastatic disease (usually to the liver or lung) in a patient who previously was treated for colorectal cancer is potentially curable by surgical resection.

Bibliography

Johnston FM, Mavros MN, Herman JM, Pawlik TM. Local therapies for hepatic metastases. J Natl Compr Canc Netw. 2013 Feb 1;11(2):153-60. [PMID: 23411382]

Item 98   Answer: C

Educational Objective: Determine preoperative staging for a patient with newly diagnosed colorectal cancer.

Contrast-enhanced CT scanning of the chest, abdomen, and pelvis is the preferred study for preoperative staging of patients with newly diagnosed colorectal cancer. This provides the most reliable means of detecting the presence of metastatic disease to the lungs, liver, intra-abdominal lymph nodes, and peritoneum, which are the most common sites of metastatic spread, and is useful in planning appropriate therapy.

A bone scan is not indicated at this time. Although bone metastases may be present in patients with several other types of cancer at presentation, this finding is extremely rare in patients with newly diagnosed colorectal cancer. Up to 10% of patients with colorectal cancer may develop bone metastases as a late complication of advanced metastatic disease, but evaluation at the time of diagnosis in the absence of specific and compelling symptoms is not warranted.

CT colonography appears to be an acceptable alternative to colonoscopy for screening of otherwise low-risk healthy individuals; however, this study is not part of the staging work-up for a patient with a known cancer diagnosis.

PET/CT scans have not been shown to improve the accuracy of preoperative staging for patients with colorectal cancer and are not recommended for either preoperative staging or postoperative surveillance.

KEY POINT

- Contrast-enhanced CT scanning of the chest, abdomen, and pelvis is the preferred study for preoperative staging of patients with newly diagnosed colorectal cancer.

Bibliography

Meyerhardt JA, Mangu PB, Flynn PJ, et al; American Society of Clinical Oncology. Follow-up care, surveillance protocol, and secondary prevention measures for survivors of colorectal cancer: American Society of Clinical Oncology clinical practice guideline endorsement. J Clin Oncol. 2013 Dec 10;31(35):4465-70. [PMID: 24220554]

Item 99   Answer: B

Educational Objective: Treat acute tumor lysis syndrome with high-volume normal saline hydration and rasburicase.

This patient requires treatment with high-volume normal saline and rasburicase because he has spontaneous tumor lysis syndrome triggered by rapid cell turnover from his acute myelogenous leukemia. Malignancies associated with rapid cell turnover can release large quantities of electrolytes and procoagulants into the circulation, causing the potentially life-threatening complication of tumor lysis syndrome. Tumor lysis syndrome may occur spontaneously with some cancers, but most often occurs after the initiation of cytotoxic therapy for tumors with a high proliferative rate, large tumor burden, or high sensitivity to cytotoxic agents. Therefore, treatment aimed at preventing tumor lysis syndrome should be considered prior to starting chemotherapy in patients at high risk. In tumor lysis syndrome, rapid cell breakdown results in hyperkalemia, hyperphosphatemia, hyperuricemia, hypocalcemia, and disseminated intravascular coagulation (DIC). Hyperuricemia can lead to urate nephropathy and acute kidney injury. Prevention or treatment involves aggressive hydration with normal saline to maintain renal perfusion and minimize uric acid or calcium phosphate deposition in the renal tubules. Because this patient already has evidence of kidney failure, hydration must be undertaken carefully to prevent significant volume overload. Hypouricemic agents are also indicated. Allopurinol is a competitive inhibitor of xanthine oxidase, which decreases the formation of new uric acid. Rasburicase is a urate oxidase (uricase) that catalyzes the breakdown of existing uric acid. Allopurinol is typically used in patients for prophylaxis for tumor lysis syndrome and in those without existing significant (>8 mg/dL [0.47 mmol/L]) elevations of serum urate. The more expensive rasburicase is usually used in patients with significantly elevated serum urate levels or in those with baseline kidney failure or in those with

CONT.

evidence of kidney injury related to tumor lysis, in order to rapidly decrease the serum urate level.

Fresh frozen plasma may be indicated if the patient develops DIC after initiating chemotherapy with resultant depletion of procoagulant. However, fresh frozen plasma would not treat tumor lysis syndrome and is only indicated when DIC is present. Based on this patient's normal serum fibrinogen level, this patient does not have DIC.

The initiation of multiagent chemotherapy prior to aggressive hydration and treatment with rasburicase is contraindicated in this patient who has acute kidney failure, likely due to tumor lysis syndrome, to prevent life threatening electrolyte abnormalities (such as hyperkalemia) associated with chemotherapy.

Platelet transfusions are indicated only for patients whose platelet count is less than 10,000/μL (10×10^9/L) or who develop spontaneous bleeding.

KEY POINT

- Patients with spontaneous tumor lysis syndrome in the setting of newly diagnosed leukemia or lymphoma should be emergently treated with high-volume normal saline prior to initiation of chemotherapy; rasburicase should also be administered in the case of kidney failure.

Bibliography

Rampello E, Fricia T, Malaguarnera M. The management of tumor lysis syndrome. Nat Clin Pract Oncol. 2006 Aug;3(8):438-47. [PMID: 16894389]

Item 100   Answer: C

Educational Objective: Manage preservation of fertility in a patient about to start chemotherapy for stage II breast cancer.

Embryo cryopreservation or other fertility preservation methods before chemotherapy should be recommended to this patient who wishes to have additional children. She has stage II breast cancer that is hormone receptor positive and *HER2* positive. Adjuvant chemotherapy with trastuzumab should be started within 4 to 6 weeks of surgery. Although infertility effects of chemotherapy are age-, dose-, and drug-dependent, with younger women being affected less often than older women, patients of any age can become infertile, particularly after taking cyclophosphamide. Starting adjuvant chemotherapy and trastuzumab now will result in infertility in a significant percentage of women and is not the best option for this patient who desires continued fertility.

Fertility preservation is almost always done with the assistance of a fertility specialist with expertise in fertility preservation procedures and can usually be completed within a few weeks. An established fertility preservation option for a woman with a partner is in vitro fertilization with embryo freezing. Newer options, often done as part of clinical trials, include freezing of unfertilized eggs and ovarian cryopreservation with future reimplantation.

Trastuzumab does not cause infertility. It is the chemotherapy itself that can result in premature menopause and infertility. Adding trastuzumab to chemotherapy as adjuvant treatment for *HER2*-positive breast cancer decreases the risk of recurrence by 50% and should be included in this patient's adjuvant regimen.

Delaying chemotherapy until after the patient completes further childbearing will result in a higher risk of distant recurrence and is not a safe option. Studies evaluating the ideal sequence of adjuvant chemotherapy and primary breast radiation showed that giving chemotherapy after radiation was associated with a higher risk of systemic recurrence. Based on these studies, a delay of more than 12 weeks in starting adjuvant chemotherapy may be detrimental and should be avoided.

There is no reason to recommend against future pregnancies in this patient. Several large retrospective studies have shown that breast cancer recurrence is not increased and survival is not decreased in breast cancer survivors who become pregnant, including patients with hormone receptor–positive cancers.

KEY POINT

- Women being treated for breast cancer who wish to preserve fertility should be referred to a fertility specialist to discuss embryo cryopreservation or other fertility preservation methods before adjuvant chemotherapy is initiated.

Bibliography

Loren AW, Mangu PB, Beck LN, et al; American Society of Clinical Oncology. Fertility preservation for patients with cancer: American Society of Clinical Oncology clinical practice guideline update. J Clin Oncol. 2013 Jul 1;31(19):2500-10. [PMID: 23715580]

Item 101   Answer: A

Educational Objective: Treat adenocarcinoma of unknown primary site predominantly below the diaphragm in the same manner as a gastrointestinal malignancy.

This patient should be treated for a gastrointestinal malignancy. He has a moderately differentiated adenocarcinoma of unknown primary site, with most of the disease occurring below the diaphragm. When adenocarcinoma of unknown primary site presents in a pattern predominantly below the diaphragm, even when upper endoscopy and colonoscopy findings are normal, empiric treatment for a gastrointestinal malignancy is appropriate.

Platinum-based chemotherapy regimens such as carboplatin plus paclitaxel or cisplatin plus etoposide would be reasonable for treating patients with a poorly differentiated cancer of unknown primary site (CUP), such as a germ cell (testicular) tumor. This patient's biopsy findings, which show adenocarcinoma with moderately differentiated histology, do not support empiric treatment for germ cell cancer.

Answers and Critiques

Empiric lung cancer regimens may be used to treat patients with CUP occurring above the diaphragm. Because this patient has no evidence of involvement of the lungs, treatment using a lung cancer paradigm is not indicated.

Platinum-based chemotherapy regimens such as carboplatin plus paclitaxel or cisplatin plus etoposide would be reasonable for treating patients with a poorly differentiated neuroendocrine CUP. However, this patient's biopsy findings do not support a diagnosis of neuroendocrine cancer.

Antiandrogen therapy, which may have potential activity against prostate cancer, may be considered in male patients with extensive bone metastases, but that is not the case in this patient.

KEY POINT

- When adenocarcinoma of unknown primary site presents in a pattern predominantly below the diaphragm, even when upper endoscopy and colonoscopy findings are normal, empiric treatment for a gastrointestinal malignancy is appropriate.

Bibliography

Petrakis D, Pentheroudakis G, Voulgaris E, Pavlidis N. Prognostication in cancer of unknown primary (CUP): development of a prognostic algorithm in 311 cases and review of the literature. Cancer Treat Rev. 2013 Nov;39(7):701-8. [PMID: 23566573]

Item 102   Answer: E

Educational Objective: Treat a patient with asymptomatic, nonbulky follicular lymphoma.

Observation is most appropriate for this 60-year-old asymptomatic patient with follicular lymphoma who has nonbulky disease, no vital organ involvement or impingement, and a normal complete blood count. Follicular lymphoma accounts for 20% of all cases of non-Hodgkin lymphoma (NHL) in the United States and Europe and 70% of all indolent NHL, ranking second in incidence to diffuse large-cell lymphoma (30%). It is characterized by surface B-cell markers (CD10, 19, 20, and 22) and small cells on morphologic analysis. The incidence increases with age, and the median age at presentation is 60 years. There is no sex predilection. Diagnosis is confirmed by biopsy of palpable lymph nodes and cytogenetic studies showing a translocation [t(11:18)] that causes overexpression of the *BCL2* oncogene. Therapy is not curative, and early initiation of treatment does not improve survival in patients with grade 1 and 2 follicular lymphoma. Treatment is therefore withheld until patients become symptomatic. Some patients do not require therapy for several decades after the initial diagnosis.

Lenalidomide, used in combination with rituximab, is a new therapy that may be effective for patients with advanced symptomatic disease, which this patient does not have.

Systemic disease–causing symptoms require multiagent therapy that traditionally includes one of three combinations: (1) rituximab plus cyclophosphamide, doxorubicin, vincristine, and prednisone (R-CHOP); (2) rituximab plus cyclophosphamide, vincristine, and prednisone (R-CVP); or (3) rituximab plus bendamustine. Radioimmunoconjugates (tositumomab and ibritumomab) have been used effectively to induce long-term remissions. Any of these approaches are suitable for patients requiring treatment.

Lymphoma causing localized symptoms can be treated effectively with involved-field radiation therapy in combination with rituximab, but such treatment is not yet needed for this patient.

KEY POINT

- Early treatment does not improve survival in patients with grade 1 and 2 follicular lymphoma.

Bibliography

Li ZM, Ghielmini M, Moccia AA. Managing newly diagnosed follicular lymphoma: state of the art and future perspectives. Expert Rev Anticancer Ther. 2013 Mar;13(3):313-25. [PMID: 23477518]

Item 103   Answer: B

Educational Objective: Diagnose human papillomavirus infection in a patient with head and neck cancer.

The most appropriate study to perform next in this patient is p16 immunohistochemistry testing. Although most squamous cell carcinomas of the head and neck were previously thought to be related primarily to tobacco and alcohol exposure, very recently, the important causative role played by human papillomavirus (HPV) has been widely recognized. HPV infection has definitively been associated with squamous cell carcinoma of the cervix for some time, and currently, it is estimated that most oropharyngeal cancers in North America and Europe are also linked to this infection. Evidence of underlying HPV infection is identified by testing for p16, which is a viral protein found in cancers that arise as a result of HPV infection. Although identifying evidence of HPV infection does not yet influence treatment decision-making, it does provide very important information regarding prognosis. The cure rate for locally advanced cancers that are linked with HPV is markedly higher than for those not linked with this virus. Because of this difference, testing for HPV is now a widely accepted intervention for any patient diagnosed with squamous cell carcinoma of the head and neck, particularly for patients with an oropharyngeal primary tumor.

A bone scan has no role in the management of this patient, as PET/CT scans have already been done. In addition, she has no indications for underlying bone metastasis based on her history.

MRI of the brain is not indicated because occult central nervous system metastases are very rare in patients with head and neck cancer, and this patient has no clinical indication of underlying brain metastasis.

Biopsy of the enlarged right cervical lymph node would provide no additional information, as the diagnosis has already been established based on biopsy of the lesion at the base of the tongue. Furthermore, because the cervical lymph node is so markedly enlarged, biopsy is not needed to establish involvement.

KEY POINT

- p16 immunohistochemistry testing to detect human papillomavirus is now a widely accepted standard-of-care intervention to help determine prognosis in patients with squamous cell carcinoma of the head and neck, particularly those with oropharyngeal primary tumors.

Bibliography

Gillison ML, D'Souza G, Westra W, et al. Distinct risk factor profiles for human papillomavirus type 16-positive and human papillomavirus type 16-negative head and neck cancers. J Natl Cancer Inst. 2008 Mar 19;100(6):407-20. [PMID: 18334711]

Item 104   Answer: A

Educational Objective: **Manage a patient with lung cancer and superior vena cava syndrome.**

Biopsy of the lung mass to obtain a histologic diagnosis is indicated. This patient has superior vena cava (SVC) syndrome, which is caused by inhibition of blood flow through the SVC or one of its major tributaries. The syndrome may occur in patients with both malignant and nonmalignant conditions. Cancers more commonly associated with SVC syndrome include lung cancer (both small cell and non–small cell lung cancer accounting for 65% of cases), aggressive lymphoma, thymoma, and primary mediastinal germ cell tumors. Nonmalignant causes include thrombosis and fibrosing mediastinitis. Presenting symptoms typically develop over weeks and include dyspnea, facial swelling, headache, and in more severe cases, stridor or mental status changes. The most common radiographic findings include mediastinal widening and pleural effusion; however, 16% of patients have a normal chest radiograph. Although in the past emphasis was placed on immediate treatment, current management emphasizes the importance of obtaining a histologic diagnosis, whenever possible, in patients with apparent malignant SVC syndrome. This allows for accurate decision-making regarding treatment of the underlying malignancy. Mediastinoscopy is routinely used to obtain tissue biopsy samples for histologic diagnosis. The complication rate from this procedure is only 5% in patients with SVC syndrome. Percutaneous transthoracic CT-guided needle biopsy appears to be a safe alternative to mediastinoscopy and has a sensitivity of 75%.

Although the patient clearly has SVC syndrome, he does not have stridor, laryngeal edema, or mental status decline. Immediate radiation therapy or stent placement is therefore not indicated.

Venography to identify a possible thrombosis is not indicated because the SVC syndrome in this patient is caused by external compression from a mediastinal mass and lymphadenopathy rather than by a thrombotic disorder.

KEY POINT

- In patients with apparent malignant superior vena cava syndrome, a histologic diagnosis should be established, whenever possible, before treatment is begun.

Bibliography

Kvale PA, Selecky PA, Prakash UB; American College of Chest Physicians. Palliative care in lung cancer: ACCP evidence-based clinical practice guidelines (2nd edition). Chest. 2007 Sep;132(3 Suppl):368S-403S. [PMID: 17873181]

Item 105   Answer: D

Educational Objective: **Manage aromatase inhibitor arthralgia in a patient with aggressive breast cancer who requires antiestrogen therapy.**

This patient should be started on tamoxifen. She has aggressive stage IIIA breast cancer with four positive axillary lymph nodes. With adjuvant chemotherapy alone, she remains at high risk for recurrence and should receive at least 5 years of antiestrogen therapy, ideally with at least 2 years of an aromatase inhibitor, if tolerated. As aromatase inhibitors may be associated with debilitating musculoskeletal symptoms, such as arthralgia in this patient, these agents should be discontinued if patients cannot tolerate them and tamoxifen should be started as an alternative antiestrogen therapy.

Approximately one third of patients taking aromatase inhibitors develop intolerable adverse effects that lead to discontinuation of these agents. In one study, 22% of all patients stopped taking these drugs following development of the aromatase inhibitor–induced arthralgia syndrome (AIIAS). Predictors of AIIAS include younger age, prior taxane chemotherapy, and a history of pre-existing joint pain. The cause of the musculoskeletal symptoms, which can occur in the upper or lower extremities, is unknown. This patient's symptoms of joint pain that are symmetric, bilateral, and worse when lying down or sitting are very typical of AIIAS.

Her symptoms are not concerning for metastases, especially because the arthralgia resolved when aromatase inhibitors were discontinued. Therefore, a PET scan is not indicated at this time.

For patients whose aromatase inhibitor–induced arthralgia does not respond to NSAIDs, treatment with duloxetine has been of benefit in clinical trials and is under further study. There is no known benefit to using prednisone for AIIAS. The Hormones and Physical Exercise (HOPE) trial showed that a regular exercise program can ameliorate arthralgia caused by aromatase inhibitors.

Restarting anastrozole will almost certainly cause the same intolerable arthralgia and is therefore not indicated. In one prospective trial of patients with AIIAS, stopping the initial aromatase inhibitor for 2 to 8 weeks and then switching to an alternate aromatase inhibitor resulted in 40% of patients being able to continue with the alternate agent. No studies to date support recommending a third attempt at use of aromatase inhibitor therapy.

KEY POINT

- In patients with aggressive breast cancer who develop severe arthralgia while on antiestrogen therapy due to an aromatase inhibitor, a second aromatase inhibitor should be tried; if the arthralgia fails to resolve, tamoxifen should be started.

Bibliography

Henry NL, Azzouz F, Desta Z, et al. Predictors of aromatase inhibitor discontinuation as a result of treatment-emergent symptoms in early-stage breast cancer. J Clin Oncol. 2012 Mar 20;30(9):936-42. [PMID: 22331951]

Item 106   Answer: A

Educational Objective: Manage metastatic colorectal cancer with K-*ras* and N-*ras* genotyping of the tumor.

This patient has metastatic colorectal cancer, and K-*ras* and N-*ras* genotyping of the tumor biopsy sample is necessary for treatment planning. The presence of multiple lung and liver metastases is not amenable to surgical resection and, as such, is incurable. In these cases, the goal of treatment is to extend survival and palliate symptoms. The increased number of chemotherapy options that are effective against metastatic colorectal cancer has prolonged median survival for patients with incurable disease from a median survival of 6 months without chemotherapy, to 12 months with 5-fluorouracil alone, to approximately 2 years with multi-agent chemotherapy. This patient will likely benefit from systemic chemotherapy; the use of multiple chemotherapy agents can be anticipated, and all agents with demonstrated activity in colorectal cancer need to be considered. One consideration in planning treatment is determining whether the epidermal growth factor receptor (EGFR) inhibitors cetuximab and panitumumab can be included in the treatment plan. Approximately 50% of colorectal cancers have a mutation in the K-*ras* or N-*ras* genes. Tumors that carry these mutations will not respond to anti-EGFR agents, and patients with these tumors are therefore not candidates for treatment with these drugs.

Dihydropyrimidine dehydrogenase (DPD) is the rate-limiting enzyme in the catabolism of 5-fluorouracil. Although assays are commercially available to measure DPD levels, these assays do not inform management and have no role in the routine treatment of patients with colorectal cancer at this time.

Patients with specific *UGT1A1* polymorphisms are more prone to irinotecan toxicity. Although commercial assays are also available to detect this polymorphism, they also do not inform management and are not indicated when treating patients with colorectal cancer at this time.

Multigene array prognostic assays are commercially available but also do not guide clinical decision making and therefore are not currently part of the routine management of patients with colorectal cancer.

KEY POINT

- Mutations in the K-*ras* or N-*ras* genes, present in approximately 50% of colorectal cancers, are associated with resistance to epidermal growth factor receptor–targeted agents (cetuximab, panitumumab).

Bibliography

Douillard JY, Oliner KS, Siena S, et al. Panitumumab-FOLFOX4 treatment and RAS mutations in colorectal cancer. N Engl J Med. 2013 Sep 12;369(11):1023-34. [PMID: 24024839]

Item 107   Answer: E

Educational Objective: Determine need for diagnostic imaging studies in a patient with low-risk prostate cancer.

No imaging studies are indicated at this time. The United States Preventive Services Task Force has concluded that the harms of screening for prostate cancer outweigh the benefits in men of any age regardless of risk factors. In contrast, the American Cancer Society and American Urological Association recommend offering both serum prostate-specific antigen (PSA) measurement and digital rectal examination to men annually beginning at the age of 50 years. The American College of Physicians and American Academy of Family Physicians both recommend that clinicians have individualized discussions with their patients regarding obtaining PSA measurements and support measuring PSA levels after such discussions in patients 50 years and older who have life expectancies of at least 10 years. This patient has low-risk prostate cancer based on the presence of a TNM stage T1c tumor (identified after an elevated screening serum PSA level is found in the absence of symptoms), a serum PSA level less than 10 ng/mL (10 µg/L), and a Gleason score less than 8. Imaging studies are currently not recommended for men with low-risk disease, as there is no evidence that such studies reliably alter management decisions.

Prostate cancer is among the most commonly diagnosed cancers in men in the United States. Most men are diagnosed with clinically occult cancer, which is identified on the basis of an abnormal serum PSA value. Most often, there are no symptoms or indicative physical findings as in the patient described here. Once the diagnosis of prostate cancer is made, the focus moves to assessment and treatment decision making. The role of imaging studies in men diagnosed with prostate cancer is to assess disease status, particularly the presence of metastatic disease. Imaging studies are indicated to evaluate symptoms suggestive of metastatic disease and also to evaluate patients at high risk for occult metastatic disease. Currently accepted parameters for imaging studies include a serum PSA level of 20 ng/mL (20 µg/L) or higher, a PSA level of 10 ng/mL (10 µg/L) or higher associated with a T2 tumor, a Gleason score of 8 or higher, or a T3 or T4 tumor.

KEY POINT

- Imaging studies are not indicated for men with newly diagnosed early-stage prostate cancer in the absence of symptoms or other high-risk features.

Bibliography

Eberhardt SC, Carter S, Casalino DD, et al. ACR Appropriateness Criteria prostate cancer-pretreatment detection, staging, and surveillance. J Am Coll Radiol. 2013 Feb;10(2):83-92. [PMID: 23374687]

Item 108   Answer: C

Educational Objective: Treat a patient with a newly diagnosed intermediate-thickness melanoma.

Sentinel lymph node biopsy is recommended for patients with melanomas of 1- to 4-mm thickness to provide accurate staging. It is also recommended for lesions less than 1 mm with certain high-risk features, such as ulceration, more than 1 mitosis/mm^2, or lymphovascular invasion. A 2-cm excision margin is appropriate for melanomas that are 1 mm thick or deeper. Metastasis to regional lymph nodes is the most important prognostic factor in early-stage melanoma and is found in 20% of patients with intermediate-thickness melanomas. Patients with intermediate-thickness melanomas have an average 5-year survival of 70% if lymph nodes are negative but only 45% if positive lymph nodes are present. If a positive sentinel lymph node is found, complete lymphadenectomy is recommended, which improves regional disease control. However, it is not known whether this procedure improves overall survival.

Adjuvant chemotherapy is not of benefit in treating melanomas. Palliative chemotherapy can be used for metastatic melanomas, although immunotherapy or targeted treatments offer improved efficacy and are usually recommended instead for advanced disease.

Whether to recommend adjuvant interferon alfa is guided by lymph node status. Adjuvant interferon alfa is an option for patients with positive lymph nodes and/or melanomas that are 4 mm or more thick. In these high-risk patients who have a 25% to 75% risk of dying of metastatic melanoma, adjuvant interferon alfa improves relapse-free survival, with less clear benefit for overall survival. Adjuvant interferon alfa would only be recommended for this patient if lymph node involvement is present.

A meta-analysis showed an improvement in disease-free and overall survival with adjuvant interferon alfa. However, in one of the largest trials, the improvement in overall survival was lost with more prolonged follow-up. Given the toxicities of interferon alfa, including fatigue, myalgia, fever, depression, and autoimmune disease, participation in clinical trials of newer agents is encouraged as an alternative option. Observation alone is also reasonable.

Because of important staging and prognostic information, as well as guidance for potential additional treatment options obtained from a sentinel lymph node biopsy in patients with intermediate-thickness melanoma, performing no further testing would be inappropriate.

KEY POINT

- Sentinel lymph node biopsy is recommended for patients with melanomas of 1- to 4-mm thickness to provide accurate staging, as metastasis to regional lymph nodes is the most important prognostic factor in patients with early-stage melanoma.

Bibliography

Wong SL, Balch CM, Hurley P, et al; American Society of Clinical Oncology; Society of Surgical Oncology. Sentinel lymph node biopsy for melanoma: American Society of Clinical Oncology and Society of Surgical Oncology joint clinical practice guideline. J Clin Oncol. 2012 Aug 10;30(23):2912-8. [PMID: 22778321]

Item 109   Answer: B

Educational Objective: Understand chemotherapy terminology.

This patient should receive conversion chemotherapy for his currently unresectable tumor. Conversion chemotherapy is given for the purpose of shrinking a tumor that is unresectable usually due to its location, often because of proximity to significant vascular structures as in this patient. Through shrinkage of the tumor with conversion chemotherapy, an adequate plane of resection between the tumor and the middle hepatic vein may become available, allowing complete removal of the tumor. This is particularly important in this patient with localized metastatic colon cancer. Although metastatic colorectal cancer is generally considered treatable but not curable, some patients with metastatic disease confined to a single organ (usually the liver or lung) may be amenable to surgical resection, and complete removal of all gross disease may be curative. Patients with a limited number of liver-only lesions, such as this patient, have been reported to have long-term disease-free survival rates of 25% to 50%.

Adjuvant chemotherapy is the term used for treatment given *after* resection of a tumor is performed with curative intent. The purpose of adjuvant chemotherapy is to eradicate any residual microscopic metastatic disease that might still be present outside of the surgical field. Adjuvant chemotherapy would not be possible in this patient with currently unresectable disease.

Neoadjuvant chemotherapy is similar to adjuvant chemotherapy in that it is given in the setting of curative-intent surgery; however, neoadjuvant therapy is given *before* surgery in an attempt to eradicate any unseen micrometastases that might be present outside of the surgical field. Although neoadjuvant chemotherapy may have the effect of tumor shrinkage, it differs from conversion chemotherapy in that it is given in patients who have resectable disease preoperatively.

Palliative chemotherapy is given to a patient with incurable, unresectable cancer and is given without realistic curative intent. Palliative chemotherapy may be administered for the purposes of possibly prolonging survival and/or controlling tumor-related symptoms.

Because chemotherapy may increase the opportunity for cure in this clinical setting, it would be inappropriate to not offer this treatment option.

KEY POINT

- Conversion chemotherapy is given to patients with unresectable tumors in an attempt to shrink the tumor to a resectable size. Neoadjuvant and adjuvant chemotherapies are given before or after curative-intent surgery, respectively, for tumors that are resectable at presentation.

Bibliography

Adam R, Wicherts DA, de Haas RJ, et al. Patients with initially unresectable colorectal liver metastases: is there a possibility of cure? J Clin Oncol. 2009 Apr 10;27(11):1829-35. [PMID: 19273699]

Answers and Critiques

Item 110   Answer: A

Educational Objective: Treat women with abdominal carcinomatosis of unknown primary site in the same manner as ovarian cancer.

Cytoreductive surgery followed by systemic chemotherapy is most appropriate in this patient with abdominal carcinomatosis due to cancer of unknown primary site (CUP). When evaluating a patient with CUP, it is important to identify whether the CUP is of a favorable or unfavorable prognostic subgroup to help guide management. Women with CUP presenting as abdominal carcinomatosis and ascites are classified as a favorable prognostic subgroup and should be assumed to have ovarian cancer until proved otherwise. Treatment is the same as for primary ovarian cancer and includes cytoreductive surgery (tumor debulking along with total abdominal hysterectomy, bilateral salpingo-oophorectomy, omentectomy, selective lymphadenectomy, and appendectomy, as well as administration of a platinum/taxane-containing chemotherapy regimen).

Ovarian cancer is unique in that its spread is mostly confined to the peritoneal cavity. The use of adjuvant intraperitoneal chemotherapy plus intravenous chemotherapy offers a survival advantage to intravenous chemotherapy alone. However, this survival advantage is associated with substantially increased toxicity. Combined intraperitoneal and intravenous chemotherapy without cytoreduction surgery is not adequate therapy for patients with CUP presenting as ovarian cancer–like disease.

Radiation therapy and concurrent chemotherapy are recommended for patients with stage IB through stage IV cervical cancer, as large randomized clinical trials have confirmed a survival advantage with this combined approach. This approach is not effective for patients with peritoneal carcinomatosis and ascites.

Systemic chemotherapy without cytoreductive surgery would be inadequate as the initial treatment of a patient with an ovarian cancer–like presentation.

Because this patient has a significant chance of meaningful benefit from treatment and has no comorbidities, providing only supportive care would be inappropriate.

KEY POINT

- Women with cancer of unknown primary site presenting as abdominal carcinomatosis and ascites are classified as a favorable prognostic subgroup and should be treated as if they have ovarian cancer.

Bibliography

Varadhachary GR. Carcinoma of unknown primary: focused evaluation. J Natl Compr Canc Netw. 2011 Dec;9(12):1406-12. [PMID: 22157558]

Item 111   Answer: B

Educational Objective: Treat recurrent superficial bladder cancer with cystectomy.

Cystectomy without prior chemotherapy is most appropriate for this patient who has superficial bladder cancer. Superficial

bladder cancer is the most common form of bladder cancer and is characterized by cancer cells confined to the mucosa, with no evidence of invasion into the muscle layer of the bladder. It is best managed by transurethral resection of the bladder tumor (TURBT), followed in most patients by either bacillus Calmette-Guérin (BCG) or mitomycin infused directly into the bladder. Although this treatment is effective in eradicating superficial bladder cancer, recurrences are common. Careful observation with serial cystoscopy is therefore essential. Many patients with recurrent superficial bladder cancer can be managed with repeat TURBT and additional intravesical infusion. However, patients who develop recurrence within 6 to 12 months of initial TURBT, or after one to two courses of BCG infusion (such as the patient described here), should undergo cystectomy. Cystectomy in this setting is associated with improved disease-specific survival. This procedure is not indicated in the initial management of superficial bladder cancer unless patients have ongoing tumor-related symptoms that cannot be managed with TURBT alone or if they are subsequently found to have muscle-invasive disease.

Systemic chemotherapy, although used prior to cystectomy for patients with muscle-invasive disease, has no role in the treatment of patients with superficial bladder cancer who are to undergo cystectomy.

External-beam radiation therapy has no established role in the treatment of superficial bladder cancer.

Repeat TURBT and BCG infusion is not indicated because this treatment has already been ineffective on two occasions.

KEY POINT

- Cystectomy is indicated for patients who develop recurrence of superficial bladder cancer within 6 to12 months of undergoing initial transurethral resection of bladder tumor or after receiving one to two courses of intravesical bacillus Calmette-Guérin.

Bibliography

Rodriguez Faba O, Gaya JM, López JM, et al. Current management of non-muscle-invasive bladder cancer. Minerva Med. 2013 Jun;104(3):273-86. [PMID: 23748281]

Item 112   Answer: C

Educational Objective: Evaluate *HER2* expression status in a patient with metastatic gastric cancer.

HER2 expression status should be determined in this patient with metastatic gastric cancer. This patient continues to have adequate caloric intake and good performance status. As such, he is an appropriate candidate for systemic chemotherapy. Approximately 20% of gastric cancers and 30% of gastroesophageal junction tumors overexpress *HER2* growth factor receptor. The anti-*HER2* monoclonal antibody trastuzumab, when added to a systemic chemotherapy regimen, is beneficial in treating patients with these tumor types. For example, an early trial of patients with gastric and gastroesophageal junction adenocarcinomas expressing *HER2* found that the median survival was statistically significantly improved by adding trastuzumab to cisplatin plus 5-fluorouracil or capecitabine (13.5 months versus 11.1 months). Use of trastuzumab is limited to those patients whose tumors overexpress *HER2*.

BRAF mutations are present in 40% of melanomas, and patients with these tumors are treated with selective *BRAF* inhibitors. However, these agents are not part of gastric cancer therapy, and knowledge of the *BRAF* mutation status of a gastric tumor would not alter treatment.

Determining the estrogen and progesterone receptor status of a tumor is important when planning treatment of patients with breast cancer but is not relevant when selecting therapy for patients with gastric cancer.

K-*ras* genotyping is needed for all patients with newly diagnosed metastatic colorectal cancer, as K-*ras* mutations inhibit activity of the anti–epidermal growth factor receptor agents cetuximab and panitumumab that are used to treat many of these tumors. However, because these agents are not active in treating upper gastrointestinal malignancies, determining K-*ras* mutation status is not indicated for this patient.

KEY POINT

- Determination of *HER2* tumor status is indicated for patients with newly diagnosed metastatic gastric cancer, as the anti-*HER2* monoclonal antibody trastuzumab, when added to a systemic chemotherapy regimen, is beneficial in treating patients whose tumors overexpress *HER2*.

Bibliography

Bang YJ, Van Cutsem E, Feyereislova A, et al; ToGA Trial Investigators. Trastuzumab in combination with chemotherapy versus chemotherapy alone for treatment of HER2-positive advanced gastric or gastro-oesophageal junction cancer (ToGA): a phase 3, open-label, randomised controlled trial. Lancet. 2010 Aug 28;376(9742):687-97. Erratum in: Lancet. 2010 Oct 16;376(9749):1302. [PMID: 20728210]

Item 113   Answer: B

Educational Objective: Determine indications for *BRCA1/2* testing in a woman with newly diagnosed breast cancer.

This patient should be offered *BRCA1/2* testing before surgical treatment is recommended. Offering *BRCA1/2* testing prior to surgery is recommended for patients younger than 45 years with either newly diagnosed breast cancer or a family history of breast or ovarian cancer. *BRCA1/2* testing is also recommended for patients with breast cancer diagnosed at any age if one or more first-, second- or third-degree relatives have been diagnosed with ovarian cancer and is recommended for women with "triple negative breast cancer" (estrogen receptor–negative, progesterone receptor–negative, and negative for *HER2* amplification) diagnosed before age 60 years. Because this patient was diagnosed with breast cancer at age 34 years and has a family history of ovarian cancer in a paternal grandmother, she has an 18% risk of having a *BRCA1/2* mutation. Offering *BRCA1/2* testing prior to breast

surgery is therefore recommended, particularly if the result will influence the patient's choice of surgery. If she tests positive for a *BRCA1* or *BRCA2* mutation, bilateral mastectomy should be considered because of the high risk for subsequent contralateral and ipsilateral breast cancers. The lifetime risk of contralateral breast cancer in women with breast cancer and a *BRCA1/2* mutation is 40% to 60%. The risk is highest in women younger than 40 years of age at diagnosis. In the United States, 50% to 70% of women with breast cancer who have a *BRCA1/2* mutation elect bilateral mastectomy, and studies suggest a survival benefit of prophylactic contralateral mastectomy in this situation.

If the patient were to test negative for a *BRCA1/2* mutation, bilateral mastectomy would not be recommended.

Left mastectomy is not usually required for a 2-cm breast cancer amenable to breast-conserving treatment, although it is an option if patients want to avoid radiation or have contraindications to radiation therapy. In addition, left mastectomy would not decrease the high risk of contralateral breast cancer for patients with a *BRCA1/2* mutation.

Lumpectomy with sentinel lymph node biopsy, followed by breast radiation therapy, is a reasonable option in patients with tumors measuring less than 5 cm that can be resected with clear margins. Survival following breast conservation therapy is equal to mastectomy in patients without *BRCA1/2* mutations.

KEY POINT

- Offering *BRCA1/2* testing prior to surgery is recommended for patients diagnosed with breast cancer before age 45 years, patients with breast cancer at any age and a family history of breast and/or ovarian cancer, and patients with triple-negative breast cancers diagnosed before age 60 years.

Bibliography

Malone KE, Begg CB, Haile RW, et al. Population-based study of the risk of second primary contralateral breast cancer associated with carrying a mutation in BRCA1 or BRCA2. J Clin Oncol. 2010 May 10;28(14):2404-10. [PMID: 20368571]

Item 114   Answer: D

Educational Objective: Determine need for screening a patient at average risk for ovarian cancer.

Ovarian cancer screening is not indicated for this patient. The lifetime risk of developing ovarian cancer is 1.4%, and this patient is of average risk. She does not have a family history suggestive of a hereditary ovarian cancer syndrome, such as family members with ovarian cancer; premenopausal breast cancer; bilateral breast cancer; the presence of both ovarian and breast cancer on the same side of the family; or the presence of Lynch syndrome cancers such as colon, endometrial, or gastric cancers. She is multiparous, has no symptoms suggestive of ovarian cancer, and has a normal pelvic examination. In addition, she used oral contraceptives for 15 years, which lowers the risk of ovarian cancer by 50%, with the protective effect lasting 30 years.

Neither serum CA-125 testing nor transvaginal ultrasound is indicated for asymptomatic women at average risk for ovarian cancer. Serum CA-125 levels are elevated in approximately 50% of women with early-stage ovarian cancer and in 80% of those with advanced ovarian cancer, but this finding is not very specific. Levels are also elevated in approximately 1% of healthy women and fluctuate during the menstrual cycle. Elevated serum CA-125 values also occur in several benign conditions, such as endometriosis, uterine fibroids, hepatitis, and peritonitis, as well as in endometrial, breast, lung, and pancreatic cancers.

The largest randomized controlled trial evaluating ovarian cancer screening in women at average risk was the Prostate, Lung, Colon, and Ovarian (PLCO) Cancer Screening Trial, in which 78,216 women were assigned to either usual care or annual serum CA-125 testing for 6 years plus annual transvaginal ultrasound for the first 4 years. After a median follow-up of 12 years, ovarian cancer was diagnosed in 5.7% of women in the screening group and 4.7% of women in the usual care group, but there was no difference between the two groups in the number of deaths due to ovarian cancer. In addition, 3285 women had false-positive results, 1080 of whom underwent surgery; 163 of the women who underwent surgery experienced at least one serious complication (15% of surgical procedures).

Patients who have a high risk of ovarian cancer, such as women with *BRCA1/2* mutations, are recommended to have semi-annual screening with pelvic examinations, serum CA-125 testing, and transvaginal ultrasound beginning at age 30 years. However, even in this high-risk group, there is no evidence that screening decreases ovarian cancer mortality. For these women, prophylactic bilateral salpingo-oophorectomy once childbearing is completed, ideally by age 35 to 40 years, is recommended.

KEY POINT

- Screening is not recommended for asymptomatic women at average risk of developing ovarian cancer.

Bibliography
Buys SS, Partridge E, Black A, et al; PLCO Project Team. Effect of screening on ovarian cancer mortality: the Prostate, Lung, Colorectal and Ovarian (PLCO) Cancer Screening Randomized Controlled Trial. JAMA. 2011 Jun 8;305(22):2295-303. [PMID: 21642681]

Item 115   Answer: D
Educational Objective: Treat a patient with localized renal cell carcinoma after surgical resection.

Close observation is the standard of care for patients following surgical resection for nonmetastatic renal cell carcinoma. The primary treatment of suspected renal cell carcinoma is surgery. Staging is predicated on tumor size as well as extension into the renal vein and into or through the Gerota fascia. Although this patient presented with symptoms suggesting an underlying process, more early-stage renal cell carcinomas are currently being identified incidentally because of the development and more frequent use of sensitive imaging techniques. Various treatment options are available for patients with advanced disease, including immunotherapy and many small-molecule tyrosine kinase inhibitors. However, at present, there is no evidence that any of these approaches is clearly associated with improved survival following resection of nonmetastatic disease, and they are therefore not used as adjuvant therapy.

The tyrosine inhibitors sunitinib and temsirolimus have shown significant activity against renal cell carcinoma and are used in patients with metastatic disease. However, they have no established role as adjuvant therapies following surgical resection. Although studies are ongoing, particularly trials of some of the tyrosine kinase inhibitors, the current standard of care following surgical resection is close observation.

Radiation therapy has no role in the management of patients following resection for localized renal cell carcinoma, even when surgical margins are positive.

KEY POINT

- Close observation is the standard of care for patients following surgical resection for nonmetastatic renal cell carcinoma, as no studies to date have identified an adjuvant therapy that improves survival in these patients.

Bibliography
Janowitz T, Welsh SJ, Zaki K, Mulders P, Eisen T. Adjuvant therapy in renal cell carcinoma-past, present, and future. Semin Oncol. 2013 Aug;40(4):482-91. [PMID: 23972712]

Item 116   Answer: D
Educational Objective: Diagnose mantle cell lymphoma.

The most likely diagnosis of this patient with diffuse lymphadenopathy, B symptoms, extranodal involvement, and cyclin D1 overexpression is mantle cell lymphoma. Overexpression of cyclin D1, a cell cycle gene regulator, is associated with a chromosomal translocation [t(11:14)] that is diagnostic of mantle cell lymphoma. Mantle cell lymphoma is a rare form of non-Hodgkin lymphoma that has a varied clinical course depending on the extent of disease at presentation. Patients usually have advanced disease at presentation, including lymphadenopathy, weight loss, and sometimes fever, and are found to have diffuse sites of involvement, including the gastrointestinal tract, bone marrow, and blood stream.

Diffuse large B-cell lymphoma can also involve multiple organs, including the bowel; however, the cells in diffuse large B-cell lymphoma are large and do not overexpress cyclin D1.

Similarly, follicular lymphoma does not usually involve the bowel and is not characterized by overexpression of cyclin D1.

Common findings in patients with Hodgkin lymphoma include palpable lymphadenopathy or a mediastinal mass. Hodgkin lymphoma is not associated with cyclin D1 overexpression or bowel involvement and is associated with a much better prognosis than mantle cell lymphoma, regardless of stage.

KEY POINT

- Mantle cell lymphoma is a rare form of non-Hodgkin lymphoma characterized by extranodal involvement and overexpression of cyclin D1, and it is associated with a poor prognosis.

Bibliography

Hoster E, Dreyling M, Klapper W, et al; German Low Grade Lymphoma Study Group (GLSG); European Mantle Cell Lymphoma Network. A new prognostic index (MIPI) for patients with advanced-stage mantle cell lymphoma. Blood. 2008 Jan 15;111(2):558-65. Erratum in: Blood. 2008 Jun 15;111(12):5761. [PMID: 17962512]

Item 117   Answer: D

Educational Objective: Diagnose a hereditary ovarian cancer syndrome.

This patient should undergo testing for Lynch syndrome (also known as hereditary nonpolyposis colon cancer). Because she has a personal history of both ovarian and endometrial cancer, as well as a family history of colon and endometrial cancer, her ovarian cancer is likely related to inheriting one of the genetic mutations present in patients with Lynch syndrome. This is an autosomal dominant cancer susceptibility syndrome caused by a germline mutation in one of the DNA-mismatch repair genes (*MLH1*, *MSH2*, and *MSH6* being the most common). Patients have an increased risk for several types of cancer, usually with early onset. The most common are a 70% risk for colon cancer, 27% to 71% risk for endometrial cancer, and 3% to 14% risk for ovarian cancer. Less common cancers include tumors of the upper urinary tract, bladder, stomach, small bowel, gallbladder, pancreas, brain, and sebaceous glands. Endometrial or, less often, ovarian cancer, can be the sentinel cancer in a patient with Lynch syndrome. Although identification of a Lynch syndrome mutation will not change the management of this patient's ovarian cancer, it will change screening for other cancers, including the need for colonoscopy every 1 to 2 years, annual skin examinations, and consideration of screening upper endoscopy. In addition, if she has Lynch syndrome, genetic testing should be offered to her first-degree relatives, with testing offered in addition to more distant relatives if first-degree relatives are unavailable or unwilling to be tested.

Based on National Comprehensive Cancer Network guidelines, all patients with ovarian cancer are eligible for *BRCA1/2* testing. Patients with *BRCA1/2* mutations are at risk for other cancers, particularly breast cancer, and additional screening and prophylaxis options should be discussed. In addition, patients with *BRCA1* mutations are eligible for clinical trials of agents that are particularly effective in *BRCA1*-related recurrent ovarian cancers, such as PARP inhibitors. If this patient does not have a Lynch syndrome–related mutation, testing for a *BRCA1/2* mutation would be recommended. However, because of her family and personal history of colon and endometrial cancers, testing for Lynch syndrome mutations is recommended first.

Serial abdominal/pelvic CT scans are not recommended to monitor patients with ovarian cancer. CT scans should be reserved for patients with symptoms or with recurrence of cancer based on clinical examination or elevated serum CA-125 levels.

Guidelines differ as to whether to monitor serum CA-125 levels in patients after treatment for ovarian cancer, and this should be discussed with individual patients. In one trial, patients with ovarian cancer treated with first-line platinum-based chemotherapy were randomized to receiving early treatment for ovarian cancer recurrence based on an increasing serum CA-125 level alone versus delaying treatment until clinical symptoms developed. Although patients in the early treatment arm started chemotherapy an average of 4.8 months earlier, there was no difference in overall survival.

KEY POINT

- Women with a personal and family history of ovarian, endometrial, and colon cancer should undergo testing for genetic mutations caused by Lynch syndrome (also known as hereditary nonpolyposis colon cancer).

Bibliography

Koornstra JJ, Mourits MJ, Sijmons RH, Leliveld AM, Hollema H, Kleibeuker JH. Management of extracolonic tumours in patients with Lynch syndrome. Lancet Oncol. 2009 Apr;10(4):400-8. [PMID: 19341971]

Item 118   Answer: C

Educational Objective: Treat a patient with stage I mycosis fungoides.

Topical glucocorticoids are most appropriate for this patient with mycosis fungoides, which is one form of cutaneous T-cell non-Hodgkin lymphoma. Lymphomas expressing T-cell surface antigens (CD4) are among the more common forms of cutaneous T-cell lymphomas. These antigens infiltrate skin and initially cause rash (mycosis fungoides) and, occasionally, also circulate in the blood (Sézary syndrome). The CD4-expressing malignant T cells are large and have classic "cerebriform"-appearing nuclei and clonal T-cell receptor gene rearrangements. Patients usually present with dry, pruritic, erythematous skin patches; mycosis fungoides confined to the skin can mimic these benign dermatologic conditions, and be undiagnosed for many years. Patients with progressive disease develop raised plaques, diffuse skin erythema, and cutaneous ulcers. In the final stages of progression, organ infiltration and evolving immunodeficiency cause recurrent bacterial infections, sepsis, and death.

Therapy is guided by disease stage. Early-stage disease (stages I and II) is limited to the skin, and patients have a median survival of over 20 years. Patients with early-stage disease are treated effectively with topical glucocorticoids. If there is no response to glucocorticoids, adding retinoids (such as bexarotene) and psoralen plus ultraviolet light (PUVA) therapy, at times combined with interferon alfa, may be effective. Patients with advanced disease (stages III and IV) have extensive skin and organ involvement and a median survival of 4 years. These patients require more aggressive therapy, including electron-beam radiation therapy; photopheresis; systemic therapy, including cyclophosphamide, doxorubicin, vincristine, and prednisone (CHOP) chemotherapy; histone deacetylase inhibitors (such as romidepsin and vorinostat); and monoclonal antibodies (such as alemtuzumab). Allogeneic hematopoietic stem cell transplantation may be curative in young patients who have advanced disease and an appropriate donor.

CHOP chemotherapy is indicated for patients with advanced disease, which this patient does not have due to absence of lymphadenopathy or organ involvement.

PUVA therapy may be effective for patients with early-stage disease who do not respond to topical glucocorticoids.

Monoclonal antibody therapy may be used in advanced stage mycosis fungoides using agents such as alemtuzumab, which is directed toward T cell surface proteins. Rituximab is a monoclonal antibody directed toward surface proteins typically found on immune system B cells and is not used in treatment of mycosis fungoides.

KEY POINT

- Patients with early-stage mycosis fungoides are treated initially with topical glucocorticoids; if glucocorticoids are ineffective, adding retinoids and psoralen and ultraviolet light therapy, sometimes combined with interferon alfa, may be effective.

Bibliography
Prince HM, Whittaker S, Hoppe RT. How I treat mycosis fungoides and Sézary syndrome. Blood. 2009 Nov 12;114(20):4337-53. [PMID: 19696197]

Item 119   Answer: D

Educational Objective: Treat stage I rectal cancer with surgical resection.

Surgical resection is indicated as the initial treatment for this patient who has stage I rectal cancer, which is defined as a tumor that invades into, but not fully through, the rectal wall, with no evidence of lymph node metastases (T2N0M0, stage I). The procedure for a tumor of the mid rectum, such as that in this patient, is a low anterior resection using the technique of total mesorectal excision to accomplish an en-bloc removal of the rectum with a fully intact mesorectum. The mesorectum is the fatty sheath that surrounds the rectum and contains the locoregional lymph nodes. Careful pathologic examination of the primary tumor and lymph nodes is necessary to confirm the disease stage. If pathology findings indicate that the tumor is a higher T stage than

expected (T3 or T4) or if any of the locoregional lymph nodes in the mesorectum are found to contain cancer (N1 or N2), postoperative chemoradiation and chemotherapy would be indicated. However, if the final pathology report confirms stage I rectal cancer, the probability of cure with surgery alone is high, and no additional treatment is indicated.

Neither chemotherapy, radiation therapy, nor combined chemotherapy plus radiation has been demonstrated to improve outcomes in patients with stage I rectal cancer, and all of them would expose these patients to unnecessary risk and toxicity.

KEY POINT

- Surgical resection is the initial treatment for patients with stage I rectal cancer (defined as a tumor that invades into, but not fully through, the rectal wall, with no evidence of lymph node metastases).

Bibliography
Garcia-Aguilar J, Holt A. Optimal management of small rectal cancers: TAE, TEM, or TME? Surg Oncol Clin N Am. 2010 Oct;19(4):743-60. [PMID: 20883951]

Item 120   Answer: B

Educational Objective: Diagnose early-stage ovarian cancer through exploratory surgery.

This patient, who has early-stage ovarian cancer (clinical stage II, with spread beyond the ovaries but confined to the pelvis), should undergo exploratory surgery. The diagnosis of ovarian cancer is usually made by surgical exploration, as there is survival benefit following intact removal of an adnexal mass in patients with early-stage disease. Survival is also improved when surgery is performed by a specialized gynecologic oncologic surgeon. If ovarian cancer is confirmed at surgery, appropriate procedures include peritoneal washings for cytology, total abdominal hysterectomy and bilateral salpingo-oophorectomy, omentectomy, full abdominal and pelvic exploration with biopsy of any masses suspicious for cancer, lymph node evaluation, and, for patients with advanced ovarian cancer, debulking of the tumor by removing as much of the cancer as possible. Optimal tumor debulking (leaving residual masses that are each less than 1 cm) improves survival.

CT-guided or ultrasound-guided biopsy of a suspected ovarian mass is contraindicated, as this may cause rupture and dissemination of cancer cells. Rupture of an ovarian mass increases the risk of peritoneal recurrence; when such rupture occurs during surgery, it is an indication for adjuvant chemotherapy, even in early stage disease.

MRI of the abdomen and pelvis is sometimes used in the preoperative staging of ovarian cancer as an alternative to CT but is unlikely to yield additional information after CT scans and ultrasound examinations are done.

Based on National Comprehensive Cancer Network guidelines, all women with ovarian cancer are eligible for *BRCA1/2* testing. Ten percent to 15% of ovarian cancers are hereditary, with *BRCA1/2* mutations being the most common. Although the initial surgical and standard adjuvant chemotherapy treatments for ovarian cancer are the same regardless of the presence of a hereditary mutation, patients with *BRCA1/2* mutations are at risk for other cancers, particularly breast cancer, and additional screening and prophylaxis options would be discussed once treatment for ovarian cancer is complete. In addition, patients with *BRCA1* mutations are eligible for clinical trials of agents that are particularly effective in *BRCA1*-related recurrent ovarian cancers, such as PARP inhibitors. However, it is not yet known whether this patient has ovarian cancer, and testing before this diagnosis is established is inappropriate.

KEY POINT

- The diagnosis of ovarian cancer is usually made by surgical exploration, as there is survival benefit following intact removal of an adnexal mass in patients with early-stage disease.

Bibliography
Engelen MJ, Kos HE, Willemse PH, et al. Surgery by consultant gynecologic oncologists improves survival in patients with ovarian carcinoma. Cancer. 2006 Feb 1:106(3);589-98. [PMID: 16369985]

Item 121   Answer: A

Educational Objective: Manage a patient with gastric mucosa-associated lymphoid tissue (MALT) lymphoma associated with *Helicobacter pylori* infection.

In this patient with a gastric mucosa-associated lymphoid tissue (MALT) lymphoma associated with *Helicobacter pylori* infection, ranitidine should be discontinued and omeprazole, metronidazole, and clarithromycin begun. MALT lines the entire gastrointestinal tract, providing immune surveillance and initiating immunologic responses to pathogens. Chronic antigen stimulation can lead to clonal expansion of MALT. Malignant transformation of MALT to lymphoma can occur, originating in the B cells of the marginal zone of MALT and expressing the CD20 surface antigen. Gastric MALT lymphoma associated with *H. pylori* infection usually presents as local disease in patients with gastric ulcers. A complete response is generally obtained following administration of combination antimicrobial therapy and a proton pump inhibitor (PPI) to treat the *H. pylori* infection. Usually, amoxicillin is combined with omeprazole and clarithromycin, but because of this patient's penicillin allergy, metronidazole is substituted for amoxicillin. A complete remission rate of nearly 80% can be expected after a full course of therapy. The duration of therapy lasts from 6 to 8 weeks to several months and is guided by treatment response as assessed by repeat upper endoscopy.

Rituximab has no role in the initial treatment of a patient with a gastric MALT lymphoma. This agent is indicated for disease that does not resolve after a complete course of combination antimicrobial therapy plus a PPI and may be combined with chemotherapy, radiation therapy, or surgery when additional treatment is required.

Bone marrow biopsy is not indicated because of the extremely low likelihood of bone marrow involvement in this setting.

A PET/CT scan is not needed because gastric MALT lymphoma usually presents as local disease, and this patient's abdominal CT scan revealed no lymphadenopathy.

KEY POINT

- The initial treatment of a patient with gastric mucosa-associated lymphoid tissue (MALT) lymphoma associated with *Helicobacter pylori* infection is antimicrobial therapy plus a proton pump inhibitor.

Bibliography
Ferreri AJ, Govi S, Ponzoni M. The role of Helicobacter pylori eradication in the treatment of diffuse large B-cell and marginal zone lymphomas of the stomach. Curr Opin Oncol. 2013 Sep;25(5):470-9. [PMID: 23942292]

Item 122   Answer: C

Educational Objective: Treat squamous cell carcinoma of the neck with chemoradiation therapy following surgical resection.

Adjuvant combined-modality treatment with chemotherapy and radiation is most appropriate for this patient with locally advanced squamous cell carcinoma. Most patients with resected squamous cell carcinoma of the head and neck will require some form of adjuvant therapy. Combined-modality chemotherapy and radiation has been shown to improve survival in patients with either positive surgical margins or lymph node metastases associated with extracapsular extension. Although several earlier studies showed a survival benefit when combined-modality therapy was used for patients with multiple positive lymph nodes without extracapsular extension, more recent studies have failed to confirm a survival benefit in that setting. Therefore, currently, either the presence of positive surgical margins at the primary resection site or of extracapsular lymph node extension is the only standard indication for combined-modality adjuvant therapy. The patient described here clearly meets these criteria.

Although cetuximab alone can be used for patients with advanced disease, it has not been associated with improved survival in the adjuvant setting.

Neither adjuvant chemotherapy alone nor adjuvant radiation therapy followed by chemotherapy has a role in the care of patients with resected squamous cell carcinoma of the head and neck.

Although not listed as an option, adjuvant radiation therapy alone is most often used for patients with earlier-stage disease and is associated with significantly decreased recurrence rates. However, it is not appropriate for patients with either positive resection margins or those with metastatic lymph nodes associated with extracapsular extension. In both of those circumstances, recurrence rates following treatment with radiation alone are clearly higher than those associated with combined chemotherapy and radiation treatment.

KEY POINT

- Adjuvant combined-modality chemotherapy and radiation has been shown to improve survival in patients with resected squamous cell carcinoma of the head and neck associated with either positive surgical margins or lymph node metastases with extracapsular extension.

Bibliography

Cooper JS, Zhang Q, Pajak TF, et al. Long-term follow-up of the RTOG 9501/intergroup phase III trial: postoperative concurrent radiation therapy and chemotherapy in high-risk squamous cell carcinoma of the head and neck. Int J Radiat Oncol Biol Phys. 2012 Dec 1;84(5):1198-205. [PMID: 22749632]

Item 123   Answer: A

Educational Objective: Manage a patient following radical inguinal orchiectomy for early-stage seminoma.

Active surveillance is appropriate for this patient with stage I seminoma following resection. Testicular germ cell tumors are divided into pure seminomas and nonseminomatous germ cell tumors (NSGCT). Recommended postsurgical treatments vary based on histologic findings and tumor stage. In general, pure seminoma is associated with a better prognosis than NSGCT. For men with stage I seminoma (disease confined to the testis), radical inguinal orchiectomy is curative in at least 80% of patients. This high cure rate with initial surgical treatment coupled with the ability to treat recurrent disease with curative intent makes active surveillance the lowest-risk approach with an expected good outcome. Active surveillance refers to a regimen of regular assessment with serum tumor marker measurement, CT scans of the abdomen and pelvis, and chest radiographic imaging. As this requires close and regular monitoring, it requires a reliable and motivated patient to be successful.

Other management options after surgery include adjuvant therapy with either single-agent carboplatin or para-aortic lymph node irradiation, although neither approach has been shown to improve overall survival. In addition, neither of these alternatives appears superior to the other, but they might be reasonable to consider in patients who wish to decline active surveillance.

Hematopoietic stem cell transplantation is used for treatment of patients with recurrent or refractory disease, usually only after treatment with multiple chemotherapeutic agents, in selected patients following adjuvant chemotherapy.

Platinum-based chemotherapy (specifically the combination of bleomycin, etoposide, and cisplatin) is the standard regimen for patients with more advanced seminoma, as well as for those with NSGCT. This regimen is not recommended for patients with stage I seminoma because of their very good prognosis and the significant potential for side effects associated with these drugs.

Retroperitoneal lymph node dissection is often used in the treatment of NSGCT but has no role in the treatment of patients with stage I seminoma.

KEY POINT

- Active surveillance is the recommended management strategy for patients with stage I seminoma diagnosed after radical inguinal orchiectomy; other options are adjuvant single-agent carboplatin or para-aortic lymph node irradiation.

Bibliography

Tandstad T, Smaaland R, Solberg A, et al. Management of seminomatous testicular cancer: a binational prospective population-based study from the Swedish norwegian testicular cancer study group. J Clin Oncol. 2011 Feb 20;29(6):719-25. [PMID: 21205748]

Item 124   Answer: C

Educational Objective: Treat a patient who responds to treatment for small cell lung cancer with prophylactic cranial irradiation.

Prophylactic cranial irradiation (PCI) is indicated. Following evaluation for pneumonia, this patient was diagnosed with limited-stage small cell lung cancer (SCLC). The definition of limited-stage disease consists of disease limited to one hemithorax, with hilar and mediastinal lymphadenopathy that can be encompassed within one tolerable radiotherapy portal. Combined chemotherapy and radiation therapy induced a significant near-complete response in this patient. At initial diagnosis and following treatment, there was no evidence of cerebral metastatic disease. Despite these results, she remains at significant risk for recurrence of small cell lung cancer. In addition, approximately one third of patients without cerebral metastatic disease at initial diagnosis will have brain metastases at the time of disease recurrence. Randomized trials assessing the role of PCI in patients with primary treatment-responsive SCLC have identified both a reduced incidence of brain metastases and an improvement in overall survival after irradiation. PCI is currently considered standard management following response to primary treatment in these patients.

Although limited-stage SCLC tumors are one of the most chemosensitive types of tumors, there are recurrences in 90% to 95% of patients. To date, attempts to improve outcomes by providing maintenance chemotherapy, adding other agents to the standard chemotherapy regimen, or by using high-dose chemotherapy with stem cell support have been unsuccessful.

PET/CT is not a standard imaging modality to assess patients with primary treatment-responsive SCLC and would provide no new information for this patient, given her CT imaging findings.

SCLC is considered a systemic disease at diagnosis, even if a potentially resectable peripheral lesion is the only finding after diagnostic studies are completed. All patients with SCLC now receive systemic chemotherapy as the mainstay of treatment. Surgery has no role in the management of patients with SCLC.

- Patients with small cell lung cancer who experience a complete or near-complete response following treatment with chemotherapy or combined chemotherapy and radiation therapy should be offered prophylactic cranial irradiation to reduce the incidence of brain metastases and improve overall survival.

Bibliography

Socha J, Kepka L. Prophylactic cranial irradiation for small-cell lung cancer: how, when and for whom? Expert Rev Anticancer Ther. 2012 Apr;12(4): 505-17. [PMID: 22500687]

Item 125   Answer: B

Educational Objective: Treat a patient with recurrent Hodgkin lymphoma who responds to salvage chemotherapy.

Autologous hematopoietic stem cell transplantation (HSCT) is the most appropriate treatment option for patients with recurrent Hodgkin lymphoma, particularly those who achieve a complete response to salvage chemotherapy. Prospective trials have consistently demonstrated a survival advantage when patients with chemotherapy-sensitive disease are treated with autologous HSCT compared with patients treated with continued salvage chemotherapy. Because this patient has achieved a complete remission following two cycles of dexamethasone, ifosfamide, cisplatin, and etoposide (DICE) chemotherapy, the next step is to administer hematopoietic growth factors, with or without chemotherapy, to mobilize, collect, and store hematopoietic progenitor cells. Once a sufficient quantity of hematopoietic progenitor cells are collected (>3 million CD34+ cells/kg patient body weight), high-dose multiagent chemotherapy followed by reinfusion of the stored progenitor cells can be completed.

Allogeneic HSCT is not indicated for patients with chemotherapy-sensitive recurrent Hodgkin lymphoma because of the significant risk of morbidity and mortality associated with allogeneic transplantation. The risk for fungal and viral infections occurring 3 months or more after transplantation is significantly greater after allogeneic than autologous transplantation. Lymphocytes derived from the donor can mount an immune response to the recipient's organs, leading to graft-versus-host disease, which may affect the skin, gastrointestinal tract, liver, ocular adnexa, lungs, bone marrow, and soft tissues. However, in patients with chemotherapy-resistant recurrent Hodgkin lymphoma, including patients who develop a relapse after autologous HSCT, allogeneic HSCT may result in prolonged disease-free survival.

Continuation of DICE chemotherapy is not optimal treatment for this patient because, as noted, patients with chemotherapy-sensitive Hodgkin lymphoma who are treated with autologous HSCT have a survival advantage compared with patients treated with continued salvage chemotherapy.

Radiation therapy in the salvage setting can be effective for patients with limited disease and may be associated with long-term disease-free survival. However, radiation therapy is much less likely to result in long-term disease-free survival in patients with advanced recurrent disease. In addition, radiation therapy would adversely affect the hematopoietic stem cells in patients being considered for autologous HSCT.

- Autologous hematopoietic stem cell transplantation is indicated for patients with recurrent Hodgkin lymphoma, particularly patients who achieve a complete response to salvage chemotherapy.

Bibliography

Rancea M, Monsef I, von Tresckow B, Engert A, Skoetz N. High-dose chemotherapy followed by autologous stem cell transplantation for patients with relapsed/refractory Hodgkin lymphoma. Cochrane Database Syst Rev. 2013 Jun 20;6:CD009411. [PMID: 23784872]

Item 126   Answer: D

Educational Objective: Manage concerns about disease recurrence in a breast cancer survivor.

Diagnostic testing is not indicated for this patient at this time. She had stage I breast cancer treated 3 years ago and has no worrisome symptoms and no abnormal findings on physical examination. In asymptomatic patients with a history of early breast cancer, routine imaging studies (excluding annual mammography) or blood tests, including tumor marker studies, are not beneficial. These tests have a 10% to 50% false-positive rate, leading to unnecessary studies and procedures. Two randomized trials showed no survival benefit from intensive screening with routine blood and imaging tests compared with clinical evaluation alone in asymptomatic patients. One of the trials showed a decreased quality of life in the group undergoing more intensive screening.

Patients with cancer in one breast are at higher risk for contralateral breast cancer (absolute risk 0.5% to 1.0% per year), although this risk is decreased by use of antiestrogen therapy. All women with a diagnosis of breast cancer should have annual mammograms. Breast MRI is only indicated for patients with *BRCA1/2* mutations or other familial breast cancer syndromes or those with a very strong family history of breast cancer. None of these high-risk situations is present in this patient.

Except for patients with familial cancer syndromes, breast cancer survivors have no increased risks for other cancers except those related to certain treatments. Patients receiving adjuvant chemotherapy with cyclophosphamide and anthracyclines have a 0.5% risk of developing myelodysplasia and acute leukemia. Tamoxifen is associated with a 1/1000 per year risk of endometrial cancer in women over 55 years of age and a smaller risk of uterine sarcoma in this age group. These risks are low, however, and routine screening blood tests and imaging studies are not recommended in asymptomatic patients.

In addition to cancer surveillance, survivor issues that should be addressed at follow-up visits include menopausal symptoms (selective serotonin reuptake inhibitors that do not interfere with tamoxifen activation or gabapentin may be helpful), sexual dysfunction including dyspareunia due to vaginal dryness (lubricants and cautious use of very low-dose vaginal estrogen are options), arthralgia from antiestrogen therapy, cognitive dysfunction, depression, fatigue, weight gain, decreased bone density, cardiovascular disease due to radiation or chemotherapy, and thrombosis in patients taking tamoxifen.

KEY POINT

- In asymptomatic patients with a history of early breast cancer, routine imaging studies (excluding annual mammography) or blood tests, including tumor marker studies, are not beneficial.

Bibliography

Hayes DF. Clinical Practice. Follow-up of patients with early breast cancer. N Engl J Med. 2007 Jun 14;356(24):2505-13. [PMID: 17568031]

Item 127   Answer: D

Educational Objective: Treat prostate cancer metastatic to bone with radium-223.

This patient, who has recurrent prostate cancer metastatic to bone, should be treated with the radiopharmaceutical agent radium-223. Patients with metastatic prostate cancer who are found to have a biochemical recurrence (a rising serum prostate-specific antigen level and no evidence of local disease progression) will typically respond to androgen deprivation therapy. However, they will also eventually develop clinical metastatic disease. Once this occurs, optimal management depends on multiple factors, including the extent and sites of metastases and the symptoms associated with the disease. One important consideration in this setting is use of a bone-seeking radiopharmaceutical agent. These agents concentrate in bone, and recent data indicate radium-223 is associated with improvement in both symptoms and overall survival. Radium-223 is indicated specifically for patients with bone-limited or bone-predominant symptomatic metastatic disease, such as that present in this patient.

Bilateral orchiectomy, while a very effective form of antiandrogen therapy, would not be indicated in a patient who has already been demonstrated to be castrate resistant.

Estrogen therapy has uncertain benefit in the treatment of castrate-resistant prostate cancer, and would not be considered an appropriate treatment option for this patient, especially given that radium-223 has been associated with both improved survival and symptom burden.

External-beam radiation to metastatic sites can be considered for treatment of patients with spinal cord compression or for those with focal symptomatic bone metastases, neither of which this patient has.

KEY POINT

- The radiopharmaceutical agent radium-223 is associated with improvement in both symptoms and overall survival when used to treat patients with bone-limited or bone-predominant symptomatic metastatic prostate cancer.

Bibliography

Parker C, Nilsson S, Heinrich D, et al; ALSYMPCA Investigators. Alpha emitter radium-223 and survival in metastatic prostate cancer. N Engl J Med. 2013 Jul 18;369(3):213-23. [PMID: 23863050]

Item 128   Answer: B

Educational Objective: Treat early-stage triple-negative breast cancer with adjuvant chemotherapy.

Anthracycline-based chemotherapy is the most appropriate treatment. Although this patient has a stage I cancer (measuring 2 cm or less and lymph node negative), it is a high-grade, triple-negative tumor (negative for estrogen receptor, progesterone receptor, and *HER2* amplification), and she is at high risk for systemic recurrence. In patients with triple-negative cancers that are 0.6 cm or greater in size, adjuvant chemotherapy, typically anthracycline-based chemotherapy, is recommended if there are no medical contraindications. Chemotherapy is the mainstay of treatment for triple-negative breast cancers, both when used as adjuvant therapy and when used for more advanced cancers. Based on retrospective analysis, adding a taxane agent to adjuvant anthracycline-based chemotherapy is of greater benefit in patients with hormone receptor–negative cancers than in patients with hormone receptor–positive cancers.

Triple-negative cancers constitute about 15% of breast cancers and are usually of high grade. They occur more frequently in young black and Hispanic women than in other ethnic groups. Patients with triple-negative cancers have a higher risk of *BRCA1/2* mutations, and *BRCA1/2* genetic testing is recommended for women diagnosed with triple-negative breast cancers before age 60 years. Most breast cancers in women with *BRCA1* mutations are triple negative.

Antiestrogen therapies such as anastrozole are not effective in hormone receptor–negative cancers and would not be used in this patient's treatment regimen.

Autologous bone marrow transplantation is not used as adjuvant treatment for breast cancer. Clinical trials on its use in both the adjuvant setting and the metastatic setting showed no improvement in survival compared to treatment with standard therapy and its use in breast cancer has been discontinued.

Epidermal growth factor receptor–targeted therapy with bevacizumab has not been found to improve disease survival or overall survival when added to adjuvant chemotherapy for patients with triple-negative breast cancers.

KEY POINT

- Adjuvant chemotherapy, typically anthracycline-based chemotherapy, is recommended for patients with triple-negative breast cancers who have no medical contraindications to this regimen.

Bibliography

Foulkes WD, Smith IE, Reis-Filho JS. Triple-negative breast cancer. N Engl J Med. 2010 Nov 11;363(20):1938-48. [PMID: 21067385]

Item 129   Answer: B

Educational Objective: Screen for breast cancer in a patient who has received chest radiation therapy.

This patient should now be screened with mammography and accompanying breast MRI on an annual basis. Women who received chest wall radiation (such as mantle radiation therapy for Hodgkin lymphoma) between the ages of 10 and 30 years are at high risk for developing breast cancer and, according to the American Cancer Society 2007 guidelines, should be screened with breast MRIs as well as annual mammograms. Such women have a 30% to 50% lifetime risk of developing breast cancer within the radiation field. A recent study from England and Wales reviewed the incidence of breast cancer in 5002 women treated with supradiaphragmatic radiation therapy for Hodgkin lymphoma before age 36 years. This study showed an increased breast cancer risk starting 10 years after radiation exposure and peaking 25 to 34 years after exposure. At the 40-year follow-up, the risk of breast cancer was 48% for patients who received 40 Gy or more of mantle radiation therapy at a young age. Breast MRI is more sensitive, although less specific, than mammography for the detection of invasive breast cancers and has been studied prospectively in women with a high risk of breast cancer. However, mammography may still detect cancers not seen on MRI; therefore, a dual imaging strategy is recommended. In one study, the combination of mammogram and breast MRI had a sensitivity of 0.94 for detecting invasive breast cancer compared with a sensitivity of 0.39 with mammogram alone.

For the reasons noted above, yearly mammograms alone are less effective than a screening program including breast MRI.

Some groups, including the American Cancer Society, recommend annual mammography starting at age 40 years for women with an average breast cancer risk, whereas the American College of Physicians and the United States Preventive Services Task Force suggest initiating discussion with patients between the ages of 40 to 49 years who are at average risk for breast cancer regarding the risks and benefits of screening to determine the appropriate screening approach. Additionally, none of these groups recommends the use of MRI in screening for breast cancer in average risk women. This woman's breast cancer risk is far above average, and delaying mammography would be an inadequate screening approach for her.

There is no evidence that breast self-examination (BSE) decreases breast mortality. Some expert groups raise concerns about increased harm with BSE, such as unnecessary distress and procedures for benign lumps. Most guidelines from expert groups recommend against BSE, with a few recommending "breast self-awareness" or education about the benefits and limitations of BSE. BSE alone as a screening strategy in this high-risk patient is inadequate.

KEY POINT

- Women who received chest wall radiation (such as mantle radiation therapy for Hodgkin lymphoma) between the ages of 10 and 30 years are at high risk for developing breast cancer and should be screened with annual mammograms and breast MRIs.

Bibliography

Swerdlow AJ, Cooke R, Bates A, et al. Breast cancer risk after supradiaphragmatic radiotherapy for Hodgkin's lymphoma in England and Wales: A National Cohort Study. J Clin Oncol. 2012 Aug 1;30(22):2745-52. [PMID: 22734026]

Item 130   Answer: A

Educational Objective: Treat non–small cell lung cancer with chemotherapy.

Chemotherapy is most appropriate for this patient with stage II non–small cell lung cancer (NSCLC). Although several combination chemotherapeutic regimens have been studied, so far only a cisplatin-based regimen has been shown to be effective in selected patients with NSCLC. Currently available studies indicate that adjuvant cisplatin-based chemotherapy, given for a total of four cycles, improves survival in patients who have undergone successful resection of stage II or stage III NSCLC, regardless of histologic type.

Erlotinib is a tyrosine kinase inhibitor with activity against tumors expressing mutations in the epidermal growth factor receptor (EGFR). Although erlotinib is effective in the treatment of EGFR mutation-positive patients with metastatic NSCLC, its effectiveness in the adjuvant treatment setting has not been established.

Although radiation therapy may decrease locoregional recurrence, it has not been shown to improve survival in patients with stage II lung cancer with clear margins after resection and therefore is not given to such patients as adjuvant treatment.

Observation alone is inappropriate because of the survival advantage associated with adjuvant chemotherapy and because this patient has no apparent contraindications to administration of chemotherapy. Potential contraindications to chemotherapy include poor performance status following surgery and the presence of medical comorbidities that predict for an increase in toxicity associated with chemotherapy treatment.

KEY POINT

- Cisplatin-based adjuvant chemotherapy improves survival for selected patients who have undergone successful resection of stage II or stage III non–small cell lung cancer, regardless of histologic type.

Bibliography

Pignon, JP, Tribodet H, Scagliotti GV, et al; LACE Collaborative Group. Lung adjuvant cisplatin evaluation: a pooled analysis by the LACE Collaborative Group. J Clin Oncol. 2008 Jul 20;26(21):3552-9. [PMID: 18506026]

Item 131   Answer: B

Educational Objective: Evaluate a patient with possible lymphoma with an excisional lymph node biopsy.

This patient most likely has lymphoma, and excisional or core needle biopsy of an enlarged lymph node should be done next to establish a tissue diagnosis. Optimally, an excisional biopsy should be performed to preserve lymph node architecture which is important in differentiating reactive lymphadenopathy from lymphoma. Core needle biopsy is able to sample some structural aspects of the lymph node, and may be used for deep lymph nodes in place of excision. This patient's presentation of asymptomatic but progressive lymphadenopathy, splenomegaly, and lymphocytosis is highly suggestive of lymphoma. To determine the subtype of lymphoma and to guide therapy, the biopsy specimen is sampled for histopathologic, cytogenetic, and fluorescence in situ hybridization (FISH) analysis, as well as immunophenotype and gene expression profiling. Routine blood studies include a complete blood count with differential, erythrocyte sedimentation rate, and serum chemistry studies, including serum urate level. Serum lactate dehydrogenase, β_2-microglobulin, and immunoglobulin levels should also be determined. Screening for viral infections, including hepatitis B and C, HIV, human T-cell lymphotrophic virus type 1, human herpesvirus-8, and Epstein-Barr virus (and, when indicated, screening for bacterial infection due to *Helicobacter pylori*), needs to be performed because these infections can be causative drivers of lymphoma. As active infections may reduce lymphoma response rates and duration, it is essential to treat both the lymphoma and any underlying infections.

Although bone marrow biopsy, generally iliac crest bone marrow biopsy, is needed to complete the evaluation, excisional or core needle biopsy should be done first to establish a tissue diagnosis prior to staging.

Fine-needle lymph node biopsy should not be used because it will not preserve the architecture of the lymph node that is required for the diagnosis of lymphoma.

Patients with aggressive lymphoma presenting with involvement of the testes, sinuses, bone marrow, and ocular sites have an increased risk of central nervous system involvement and require lumbar puncture for cerebrospinal fluid examination. This procedure is only appropriate following the diagnosis and staging of non-Hodgkin lymphoma.

PET scanning is performed to complete staging but, again, should not be done until a tissue diagnosis is established. Early repeat PET scanning (after two to three cycles of chemotherapy) provides important prognostic information for patients with Hodgkin lymphoma but not for those with non-Hodgkin lymphoma.

KEY POINT

- Excisional biopsy of an adequate tissue sample that preserves the architecture of the lymph node is required for the diagnosis of lymphoma.

Bibliography

Amador-Ortiz C, Chen L, Hassan A, et al. Combined core needle biopsy and fine-needle aspiration with ancillary studies correlate highly with traditional techniques in the diagnosis of nodal-based lymphoma. Am J Clin Pathol. 2011 Apr;135(4):516-24. [PMID: 21411774]

Item 132   Answer: E

Educational Objective: Manage early-stage prostate cancer in an elderly man with medical comorbidities.

Observation, or watchful waiting, is most appropriate for this elderly man with newly diagnosed prostate cancer and medical comorbidities after the benefits and risks of this approach are discussed with the patient. Observation is based on an assessment that a patient would not benefit from definitive treatment of prostate cancer, either because of significant comorbidities or a shortened life expectancy, with the expectation that palliative treatment could be provided if the disease progresses. This patient's prostate-specific antigen (PSA) level, extent of disease based on biopsy findings, and Gleason score are all predictors of low-risk disease. Furthermore, he has a significant medical history, including worsening heart failure. Given that this patient has very low-risk prostate cancer and a life expectancy most likely less than 10 years, observation is the most appropriate management option for this patient.

Active surveillance, in contrast to observation, is the postponement of definitive therapy with the intent to pursue treatment of curative intent if there is evidence of disease progression. Active surveillance involves a program of regular assessment with physical examination, PSA testing, and prostate biopsy. It would not be appropriate for this patient, given his life expectancy related to significant medical comorbidities.

Cryotherapy is a technique that freezes prostatic cancer cells to treat localized prostate cancer. However, its role as a treatment option for localized prostate cancer has not been established at present.

Both external-beam radiation therapy and radical prostatectomy are reasonable alternatives for definitive treatment in patients considered appropriate candidates for therapy. However, the risks of either would likely outweigh the benefits of treatment in this patient with low-risk disease and significant medical comorbidities.

- Observation is the appropriate management for an elderly man with newly diagnosed, low-risk prostate cancer and medical comorbidities that significantly limit life expectancy.

Bibliography

Shappley WV 3rd, Kenfield SA, Kasperzyk JL, et al. Prospective study of determinants and outcomes of deferred treatment or watchful waiting among men with prostate cancer in a nationwide cohort. J Clin Oncol. 2009 Oct 20;27(30):4980-5. [PMID: 19720918]

Item 133   Answer: D

Educational Objective: Determine the prognosis in a patient with newly diagnosed colon cancer.

Tumor stage is usually the most important prognostic factor in determining a patient's outcome. Staging typically involves ordering appropriate tests to identify the local extent of the primary tumor and to determine whether the disease has spread beyond the site of origin. Although specific staging will vary according to the unique anatomic and biologic features of the primary site, there are many common steps to the staging process. Most solid tumors are staged according to the American Joint Commission on Cancer (AJCC) TNM classification. "T" indicates the extent of the tumor (size and/or depth of penetration), "N" represents the number of locoregional lymph nodes that contain cancer, and "M" indicates whether metastases are present or absent. TNM scores are then classified on a scale of stage I to IV, with stage I tumors having the best prognosis and stage IV having the worst.

Although poorly differentiated tumors generally have a worse prognosis than well-differentiated tumors, this is a modest prognostic factor compared with staging.

Performance status, which is a designation of the patient's overall medical "wellness" and ability to perform routine daily activities, may have important prognostic implications within a particular stage of disease but is far less significant prognostically than the stage itself.

Tumor size may be a component of the "T" stage, but by itself has only modest prognostic significance relative to overall stage. Generally, the degree of lymph node involvement has a greater negative impact on prognosis than does a higher T stage, and the presence of metastatic disease beyond lymph node involvement has the worst prognosis.

- Tumor stage is usually the most important prognostic factor in determining outcome in a patient with newly diagnosed cancer.

Bibliography

Edge S, Byrd DR, Compton CC, Fritz AG, Greene FL, Trotti A, eds. *AJCC Cancer Staging Manual*. 7th ed. New York, NY: Springer; 2010.

Item 134   Answer: B

Educational Objective: Treat locally advanced anal cancer with radiation and concurrent chemotherapy.

This patient, who has locally invasive squamous cell carcinoma of the anus, requires pelvic radiation therapy and concurrent systemic chemotherapy, a regimen that is appropriate for patients with stage I, II, and III anal cancer. Compared with rectal cancer, which is typically adenocarcinoma for which resection is the initial therapeutic step, anal cancers are usually of squamous cell origin, with chemoradiation the primary treatment modality owing to increased cure rates. Mitomycin plus 5-fluorouracil (5-FU) has been used to treat patients with anal cancer since the 1970s and remains the standard chemotherapy regimen. Randomized clinical trials have demonstrated that radiation therapy plus chemotherapy is superior to radiation therapy alone and that the combination of 5-FU plus mitomycin is superior to use of 5-FU alone.

Radiation therapy alone is inadequate for treatment of anal cancer.

If radiation therapy and chemotherapy fail to eradicate this patient's anal cancer, surgery can be performed as salvage treatment. However, the procedure required to excise an anal cancer also requires removal of the anal sphincter and placement of a permanent colostomy. Consequently, surgery as either initial treatment or as a planned procedure following initial radiation therapy and chemotherapy without documentation of continuing metastases would not be appropriate because of the unacceptable level of morbidity.

Anal cancer is a squamous cell carcinoma that arises in the squamous epithelium of the anus and is typically associated with human papillomavirus exposure. It is a distinct entity from rectal cancer, which arises in the columnar epithelium of the rectum, is an adenocarcinoma, and is typically treated with a combination of radiation therapy, chemotherapy, and definitive surgery.

- The standard treatment regimen for patients with stage I, II, or III anal squamous cell carcinoma is radiation therapy with concurrent chemotherapy consisting of mitomycin plus 5-fluorouracil.

Bibliography

James RD, Glynne-Jones R, Meadows HM, et al. Mitomycin or cisplatin chemoradiation with or without maintenance chemotherapy for treatment of squamous-cell carcinoma of the anus (ACT II): a randomized, phase 3, open-label, 2×2 factorial trial. Lancet Oncol. 2013 May;14(6):516-24. [PMID: 23578724]

Item 135   Answer: D

Educational Objective: Manage a patient with a low-grade metastatic carcinoid tumor.

Repeat abdominal imaging with a contrast-enhanced CT scan of the abdomen in 3 to 4 months is most appropriate. This patient has an incidental finding of a metastatic low-grade carcinoid tumor that is asymptomatic and hormonally nonfunctional. It is impossible to know how long the tumor has been present. However, given the benign presentation and near-normal liver function studies, the tumor has probably been present for many years. Because urgent intervention is unlikely to be needed, expectant observation and repeat imaging studies in 3 to 4 months will be useful in establishing disease progression. For many patients, little or no change is seen on serial scans, and these patients may be followed with serial imaging studies two to three times each year. If substantial tumor progression or tumor-related symptoms develop, intervention should be considered.

Hepatic artery embolization may be effective in decreasing tumor volume in the liver or decreasing hormone production in patients with neuroendocrine tumors. However, this is an invasive procedure that carries risks of morbidity and mortality and would not be appropriate for an asymptomatic patient with small-volume, hormonally nonfunctional disease.

This patient does have a positive radiolabeled octreotide scan, indicating that somatostatin receptors are present on the tumor (as they are in most neuroendocrine tumors). Therefore, treatment with octreotide, a somatostatin analogue, could be considered in the future if the disease progresses. Although actual tumor regression following octreotide administration is rare, octreotide has been demonstrated to stabilize and delay progression of carcinoid tumors and would be an appropriate consideration if progression of this patient's tumor is seen on serial imaging.

Radiofrequency ablation is another invasive procedure that can be used to treat patients with a small number of liver lesions. However, it has no role in the treatment of patients with numerous lesions, such as the patient described here.

Systemic chemotherapy would also not be indicated in a patient with an asymptomatic neuroendocrine tumor in the absence of disease progression or disease-related symptoms.

KEY POINT

- Appropriate management for a patient with an incidental finding of a metastatic low-grade carcinoid tumor that is asymptomatic and hormonally nonfunctional consists of expectant observation and repeat imaging studies several times each year to determine whether the disease is progressing.

Bibliography

Kulke MH, Siu LL, Tepper JE, et al. Future directions in the treatment of neuroendocrine tumors: consensus report of the National Cancer Institute Neuroendocrine Tumor clinical trials planning meeting. J Clin Oncol. 2011 Mar 1;29(7):934-43. [PMID: 21263089]

Item 136   Answer: D

Educational Objective: Diagnose and stage pancreatic adenocarcinoma.

The most appropriate management is surgical resection of the pancreatic mass. This patient likely has localized and potentially resectable pancreatic adenocarcinoma. Strong

supportive data include clinical risk factors (age ≥50 years, cigarette smoking, new-onset diabetes mellitus), symptoms (weight loss, dyspepsia), and CT imaging findings (a discrete, solid, low-attenuating mass with dilation of the upstream pancreatic duct and common bile duct ["double-duct sign"]).

Percutaneous or endoscopic ultrasound-guided tissue sampling is generally not recommended in patients who are operative candidates with potentially resectable (localized) pancreatic cancer because negative results may simply represent sampling error and are insufficient to rule out the presence of cancer. Thus, they entail risk and do not affect management.

The tumor marker CA 19-9 has variable sensitivity and specificity for pancreatic cancer and is generally not recommended as a screening test; management will not be changed by the results of this test at this time, however, it can add prognostic value for patients diagnosed with metastatic pancreatic cancer.

KEY POINT

- In patients who have imaging that is characteristic of resectable pancreatic cancer, tissue sampling prior to potential curative resection is not appropriate, and definitive resection without prior tissue confirmation should be pursued.

Bibliography

Muniraj T, Jamidar PA, Aslanian HR. Pancreatic cancer: a comprehensive review and update. Dis Mon. 2013 Nov;59(11):368-402. [PMID: 24183261]

Item 137   Answer: B

Educational Objective: Diagnose metastatic breast cancer through biopsy of a suspicious lesion.

Patients with a history of early breast cancer who develop findings suspicious for metastatic breast cancer should first have a biopsy of one of the suspected metastatic sites to confirm the diagnosis and to assess hormone receptor and *HER2* status, as these may differ from the original cancer. A study of suspected metastatic lesions in 121 women with newly metastatic breast cancer showed discordance between the primary and the metastatic site in 16% of specimens for estrogen receptor, 40% for progesterone receptor, and 10% for *HER2*. Biopsy led to a change in management in 14% of patients. Since bone biopsy specimens cannot be assessed for *HER2* status unless there is a soft tissue component, biopsy of an area other than bone is preferred, if possible.

Beginning chemotherapy is inappropriate before the diagnosis of metastatic breast cancer and its hormone receptor and *HER2* status are confirmed by biopsy.

Beginning antiestrogen therapy (for example, exemestane combined with everolimus) is also inappropriate before biopsy confirmation of metastatic breast cancer.

Although a PET/CT scan may be useful for staging disease and following response to treatment in patients with metastatic breast cancer, it is important first to establish the diagnosis by biopsy. In this patient, the ultrasound and

CT scans have already identified an accessible location for biopsy, and a PET scan is not needed before proceeding to biopsy of one of the liver lesions.

KEY POINT

- Patients with a history of early breast cancer who develop findings suspicious for metastatic breast cancer should undergo biopsy of one of the suspected metastatic sites to confirm the diagnosis and to assess hormone receptor and *HER2* status, as these may differ from the original cancer.

Bibliography

Amir E, Miller N, Geddie W, et al. Prospective study evaluating the impact of tissue confirmation of metastatic disease in patients with breast cancer. J Clin Oncol. 2012 Feb 20;30(6):587-92. [PMID: 22124102]

Item 138   Answer: A

Educational Objective: Manage a patient with metastatic lung cancer and poor performance status.

Recommending comprehensive palliative care assessment for possible hospice care is indicated. Stage IV (metastatic) non–small cell lung cancer (NSCLC) is incurable. Because metastatic NSCLC is a systemic process, systemic chemotherapy is typically used as the primary treatment modality. Chemotherapy for stage IV NSCLC has been shown to prolong survival and improve quality of life. However, patients with poor performance status and advanced disease have a limited prognosis (less than 4 months) despite therapy. Goals of therapy for these patients are symptom palliation and possible prolongation of survival. This patient has progressive metastatic lung cancer based on imaging studies that were obtained after she completed four cycles of chemotherapy. She also has a clear decline in functional status. Based on these findings, hospice care would be most appropriate.

The response rate to second-line chemotherapy is very low in patients with NSCLC. In addition, all available evidence indicates that patients with an Eastern Cooperative Oncology Group/World Health Organization performance status of 2 or worse do not derive benefit from chemotherapy.

Providing artificial nutrition for patients with advanced cancer has not been shown to improve outcomes and is not usually recommended.

The pleural effusion identified on the most recent imaging studies is small and is not causing respiratory compromise. Thoracostomy tube drainage is therefore not indicated.

Radiation therapy should be considered to relieve pain, particularly bony pain, visceral pain (when secondary to capsular distension), or pain due to nerve/nerve root compression. Although this patient has pain due to a metastatic lesion involving the L3 vertebral body, the pain is mild, managed with a NSAID, and there is no evidence of cord compression; consequently, radiation treatment is not needed for palliation.

KEY POINT

- Patients with lung cancer and poor performance status do not benefit from chemotherapy and should undergo a palliative care assessment.

Bibliography

Weissman DE, Meier DE. Identifying patients in need of a palliative care assessment in the hospital setting: a consensus report from the Center to Advance Palliative Care. J Palliat Med. 2011 Jan;14(1):17-23. [PMID: 21133809]

Item 139   Answer: B

Educational Objective: Diagnose renal cell carcinoma in a patient with erythrocytosis and a high serum erythropoietin level.

This patient requires CT of the abdomen and pelvis to detect possible renal cell carcinoma. The findings of a markedly elevated serum erythropoietin level due to secondary erythrocytosis plus vague midback pain and microscopic hematuria suggest the presence of an underlying renal cell carcinoma. Renal cell carcinoma is associated with secondary erythrocytosis in about 1% to 3% of patients. Polycythemia vera (PCV), a myeloproliferative neoplasm that results in excessive and unregulated erythrocyte production, is associated with very low serum erythropoietin levels. In contrast, an elevated serum erythropoietin level indicates the presence of secondary erythrocytosis. Although the most common causes of secondary erythrocytosis are chronic hypoxia and elevated carboxyhemoglobin concentrations due to tobacco use, an important cause is an erythropoietin-producing tumor. Other tumors commonly associated with secondary erythrocytosis include hepatocellular carcinoma and pheochromocytoma.

Bone marrow biopsy is not indicated because of this patient's markedly elevated serum erythropoietin level, which suggests external erythropoietin production and not a bone marrow disorder as a cause of this patient's polycythemia.

JAK2 mutation testing, which would be appropriate to rule out PCV in a patient with a very low serum erythropoietin level, is not indicated for this patient who has a markedly elevated level that is not compatible with a diagnosis of PCV.

Peripheral blood flow cytometry would not add useful information because this patient has isolated polycythemia and no evidence of abnormal lymphocytes. Flow cytometry is best used to help establish a diagnosis when evaluating for a malignancy that would reveal a monoclonal population of cells with a specific phenotype.

KEY POINT

- The finding of a markedly elevated serum erythropoietin level in a patient with vague midback pain and microscopic hematuria suggests the presence of an underlying renal cell carcinoma.

Bibliography

Kremyanskaya M, Mascarenhas J, Hoffman R. Why does my patient have erythrocytosis? Hematol Oncol Clin North Am. 2012 Apr;26(2):267-83, vii-viii. [PMID: 22463827]

Item 140   Answer: B

Educational Objective: Treat a localized gastrointestinal stromal tumor with imatinib after surgical resection.

Imatinib for 3 years is the most appropriate adjuvant treatment for this patient, who has a localized gastrointestinal stromal tumor (GIST) associated with a relatively higher risk for recurrence. GISTs, although rare, are the most common sarcoma of the gastrointestinal tract. The most common site is in the stomach, but GISTs can arise anywhere in the digestive tract. Location outside the stomach, larger size, and higher mitotic index constitute relative high-risk factors for recurrence after resection. Patients with small gastric GISTs with low mitotic indices may often be managed with surgery alone. Higher-risk tumors, such as in this patient, require further treatment. A 3-year course of the oral tyrosine kinase inhibitor imatinib has been shown to improve outcomes when used as adjuvant therapy after surgical resection of localized higher-risk GISTs. Imatinib has also been shown to be highly active in treating patients with metastatic GISTs, in whom lifelong therapy is recommended. Finally, randomized clinical trials have shown a superior outcome for those patients with localized higher-risk GISTs who receive imatinib for 3 years compared with those receiving 1 year of treatment.

The MAGIC trial demonstrated the superiority of preoperative and postoperative chemotherapy (epirubicin, cisplatin, and 5-fluorouracil) compared with surgery alone for treatment of gastric and esophageal/gastroesophageal junction adenocarcinomas. In patients who undergo surgery as initial therapy, postoperative 5-fluorouracil and leucovorin plus radiation therapy have been shown to confer a survival benefit compared with postoperative observation alone. These therapies are not effective treatments for GISTs.

GISTs are relatively resistant to radiation, and adjuvant radiation therapy is not routinely indicated.

Observation following surgical resection is appropriate only for patients with GISTs associated with favorable risk factors, whereas this patient has a higher-risk tumor.

KEY POINT

- Patients with a localized gastrointestinal stromal tumor with a relatively higher risk for recurrence should be treated with imatinib for 3 years following resection of the tumor.

Bibliography

Joensuu H, Eriksson M, Sundby Hall K, et al. One vs three years of adjuvant imatinib for operable gastrointestinal stromal tumor: a randomized trial. JAMA. 2012 Mar 28;307(12):1265-72. [PMID: 22453568]

Item 141   Answer: C

Educational Objective: Manage neutropenia and fever in a patient with leukemia.

This patient requires immediate parenteral administration of a broad-spectrum antibiotic such as piperacillin-tazobactam while blood and urine cultures are pending. Neutropenia is defined as an absolute neutrophil count less than 1000/µL (1.0×10^9/L). Monotherapy with a β-lactam agent with broad coverage of gram-positive and gram-negative organisms with antipseudomonal activity has been shown to be effective in treating neutropenic fever and is the most commonly used approach. Although combination antibiotic therapy is often used (such as the addition of an aminoglycoside for additional antipseudomonal coverage), no specific regimen has been shown to be superior to broad-spectrum monotherapy. It is also reasonable to further broaden directed antimicrobial therapy if a specific source is suspected, such as adding gram-positive coverage (for example, vancomycin) if a central catheter infection is considered likely. Antifungal agents are usually considered only for patients with mucosal barrier inflammation and prolonged neutropenia (>1 week), and antiviral agents are used only in patients whose disease or therapy is associated with immunosuppression. Antimicrobial therapy should be narrowed if a specific organism or organisms are identified on culture.

Because of resistance, fluoroquinolones are not frequently used as initial monotherapy for patients with neutropenic fever. However, they may have a role in selected low-risk patients with stable vital signs and an unremarkable physical examination who might be eligible for outpatient oral therapy at experienced centers with close monitoring capability. They may also be used as add-on therapy for specific infections or for directed therapy based on culture results.

Hematopoietic growth factors, including granulocyte-macrophage colony-stimulating factors, are effective in preventing neutropenia and allowing for continued full-dose chemotherapy when appropriate. These agents also may reduce the duration of neutropenia and the length of hospitalization for patients admitted if fever develops in the setting of neutropenia. However, hematopoietic growth factors are not a replacement for immediate antimicrobial therapy in patients with fever and neutropenia and do not have a clear role in treatment.

Waiting for culture results before administering antimicrobial agents in patients with neutropenia and fever is never appropriate. If patients do not receive parenteral antimicrobials immediately after cultures are taken, their condition can rapidly deteriorate over 12 to 24 hours, and they can experience sepsis, shock, and death.

Although gram-positive organisms are the most commonly identified cause of neutropenic fever, initial monotherapy with vancomycin is not appropriate because of the potential virulence of gram-negative organisms. Vancomycin is usually not a routine component of empiric

CONT.

broad-spectrum antibiotic therapy for neutropenic fever without a specific indication.

KEY POINT

- Patients with a neutrophil count less than 500/µL $(0.5 \times 10^9/L)$ or at any level in the presence of fever or other signs of infection require rapid administration of broad-spectrum antibiotics.

Bibliography

Paul M, Yahav D, Fraser A, Leibovici L. Empirical antibiotic monotherapy for febrile neutropenia: systematic review and meta-analysis of randomized controlled trials. J Antimicrob Chemother. 2006 Feb;57(2):176-89. [PMID: 16344285]

Item 142   Answer: A

Educational Objective: **Manage a patient with prostate cancer recurrence following radical prostatectomy.**

Androgen deprivation therapy is indicated for this patient with possible metastatic prostate cancer. Following surgery for early-stage prostate cancer, the serum prostate-specific antigen (PSA) level should be undetectable. A postoperative serum PSA level of 0.2 ng/mL (0.2 µg/L) or greater is therefore diagnostic of residual or recurrent prostate cancer. Although this finding can represent either locally recurrent or distant metastatic disease, timing is an important discriminating factor in ascertaining the likelihood of local versus distant recurrence. Men who have a persistently elevated PSA level, particularly a rising level immediately following surgery (such as the patient described here), have a high likelihood of harboring distant metastatic disease. Androgen deprivation therapy is therefore indicated for this patient. Prostate cancer cells usually need testosterone to grow. Surgical or chemical castration is highly effective in reducing serum testosterone levels and suppressing prostate cancer cell growth.

Patients with metastatic prostate cancer are first treated with androgen deprivation therapy. Although prostate cancer initially is androgen dependent, over time, cancer cells become androgen independent. Chemotherapy has recently been shown to prolong life expectancy in many of these patients. Since this patient has not yet been treated with androgen deprivation therapy, chemotherapy is not indicated.

A rising PSA level indicates biochemical recurrence, and estimates of survival can be made from the time of completion of treatment to the rise in the PSA, the rate of that rise, and the initial Gleason score. Although recurrent disease after definitive therapy of early-stage prostate cancer is incurable, significant palliation can be achieved with hormone deprivation therapy and chemotherapy. Continuing to monitor the PSA level without initiating therapy is not recommended.

Identification of biochemical recurrence 2 or more years after surgery is more consistent with local recurrence. Studies have shown that salvage radiotherapy is beneficial for men diagnosed with a biochemical recurrence 2 or more years after surgery. In contrast, radiotherapy does not seem to benefit men in whom a PSA level remains detectable following surgery.

KEY POINT

- Men who have a persistently elevated serum prostate-specific antigen level immediately following surgery for prostate cancer have a high likelihood of harboring distant metastatic disease and should be started on androgen deprivation therapy.

Bibliography

Zaorsky NG, Raj GV, Trabulsi EJ, Lin J, Den RB. The dilemma of a rising prostate-specific antigen level after local therapy: what are our options? Semin Oncol. 2013 Jun;40(3):322-36. [PMID: 23806497]

Item 143   Answer: D

Educational Objective: **Treat locally advanced squamous cell carcinoma of the neck with radiation therapy or surgery alone.**

Either radiation therapy or surgical resection is the most appropriate treatment for this patient with early stage squamous cell carcinoma of the oropharynx. Because head and neck cancers tend to recur locally rather than spread systemically, radiation therapy and surgical resection are the primary treatment modalities for stage I and II disease (without lymph node involvement) of the oropharynx. These tumors are highly curable with either modality, with the specific treatment typically selected based on factors such as surgical accessibility of the tumor and the expected morbidity and functional outcomes anticipated with either approach. In patients treated with surgery as the initial approach, adjuvant radiation or combined chemotherapy and radiation may also be indicated for follow-up treatment based on findings at surgery such as close or positive surgical margins, the presence of lymphovascular or perineural invasion, or identification of more advanced (T3 or T4) disease. An important exception to this general treatment approach for early stage head and neck squamous cell malignancies is nasopharyngeal cancer, which is treated with radiation alone for stage I disease and combined chemotherapy and radiation for stage II and higher disease because of a higher risk of distant disease occurrence with these tumors.

Because of their higher rate of locoregional recurrence, more locally advanced tumors (lymph node involvement) are usually treated with surgery (for accessible oral cavity tumors) or combined modality therapy (for other oropharyngeal anatomic sites) that includes radiation along with concurrent chemotherapy with a radiation sensitizer; cisplatin is the most commonly used agent for this purpose. Multiple studies have found that use of combined modality therapy results in significantly improved patient outcomes. However, treatment for locally advanced disease with cisplatin chemotherapy and radiation in this patient with early stage cancer would not be indicated.

Radiation therapy is considered definitive treatment for early stage head and neck cancer. Therefore, adjuvant chemotherapy following radiation therapy is not indicated and would not be an appropriate treatment in this patient.

Cetuximab, a monoclonal antibody directed against the epidermal growth factor receptor, also has an established role in the treatment of locally advanced squamous cell carcinoma of the head and neck when given with radiation therapy. The addition of either cisplatin or cetuximab has been shown to improve survival when compared with radiation therapy alone in patients with locally advanced disease. However, this is not the standard of care treatment for patients with early stage disease who have a much better prognosis and who can be effectively treated with either primary radiation therapy or surgery alone.

KEY POINT

- Patients with early stage head and neck cancer should be treated with either surgery or primary radiotherapy; use of combined chemotherapy and radiation is not indicated.

Bibliography

Gunn GB, Frank SJ. Advances in radiation oncology for the management of oropharyngeal tumors. Otolaryngol Clin North Am. 2013 Aug;46(4):629-43. [PMID: 23910474]

Item 144   Answer: A

Educational Objective: Treat metastatic pancreatic cancer with multiagent systemic chemotherapy.

Multiagent systemic chemotherapy, with a preferred regimen of 5-fluorouracil, leucovorin, irinotecan, and oxaliplatin (FOLFIRINOX), is most appropriate for this patient, who has a history of stage II pancreatic cancer and now has developed a metastatic recurrence. Patients with pancreatic cancer remain at substantial risk of developing a metastatic recurrence within the first 2 years after undergoing appropriate surgical resection (Whipple procedure). For such patients who are otherwise medically fit and have good performance status, FOLFIRINOX chemotherapy is associated with improved outcomes compared with single-agent chemotherapy. More recently, the combination of nab-paclitaxel and gemcitabine has been shown to be modestly superior to gemcitabine alone.

Gemcitabine as single-agent therapy would be suitable for a patient with metastatic pancreatic cancer who is more debilitated (poor performance status) than the patient described here.

Radiation therapy to the liver might be appropriate for treatment of locally symptomatic liver disease but would not be effective for management of metastatic pancreatic cancer in a patient who is otherwise a good candidate for systemic chemotherapy.

Transarterial chemoembolization is used for treatment of metastatic lesions to the liver associated with a number of different cancers. It is most effective in treating larger, symptomatic metastatic lesions, but does not address systemic disease and would not be expected to be as effective as multiagent systemic chemotherapy.

KEY POINT

- Multiagent systemic chemotherapy with 5-fluorouracil, leucovorin, irinotecan, and oxaliplatin (FOLFIRINOX) is appropriate treatment for metastatic recurrence of pancreatic cancer in patients with good performance status.

Bibliography

Conroy T, Desseigne F, Ychou M, et al; Groupe Tumeurs Digestives of Unicancer; PRODIGE Intergroup. FOLFIRINOX versus gemcitabine for metastatic pancreatic cancer. N Engl J Med. 2011 May 12;364(19):1817-25. [PMID: 21561347]

Item 145   Answer: C

Educational Objective: Treat Burkitt lymphoma with hyperfractionated cyclophosphamide, vincristine, doxorubicin, and dexamethasone (R-hyper-CVAD).

Combination chemotherapy consisting of rituximab plus hyperfractionated (rapidly cycled) cyclophosphamide, vincristine, doxorubicin, and dexamethasone (R-hyper-CVAD) is most appropriate for this patient with CD20-positive Burkitt lymphoma. The most aggressive forms of large cell lymphoma include Burkitt lymphoma and lymphoblastic lymphoma. Onset of disease is acute, and patients usually present with life-threatening metabolic and structural abnormalities (this patient has early tumor lysis syndrome and impending airway obstruction). Treatment with R-hyper-CVAD, which is also used to treat acute lymphoblastic leukemia, is associated with high response rates (80%) and is curative in nearly 50% of patients with CD20-positive disease. The International Prognostic Index (IPI) score was developed to assist in determining prognosis before therapy. The IPI score is based on the patient's age, serum lactate dehydrogenase level, number of extranodal sites, disease stage, and performance status. Patients with Burkitt lymphoma have high IPI scores and always warrant aggressive and immediate therapy. Careful monitoring is required when treating patients with Burkitt lymphoma because rapid cell turnover and cell death are exacerbated by initiation of chemotherapy. Aggressive intravenous hydration, urine alkalinization, and administration of allopurinol or rasburicase are indicated in addition to chemotherapy.

Although Burkitt lymphoma can be localized in presentation, it is considered a generalized disease process and is treated with systemic agents. Therefore, neither surgery nor involved-field radiation therapy is indicated as primary treatment.

Because of their association with *Helicobacter pylori* infection, gastric mucosa-associated lymphoid tissue lymphomas can often be induced into complete and durable remission with the combination of antimicrobial agents and a proton pump inhibitor such as amoxicillin, clarithromycin, and omeprazole without the need for additional chemotherapy. This

H
CONT.

regimen is not effective for patients with aggressive large B-cell lymphoma, such as Burkitt lymphoma.

KEY POINT

- Patients with Burkitt lymphoma always warrant aggressive and immediate therapy with combination chemotherapy and aggressive intravenous hydration, urine alkalinization, and administration of allopurinol or rasburicase.

Bibliography

Molyneux EM, Rochford R, Griffin B, et al. Burkitt's lymphoma. Lancet. 2012 Mar 31;379(9822):1234-44. [PMID: 22333947]

Item 146   Answer: A

Educational Objective: Treat advanced chronic lymphocytic leukemia that is resistant to standard therapy.

Hematopoietic stem cell transplantation (HSCT) is most appropriate for this patient who has aggressive B-cell chronic lymphocytic leukemia (CLL) refractory to therapy. CLL is the most common form of adult leukemia, accounting for 10% of all hematologic malignancies. Patients with CLL are usually diagnosed at a median age of 70 years. Many of these patients are asymptomatic at the time of diagnosis and are identified after detecting lymphocytosis on a complete blood count obtained for other purposes. The disease course is often indolent with many patients not requiring treatment. For those who do, newer therapies have improved the median survival for patients with CLL nearly to that of age-matched healthy controls. Although younger patients develop CLL less often, they usually have more aggressive disease as in this patient who had systemic symptoms at presentation in addition to significant lymphadenopathy and splenomegaly. In addition, his disease resistance to standard rituximab and multiagent chemotherapy, the presence of immune thrombocytopenia, and a 17p deletion together confer a limited likelihood of survival (median survival less than 3 years). Because of this, HSCT is the only therapeutic option for this patient that is associated with the potential for cure, and he has siblings who might serve as possible HLA-matched donors.

Leukapheresis is the selective removal of leukocytes from the blood and is typically used in patients with acute leukemias, particularly acute myelogenous leukemia, in which myeloblast counts typically exceeding 100,000/µL (100×10^9/L) result in leukostasis with resulting respiratory failure and central nervous system symptoms. Leukapheresis rapidly lowers the leukocyte count, decreasing leukostasis. However, leukostasis is rarely associated with CLL, and even with very high leukocyte counts, leukapheresis is not indicated in this patient without an extreme elevation of his leukocyte count or evidence of hyperviscosity.

The lymphocytes associated with CLL are usually exquisitely radiosensitive, and radiation of bulky lymph nodes may be helpful in managing symptoms associated with lymphadenopathy. It is frequently used in conjunction with other more definitive treatments or palliatively.

However, this patient does not have significant symptoms related to his lymphadenopathy, and radiation therapy would also not address the underlying hematologic malignancy in this patient.

Splenectomy has been shown to be beneficial in patients with CLL who have marked splenomegaly or profound cytopenias in which splenomegaly may be a contributing factor. However, it is usually reserved for patients whose disease does not respond to chemotherapy or other treatments. Although this patient has evidence of splenomegaly and a low platelet count, he has no evidence of organ impingement from his enlarged spleen or bleeding from his thrombocytopenia. Therefore, there is no current indication for splenectomy at this time.

KEY POINT

- Allogeneic hematopoietic stem cell transplantation, a potentially curative therapy option, should be considered for a young patient with advanced chronic lymphocytic leukemia associated with a high risk of disease progression.

Bibliography

van Besien K, Keralavarma B, Devine S, Stock W. Allogeneic and autologous transplantation for chronic lymphocytic leukemia. Leukemia. 2001 Sep;15(9):1317-25. [PMID: 11516091]

Item 147   Answer: C

Educational Objective: Treat a high-grade neuroendocrine tumor of unknown primary site with platinum-based chemotherapy.

This patient has a high-grade poorly differentiated neuroendocrine tumor of unknown primary site; such tumors often respond rapidly to systemic platinum-based chemotherapy, such as the regimens used to treat small cell lung cancer. Although these regimens can have substantial side effects, the potential for clinical benefit, including improved symptom control and prolonged survival, is significant. Bone metastases are also likely to respond to this chemotherapy regimen.

Hepatic artery embolization is a locoregional therapy that is often used to treat patients with low-grade neuroendocrine tumors, but this technique is not effective for treating patients with high-grade neuroendocrine tumors and would not provide therapy for the bone metastases.

Octreotide is useful for treating patients with low-grade neuroendocrine tumors and for managing hormonal symptoms caused by hormonally functional tumors, but it is not effective for treating patients with high-grade neuroendocrine tumors.

Radiation therapy for bone metastases is inappropriate because it would delay chemotherapy for the visceral metastases, which are clinically more important. In addition, chemotherapy may also treat the bone metastases.

Radiofrequency ablation is useful for treating patients with a limited number of small metastases of low-grade neuroendocrine tumors but would not be appropriate for

Answers and Critiques

treating patients with high-grade neuroendocrine tumors or for managing patients with bulky liver metastases.

KEY POINT

- High-grade poorly differentiated neuroendocrine tumors of unknown primary site often respond rapidly to systemic platinum-based chemotherapy, such as the regimens used to treat small cell lung cancer.

Bibliography

Reidy DL, Tang LH, Saltz LB. Treatment of advanced disease in patients with well-differentiated neuroendocrine tumors. Nat Clin Pract Oncol. 2009 Mar;6(3):143-52. [PMID: 19190591]

Item 148   Answer: B

Educational Objective: Treat a premenopausal patient who has completed breast cancer therapy with antiestrogen therapy.

This patient, who has completed breast surgery, adjuvant chemotherapy, and primary breast radiation, should now be started on antiestrogen therapy. Tamoxifen has been the standard treatment in premenopausal women. As her breast cancer is estrogen receptor positive, adjuvant antiestrogen therapy will reduce her risk of distant recurrence by 40% to 50%. For premenopausal women with hormone receptor-positive early-stage breast cancer, tamoxifen should be used for at least 5 years–preferably 10 years based on the Adjuvant Tamoxifen: Longer Against Shorter (ATLAS) and Adjuvant Tamoxifen Treatment Offers More (aTTom) trials.

Exemestane is an aromatase inhibitor that blocks peripheral conversion of androgens to estrogens. Aromatase inhibitors are therefore used only in postmenopausal women in whom the primary source of estrogen is peripheral conversion of adrenal androgens; therapy with exemestane alone would therefore not be appropriate in the woman with residual ovarian function. However, exemestane has recently been compared with tamoxifen in conjunction with ovarian suppression in premenopausal women. The Tamoxifen and Exemestane Trial (TEXT) and Suppression of Ovarian Function Trial (SOFT) trials have shown improved disease-free survival at 5 years for exemestane with ovarian suppression compared to tamoxifen with ovarian suppression, and this is now an option that can be discussed with premenopausal patients, particularly those at high risk of recurrence. There is at present no difference in breast cancer mortality between these two treatments and the toxicity analysis of these treatments with ovarian suppression compared to tamoxifen alone has not yet been done.

There is no evidence that maintenance chemotherapy is effective in early stage breast cancer and it has not been used outside of a clinical trial.

Without antiestrogen adjuvant therapy, the patient's risk of distant recurrence will increase. As above, antiestrogen therapy reduces the risk of breast cancer distant recurrence by 40 to 50% and also decreases the risk of contralateral breast cancers by 50%. Its use should be recommended in this patient with hormone receptor–positive early-stage breast cancer.

KEY POINT

- The recommended adjuvant endocrine therapy following breast cancer treatment for a premenopausal patient is tamoxifen for at least 5–preferably 10–years.

Bibliography

Burstein HJ, Temin S, Anderson H, et al. Adjuvant endocrine therapy for women with hormone receptor-positive breast cancer: american society of clinical oncology clinical practice guideline focused update. J Clin Oncol. 2014 Jul 20;32(21):2255-69. [PMID: 24868023]

Item 149   Answer: A

Educational Objective: Manage non–small cell lung cancer and poor performance status with palliative care.

The most appropriate management for this patient with metastatic non–small cell lung cancer (NSCLC) and a poor performance status is a comprehensive palliative care assessment. While systemic chemotherapy treatment with a platinum-based doublet regimen has been shown to improve both overall survival and quality of life, this has only been shown for patients with good performance status (Eastern Cooperative Oncology Group/World Health Organization performance status of 2 or better). Patients with a performance status of 2 can carry out all self-care activities and they are also active more than 50% of waking hours. This patient clearly does not meet that definition, as he is spending significant time in bed and requires help with self-care activities. For a patient such as this, chemotherapy treatment has no benefit and instead is associated with potential harm and significant negative impact on quality of life. In contrast, palliative care instituted early in the disease course for patients with metastatic NSCLC has shown to improve symptom control and improve survival.

Pleurodesis, or obliteration of the pleural space, may be helpful in managing recurrent malignant pleural effusion. However, this patient has undergone thoracentesis without evidence of recurrent effusion. Therefore, pleurodesis would not be indicated in this patient.

Radiation treatment to sites of osseous metastases is indicated only for symptom control or for stabilization of a suspected impending fracture. Neither of these is indicated to be an issue for this patient.

KEY POINT

- Early palliative care has shown to improve symptom control and survival in patients with non–small cell lung cancer and associated poor performance status.

Bibliography

Temel JS, Greer JA, Muzikansky A, et al. Early palliative care for patients with metastatic non-small-cell lung cancer. N Engl J Med. 2010 Aug 19;363(8):733-42. [PMID: 20818875]

Index